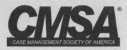

second edition

Core Curriculum for Case Management

Suzanne K. Powell, RN, BSN, MBA, CPHQ, CCM

Director, Acute Care Quality Improvement Program
Health Services Advisory Group
Phoenix, Arizona

Editor-in-Chief
*Professional Case Management: The Leader
  in Evidence-Based Practice*

Hussein A. Tahan, RN, DNSc, CNA

Executive Director of Quality and Performance Excellence
  International
New York Presbyterian Hospital
New York, New York

Wolters Kluwer | Lippincott Williams & Wilkins
Health

Philadelphia · Baltimore · New York · London
Buenos Aires · Hong Kong · Sydney · Tokyo

Senior Acquisitions Editor: Margaret Zuccarini
Production Project Manager: Cynthia Rudy
Director of Nursing Production: Helen Ewan
Senior Managing Editor / Production: Erika Kors
Design Coordinator: Holly Reid McLaughlin
Cover Designer: Christine Jenny
Manufacturing Coordinator: Karin Duffield
Production Services / Compositor: Techbooks
Printer: R. R. Donnelley–Crawfordsville

9 8 7 6 5 4 3 2 1

Library of Congress Cataloging-in-Publication Data

CMSA core curriculum for case management / [edited by] Suzanne K. Powell, Hussein A. Tahan. — 2nd ed.
    p. ; cm.
Includes bibliographical references and index.
ISBN-13: 978-0-7817-7917-3 (alk. paper)
ISBN-10: 0-7817-7917-0 (alk. paper)
    1. Nursing care plans–Outlines, syllabi, etc. 2. Primary nursing–Administration–Outlines, syllabi, etc. 3. Hospitals–Case management services–Outlines, syllabi, etc. I. Powell, Suzanne K. II. Tahan, Hussein A. III. Case Management Society of America. IV. Title: Core curriculum for case management.
    [DNLM: 1. Case Management–Outlines. 2. Nursing Care–organization & administration–Outlines. WY 18.2 C649 2008]
    RT90.7.C636 2008
    362.1'73068—dc22

2007000282

**To case managers everywhere . . .
and their patients**

Contributors
and Reviewers

CONTRIBUTORS

Elizabeth Alvarado, LCSW-R, CCM
Social Work Manager, Discharge Planning
New York Presbyterian Hospital/CUMC
New York, New York
Chapter 5

John Banja, PhD
Assistant Director for Health Sciences
and Clinical Ethics
Associate Professor of Rehabilitation Medicine
Center for Ethics
Emory University
Atlanta, Georgia
Chapter 27

Becky Bigio, NP-P/PhD
Director, The Senior Source Care Management
Program
Selfhelp Community Services, Inc.
New York, New York
Chapter 23

Jackie Birmingham, RN, BSN, MS, CMAC
Vice President of Professional Services,
eDischarge™
Curaspan, Inc.
Newton, Massachusetts
Chapter 10

Lyla J. Correoso, MD
Medical Director, Bronx Hospice and Palliative Care
Visiting Nurse Service of New York
Bronx, New York
Chapter 7

Beverly Cunningham, MS, RN
Associate Administrator Clinical Performance
Improvement
Medical City Dallas Hospital
Dallas, Texas
Chapter 2

Stefani Daniels, MSNA, RN, ACM, ACMA
Managing Partner
Phoenix Medical Management
Pompano Beach, Florida
Chapter 4

Lori A. Davis, RN, CCM, CLCP, MSCC
Life Care Planner
MedAllocators, Inc.
Duluth, Georgia
Chapter 21

Deborah V. DiBenedetto, BSN, MBA, RN, COHN-S/C, ABDA, FAAOHN
Practice Leader
Integrated Health and Productivity Management
(IHPM)
Risk Navigation Group LLC
Battle Creek, Michigan
Chapter 18

Michael B. Garrett, MS, CCM
Vice President, Business Development
Qualis Health
Seattle, Washington
Chapters 11, 25

iv

Elizabeth Bodie Gross, RN, APN, FNP, MS, MBA, CCM
Principal
Quality Health Unlimited, PC
Barrington, Illinois
Chapter 8

Cheri Lattimer, RN, BSN
Executive Director
Case Management Society of America
Little Rock, Arkansas
Chapter 11

Sandra Lowery, RN, BSN, CRRN, CCM, CNLCP
President
CCMI Associates
Francestown, New Hampshire
Chapter 1

Kathleen G. Mastrian, RN, PhD
Associate Professor and Program Coordinator, Nursing
The Pennsylvania State University, Shenango Campus
Sharon, Pennsylvania
Chapters 15, 16

Patricia McCollom, MS, RN, CRRN, CDMS, CCM, CLCP, FIALCP
Nurse Consultant
Management Consulting and Rehabilitation Services, Inc.
Ankeny, Iowa
Chapter 17

Dee McGonigle, PhD, RN, FACCE, FAAN
Associate Professor of Nursing and Information Sciences and Technology
The Pennsylvania State University, New Kensington Campus
New Kensington, Pennsylvania
Chapters 15, 16

Mary Jane McKendry, RN, MBA, CHE, CCM
Vice President, Disease Care Management Operations
Renaissance Health Care/Fresenius Medical Care North America
Waltham, Massachusetts
Treasurer, Case Management Society of America
Chapter 14

Lynn S. Muller, RN, BS, CCM, JD, JMC
Nurse Attorney and Partner
Muller & Muller, Attorneys at Law
Bergenfield, New Jersey
Chapter 26

Suzanne K. Powell, RN, BSN, MBA, CPHQ, CCM
Director, Acute Care Quality Improvement Program
Health Services Advisory Group
Editor-in-Chief
Professional Case Management: The Leader in Evidence-Based Practice
Phoenix, Arizona
Chapters 6, 12, 20, 24

Karen N. Provine, MS, CRC, CCM, CDMS, LPCC
Staff Development Specialist
New Mexico Division of Vocational Rehabilitation
Albuquerque, New Mexico
Chapter 19

Robert Pyke, Jr., RN, CPNP
Co-administrator, Telehealth Listserv and E-health Listserv
North American Coordinator, Med-e-Tel—The International Educational and Networking Forum for eHealth, Telemedicine and Health ICT
Chapter 16

Mary Rosedale, PhD-C, **APRN-BC, CNAA**
Coordinator, Master's/Post-Master's Nursing
   Administration Program and Master's/
   Post-Master's/Joint MS Program
New York University
New York, New York
Chapter 23

Linda Santiago, RN, BSN
Health Team Manager
VNSNY Hospice
Bronx, New York
Chapter 7

Linda N. Schoenbeck, RN, BS, C, CCM
Director, Utilization Services
Health Services Advisory Group
Phoenix, Arizona
Chapters 6, 22

Marietta P. Stanton, PhD, RN, **CX, CNAA, BC, CMAC, CCM**
Professor and Director of the Graduate Program
University of Alabama
Capstone College of Nursing
Tuscaloosa, Alabama
Chapter 13

Edward Sunderland, LCSW
Clinical Coordinator of the Street to Home
   Initiative
Common Ground Community
New York, New York
Chapter 5

Hussein A. Tahan, DNSc, RN, **CNA**
Executive Director of Quality and Performance
   Excellence International
New York Presbyterian Hospital
New York, New York
Chapters 3, 6, 8, 9, 13, 20

Lewis E. Vierling, MS, CCM, CRC, NCC, NCCC
Vocational Rehabilitation Consultant
Management Consulting & Rehabilitation
   Services, Inc.
Ankeny, Iowa
Chapter 19

REVIEWERS

Kaye S. Admire, RN, MSN, **RNCS**
Senior Clinical Project Coordinator
Presbyterian Health Plan
Albuquerque, New Mexico

Patricia Agius, RN, BS, A-CCC, **CCM, CPHQ**
Nurse Case Manager
Independent Consultant and Bethel
   Health Care Center
Chapter President, NJCMSA &
   CPC CMSA Rep 06-07
Bethel, Connecticut

Rebecca A. Brotemarkle, MSN, MBA, RN, ACRN
Advanced Practice Case Manager
Johns Hopkins HealthCare, LLC
Glen Burnie, Maryland

Jean Calhoun, RN, BSN, MS, **MSN, CCM**
Clinical Director, Case Management
Albuquerque, New Mexico

Dana Derevin Carr, RN, CM, CCM, MS/MPH
Care Manager—Acute Rehab/Surgical Step Down
Jacobi Medical Center
Bronx, New York

Crystal C. Carvotta-Brown, RN, BSN, MMHCA, CCM, CRRN, CMAC, CPHQ
Director, Quality & Regulatory Compliance
MES Solutions
Norwood, Massachusetts

Paula D. Casey, MSN, RN, ONC, CCM
Manager, Health Services
Presbyterian Health Plan
Albuquerque, New Mexico

Connie Commander, RN, BS, CCM, CPUR, ABDA
President, Commander's Premier
    Consulting Corp
Pearland, Texas

Sydney S. Denius, RN
Case Manager, Long Term Acute Select
    Specialty Hospital
Denver, Colorado

Kathleen Ward Douglas, RN, MPA, CCM
President, K.A. Shannon Consulting, LLC
Phoenix, Arizona

Marsha Ellefson, RN, BA, CCM, CPUR
Team Lead/ Case Management
Premera Blue Cross
Spokane, Washington

Pat Trefny Ford, RN, BS, CPHQ, CCM
President/Owner
Pat Ford HealthCare Consulting
Edmonds, Washington

Mary F. Gambosh, RN, CCM
Independent Consultant
Charlotte, North Carolina

Carol A. Gleason, MM, RN, CRRN, CCM, LRC
Director of Admissions
Radius Specialty Hospital
Boston, Massachusetts

Deborah A. Gutteridge, MS
Clinical Evaluator/Admissions Coordinator
Mentor ABI/Center for
    Comprehensive Services
Kansas City, Missouri

Tierney Davis Hogan, RN, BS, CCM
Medical Management Coordinator
Regence BlueShield
Seattle, Washington

Diane L. Huber, PhD, RN, FAAN, CNAA, BC
Professor, College of Nursing and
    College of Public Health
University of Iowa
Iowa City, Iowa

Michele Y. Jones, RN, CCM
Disease Management Case Manager
Johns Hopkins Health Care
Baltimore, Maryland

Shelly Kinney, RN, CCM
Case Management Supervisor
GENEX Services, Inc.
Omaha, Nebraska

Margaret Leonard, MS, RN, C, FNP, CM
Vice President for Clinical Services
Hudson Health Plan
Adjunct Instructor
College of New Rochelle School of Nursing
Tarrytown, New York

Victoria E. Loner, RN, CCM, CMCN, CPUR
Manager, Utilization Management
MVP Health Care
Williston, Vermont

Sandra L. Lowery, BSN, RN, CRRN, CCM
President, CCMI Associates
Adjunct Faculty, Granite State College
Francestown, New Hampshire

Nancy Martin, RN, MS, CCM
Case Manager, Johns Hopkins Health Care
Glen Burnie, Maryland

Carla D. McPherson, MS, RN
Clinical Nurse Educator Medical–Surgical
Nursing
University of Arizona College of Nursing
Tucson, Arizona

Peter Moran, RN C, BSN, MS, CCM
ED Case Manager, President-Elect
CMSA 2006–2007
Massachusetts General CMSA
Newburyport, Massachusetts

Mary Beth Newman, MSN, RN, A-CCC, CMAC
Program Manager, Care Management
Anthem Blue Cross and Blue Shield
Mason, Ohio

Rebecca Perez, RN, CCM, CPUR, CPUM
Health Services Coordinator
Carpenters' Health & Welfare Trust Fund
St. Louis, Missouri

Michelle Robbins, RN, BSN, CCM
Case Manager/Complex Medical Team/
Telewatch
Johns Hopkins HealthCare
Ocean City, Maryland

Susan A. Rogers, RN, BSN, CCM
President, Rogers Professional Guidance
Overland Park, Kansas

Carolyn Simon, MSN, RN, CPUR, CCM
Case Management Coordinator
Blue Cross Blue Shield of New Mexico
Secretary, CMSA
Albuquerque, New Mexico

Nancy E. Skinner, RN, CCM
Principal Consultant
Riverside Healthcare Consulting
Whitwell, Tennessee

Viki Solomon, RN, BA, BSN, CRRN, CCM, ABDA
President, Viki Solomon and Associates, Inc.
Ft. Lauderdale, Florida

Lorraine Phyllis Theodos, CCM, BSN, MSN, MBA, MPH
Interim Director of Care Management
Victory Memorial Hospital
Waukegan, Illinois

Marilyn Van Houten, RN, MS, CDMS, CCM
President/Case Management Consultant
Rehabilitation Case Management, Inc.
Miami, Florida

Cynthia E. Whitaker, RN, BSN
URAC Accreditation Consultant
Victor, Montana

Alison B. White, RN, MHA, CCM, CPHQ
Director, Regional Care Management and
Quality Improvement
Dartmouth-Hitchcock Alliance
Lebanon, New Hampshire

John A. Zeier, RN, MSN, CFNP
Clinic Director/Family Nurse Practitioner
Yachats Community Health Clinic
Yachats, Oregon

Foreword

There could never be a better time for case management than today! CM has become a core element of the health care delivery system or model in almost every organization, any setting across the continuum of care, and all levels of care. Research findings support the value CM adds to health care outcomes for all: the recipient of care (consumer), the payer, and the provider. Most importantly, CM is known today to be an effective strategy for safe care—an area of grave concern that has surfaced recently. In this regard, case managers are gaining a progressively more significant role and status in assuring the safe, quality, and effective delivery of care, and have become the nucleus of multidisciplinary health care teams.

For these reasons and many others discussed in this second edition of the *CMSA Core Curriculum for Case Management*, the practice of CM will continue to flourish and to be "part and parcel" of the health care delivery system for years to come. In addition, case managers will remain the linchpins of the multidisciplinary health care teams of providers and the advocates of the consumers of care. Within the context of CM practice, they are key players in the process of integrating the various health care professional disciplines for the benefit of the consumers, providers, and payers. This integration works to decrease duplication, fragmentation, and silos in care delivery and replace them with efficiency, effectiveness, accountability, and collaboration.

The Case Management Society of America (CMSA), a multidisciplinary organization that is dedicated to the support and development of CM professionals, is proud to present the *CMSA Core Curriculum for Case Management* to all of those directly or indirectly involved in CM practice. CMSA believes that case managers (including nurses, social workers, rehabilitation counselors, life care planners, therapists, pharmacists, physicians, and others) are pioneers of health care transformation and need an invaluable resource that helps them keep their CM expertise, knowledge, skills, and competencies current. Better yet, this resource will assist case managers to be ready and able to meet the future, and perhaps unforeseen, demands of effective health care delivery. Through the combined efforts of CMSA, the authors, and the editors, the *Core Curriculum* is an educational resource written to identify basic to advanced components, interventions, delivery models, roles, and concepts of case management.

CMSA would like to acknowledge the dedication of Suzanne K. Powell and Hussein A. Tahan for their commitment to produce a comprehensive and cutting edge *Core Curriculum*, and for ongoing support of our vision of "case managers as pioneers of health care change. . ." and our mission to "positively impact and improve patient wellbeing and health care outcomes." The contents of this book provide a road map toward understanding the various services, requirements, standards, and tools of a case manager, yet they acknowledge the unity through diversity that attracts clinicians and others to CM.

CMSA encourages you to continue to evolve CM with new research, evidence, performance measures, technology, and models of practice—moving our interactions with the health care community (including legislators, regulators, and especially consumers) to a fully integrated collaborative approach to care that will ensure positive outcomes and mark our place in the health care industry as dynamic leaders for effective change.

Cheri Lattimer, RN, BSN
Executive Director, Case Management Society of America

Preface

Change. The generation alive today has experienced perhaps more change than any one before. Change is inevitable and is happening every day—and every moment—of our lives. In our own world of health care, professionals have seen the devastation of diseases that attack the core of human survival (the immune system); we also have seen health care "management" techniques that attack the core of the provider–patient relationship. The health care system rapidly and insidiously became more complex—so complex, in fact, that the average person could no longer navigate its course. This offered a great opportunity for a special health care professional—the *case manager*—to partner with the patient in making the "course" manageable.

In the 1980s, a group of health care professionals of various credentials intuitively knew that strict utilization review techniques were not addressing the major economic, quality, and ethical problems of our health care system. The methods some organizations employed to "review" patients' conditions for "medical necessity" became an additional barrier between the patient and his or her medical needs. They also resulted in another significant barrier between the payer and the provider of care. Therefore, in grassroots fashion and on a case-by-case basis, case management models of patient care delivery were implemented. Today, they have become popular and necessary strategies to counteract these barriers and problems. Case managers began managing out-of-control resource utilization while helping to ensure quality of care and patient safety and satisfaction. At that point, most case managers were learning the job through trial-and-error (or, less eloquently, by the "seat of their pants"). Published information to help chart the way was lacking.

Case management continued to grow and managed care organizations (MCOs) and other insurers, realizing its fiscal possibilities, encouraged the concept. Case managers were now working throughout the continuum to coordinate patient care. Population-specific case management, or disease management, evolved, thus expanding the scope of case management from a case-by-case event to one in which entire groups of people could benefit. Today its impact is seen worldwide. The number of case managers practicing in the U.S. has grown to exceed 100,000 professionals, of which approximately one third are credentialed as "certified case managers." This workforce is not limited to a specific discipline or specialty; on the contrary, the practice of case management is multidisciplinary in nature, with nurses, social workers, vocational rehabilitation counselors, physical and occupational therapists, and other licensed professionals all assuming the role of case manager. This unique diversity makes the practice of case management dynamic, popular, attractive, and influential.

There is no better time for case management to be "part and parcel" of health care delivery systems, both domestically and internationally. Because of the increased complexity and chronicity of individuals' health conditions, the growing proportion of the elderly in our population, and the great number of recent diagnostic and therapeutic innovations, patients are receiving care in various settings, especially during a single episode of illness, and they are cared for by many health care professionals (generalists and specialists). Such care transitions and hand-offs may leave patients at increased risk for medical errors and unsafe situations. Case management provides a strategy for addressing such concerns; in fact, it prevents medical errors and ensures that patients experience safe and quality services. In addition, case managers enhance open communication among direct and indirect care providers, both internal and external to a health care organization; advocate for patients and their families; facilitate positive and desirable outcomes; and ensure cost-effective care and use of resources.

Today, the knowledge of case management has grown so exponentially that there are many books and periodicals about its various aspects of practice. In addition, the Case Management Society of America (CMSA), founded in 1990, continues to promote the development of professional case management through annual conferences, through the Standards of Practice for Case Management, and the Ethics Statement on Case Management Practice. Its other activities include several critical task forces to enhance research and knowledge pertinent to the case management profession. Case Management Society International (CMSI) communicates with members in countries such as Australia, Canada, Germany, New Zealand, Puerto Rico, South Africa, and the United Kingdom. Interested groups have also been formed in China, Japan, Singapore, South Korea, and Spain.

This Core Curriculum, sponsored by CMSA, represents a synthesis of the case management evolution and a forecast about its future. The chapters, which have been written by renowned experts in the field, address important topics of case management practice, such as background and overview of case management, practice settings, roles and functions of case managers, case management tools and protocols, specialty practices, effectiveness of case management, and legal and ethical obligations. This second edition of the Core Curriculum expands on the original content and includes new materials, particularly in the areas of legal, ethical, and safe case management practice; description of roles and functions of case managers as they relate to the various care settings and patient populations; telemedicine; and the training, education, and credentialing of case managers. The additional information is necessary to keep case managers informed about the current state of case management practice and to arm them with the skills, knowledge, and competencies needed for effective delivery of case management services.

It is important to note that this Core Curriculum is essentially an overview of the topics necessary for competent practice. Although written in an outline format, the text contains a great deal of useful information, charts, graphs, examples, tables, references, and supporting material for further study. The broad scope of case management issues presented serves as a teaching tool and reference for:

- Development of college and university curriculum
- Orientation and training of case managers within an organization or a facility and practice setting
- Study parameters for various credentials, such as case management certifications
- Accreditation basics
- Self-orientation when beginning a "new" case management career
- Case management model design or re-design
- Development of job descriptions for case managers
- Evaluation of performance and productivity of case managers
- Evaluation of effectiveness (or return on investment) of case management programs and models

Case management is an important solution to a major economic and humanitarian problem. It will continue to grow in importance, because it works! Current research-based evidence supports it. Core Curriculum reflects the most up-to-date knowledge in case management practice, and prevents case managers from having to learn their role by "flying by the seat of their pants." We would like to thank CMSA and all the contributors for their expertise and dedication to this project. They are truly a group of special individuals who shared their knowledge for the growth of the case management profession and for the good of health care.

Suzanne K. Powell
Hussein A. Tahan

Acknowledgments

The authors would like to thank the contributors who dedicated so much of their time and expertise to this important work. Your devotion to case management is evident in your work, and we thank you!

We would also like to thank the Board of the Case Management Society of America for all of their input and encouragement throughout the writing process, and for putting their faith in us and our abilities.

Last, but certainly not least, we would like to thank Senior Acquisitions Editor Margaret Zuccarini for all of her support and guidance during this project. Thank you!

Contents

chapter 4
Case Management in the Acute Care Setting   74
Stefani Daniels   74

chapter 5
Case Management in the Home Care Setting   97
Elizabeth Alvarado
Edward Sunderland

chapter 6
Case Management in the Long-Term Care and Rehabilitation Settings   111
Linda N. Schoenbeck
Hussein A. Tahan
Suzanne K. Powell

chapter 7
Case Management in the Palliative Care and Hospice Settings   142
Lyla J. Correoso
Linda Santiago

section two
Roles and Functions of Case Managers

chapter 8
The Case Manager   159
Elizabeth Bodie Gross
Hussein A. Tahan

chapter 9
The Case Management Process   177
Hussein A. Tahan

chapter 10
Transitional Planning   190
Jackie Birmingham

chapter 11
Utilization Management and Resource Management   208
Cheri Lattimer
Michael B. Garrett

chapter 12
Leadership Skills and Concepts   223
Suzanne K. Powell

chapter 13
Education, Training, and Certification of Case Managers   240

Marietta P. Stanton
Hussein A. Tahan

section three
Case Management Tools

chapter 14
Case Management Plans, Clinical Pathways, and Protocols   273

Mary Jane McKendry

chapter 15
Information Systems in Case Management   292

Dee McGonigle
Kathleen Mastrian

chapter 16
Telehealth and Telemedicine in Case Management   324

Dee McGonigle
Kathleen Mastrian
Robert Pyke

section four
Specialty Practices in Case Management   347

chapter 17
Life Care Planning and Case Management   349

Patricia McCollom

chapter **18**
Workers' Compensation Case Management   364
Deborah V. DiBenedetto

chapter **19**
Disability and Occupational Health Case Management   400
Karen N. Provine
Lewis E. Vierling

chapter 26

Legal Issues in Case Management Practice   571

Lynn S. Muller

chapter 27

Ethical Issues in Case Management Practice   594

John Banja

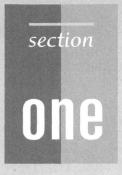

section

one

Background and Overview

History and Evolution of Case Management

Sandra Lowery

Upon completion of this chapter, the reader will be able to:

1. Recognize the history of case management over the past century.
2. Discuss the impetus for its rapid growth over the past two decades.
3. Relate the professional development of case management practice.
4. List the purposes and goals of case management.
5. Understand the philosophical tenets of case management practice.
6. Define the domains of case management.
7. Describe case management, primary care case management, and care management.
8. Identify the national standards of practice and conduct for case managers.

IMPORTANT TERMS AND CONCEPTS

American Nurses Association (ANA)
American Nurses Credentialing Center (ANCC)
Association of Rehabilitation Nurses (ARN)
Care Management
Case Management
Certified Case Management (CCM)
Commission for Case Management Certification (CCMC)
Case Management Society of America (CMSA)

Domains of Case Management
National Association of Rehabilitation Professionals in the Private Sector (NARPPS, now IARP)
National Association of Social Workers (NASW)
National Council on Aging (NCOA)
Primary Care Case Management
Standards of Practice

■ INTRODUCTION

A. Historical perspective
1. Early 1900s—Public health nurses and social workers coordinated services through the Department of Public Health.
2. 1920s—Psychiatry and social work focused on long-term, chronic illnesses, managed in the outpatient community setting.
3. 1930s—Public health visiting nurses used community-based case management approaches in their patient care.
4. 1943—Liberty Mutual used in-house case management/rehabilitation as a cost-management measure for workers' compensation insurance.
5. Post–World War II—Insurance companies employed nurses and social workers to assist with the coordination of care for soldiers returning from the war who suffered complex injuries requiring multidisciplinary intervention.
6. 1966—Insurance Company of North America (INA, now CIGNA), led by George Welch, developed an in-house program that incorporated vocational rehabilitation and nurse case management, which later became known as Intracorp.
7. 1970s—Due to the success of Liberty Mutual and INA in managing medical costs and returning workers to work, other workers' compensation insurers developed case management programs.
8. 1970s—Medicaid and Medicare demonstration projects employed social workers and human service workers to arrange for and coordinate medical and social services to defined patient populations in the community.

This chapter is a revised version of Chapter 1 in the first edition of *CMSA Core Curriculum for Case Management*. The contributor wishes to acknowledge Marlys A. Severson, as some of the timeless material was retained from the previous version.

    a. Spurred by the federally legislated deinstitutionalization of the mentally ill and mentally retarded population (now identified as the developmentally disabled)

    b. National Long Term Care Channeling Demonstration Projects were funded by government community-based programs for the low-income and frail elderly, designed to maintain this population in the community.

9. 1978—The Older Americans Act authorized case management for elders through area agencies on aging throughout the United States.

10. 1980s—Health insurers developed case management programs, targeted at the catastrophically injured and ill population. Focus was on cost containment due to the double-digit inflation rate for medical costs.

    a. Some programs were designed similarly to the workers' compensation insurance models, with a focus on quality and cost of care to achieve results.

    b. Some programs implemented a utilization management approach, with a focus on cost outcomes.

11. Late 1980s–2000—Provider-based programs proliferated in acute care hospitals; home care agencies, rehabilitation facilities, and skilled nursing facilities were established.

    a. Often these case management models combined utilization review and discharge planning functions into a case management role.

    b. Both nurses and social workers were hired for provider-based case management positions.

    c. Growth of provider-based case management was spurred by the shifting of financial risk to provider organizations, as well as by external quality and cost demands by payers and accreditation bodies.

12. 1990s–2006—Number of case managers increased to an estimate of greater than 100,000. Although cost containment remained important, the realization that quality care is an essential element to achieve this became a primary driver.

B. Impetus for the explosive growth of case management

1. Cost of health care—Increasing amount of the gross domestic product (GDP) goes toward health care, as compared with global competitors. In early 1990s, one-seventh of the United States GDP went toward payment for health care (Cohen, 1996). By 2004, this reached 15% and was still increasing (CMS).

2. Increasing consumerism secondary to more accessible information, increased expectations of patient involvement on the part of health plans, shift of health care financing to consumers, and negative repercussions of managed care

3. New emphasis on complementary and alternative medicine, with limited reimbursement by health plans

4. Information explosion through expansive use of electronic communication technology

5. Rapid development of genetic and medical advances

6. Growing emphasis on results, the value of health care dollars, and accountability for end outcomes
7. Significant changes in the health care delivery system and reimbursement for care
   a. Increased fragmentation of care delivery
   b. Increased level of consumer financial responsibility with decreased benefits, more co-pays and deductibles
   c. Multiple levels and settings of care delivery, leading to much confusion, poorly coordinated care, poor care accountability, and cost shifting
8. Public awareness of the fallibility of the health care system
   a. National reports such as "To Err is Human" and "Crossing the Quality Chasm" by the Institute of Health identifying safety problems from medical errors
   b. Public report cards on providers, with comparative quality and cost data
   c. Published data showing great variability in treatment, with inconsistent adherence to medical evidence, from the Dartmouth Atlas of Health Care and other national reports
9. Demands for quality care as well as cost effectiveness by private and public payers, through accreditation and pay-for-performance measures
10. Increased recognition of case management as beneficial for cost and quality outcomes
11. Demographics, including increased longevity, a growing aging population, geographic separation of extended families, and increased reliance on institutions for long-term care

C. Professional development and standards of practice became a necessity in order to set forth meaningful and relevant guidelines.
   1. National standards for professional practice
      a. Individual practitioner standards
         i. Case Management Society of America (CMSA), 1995, revised 2002
         ii. National Association of Social Workers (NASW)
         iii. American Nurses Association (ANA)
         iv. National Association of Rehabilitation Professionals in the Private Sector (NARPPS)
         v. National Council on Aging (NCOA)
         vi. Association of Rehabilitation Nurses (ARN)
         vii. National Association of Professional Geriatric Care Managers (NAPGCM)
      b. Organizational standards
         i. Utilization Review and Accreditation Commission (URAC), v. 1.0 through 2.0
         ii. Commission on Accreditation of Rehabilitation Facilities (CARF)
         iii. Joint Commission on Accreditation of Healthcare Organizations (JCAHO)

2. National certification in case management
    a. Certified Case Manager (CCM), CCMC, testing/credentialing began in 1993
    b. Nurse Case Manager (RN, CM), ANA
    c. American Nurses Credentialing Center (ANCC)
    d. Certification in Continuity of Care, Advanced (A-CCC), American Association for Continuity of Care (AACC)
    e. Certified Social Worker Case Manager (CSWCM), NASW
    f. Certified Occupational Health Nurse Case Manager (COHN-CM), AOHN
    g. Certified Rehabilitation Nurse, (CRRN), ARN
    h. Certified Rehabilitation Counselor (CRC), Commission for Certified Rehabilitation Counselors
    i. Care Manager, Certified (CMC), National Academy of Certified Case Managers
    j. Commission for Case Management Certification (CCMC)
3. National journals and publications
    a. *Professional Case Management: The Leader in Evidence-Based Practice* (Lippincott)
    b. *The Case Manager* (Elsevier)
    c. *Care Management* (Mason Medical)
    d. *Case Management Advisor* (American Health Consultants)
    e. *Care Management Journals* (Springer)
4. Education
    a. Academic
        i. Graduate degree programs in nursing case management
        ii. Certificate programs
        iii. Core curriculum for social work includes the core principles of case management
    b. Continuing education
    c. Online forums
5. Legislation affecting case management
    a. Private sector
        i. Workers' compensation insurance
        ii. Laws for utilization review in some states
        iii. Varying laws in each state
    b. Public sector
        i. Medicaid waiver programs
        ii. Medicare waiver programs
        iii. Community human service agencies serving the mentally ill/developmentally disabled population
6. Professional associations
    a. CMSA, international with local affiliates
    b. NAPGCM, national with local affiliates

    c. International Association of Rehabilitation Providers (IARP, formerly NARPPS), international with local affiliates

    d. Association of Certified Case Managers (ACCM), national

    e. American Case Management Association (ACMA), national with local affiliates

■ KEY DEFINITIONS

A. ADL—Activities of daily living, which include activities carried out for personal hygiene and health.

B. Assessment—The process of collecting in-depth information about a person's health and functioning to identify needs in order to develop a comprehensive case management plan that will address those needs. Information should be gathered from all relevant sources, as well as from client contact.

C. Autonomy—A form of personal liberty in which the client holds the right and freedom to make decisions regarding his or her own treatment and course of action, and to take control of his or her health, fostering independence and self-determination.

D. Case manager—A health care professional who is responsible for utilizing the case management process for individuals with health-related needs, with the goal of maximizing their wellness, autonomy, and appropriate use of resources.

E. Catastrophic case—Any medical condition that has heightened medical, social, and financial consequences.

F. Coordination—The process of organizing, securing, integrating, and modifying the resources necessary to accomplish the goals set forth in the case management plan.

G. Developmental disability—Any mental and/or physical disability that has an onset before age 22 and may continue indefinitely. It can limit major life activities.

H. Disability case management—A process of managing occupational and nonoccupational health conditions with the goal of returning a disabled employee to health, productivity, and employment.

I. Discharge planning—The process of assessing the individual's care needs upon discharge from a health care facility or agency and ensuring that the necessary services are in place before discharge.

J. Implementation—The process of executing specific case management activities and/or interventions that will lead to accomplishing the goals identified in the case management plan.

K. Mental retardation—Subaverage general intellectual functioning manifested during the developmental period and existing concurrently with impairment in adaptive behavior.

L. Monitoring—The ongoing process of gathering sufficient information from all relevant sources regarding the effectiveness of the case management plan implemented.

M. Planning—The process of determining specific needs, goals, and actions designed to meet the client's needs as identified through the assessment process.

N. Primary care—A process of assessing, planning, coordinating, and providing health care from a consistent practitioner who serves as the central point of contact for all other practitioners.

O. Provider—A person, facility, or agency that provides health care services.

P. Social work—A health care profession that promotes social change, problem solving in human relationships, and the empowerment and liberation of people to enhance well-being.

Q. Standards of practice—Statements of the acceptable level of performance or expectation for professional intervention or behavior associated with a professional practice.

R. Utilization review—A mechanism used by some insurers and employers to evaluate health care on the basis of medical appropriateness, necessity, and quality. Typically, it is used to determine access to an insurance benefit.

S. Vocational rehabilitation—A process whereby a skilled professional utilizes the case management process to address the medical and vocational services necessary to facilitate a disabled individual's expedient return to suitable employment.

■ CASE/CARE MANAGEMENT DEFINITIONS

A. Case management
  1. Case management is a collaborative process of assessment, planning, facilitation, and advocacy for options and services to meet an individual's health needs through communication and available resources to promote quality and cost-effective outcomes (CMSA, 2002).
  2. Case management is a set of logical steps and a process of interaction within a service network that assure that a client receives needed services in a supportive, effective, efficient, and cost-effective manner (Weil and Karls, 1985).
  3. Case management is a health care delivery process whose goals are to provide quality health care, decrease fragmentation, enhance the client's quality of life, and contain costs (ANA, 1994).
  4. A case manager tracks the patient through the various units of the system. Case management roles vary widely among systems and organizations. One approach to case management is to use patient care plans developed during this process that identify "critical pathways" of key events that must occur in order to achieve the desired outcome in a timely manner. The nurse case manager oversees these critical paths and facilitates interventions to ensure that the patient progresses through the desired events appropriately and satisfactorily. In some managed care organizations, a case manager addresses the long-term needs of the enrolled members, not just their current interaction within the system (ANA, 1994).

5. Case management is the process of planning, organizing, coordinating, and monitoring the services and resources needed to respond to an individual's health care needs (ARN, 2006).

6. Social work case management is a method of providing services whereby a professional assesses the needs of the client and family, and arranges, coordinates, monitors, evaluates, and advocates for a package of multiple services to meet the specific client's complex needs (NASW, 1992).

7. Medical case management is defined as the process of assessing, planning, coordinating, monitoring, and evaluating the services required to respond to an individual's health needs to attain the goals of quality and cost-effective care (NARPPS, 1995).

8. Case management is a systematic process that serves individuals with disabilities through ongoing coordination and referral among human service systems. This process centers on the person served, is goal oriented, and promotes the individual's optimum level of independence and functioning (CARF, 1989).

9. Case management is a method of managing the provision of health care to members with catastrophic or high-cost medical conditions. The goal is to coordinate the care so as to improve continuity and quality of care as well as lower costs (Kongstvedt, 2003).

10. Case management is a collaborative practice that assesses, plans, coordinates, implements, monitors, and evaluates the options and services required to meet the client's health and human services needs. It is characterized by advocacy, communication, and resource management and promotes quality and cost-effective interventions and outcomes (CCMC, 2005).

11. Nursing case management is an approach that focuses on the coordination, integration, and direct delivery of patient services, and places internal controls on the resources used for care—a nursing care delivery system that supports cost-effective, patient outcome-oriented care (Cohen and Cesta, 1997).

12. Case management is a coordination of a specific group of services on behalf of a specific group of people. Case management can also be defined by listing its component processes. By widespread agreement, these processes include screening or case finding, comprehensive multidimensional assessment, care planning, implementation of the plan, monitoring, and reassessment (Powell, 2000).

B. Care management
The terms *case management* and *care management* traditionally are used interchangeably when the role is consistent in definition and concept.

1. Care management is a component of the community care system. Its process includes assessing a person's functional level and impairments—physical, cognitive, social, emotional—in order to identify what needs and problems are present, as well as the individual's current capacity and support—family, friends, financial, and environmental; developing a plan of care that addresses the needs and prob-

lems presented and incorporates the services that are needed to enhance the current support system; identifying and arranging for coordinated delivery of those services; monitoring changes in the person's condition and circumstances, and in the provision of services; and reassessing the person's needs on a regular basis (NCOA, 1988).

2. Care management is the coordination of treatment needs with available resources to ensure quality care and positive outcome utilizing cost-effective methods (American Congress of Rehabilitation Medicine, 1988).

3. Many terms have been used to describe the case management role and process: *care management, case or care coordination, service coordination, service management,* or *case management.* The National Council on Aging uses "care management" because it conveys the management of care as opposed to the management of the client, recognizing the right to the self-determination of the person receiving care (NCOA, 1988).

4. "Care Management" is sometimes used as a department title that includes multiple functions, such as case management, utilization review, benefit denial management, quality management, and others.

5. "Care management," as well as other terms such as *care coordination,* has evolved in recent years to provide some distance from the managed care backlash, in which case management was often perceived to be a negative aspect.

6. The term *care management* is often used instead of *case management* for the chronic, elderly, and long-term care client populations.

C. Primary care case management
   1. Involves dual roles—caregiving and case management
   2. Creates potential ethical and conceptual conflict—"Severe conflicts of interest can emerge when case managers are also service providers rather than relatively disinterested allocators of service" (Kane, 1988, p. 29).
   3. Federally legislated model of case management for certain states' Medicaid risk plans
   4. Often the model for home care agencies and skilled nursing facilities

■ **TARGET PATIENT POPULATIONS**

Client selection criteria are determined by the purchaser/employer of the case manager. Populations may be targeted for the following reasons or conditions:

A. Diagnostic categories ✓
   1. Acute injury or illness
   2. Chronic illness or injury
   3. Multiple diagnoses
   4. End stage diseases (e.g., renal, COPD)

B. Potential for large consumption of resources✓
   1. Financial
   2. Service

C. Frail and elderly

D. Those experiencing frequent or prolonged hospitalizations and/or emergency department visits

E. Procedure (e.g., organ transplant)

F. Multiple psychosocial factors, i.e., need for support system, transportation, financial resources, decision support, habilitation, residential

G. Vocational support (disability case management)

H. Functionally impaired, i.e., dependency for ADLs and IADLs

I. Individuals who are eligible by law, e.g., those with mental retardation/developmental disabilities

■ CASE MANAGEMENT PHILOSOPHY

A. All individuals, particularly those experiencing catastrophic and high chronicity injuries and illnesses, should be evaluated for case management services. The components of case management address care that is holistic and client-centered, with mutual goals, allowing stewardship of resources for the client and health care system. Through these efforts, case management focuses simultaneously on achieving health and wellness, and all parties benefit. Taken collectively, services offered by a professional case manager can enhance a client's safety, well being, and quality of life while reducing total health care costs. Thus, effective case management can directly and positively affect the social, ethical, and financial health of the country and its population (CMSA, 2002).

B. Each person is unique, with specific needs, goals, and preferences. All individuals have a right to autonomy, a right to make their own choices and decisions, and a right to exercise control over their own lives. Care management does not replace family assistance, but aids and improves the family's ability to care for its dependent relative. It maximizes the capacity of the person and his or her caregiver to make informed and independent decisions in arranging for needed care (NCOA, 1988).

C. Case management is a specialty practice within one's health and human services profession. It functions best when it is practiced in an environment where there is open communication between the client, providers, and pertinent parties (CCMC, 2005).

D. Case management rests on a foundation of professional values, knowledge, and skills. It follows basic ethical tenets, including recognition of the inherent worth and capacity of the individual and of the individual's right to self-determination and confidentiality. It is based on the recognition that a trusting and empowering direct relationship between the case manager and the client is essential to achieve the goals of case management (NASW, 1992).

E. Five principles serve as the basis of case management practice (Cohen, 1996):
   1. The focus is on the client and family.
   2. It involves negotiating, coordinating, and procuring services and resources needed.
   3. It entails using a clinical reasoning process.

4. It involves developing various relationships.
5. It is episode- or continuum-focused.

■ PURPOSES AND GOALS OF CASE MANAGEMENT

A. Purposes
1. To interject objectivity and information where it is lacking in order to promote informed decision making by the client and others
2. To maximize efficiency in use of available resources
3. To work collaboratively with the patient, physician, family/significant other, and the health care provider to implement a plan of care that meets the individual's needs
4. To promote quality, safe, and cost-effective care; ensure appropriate access to care; work collaboratively with the client and all pertinent parties (CMSA, 2002)
5. To make the system work more effectively in order to ensure that individuals receive assistance that is responsive to their needs (NCOA, 1988)
6. To work directly with clients and families over time to assist them in arranging and managing the complex set of resources that the client requires to maintain health and independent functioning. Care coordination seeks to achieve the maximum cost-effective use of scarce resources by helping clients get the health, social, and support services most appropriate for their needs at a given time. It guides the client and family through the maze of services, matches service needs with funding authorization, and coordinates with clinician and provider organizations (Williams and Torrens, 1993).
7. To move the client toward successful meeting of planned outcomes where interventions are tied to a sense of movement, and constant evaluation occurs to measure progress (Cohen, 1996)

B. Goals
Regardless of practice setting, the goals of case management are to *simultaneously* promote the client's wellness, autonomy, and appropriate use of service and financial resources.
1. Through early assessment, ensure that services are generated in a timely and cost-effective manner.
2. Assist patients to achieve an optimal level of wellness and functioning by facilitating and coordinating timely and appropriate health services.
3. Assist patients to self-direct care appropriately, self-advocate, and make informed decisions to the degree possible.
4. Facilitate the organization and sequencing of appropriate health care services in the most cost-effective manner, without compromising quality of care in order to promote optimal outcomes for all parties involved (NARPPS, 1989).
5. Maintain the greatest amount of independence and human dignity for the client; enable the client to reside in the most appropriate environment; provide an appropriate, comprehensive, and coordinated response to the client's needs that addresses prevention as

well as rehabilitation and maintenance; build and strengthen family and community support; serve as an integral line (NCOA, 1988).

6. Enhance client safety, productivity, satisfaction, and quality of life; assist clients to appropriately self-direct care, self-advocate, and make informed and timely health care decisions (CMSA, 2002).

7. Provide quality health care along a continuum, decrease fragmentation of care across many settings, enhance the client's quality of life, and contain costs.

8. Return the patient to work or assess the patient's ability to return to work and develop a plan that will assist the patient in returning to work or becoming employable.

9. Enhance the developmental, problem-solving, and coping capacities of people; promote the effective and humane operation of systems that provide resources and services to people; link people with systems that provide them with resources, services, and opportunities; and contribute to the development and improvement of social policy (NASW, 1992).

10. Enhance quality of care (Siefker et al., 1995).

■ CASE MANAGEMENT DOMAINS

A. The six knowledge domains for effective case management practice (CCMC, 2005) and their content describe the knowledge and expertise that case managers must possess in order to carry out the essential activities of case management.

1. Case management concepts
   a. Accreditation standards and requirements
   b. Case management models
   c. Case management process and tools
   d. Case recording and documentation
   e. Goals and objectives of case management
   f. Program evaluation and research methods
   g. Quality and performance improvement concepts

2. Case management principles and strategies
   a. Confidentiality
   b. Conflict resolution strategies
   c. Negotiation
   d. Ethics
   e. Health care and disability-related legislation
   f. Interpersonal communication
   g. Legal and regulatory requirements
   h. Risk management
   i. Standards of practice

3. Psychosocial and support systems
   a. Behavioral health and psychiatric disability concepts

    b. Psychological and neuropsychological assessment
    c. Management of clients with substance use/abuse/addiction
    d. Wellness and illness prevention concepts and strategies
    e. Community resources
    f. Support programs
    g. Family dynamics
    h. Multicultural issues as they relate to health behavior
    i. Psychosocial aspects of chronic illness and disability
    j. Spirituality
    k. Management of complementary alternative medicine practices
    l. Concepts related to working with clients who have been abused
    m. Crisis intervention strategies

4. Health care management and delivery
    a. Management of acute and chronic illness and disability
    b. Assessment of physical functioning
    c. Assistive technology
    d. Continuum of care
    e. Critical pathways, standards of care, practice guidelines
    f. Health care delivery systems
    g. Levels of care
    h. Management of medication use
    i. Rehabilitation service delivery systems
    j. Roles and functions of providers
    k. Health care providers
    l. Roles and functions of case managers in various settings

5. Health care reimbursement
    a. Managed care concepts
    b. Cost containment principles
    c. Health care insurance principles
    d. Managed care reimbursement methodologies
    e. Prospective payment system
    f. Private benefit programs
    g. Public benefit programs
    h. Utilization management
    i. Cost–benefit analysis

6. Vocational concepts and strategies
    a. Ergonomics
    b. Job analysis, modification and accommodation, and vocational assessment
    c. Disability compensation systems
    d. Job development and placement
    e. Life care planning
    f. Vocational aspects of chronic illness and disability

      g. Work adjustment and work transition

      h. Workers' compensation principles

      i. Work-hardening resources and strategies

REFERENCES

American Congress of Rehabilitation Medicine (ACRM). (1988). *White Paper on Case Management.* Chicago: ACRM.

American Nurses, Association (ANA). (1994). *Nursing Case Management.* Kansas City, MO: ANA.

Association of Rehabilitation Nurses (ARN). (2006). Role descriptions: The rehabilitation nurse case manager. Website: *www.rehabnurse.org/profresources/casemgr.html.* Retrieved February 20, 2006.

Case Management Society of America (CMSA). (2002). *Standards of practice for case management.* Little Rock, AR: CMSA.

Cohen, E. (1996). *Nurse case management in the 21st century.* St. Louis: Mosby Year Book.

Cohen, E., Cesta, T. (1997). *Nursing case management. From concept to evaluation,* 2nd ed. St. Louis: Mosby Year Book.

Commission on the Accreditation of Rehabilitation Facilities (CARF). (1989). *Case Management Standards.* Tucson, AZ: CARF.

Commission for Case Manager Certification (CCMC). (2005). Website: *www.ccmcertification.org.*

Kane, Rosalie. (1988). Case management: Ethical pitfalls on the road to high-quality managed care. *Quality Review Bulletin,* Joint Commission on Accreditation of Healthcare Organization.

Kongstvedt, Peter. (2003). *Essentials of managed health care with study guide,* 4th ed. Aspen.

National Association of Professional Geriatric Care Managers (NAPGCM). (1997). *Standards of practice for professional geriatric care managers.* Tucson, AZ: NAPGCM.

National Association of Rehabilitation in the Private Sector (NARPPS). (1995).

National Association of Social Workers (NASW). (1984). *NASW standards and guidelines for social work case management for the functionally impaired.* Silver Springs, MD: NASW.

National Association of Social Workers (NASW). (1992). *NASW standards for social work case management.* Washington, DC: NASW.

National Council on Aging (NCOA). (1988). *Care management standards.* Washington, DC: NCOA.

Powell, S. (2000). *Advanced Case Management: Outcomes and Beyond.* Philadelphia, Pa: Lippincott, Williams & Wilkins.

Siefker, J. M., et al. (Eds.) (1995). *Fundamentals of case management.* St. Louis: Mosby.

Utilization Review and Accreditation Commission (URAC). (2002). *Case management standards, v.2.0.* Washington, DC: URAC.

Weil, M., & Karls, J. M. (1985). *Case management in human service practice.* San Francisco: Jossey-Bass.

Williams S. J., Torrens P. R. *(1993). Introduction to Health Services,* 4th ed. Albany, NY: Delmar Publishers.

SUGGESTED READING

American Hospital Association (AHA). (1987). *Case management: An aid to quality and continuity of care.* Chicago: AHA.

Cesta, T., Tahan, H., & Fink, L. (1998). *The case manager's survival guide: Winning strategies for clinical practice.* St. Louis: Mosby Year Book.

Chan, F., et al. (1999). Foundational knowledge and major practice domains of case management. *Journal of Care Management, 5*(1), 10–11, 14, 17–18, 26–28, 30.

Henderson, Mary G. (1988). Measuring quality in medical case management programs. *Quality Review Bulletin,* Chicago, IL. Joint Commission on Accreditation of Healthcare Organizations.

Mullahy, C. (2004). *The case manager's handbook,* 3rd ed. Sudbury, MA: Jones and Bartlett.

National Center for Cost Containment, Department of Veterans Affairs. (1995). *Social work service practice guidelines, number 2: Social work case management.* Milwaukee, WI: Department of Veterans Affairs.

Roberts-DeGennaro. (1992). Generalist model of case management practice. *Journal of Case Management, 2*(3).

Stolte Upman, C. (2003). The evolution of case management: Where we are today. *Care Management,* June.

Tahan, H. (1999). Clarifying case management: What is in a label? *Nursing Case Management, 4*(6), 268–276.

Health Care Insurance, Benefits, and Reimbursement Systems

Beverly Cunningham

LEARNING OBJECTIVES

Upon completion of this chapter, the reader will be able to:

1. Define important terms and concepts related to the health care delivery system, health care insurance, and reimbursement.
2. Name four types of health care delivery systems.
3. Name three challenges facing managed care and health care delivery systems.
4. Name the different types of reimbursement methods and describe each.
5. Name the types of insurance.
6. Identify the role of the case manager in health care reimbursement.

IMPORTANT TERMS AND CONCEPTS

All Patient Related Diagnosis Related Group (APR-DRG)
Ambulatory Payment Classification (APC)
Capitation
Carve-Out
Commercial Insurance

Concurrent Review
Continuum of Care
Co-insurance
Co-pay
Credentialing
Deductible
Denial of Payment

17

Diagnosis Related Group (DRG)
Fee for Service
Gatekeeper
Health Care Reimbursement
Health Maintenance Organization
  (HMO)
Indemnity
Lifetime Maximum
Managed Care
Medicaid
Medical Necessity
Medicare
Minimum Data Set (MDS)
Out-of-Pocket Maximum

Per Diem
Point of Service Plan
Preauthorization
Predictive Modeling
Preferred Provider Organization
  (PPO)
Primary Care Physician (PCP)
Prospective Payment System
Resource Utilization Groups (RUGs)
Retrospective Review
Risk Sharing
Stop Loss
Third Party Administrator (TPA)
Utilization Review and Management

■ INTRODUCTION

   A. The increased costs of health care services and the consumers' demand for high quality and safe care have given rise to new methods of health care reimbursement. They have also made old ways of reimbursement either obsolete or more popular.

   B. Changes in payment structures have taken place in almost every sector of the health care industry. However, the most dominant driver for these changes has been cost containment.

     1. Managed care type health plans have become popular over the past two decades and regulatory attempts to contain health care costs continue to grow through the implementation of various managed care strategies and federally funded demonstration projects.

     2. The Centers for Medicare and Medicaid Services (CMS) have extended the prospective payment system (PPS) methods to almost all care settings of health care delivery. In addition to acute care, PPS is now applied in ambulatory, long-term, and home care settings, among others.

   C. Reimbursement methodologies for health care services vary widely. They are determined by the reimbursement source/payer: PPS, managed care, capitation, fee for service, and so on.

   D. Managed care encompasses a wide variety of terms and concepts, from the structure and purpose of the health care organization itself, to the tools used in a health care delivery system or insurance plan.

   E. Government-based insurers/payers, such as Medicare and Medicaid benefit programs, often influence the processes used by managed care organizations and plans.

This chapter is a revised version of what was previously published in the first edition of *CMSA Core Curriculum for Case Management*. The contributor wishes to acknowledge Penny M. Burman, as some of the timeless material was retained from the previous version.

F. Benefit systems and reimbursement amounts are determined by payer source, which can be classified into two broad groups: commercial insurance and government payers.
  1. Benefits are usually received only by those who are covered by a health insurance plan.
  2. Federal government assumes health care responsibility for older citizens and those with specified long-term disabilities.
  3. State government assumes health care responsibility for children and indigent adults meeting specific state guidelines.

G. Health care responsibility varies by state policies. For example, federal and state programs may assign responsibility for management of health care benefits to a third party—known as Managed Medicare or Managed Medicaid plans.

H. The case manager's involvement with health care reimbursement, especially managed care, varies based on the degree and complexity of the:
  1. Health care services offered,
  2. Needs of the patient and family served,
  3. Benefits as defined in the health insurance plan, and
  4. The payer/insurer and its contract.

■ KEY DEFINITIONS

A. Capitation—A set amount paid to a provider (individual or agency) on the basis of per member "per year" or "per month," no matter what type of care/services is provided or not provided. Rates may vary widely with age and gender of members. Amount is predetermined and stipulated in a managed care contract between the insurer/payer and the health care provider (individual or agency).

B. Co-insurance—Percentage of allowed charges of a covered service for which a member in the health plan is responsible.

C. Commercial insurance—Payers that are not related to, or sponsored by, state or federal health insurance programs.

D. Co-pay—Predetermined dollar amount for which a member of a health plan is responsible each time a specific service is rendered (i.e., office visit, emergency department visit, prescription).

E. Deductible—Fixed amount of money a member in a health plan must pay each year before insurance benefits are paid by the insurance company. This is usually disbursed at the time the member accesses health care services.

F. Diagnosis related groups (DRGs)—The DRG system is a patient classification scheme that provides a means of relating the type of patient a hospital treats (i.e., the medical/clinical condition, acuity, and diagnosis) to the costs incurred by the hospital during care provision (i.e., resource utilization and intensity).

G. Gatekeeper—A primary care physician (usually a family practitioner, internist, pediatrician, or nurse practitioner) to whom a plan member is assigned. Responsible for managing all referrals for specialty care and other covered services used by the member.

H. Government payers—Payers that are related to, or sponsored by, state or federal health insurance programs such as Medicare and Medicaid benefit programs.

I. Health care delivery system—A comprehensive model or structure used in the delivery of health care services to individuals—for example, integrated delivery system (IDS).

J. Health care reimbursement—Payment regarding health care and services provided by a physician, medical professional, or agency to individuals in need of such services.

K. Managed care—A system of health care delivery that aims to provide a generalized structure and focus when managing the use, access, cost, quality, and effectiveness of health care services. It links the patient to provider services.

L. Minimum data set (MDS)—The assessment tool used in skilled nursing facility settings to place a patient into a resource utilization group (RUG), which determines the facility's reimbursement rate.

M. Network model—A group of physicians and related health care providers (may include health care facilities), contracted with a health insurance plan, from which a member should seek services. In this model, members have the option to go out of network for services. However, should the member select an out-of-network provider, out-of-pocket expenses may be higher than those incurred had the member remained within the network.

N. Out-of-pocket maximum—Maximum per calendar year for which a health plan member is responsible. Co-insurance, deductible, and co-pay payments accumulate toward this maximum.

O. Predictive modeling—A process used by managed care organizations to identify which of their members will have the highest future medical costs and will be in need of an increased amount of health care services. This tends to be based on clinical and demographic patient information and past expenditure.

P. Prospective payment system (PPS)—A health care payment system used by the federal government for reimbursing health care providers and agencies for medical care provided to individuals who belong to a governmental insurance plan.

Q. Re-insurance—Insurance to cover any losses incurred while covering claims that exceed a specified dollar threshold. This is most frequent with health maintenance organization (HMO) type plans.

■ DRIVING FORCES BEHIND HEALTH CARE REIMBURSEMENT SYSTEMS

A. There are several factors that impact the nature of the health care delivery system and its reimbursement structures.

B. As the health care industry continues to be dynamic and constantly changing, and innovations in diagnostics and therapeutics occur, the cost of health care services will continue to rise prompting necessary modifications in the reimbursement systems. Below are some important factors that affect such changes.

C. Commercial payers

   1. Technology and innovations are more popular today in the health care market than ever before.

     a. Are evident in the increased use of web-based products, including systems used for verification, authorization, approval of benefits, and claims payments or denials

     b. Are used to improve the efficiency and effectiveness of health care services

     c. Have resulted in a surge of expensive and complex technological advances in health care services, including diagnostic and therapeutic modalities

     d. Also include clinical trials, especially in the area of pharmaceuticals

   2. Need to reduce the increased costs of care. Some of the reasons behind the increased costs are:

     a. Aging population

     b. Complexity and chronicity of patients' health conditions, including the increased number of comorbidities and need for polypharmacy

     c. Need for post–acute medical care management; for example, durable medical equipment (DME), home health services, and lower level of care facilities

     d. Pharmaceutical costs

     e. Implants and prostheses costs

     f. Inpatient versus outpatient medical management

   3. Consumer demand for lower costs and higher quality

   4. Malpractice insurance claims

   5. Insurance premiums—For insurance plans, single individuals, and employers

   6. Opportunity for managed care to administer federal or state plans, such as Medicare Managed Care, Medicaid Managed Care, Child Health Plus, and Family Health Plus

   7. Leapfrog initiatives—Coalition of public and private organizations (including employers and insurance plans) setting standards for hospitals to avoid preventable patient care errors

     a. Examples of such standards include the use of intensivists and computerized order entry systems.

   8. Accreditation agencies—Agencies setting health care standards and expectations, such as the:

     a. National Committee for Quality Assurance (NCQA)

     b. Joint Commission on Accreditation of Healthcare Organizations (JCAHO)

      c. Utilization Review Accreditation Commission (URAC)

      d. Commission on Accreditation of Rehabilitation Facilities (CARF)

   9. Federal rules, laws, and regulations

  10. Employer costs

D. Government payers

   1. Are affected by the Balanced Budget Act (BBA) of 1997, which was a response to concern of potential insolvency of Medicare Hospital Insurance Trust Fund. The primary goal of BBA was to reduce Medicare spending as follows:

      a. Reduced Medicare beneficiary health care benefits

      b. Eliminated cost-based reimbursement for post–acute care services

   2. Desire to balance cost with payment

      a. Pay for performance (P4P)

      b. Potential move from payment by DRG to payment using APR-DRG reimbursement system

   3. The prospective payment system (PPS), which was originally defined by Social Security amendment of 1983 and focused on reimbursement for hospital care

      a. Uses the diagnosis related group (DRG), a financial tool, as the reimbursement method for health care services rendered in the hospital setting and is characterized by the following:

         i. Payment is fixed and based on the operating costs of the patient's diagnosis.

         ii. Predetermined case rate that is paid regardless of the actual costs incurred by the provider of services.

         iii. Uses the DRG to establish amount of reimbursement

      b. DRGs demonstrate groups of patients using similar resources and experiencing similar length of hospital stay.

      c. DRGs developed based on research conducted by a team of health care providers and researchers at Yale University, CT.

   4. The ambulatory payment classification (APC) system, which was rolled out in 2000 and is described as follows:

      a. A prospective payment fee schedule for bundled outpatient services

      b. An encounter-based outpatient reimbursement system that is similar in philosophy to the DRG system

      c. Unlike DRGs, a single outpatient encounter may result in the payment of one or more APCs

   5. Rehabilitation prospective payment system

      a. A prospective payment system for rehabilitation facilities, similar to that of acute care/hospital-based care (i.e., the DRG system)

      b. Includes a patient assessment instrument (PAI) that captures a score that is used to place a patient in a case mix group (CMG) and to establish the reimbursement rate

      c. CMGs function similar to the DRG and APC systems

d. In the CMG system, rehabilitation patients are classified into groups based on clinical/medical characteristics and expected resource consumption

6. Resource utilization groups (RUGs)

a. A prospective payment system for skilled nursing facilities, similar to that of acute care/hospital-based care (i.e., the DRG system)

b. Classifies skilled nursing facility patients into 7 major hierarchies and 44 resource utilization groups based on information from the minimum data set (MDS)

c. The MDS includes data that reflects the patient's medical/clinical condition and resources/services required for care.

d. Reimbursement is based on the assigned hierarchy and RUG.

■ TYPES OF INSURANCE

A. Commercial programs

1. Liability insurance—Benefits paid for bodily injury, property damage, or both

2. No-fault insurance—Includes auto and workers' compensation

a. Auto

i. Benefits for injuries, property damage, or both, incurred while driving, or being present in, a vehicle

ii. Policy regulations vary from state to state.

b. Workers' compensation

i. An insurance program that provides medical benefits and replacement of lost wages for persons suffering from injury or illness that is caused by or occurred in the workplace

ii. An insurance system for industrial and work-related injury. It is regulated primarily among the separate states; however, in certain specified occupations it is regulated by the federal government.

iii. Often requires the employee to follow a specific process/procedure for the medical services and benefits to be paid

iv. Is a heavy user of the case manager's role

v. Focuses on timely return to work to minimize outlay of lost wages

3. Accident and health insurance

a. Includes payment for health care–related costs

b. Often has a lifetime maximum benefit

c. May include long- or short-term disability insurance to provide replacement of salary when the member is unable to work, due to illness or injury

4. Insurance plans

a. Indemnity—Security against possible loss or damages. Reimbursement for loss that is paid in a predetermined amount in the event of covered loss.

      i. Fee for service structure

      ii. Consumer has freedom to choose care provider

      iii. Payment by predetermined contract

      iv. May also be a managed plan, with some degree of control

      v. Benefits are in the form of payments rather than services. In most cases after the provider has billed the individual, the insured person is reimbursed by the company.

   b. Group medical

      i. Of varying terms. For example, employment status of the enrollee may change benefits; i.e., active, retired, or terminated employee—Consolidated Omnibus Budget Reconciliation Act of 1986 (COBRA).

      ii. Length of service may also affect benefits.

      iii. Disability

         a. Could be short-term or long-term

         b. May be a wage replacement only and may lack health care intervention

   c. Consumer driven

      i. Consumer determines how health care dollars will be spent

      ii. High deductibles

      iii. Varying strategies, including online menus of benefits

      iv. Premiums set according to benefits selected by employees

      v. High interest, but low enrollment

   d. Diagnosis-specific benefits

      i. Additional funding by regulatory agencies (state, federal, local)

      ii. Examples—Cystic fibrosis, premature babies, crippled children, Easter Seals, Shriners

      iii. Variation in funding from private sector and regulatory agencies

   e. Stop-loss insurance

      i. Large dollar cases only

      ii. Increased value of case management

   f. Managed care plans

      i. A system designed to maintain the quality of health care in a cost-effective manner with a focus on delivery of health care services and payment for those services.

      ii. Also refers to both an organization that coordinates the purchase and/or delivery of health care services and a set of techniques used to ensure the efficiency and effectiveness of the use of these services (Redman, in Cohen and Cesta, 2005).

      iii. The primary goal is to have a system that delivers value by giving access to quality, cost-effective health care.

B. Government programs

  1. Medicare

    a. Created in 1966, Title 18 of the Social Security Act, to finance medical care for persons aged 65 years or older, and the disabled who are entitled to social security benefits

    b. Is under the administrative oversight of CMS

    c. Identifies mandated hospital services through conditions of participation for hospitals

    d. Traditional Medicare

        i. Part A covers hospitalization and Part B covers mainly physician services and emergency department visits.

    e. Medicare Choice plan (M+C)

        i. Created by the Balanced Budget Act of 1997

        ii. HMO plans that contract with government to administer Medicare benefits to its members

    f. Managed Medicare

        i. Is an option afforded to Medicare enrollees and is similar to a health maintenance organization (HMO) in structure

        ii. Provides all services that a Medicare recipient would normally receive

        iii. Provides health care services on a prepaid capitation basis

2. Medicaid

    a. Created in 1966, Title 19 of the Social Security Act, to finance health care of the indigent

    b. Jointly financed by federal and state governments through the tax structure

    c. States may impose nominal deductibles and co-payments on Medicaid recipients for certain services.

    d. Eligibility criteria vary from state to state and are based on the person's income and assets.

    e. Managed Medicaid

        i. Similar to Managed Medicare, afforded to the recipients of Medicaid benefits

        ii. Focuses on cost containment, improved access to care, and quality of care

        iii. Provides all services that a Medicaid recipient would normally receive

        iv. Provides health care services on a prepaid capitation basis

3. Military insurance

    a. Tricare

        i. Managed care insurance plan for active duty and retired members of the military, their families, and survivors

        ii. Formerly called CHAMPUS

        iii. U.S. Family Health Plan

    b. Veteran administration

        i. Insurance plan for active duty and retired members of the military, their families, and survivors

■ COMPONENTS OF HEALTH CARE REIMBURSEMENT

A. Limits
   1. Define access to care for many plans including types of services covered
   2. Include list of providers an enrollee may use for health care services
   3. Delineate consumer choice for services; e.g., within or out-of-network
   4. Explain the cost and premium

B. Reimbursement mechanism—The method applied for payment for care rendered. This could be in the form of case rate, capitated rate, fee for service, discounted, per diem, and others.

C. Quality management program/model
   1. A formal and planned, systematic, organizationwide (or network-wide) approach to the monitoring, analysis, and improvement of the organization's performance; thereby continually improving the extent to which providers conform to defined standards, the quality of patient care and services provided, and the likelihood of achieving desired outcomes.
   2. May focus on measuring outcomes on certain quality metrics (e.g., immunization rates, mammography and cervical cancer rates, and so on), provider profiles on resource utilization, and enrollee satisfaction with care.
   3. Government payers such as Medicare and Medicaid examine quality improvement through the use of peer review organizations (PROs); in some states they are called quality improvement organizations (QIOs).
      a. Medicare and Medicaid oversight for appropriateness and quality of care
      b. Establish medical necessity criteria
      c. Tie financial risk to quality of care
      d. May focus on measuring outcomes on certain metrics. For example, core measures of certain diagnoses (also known as *appropriate care measures*), such as heart failure, acute coronary syndrome, and pneumonia, and patient satisfaction with care.

D. Risk sharing—The process whereby an HMO and contracted provider each accept partial responsibility for the financial risk and rewards involved in cost effectively caring for the members enrolled in the plan and assigned to a specific provider.

E. Credentialing—The review process applied to approve a health care professional, such as a physician as a provider of care and participant in a health plan.
   1. Specific criteria are used in the review and approval process.
   2. Criteria may include, but are not limited to, the following:
      a. References
      b. Training and education, including diplomas
      c. Licensure

    d. Board certifications, if any

    e. Experience record

    f. Malpractice insurance

F. Continuum of care—Matching ongoing needs of the individuals being served by the case management process with the appropriate level and type of health, medical, financial, legal, and psychosocial care for services within a setting or across multiple settings (CCMC, 2005).

G. Medical management—Includes case management and disease management.

   1. Case management—A collaborative process that assesses, plans, implements, coordinates, monitors, and evaluates the options and services required to meet an individual's health needs, using communication and available resources to promote quality, cost-effective outcomes (CCMC, 2005).

   2. Factors that indicate need for intensive case management and/or medical management include, but are not limited to, the following:

    a. High dollar patient (high expense)

    b. Specific diseases, especially those that are complex and at risk for intense progression and deterioration

    c. Complex and/or costly interventions/procedures, such as transplant

    d. Investigational procedures/treatments

   3. Disease management—A system of coordinated health care interventions and communications for populations with chronic conditions in which patient's self-care efforts are significant.

    a. Supports the physician or practitioner/patient relationship

    b. Uses disease management plans of care that emphasize prevention of exacerbations and complications of medical condition

    c. Employs evidence-based practice guidelines

    d. Focuses on patient empowerment strategies with the goal of improving overall health

    e. Focuses mainly on chronic disorders

    f. May include risk assessment of members

    g. Population management

    h. Management of acute phase of disease, with a focus on disease-specific complication management

H. Utilization management—Review of health care services to ensure that they are medically necessary, provided in the most appropriate care setting, and at or above quality standards.

   1. Prior approval requirements for specific procedures, such as transplants, potentially cosmetic procedures, investigational procedures

   2. Precertification, also known as *prior authorization*, most often related to medical necessity

    a. Focus may be primarily on inpatient verses outpatient

    b. Goal is to reduce inpatient/hospital days to those necessary

      c. Hospital days per member, per month reports are reviewed by the plan's oversight group as a measure of utilization and resource consumption

   3. Concurrent review (continued stay review)—Reviews to approve continued treatments, such as inpatient hospitalization, rehabilitation, home care, DME, long-term care.

   4. Retrospective review—A form of review of a patient's medical record, conducted after health care services (including hospital stay) have been rendered and the patient is released; used to track appropriateness of care and consumption of resources.

   5. Transitional/discharge planning—Transitioning patients from one level of care to another, usually from most to least acute; however it may happen in the reverse way as well.

I. Outcomes reporting

   1. Feedback to compare providers with other providers. Outcome metrics may include, for example:

      a. Physician practice patterns

      b. Hospital length of stay, complication rate, mortality rate, readmission rate

      c. Home care outcomes

      d. CMS metrics, such as the core measures or appropriateness of care measures (e.g., those for pneumonia, heart failure, and acute myocardial infarction) and patient satisfaction with services

      e. Often includes benchmarking

   2. Health Plan Employer Data and Information Set (HEDIS)

      a. Performance measurement set for managed care organizations; focuses on the quality of the systems, processes, and services offered by the plan to enrollees. Also includes access to services and effectiveness of care.

      b. Developed by National Commission on Quality Assurance (NCQA)

      c. Data are made available to both consumers and providers.

      d. Data may include effectiveness of care, access to care, consumer satisfaction, cost, utilization management, and credentialing of providers.

   3. Benchmark opportunity for plans, providers, facilities

   4. Member satisfaction with care/service

J. Pharmaceutical services—Medications-related services and options offered by the health insurance plan.

   1. Mail-order services for lower costs

   2. Prescription cards for decreased costs for formulary medications (members are generally responsible for a co-pay, co-insurance, or both)

   3. Pharmaceutical benefits manager (PBM)

K. Centers of Excellence

   1. Service lines—such as cardiology—where the member, if receiving care by the provider, can receive discounted services

2. Encourage best-practice outcomes, such as length of stay, readmission rates, cost per case, clinical outcomes, and member satisfaction

■ HEALTH CARE DELIVERY SYSTEMS

A. Health maintenance organization (HMO)—An organization that provides or arranges for coverage of designated health services needed by plan members for a fixed prepaid premium.

1. There are four basic models of HMOs: group model, individual practice association (IPA), network model, and staff model.

2. Under the federal HMO Act, an organization must possess the following to call itself an HMO:
   a. An organized system for providing health care in a geographical area,
   b. An agreed-on set of basic and supplemental health maintenance and treatment services, and
   c. A voluntarily enrolled group of people.

3. Set of designated health care providers who receive a predetermined payment

4. Special attention is paid to access to specialists' care to influence appropriate utilization of specialty care or services; i.e., those necessary due to patient's condition and choice of the most relevant treatment approach.

5. PCP serves as gatekeeper.

6. Coverage for services out of network is limited and carefully determined.

7. May be combined with health care delivery system and various insurance plans such as a preferred provider organization (PPO)

8. HMO models include the following:
   a. Group
      i. Contract with multispecialty physician group organized in partnership or cooperation
      ii. Physicians are employed directly by the group practice
      iii. HMO and group share risk
      iv. Also called *closed model*
   b. Individual/Independent Practice Association (IPA)—An HMO model that contracts with a private practice physician or health care association to provide health care services in return for a negotiated fee.
      i. The IPA contracts with physicians to provide services; however, they continue in their existing individual or group practice.
      ii. Physicians may provide care to HMO and non-HMO patients and have control over the way their offices are run.
      iii. IPA compensates the physicians on a fee schedule or a fee-for-service basis.

      iv. May be more cost effective, with fewer limits than traditional HMO

      v. May apply varying reimbursement methods

    c. Staff model—An HMO model where physicians are employed by the HMO to provide services to its beneficiaries.

      i. Salaried physicians and HMO-owned group practice

      ii. Greatest control

      iii. Performance/production financial incentives

      iv. Also called *closed panel*

      v. Comprehensive services at one site

      vi. Administrative functions are the responsibility of the HMO

    d. Network model—A model where the HMO contracts with a variety of groups of physicians and other providers in a network of care with organized referral patterns.

      i. Networks allow providers to practice outside the HMO.

      ii. Similar to group model, except involves more than one physician group

      iii. May be open or closed model, depending on number of group practices or specialties in contract

    e. Mixed model—A combination of some or all of the different models structures.

    f. Open panel

      i. Primary care provider (PCP) acts as the gatekeeper.

      ii. Patients may seek care of specialist providers without a referral from the PCP.

      iii. Co-pay is higher for self-referrals.

    g. Closed panel

      i. PCP acts as the gatekeeper.

        a. Patients may *not* seek care of specialist providers without a referral or authorization from the PCP.

      ii. Co-pay is less than that of an open panel model.

B. Preferred provider organization (PPO)

  1. An insurance structure in which contracts are established with providers of medical care.

  2. Providers under a PPO contract are referred to as *preferred providers*.

  3. Usually the contract provides significantly better benefits for services received from preferred providers, thus encouraging members to use these providers.

  4. Covered persons are generally allowed benefits for nonparticipating provider services, usually on an indemnity basis with significant copayments.

  5. Contracts with providers for discounted fee for service

  6. Allows self-referral

  7. May be higher co-pay for out-of-network referrals

C. Point of service (POS)
1. A type of health plan allowing the covered person to choose to receive a service from a participating or a nonparticipating provider.
2. Different benefit levels associated with the use of participating providers.
3. Members usually pay substantially higher costs in terms of increased premiums, deductibles, and coinsurance.
4. Allows a blend of HMO and PPO

D. Exclusive provider organization (EPO)
1. A managed care plan that provides benefits only if care is rendered by providers within a specific network
2. Limited use of providers (like HMOs), but much less regulated

E. Integrated delivery system (IDS)
1. Partnership formed among physicians, physician groups, hospitals, and other providers to manage health care (often involves contract with payer organization)
2. System of health care providers organized to provide span of services across the continuum of care and settings

■ **REIMBURSEMENT METHODS**

A. Fee for service—Providers are paid for each service performed.
1. Set fee for service provided
2. Fee schedules are an example of fee for service.
3. No discounts given

B. Discounted fee for service
1. Providers are paid set fee for specific service, but at a previously agreed-upon discount

C. Per diem
1. All services provided for a specific amount per day regardless of actual costs
2. Based on averaging costs and number of days of service

D. Percent of charges
1. Fixed percentage of charges paid to hospitals, based on charges on patient's bill
2. Percent may vary based on contractual agreements

E. Risk sharing
1. The process whereby an HMO and contracted provider each accept partial responsibility for the financial risks and rewards involved in caring for the members enrolled in the plan
2. Focuses on target payment for health care costs per member per month between a plan and a provider or a network of providers
3. Evaluation at end of year determines gains/losses that are shared, with the goal being decreased costs

F. DRG/Case rate
   1. Rate of reimbursement that packages pricing for a certain category of services. Typically combines facility and professional practitioner fees for care and services.
   2. Specific dollar amount paid based on classification of illness, diagnosis, or procedure
   3. Audits may be done to ensure accurate coding.

G. Capitation
   1. A fixed amount of money, per member per month (PMPM), paid to a care provider for covered services rather than based on specific services provided.
   2. The typical reimbursement method used by HMOs.
   3. Whether a member uses the health service once or more than once, a provider who is capitated receives the same payment.

H. Carve-out services
   1. Usually refers to payers
   2. Services excluded from a provider contract that may be covered through arrangements with other providers
   3. Separate negotiations for unusually complex or high-cost services, such as organ transplant or bone marrow transplant
   4. Could be services required in a complicated case. For example, additional home care services that exceed expected care, such as additional physical therapy services.
   5. Providers are not financially responsible for services carved out of their contract. Examples of these services are mental/behavioral health and substance/chemical dependency.

I. Pay-for-performance (P4P)
   1. Pay based on outcomes of specific diseases or DRGs
   2. May be managed through a Center of Excellence, such as cardiovascular or orthopedic
   3. Outcomes may include mortality and morbidity rates, Core Measures, clinical outcomes, patient/family health-related teaching, length of stay, costs, readmission and complications rates, and satisfaction with care

J. Global payment and package pricing
   1. A predetermined all-inclusive payment structure for a specific set of related services, treated as a single unit for billing or reimbursement purposes
   2. Combines reimbursement for both facility and professional services into one lump sum payment
   3. Commonly seen in transplants
   4. Usually includes both preoperative and postoperative care, perinatal care, including delivery services

K. Stop loss
1. Used to share risk in complex patients
2. Payment may increase after a specified dollar threshold is met. For example, hospital payment would convert from DRG payment to percent of charges once charges reach a specified dollar amount

L. Managed government plans
1. Payment by a plan that agrees to pay health care benefits for specific populations, such as Medicare or Medicaid
2. Managed Medicare plans are selected by patients and are optional.
3. Managed Medicaid plans may be either selected by patients or, most often, mandated by a state.
4. Provider follows government rules and regulations for these payment groups; that is, at a minimum, providers must offer the same services offered under the government plans (mainly Medicare and Medicaid).
5. Plan assumes risk for member, who relinquishes traditional coverage (either voluntary or assigned, depending on state regulations).

M. Third party administrator/administration (TPA)
1. Administration of a group insurance plan by some person or firm other than the insurer of the policyholder
2. A third party administration is an organization outside of the insuring organization that handles only administrative functions, such as utilization review and processing of claims.
3. A third party administrator is used by organizations that actually fund the health benefits but do not find it cost effective to administer the plan themselves.

N. Government payers
1. Medicare and Medicaid benefit plans
2. Future plans for reimbursement
   a. Medicare demonstration projects
   b. Refined DRGs
   c. Other care settings with impending PPS-type reimbursement method

■ CHALLENGES WITH HEALTH CARE REIMBURSEMENT

A. Financial—Concern that financial incentives may compromise quality of care

B. Patient choice of physicians/care providers and facilities limited unless patient pays out-of-network fees

C. Benefits mandated by various state regulations; i.e., one state might require a certain number of mammograms be covered for women in certain age groups, whereas another state may require something different be covered

D. Workers' compensation
   1. Compensation laws vary from state to state, requiring case managers to have knowledge of the varying state laws. State workers' compensation guidelines take precedence over the funding source's guidelines.
   2. Some are in the form of managed care plans and are not required to follow the requirements of traditional state plans.
   3. Often more legal risk is involved and potentially more litigious than medical cases.
   4. Case management services are offered based on the requirements of the workers' compensation–related regulations and state legislation.
   5. Increased value in, and greater acceptance of early return-to-work programs

E. Patient and provider education is essential.

F. Varying communication with payer; for example, telephone, fax, web-based

G. Often minimum flexibility, especially when it comes to:
   1. Nontraditional treatments,
   2. Uncovered benefits, and
   3. Post-acute levels of care.

H. Focus on technical denials, rather than payment for services provided. For example, lack of notification for hospital admission

I. Off-shore outsourcing of utilization management services (through TPA)

J. Underinsured patients
   1. Minimum payment per hospitalization
   2. Severely restricted lifetime maximum
   3. Carve out of specific diseases
   4. Extremely high co-pay or deductible structure

K. Medicare demonstration projects and their effects on reimbursement systems will result in renewed reimbursement methods such as pay-for-performance or global funding for certain procedures or diseases.

■ LEGAL ISSUES IMPACTING MANAGED CARE

A. Government and legislative issues
   1. Employee Retirement Income Security Act Guidelines (ERISA)—Self-insured companies not required to hold to same minimum benefit regulations; e.g., some groups may limit benefits for HIV-related treatments

B. Clinical practice guidelines, often used in managed care, may put the plan at risk for litigation. This may be seen as limiting care for the benefit of decreasing costs.

C. Increased complaints about decisions to withhold treatment

D. Increased concern about ethical decisions impacting patient care

E. Consolidated Omnibus Budget Reconciliation Act of 1986 (COBRA)—Law requiring certain employers to allow qualified employees, spouses, and dependents to continue health insurance coverage when it would otherwise stop; for example, when one resigns from employment.

F. Health Information Portability and Accountability Act (HIPAA) of 1996
  1. Came about with the advent of electronic medical records and the transfer of information electronically from one health plan to another or care provider to another
  2. Privacy rule protects individual medical records and personal health information (PHI).
  3. Limits the release of information to the minimum reasonably needed for the purpose of disclosure
  4. In addition to privacy, HIPAA makes health insurance more portable from job to job and ensures continuity of coverage/benefits.
  5. Can decrease waiting periods for insurance to be effective
  6. Includes a variety of regulations, such as fraud and abuse, minimum maternity hospital stays, and medical spending accounts
  7. Gives patients the right to obtain copies of their own health records

■ STRATEGIES IN MANAGED CARE

A. Managed care practices have resulted in the addition or reinforcement of many strategies that ensure quality of care and assist in controlling health care costs. Some of the strategies case managers must be aware of are the following:
  1. Credentialing and re-credentialing of physicians
  2. Medical management practices that are part and parcel of managed care—utilization management, case management, quality management, disease management
  3. Claims processing and the use of information systems
  4. Keeping costs at a minimum by applying the following strategies:
     a. Complying with the procedures and practices stipulated in the contractual agreement between health plans and providers/agencies
     b. Ensuring that bed days in hospitals are appropriate and as indicated by the patient's conditions
     c. Using the demand management programs/services offered by the health plan
     d. Employing health promotion and illness prevention strategies such as patient and family education, risk-reduction programs, etc.
  5. Managed care/insurance contracts that are specific about reimbursement, utilization management, and the denials and appeals processes/procedures
     a. Utilization management practices
        i. Precertification
        ii. Authorization
        iii. Level of care

b. Definitions of medical necessity for care and treatment applying evidence-based guidelines and protocols

c. Reimbursement methods, such as per diem or case rate

d. May be very detailed, including reimbursement terms and criteria by service line, or time of day for communication requirements

e. Denial and appeal processes

f. Often stipulate billing mechanism and process

6. Shifting from inpatient care to outpatient care, when possible

a. Insurance plans may try to decrease hospital bed days by shifting inpatients to observation status

b. Decisions regarding best care setting for treatment are made based on the clinical condition of the patient and the treatment options to be implemented

7. Tracking the duration/length of treatment, especially length of hospital stay; lifetime maximum, episode-of-care maximum payment

8. Complying with NCQA standards and the HEDIS national indicators and performance measures

a. NCQA is a national organization comprised of health care quality management professionals

b. Offers an accreditation program for managed health care plans

c. Focus on the quality of the systems, processes, and services a managed care/health plan delivers to its enrollees

d. Performance of health plans on the HEDIS measures is in the public domain and accessible to health care consumers

e. HEDIS targets the following quality areas:

i. Effectiveness of care

ii. Access to and availability of services

iii. Consumer satisfaction with care

iv. Health plan stability

v. Consumer health choice

vi. Cost of services

vii. Utilization management

viii. Credentialing of health care professionals

■ IMPLICATIONS OF REIMBURSEMENT FOR CASE MANAGERS

A. For effective practice and performance, case managers must be knowledgeable in the following areas:

1. The health plan or the managed care contract

a. Payer contact information

b. Reimbursement method(s)

c. Utilization review and management

d. Medical necessity criteria

e. Post–acute care approved panel of providers (individuals and facilities/agencies)

    f. Contract writing and input

    g. Denials and appeals processes/procedures

2. The relationships with the insurance-based case manager

    a. Be aware of the implications of the role of the case manager in insurance companies and the complexity of said role, especially in large companies and when there is a need for plan dollars to be utilized in a nontraditional fashion.

    b. Provide advocacy when patients' needs may not be considered in the typical premium structure. These situations result in the need for case managers to ensure advocacy for their patients' benefits.

    c. Be aware of the layers of fiduciaries, administrators, and claims adjustors involved in approval processes.

    d. Special attention should be paid to untimely decisions, which delay case manager interventions and patient treatment. The case manager must be aware of the contractual and legislative time frames that must be adhered to.

    e. Size of insured groups can impact the timeliness of appropriate cost-effective care.

    f. Case managers must know state regulations for plan coverage to ensure timely coordination of benefits.

    g. Optimize communication opportunities with insurance company staff.

    h. Understand case management role, as defined by the health plan.

3. The use of medical necessity and appropriateness of services criteria to ensure approval of benefits and reimbursement

    a. Be knowledgeable of the utilization review/management criteria used by payers.

    b. Gain a comprehensive understanding of benefits based on specific health plans; for example, lifetime maximums and use of Medicare days for hospitalized patients.

    c. Be able to develop effective plans of care for patients and broker appropriate services as needed and across the continuum of care.

    d. Ensure optimal use of available benefits.

    e. Focus on efficiency and effectiveness of service delivery.

    f. Coordinate care and services with patients, families, and other care providers.

    g. Negotiate the availability of services, especially those not covered in the benefits; however, focus on being cost effective and on ensuring optimal quality outcomes.

4. Building partnerships with physicians

    a. Function as an effective leader or facilitator of the multidisciplinary team.

    b. Work closely with physicians on establishing appropriate plans of care for patients, including discharge plans, reimbursement plans, and procurement of resources.

    c. Collaborate with physicians when addressing reimbursement denials.

    d. Educate physicians about the dynamics of health care delivery systems, including the various types of health plans and their related utilization management procedures.

5. How to identify nonmedical challenges that influence patient care outcomes and transitions of care

    a. Understand the impact of underinsurance (and lack of insurance altogether) on patient care delivery, access to services, and outcomes of care.

    b. Identify the presence of psychosocial and financial barriers that impact care delivery, decision making regarding treatment options, and patient's adherence to treatment regimen.

    c. Be aware of the reasons that patients may exhibit behaviors of noncompliance with the plan of care, identify such behaviors, and address them to prevent undesired outcomes.

    d. Be sensitive to cultural factors that may negatively or positively affect patient's behaviors and adherence to the plan of care.

6. How to manage conflict and resolve problems when they arise

    a. Coordinate patient care activities when patient choices do not match recommendations by health care providers, such as the patient or family who chooses to take a patient home when a skilled nursing facility is recommended and necessary.

    b. Hold a case conference when conflicts regarding the development of the plan of care or making decisions regarding treatment options arises between patients and their families or between patients and their health care providers.

    c. Be able to assume the role of the patient advocate when needed.

    d. Seek the counsel of a third party, such as a patient representative, when unable to resolve conflict.

    e. Call for an ethics consult when the need arises.

REFERENCES

Cohen, E. L., & Cesta, T. G. (2005). *Nursing case management*, 4th ed. St. Louis, MO: Mosby.

Commission for Case Manager Certification (CCMC). (2005). *CCMC glossary of terms*. Rolling Meadows, IL: Author. Website: *www.ccmcertification.org/pages/22frame_set.html*. Retrieved March 23, 2006.

SUGGESTED READING

Cesta, T. G. (2002). *Survival strategies for nurses in managed care*. St. Louis, MO: Mosby.

Cesta, T. G., & Tahan, H. A. (2003). *The case manager's survival guide*, 2nd ed. St. Louis, MO: Mosby.

Daniels, S., & Ramey, M. (2005). *The leader's guide to hospital case management*. Sudbury, MA: Jones and Bartlett.

Kongstvedt, P. (2003). *Essentials of managed health care*, 4th ed. Gaithersburg, MD: Aspen.

Mullahy, C. (2004). *The case manager's handbook*, 3rd ed. Sudbury, MA: Jones and Bartlett.

William, C. (2002). *Financial strategy for managed care organizations: Rate setting, risk adjustment, and competitive advantage*. Health Administration Press: ACHE.

3

Case Management Practice Settings and Throughput

Hussein A. Tahan

Upon completion of this chapter, the reader will be able to:

1. Identify the various health care settings that constitute the continuum of care.
2. Define the continuum of care.
3. List the practice settings of case management.
4. Describe the role of the case manager in relation to the continuum of care and practice settings.
5. Define what throughput is and describe its relationship with case management.
6. Describe the role of the case manager in throughput and patient flow.

Beyond-the-Walls Case Management
Continuum of Care
Independent Case Management
Input
Level of Care

Outcome
Output
Patient Flow
Payer-Based Case Management
Practice Setting

Private Case Management
Process
Structure
Telephonic Case Management

Throughput
Transition of Care
Within-the-Walls Case Management

■ INTRODUCTION

A. Case management has been applied as a strategy or a model for care delivery in every setting of the health care continuum.

B. There are many reasons for the implementation of case management models in various care settings. Some of these are the following:
1. Rising number of the elderly, especially those with chronic and complex health conditions.
2. Use of innovative and sophisticated health care technology that tends to be costly, including biomedical informatics.
3. Increase in the use of minimally invasive and robotic surgery and the likelihood of performing surgical procedures in the ambulatory care setting.
4. Rising number of newer and rare diseases especially those that are infectious in nature and that require costly health care resources.
5. Popularity of life-prolonging treatments such as organ transplantation.
6. Changes in health care reimbursement methods, particularly those that place the provider of care or the consumer at higher financial risk. For example, managed care, capitation, and prospective payment systems.
7. Prospective payment systems being applied by federal and state governments reaching almost all settings of care delivery such as long-term care, home care, acute care, rehabilitation, and skilled care environments.
8. Educated consumers of health care.
9. Pressures to cut the forever rising cost of health care services.
10. Shortages in health care workforces including nursing; pharmacy; and physical, occupational, and respiratory therapy.
11. Rising ethical concerns and legal liability resulting in the practice of defensive medicine.
12. Shift of health care delivery and services from the acute to the non–acute care settings such as home care, long-term care, and rehabilitation care settings.
13. Increased demand for quality of care that is supported or evidenced by measurable outcomes.
14. Changes in the standards of accreditation and regulatory agencies, particularly those that impact on case management practice such as those that address continuity of care, care across the continuum, discharge planning, safety, and patients' rights.

C. Case management is not a new approach to managing patient care. It has reached every health care setting across the continuum (Cesta and Tahan, 2003).

   1. 1880s: Outpatient and community settings, particularly the care of the poor
   2. 1920: Outpatient and community care settings, particularly the care of psychiatric patients and individuals with chronic and long-term illnesses
   3. 1930: Public health/community care settings
   4. 1950: Behavioral health across the continuum of care
   5. 1970s and 1980s: Long-term care settings through demonstration projects funded by Medicare and Medicaid waivers
   6. 1985: Acute care settings, particularly as nursing case management programs
   7. 1990s: Virtually all health care settings including managed care organizations

D. The use of case management varies from one practice setting to another, with its identifying characteristics dependent on the discipline that applies it, the professional who assumes the role of the case manager, the staffing mix, and the context of the setting where it is implemented including its related reimbursement method(s).

E. The main characteristics of case management, regardless of care or practice setting, include the following:

   1. Outcomes-oriented care delivery that focuses on monitoring and measurement of patient safety, continuity, and quality of care
   2. Appropriate resource allocation and utilization that is justified by the patient's condition and the required treatment, with cost effectiveness as the ultimate outcome
   3. Comprehensive care planning including early assessment, intervention, and linking patients and their families to needed services
   4. Integration and coordination of care delivery to eliminate fragmentation and/or wastes
   5. Collaboration across care providers and care settings
   6. Advocacy to ensure that needed services are obtained and expected outcomes are met
   7. Use of a licensed professional as the case manager
   8. Compliance with the standards of accreditation and regulatory agencies
   9. Open lines of communication and sharing of important information across care providers, care settings, and the patient/family
   10. Consumer and staff satisfaction

F. Case management allows the integration and coordination of health care services across consumers of health care, providers of care, payers for services, and care settings; that is, across persons, space, and time. This is most effective because case management:

   1. Opens lines of communication about needed and important information among providers, consumers, and payers

    2. Facilitates an environment of collaboration among providers, consumers, and payers. Such is most evident in the presence of shared goals, effective communication, and shared decision making

    3. Promotes a patient-centered approach to care by meeting all the patient's and family's needs and interests

    4. Ensures continuity of care over time and across care settings or providers

G. Case management gained more momentum when the health care delivery system began to gradually shift away from the inpatient care setting (hospital). Owing to numerous technological advances in diagnostics, medications, and procedures, and the evolution of reimbursement plans that limit inpatient hospital stays (e.g., Medicare's prospective payment system, and managed care health plans), most health care needs can be handled on an outpatient basis.

H. Case management has been described as "within the walls" and "beyond the walls" (Cohen and Cesta, 2005).

    1. Within-the-walls—Case management models in the acute care/hospital settings

    2. Beyond-the-walls—Case management models in the outpatient, community, long-term, and payer-based settings

I. Case management has also been implemented as a core strategy of population-based disease management programs.

J. Recently, case management became an essential strategy for ensuring patient safety, especially in reducing or preventing the risk for medical errors during transitions of care (handoffs), patient flow through the system of health care services, and throughput.

■ KEY DEFINITIONS

A. Beyond-the-walls case management—Models of case management that are implemented outside the acute care/hospital setting; that is in the community, outpatient, long-term, and payer settings.

B. Boarding—Occurs as a result of situations when a patient remains in an area such as the emergency department (ED) or post-anesthesia care unit for a period of time, usually 2 hours or longer, after a decision has been made to admit the patient to an inpatient bed.

C. Crowding—Increased number of patients who are awaiting care or are in the process of receiving care in an area (i.e., care setting such as the ED) beyond the capacity the area can handle. An example is ED crowding as a result of inability to move patients out of the ED and into inpatient beds when these patients must be admitted rather than released.

D. Diversion—Occurs when hospitals request that ambulances bypass their EDs and transport patients to other health care facilities who otherwise would have been cared for at these EDs. This event happens as a result of ED crowding and situations where EDs cannot safely handle additional ambulance patients.

E. Handoff—The act of transferring the care of a patient from one provider to another, from one care setting to another, or from one level of care to another.

F. Health care continuum—Care settings that vary across a continuum based on levels of care that are also characterized by complexity and intensity of resources and services.

G. Input—Elements or characteristics taken into consideration when providing care to a patient. It also may mean the patient's condition at the time he or she presents for care in a particular care setting such as a clinic, emergency department, or hospital. Examples may include age, gender, health status, social network, reason for accessing health care services, or insurance status.

H. Left before a medical evaluation—Occurs when a patient who presents to the ED for care, but leaves the ED after triage and before receiving a medical evaluation. Generally this happens with nonemergent conditions where patients need to wait for treatment.

I. Level of care—The intensity of resources and services required to diagnose, treat, preserve, or maintain an individual's physical and/or emotional health and functioning. Levels of care vary across a continuum of least to most complex resources and/or services—that is, from nonacute, to sub-acute, to acute, to critical.

J. Level of service—The delivery of services and use of resources that are dependent on the patient's condition and the needed level of care. Assessment of the level of service is used to ensure that the patient is receiving care at the appropriate level.

K. Outcome—The result, output, or consequence of a health care process. It may be the result of care received or not received. It also represents the cumulative effects of one or more processes on an individual at a defined point in time. Outcome can also mean the goal or objective of the care rendered.

L. Output—Results or outcomes of care provision. It also may mean the patient's condition at the time he or she exits a health care setting or transitions to another level of care or location. Examples may include death, discharge to home with home care or no services, or discharge to a skilled nursing facility.

M. Patient flow—The movement of patients through a set of locations in a health care facility. These locations are the levels of care required by the patient based on health condition and clinical treatment. Patient flow entails the transitioning of an individual from point A to point B of a health care facility or setting; that is, from the patient's entry point to the checkout point of the health care facility where care is being provided.

N. Practice setting—A care setting in which a case manager is employed and is able to execute his or her responsibilities. Care settings vary across homogeneous populations of patients such as organ transplant, pediatrics, and geriatric; or across physical care delivery areas such as ambulatory/clinics, acute/hospital, long-term, skilled care facilities, or sub-acute rehabilitation.

O. Process—The methods, procedures, styles, and techniques rendered in the delivery of health care services. These relate to the roles, responsibilities, and functions of the various health care providers and how they go about fulfilling them.

P. Structure—The characteristics of the system/environment of care or health care organization including those associated with the providers of care and the patients/families who are the recipients of care. It relates to the level of care or setting; the nature of the care delivery model; the health status of the patients; and the skills, knowledge, education, and competencies of the health care providers.

Q. Throughput—The actual operations of a care setting. It also refers to the clinical and administrative processes applied in the setting to deliver quality patient care and services. Processes may include the use of a case manager; availability of ancillary services such as pharmacy, laboratory, and radiology; and the type of treatments implemented for the care of a patient.

R. Transition of care—The process of moving patients from one level of care to another, usually from most to least complex; however, depending on the patient's health condition and needed treatments, the transition can occur from least to most complex.

S. Within-the-walls case management—Models of case management that are implemented in the acute care/hospital-based setting.

■ CASE MANAGEMENT PRACTICE SETTINGS

A. Case management is practiced across all settings of the health care continuum in varying degrees of complexity and intensity and is dependent on the following four factors:
  1. The context of the care setting (e.g., ambulatory versus acute/hospital);
  2. The patient's health condition and needs (e.g., critical/acute episode of illness versus long-term and chronic condition);
  3. The reimbursement method applied (e.g., managed care or capitation versus prospective payment system); and
  4. The type of care provider(s) needed for care provision (e.g., generalist versus specialist physician, individual provider versus a multidisciplinary team).

B. The role of the case manager also varies based on the care/practice setting and the above four factors. It tends to be more complex as the needs and services a patient requires intensify. The role also is more necessary and valuable when a multidisciplinary team of providers is involved in the care of a patient compared to a single or primary care provider alone.

C. The best and most effective models of case management are those that focus on the continuum of care and settings. Regardless of the setting in which the model is implemented, it is most beneficial if it facilitates (specifically in the role of the case manager) open lines of communication and collaborations/partnerships with health care providers practicing in other settings, emphasizes a patient- and family-centered approach to care provision, and ensures that the patient/family needs are addressed even beyond the setting the patient accesses for care.

D. According to Cesta and Tahan (2003), the health care continuum can be divided into three major settings based on the scope, type, and cost of services provided. These are:

1. Pre-acute setting

a. Focus is on the prevention of illness or deterioration in an individual's health condition

b. Least complex services; primarily proactive approach to care provision that can be self-directed or that may not require the attention of a health care provider

c. Cost is low; in some instances may be free

d. Examples may include primary prevention of illness in the form of health promotion, risk assessment, and screening; fitness; counseling; lifestyle changes; and behavior modification

e. Provision of care does not require admission to a health care facility; care may be limited to a clinic or outpatient setting including a physician's office, a managed care organization, and community-based health centers

f. Case management services are minimal and include telephonic health promotion services and advice lines, health appraisals, and risk-reduction strategies

2. Acute setting

a. Focus is on treating an acute episode of illness such as medical or surgical management, and trauma or emergency care

b. Most complex services; primarily reactive approach to care provision and requires the attention of a health care provider(s)

c. Cost is high; care provision may require the authorization of the payer or insurer

d. Examples may include secondary and tertiary prevention of illness, major diagnostic and therapeutic modalities, surgical/operative procedures, medical management, acute or intensive/critical care, emergency care, specialty care

e. Provision of care requires admission to an acute care facility/hospital, acute rehabilitation facility, post-anesthesia and intensive care area, or emergency department

f. Case management services are intensive and comprehensive in nature including primarily care coordination and management

3. Post-acute setting

a. Focus is on the provision of services needed by patients after an acute episode of illness that may have required an acute care/hospital admission

      b. Moderate complexity services; primarily reactive approach to care provision and requires the attention of multiple health care professionals such as physical and occupational therapists

      c. Cost is moderate to high; care provision may require the authorization of the payer or insurer

      d. Examples may include home care, palliative and end-of-life care, rehabilitative and restorative services, long-term care including custodial and skilled care

      e. Provision of care may occur in the home or community setting or may require admission to a health care facility such as a sub-acute rehabilitation or nursing home, assisted living, hospice, day care centers

      f. Case management services are moderate to complex including primarily transitional planning activities such as placement of patients in appropriate level of care/setting

E. The pre-acute case management practice settings include:
1. Telephonic
2. Payer-based or managed care organization
3. Ambulatory or clinic/outpatient
4. Community care
5. Disease management (see Chapter 20)

F. The acute case management practice settings include:
1. Hospital (see Chapter 4)
2. Acute rehabilitation (see Chapter 6)
3. Emergency department
4. Transitional hospitals, also known as sub-acute care facilities (see Chapter 6)
5. Disease management (see Chapter 20)

G. The post-acute case management practice settings include:
1. Sub-acute (see Chapter 6)
2. Home care (see Chapter 5)
3. Long-term care (see Chapter 6)
4. Palliative or hospice (see Chapter 7)
5. Respite care (see Chapter 6)
6. Residential (see Chapter 6)
7. Custodial (see Chapter 6)
8. Assisted living (see Chapter 6)
9. Day care (see Chapter 6)
10. Independent or private case management agency
11. Workers' compensation (see Chapter 18)
12. Disability management (see Chapter 19)
13. Occupational health (see Chapter 19)
14. Life care planning (see Chapter 17)
15. Disease management (see Chapter 20)

■ TELEPHONIC CASE MANAGEMENT

A. *Telephonic* case management is defined as the delivery of health care services to patients and their families or caregivers over the telephone or via the use of various forms of telecommunication methods such as fax, e-mail, or other forms of electronic communication methods.

B. Most commonly used in the managed care organization (MCO) setting. It takes place in the form of communication between the MCO representatives (mostly MCO-based case managers) and its members.

C. Became more popular in the 1990s with the increased infiltration of managed care health plans. It was viewed as an essential strategy for cost containment.

D. MCOs provide telephonic case management services as an additional benefit to their members. Through this strategy telephonic triage and the provision of health advice have become more common. Through these approaches, case managers ensure the appropriate use of health care resources and allocated such resources based on the needs of the individual member.

E. Telephonic case management is considered a cost-effective and proactive approach to preventing catastrophic health outcomes or deterioration in a patient's condition that requires acute care or a hospital stay.

F. Case managers provide telephonic case management services on a 24 hours/7 days-a-week basis. The main focus is triage services and utilization management of health care resources.

G. Case managers in the telephonic case management practice setting engage in the following activities:
   1. Telephonic triage
   2. Easing the access of patients to health care services
   3. Facilitating the access of the patient to the appropriate level of care, health care provider, and service
   4. Intervening in a timely manner and sharing real time information
   5. Empowering the patient/family/caregiver to assume responsibility for self-care and health management
   6. Identifying the patient's health risk and instituting appropriate action or referral for services
   7. Engaging in cost-reduction activities by promoting access to health services that are appropriate to the patient's condition; for example, preventing the provision of care in the emergency department setting when the patient's condition does not warrant such services, rather directing the patient to seek health services by the primary care provider
   8. Educating patients and their families about health regimen and encouraging them to adhere to it
   9. Following up with patients and/or their families post-discharge from a hospital or ED to ensure safety and adherence to medical regimen, answer their questions, and provide counseling and emotional support

    10. Coordinating and integrating services using evidence-based algorithms, protocols, or guidelines, which include decision trees that are based on certain criteria or assessment cues/data

    11. Assessing and evaluating the patient's condition over the telephone; identifying problems; and directing appropriate action. The assessment is guided by the relevant protocol, and depending on the findings, the case manager determines the urgency of the situation and decides on the necessary type of intervention or advice

    12. Counseling patients regarding their health benefits and answering their questions

    13. Providing health advice

    14. Explaining claims

    15. Authorizing services

    16. Brokering services or directing other case managers to arrange for community-based services with participating agencies or providers

H. Case managers in the telephonic case management practice setting also apply the case management process, however, without a face-to-face interaction with the patient or family. In this process, they:

    1. Interview the patient and/or family member/caregiver

    2. Complete an assessment or evaluation of the patient's condition, situation, or the reason for the call

    3. Analyze the findings using an algorithm or a guideline (usually automated)

    4. Determine the urgency of the situation and plan care (i.e., triage or advice) accordingly

    5. Implement necessary action or care strategy (e.g., refer to ED or the primary care provider)

    6. Evaluate outcomes

    7. Document episode of service

I. Telephonic case management is known to apply two main strategies to ensure cost effectiveness and the provision of care in the most appropriate setting and by the necessary care provider. These are:

    1. Demand management

       a. The main focus is on the appropriate utilization of resources and services

       b. Case managers provide patients with information about their disease, disease process, medical regimen, and desired outcomes

       c. Case managers also encourage patients to participate in self-care and in making decisions regarding their health care needs

       d. The primary outcome is reduction in unnecessary use of EDs, urgent care settings, or acute care facilities

    2. Telephone triage

       a. The main focus is sorting out requests for services based on severity, urgency, and complexity

J. In deciding on the urgency of need for access to health care services, case managers place patients into three categories based on the findings of the telephonic assessment and evaluation. These are:
  1. Emergent
     a. Need to be seen by a health care provider immediately (e.g., acute chest pain)
     b. Usually the patient is referred to the ED
     c. May need the help of emergency medical services personnel
  2. Urgent
     a. Need to be seen within 8 to 24 hours (e.g., vomiting)
     b. Usually the patient is referred to the primary care provider
     c. Health advice may be given to be followed while the patient is waiting to see the primary care provider (e.g., drink extra fluids)
  3. Nonurgent
     a. Can be seen routinely by a primary care provider or treated at home with appropriate follow up (e.g., minor bruise or abrasion)
     b. Health advice is given and the patient is directed to see the primary care provider within a certain number of days if symptoms are not improved

K. In making triage decisions, case managers also use other information such as age, gender, past medical history, medications intake, and primary care provider. In addition, they may ask for health plan–related information such as plan/account number, location of residence, and so on.

L. A rule of thumb for the case manager in telephonic triage is referring those who require care to the appropriate care provider and optimal setting.

■ CASE MANAGEMENT IN THE PAYER-BASED SETTING OR INSURANCE COMPANIES

A. Case managers in the payer-based setting are employees of the insurance company (i.e., health maintenance and managed care organizations).

B. In this setting, the main focus of case management is the health and wellness of the enrollee and the role of the case manager as a liaison between the providers of care—whether an individual or an agency/facility—and the insurance company.

C. Case managers are not the "claims police" despite the fact that they ensure cost-effective treatment plans. Rather, they are:
  1. Coordinators of care, problem solvers, advocates, and educators;
  2. Professionals who collaborate with physicians and other care providers (including the provider-based case manager) to ensure the provision of appropriate and safe care;
  3. Negotiators of services such as home care, durable medical equipment, and physical therapy;
  4. Counselors in that they ensure that the patient follows the prescribed treatment plan; and

     5. Liaisons with insurance claims staff. In this regard, they clarify insurance claims information (Mullahy, 2001).

D. In the payer-based setting, case managers build programs or systems that make it feasible to identify enrollees who are at risk for illness, and those who are considered the "high-risk, high-cost" cases.

     1. Examples of such cases are: cancer, AIDS, organ transplantation, head/brain injury, spinal cord injury, severe burns, high-risk pregnancy, neuromuscular problems, and others.

     2. Case managers work closely with these types of enrollees to ensure they receive the services they need in the appropriate level of care/setting and by the necessary provider(s).

     3. The main goal is provision of quality and cost-effective care.

E. Mullahy (2001) also identified four major areas of activities for case managers in the insurance/managed care practice setting. Some of these activities are applied based on the need and the situation or the job description designed by the insurance company. The areas of activities are described below.

     1. Medical activities—to ensure that the enrollee receives the most effective medical/health care

       a. Keeping contact with the patient while at home or in a health care facility receiving care

       b. Assessing the patient's condition and working closely with the health care team to discuss the enrollee's course of treatment, progress, and needs

       c. Arranging for services required or working closely with the internal or hospital-based case manager on such. Services may include transportation, home care, durable medical equipment, home utilities, psychosocial counseling, and therapy

       d. Coordinating activities closely with the health care team (especially the case manager and the social worker of the facility where an enrollee is being treated) to eliminate duplication or fragmentation of services, and to conserve benefit dollars

       e. Providing health education and psychosocial counseling services to the enrollee and his or her family

       f. Assisting in obtaining payer authorizations for modalities of treatment recommended or indicated

       g. Acting as a liaison between the insurance company and the health care team including the physician

     2. Financial activities—to ensure cost-effective treatments

       a. Assessing the enrollee's medical benefits plan for coverage, out-of-pocket expenses, out-of-plan coverage, and other limitations

       b. Suggesting to the health care team medically appropriate alternative treatment settings and options

       c. Counseling the enrollee and family about benefits and budgeting, sorting out bills

    d. Educating the insurance company about the risk of noncompliant, untreated, or unmanaged cases

3. Behavioral/motivational activities—to ensure adherence to medical regimen and to reduce stress or frustration

    a. Exploring the enrollee's (and family's) feelings about himself or herself and the illness or injury

    b. Supporting the enrollee and family in dealing with the illness and the treatment by providing psychosocial counseling and behavioral modification activities

    c. Offering reassurance and information about the enrollee's illness and treatment

    d. Encouraging the enrollee to pursue a healthy lifestyle—smoke cessation, exercise, healthy eating

    e. Referring the patient for counseling by a specialist (psychologist or psychiatrist)

4. Vocational activities—to ensure continued employment and facilitate return to work

    a. Overseeing psycho-vocational testing, work evaluation, and on-the-job training as appropriate

    b. Assessing the enrollee's past education, employment history, work experiences, job skills, and vocational interests

    c. Assisting the enrollee in using the recuperative period in a constructive manner

    d. Communicating with the enrollee's employer or employment supervisor especially to discuss expectations, options, and the enrollee's needs

    e. Completing a job analysis and discussing the possibility of returning to the same job/work setting or another modified job/work setting

F. The insurance company–based case manager may engage in activities either telephonically or face to face/on site in the health care organization where an enrollee is being treated.

G. Many insurance companies employ case managers to assume responsibility for their utilization management programs. Examples of utilization management activities include (for more details, see Chapters 2 and 11):

1. Authorizations or certifications for services

2. Preadmission, concurrent and retrospective reviews

3. Denials and appeals management

4. Reporting on utilization management activities and outcomes

H. Payer-based case managers may execute their roles either onsite where the provider of care is or via the telephone in the form of telephonic case management.

I. The telephone-based case manager's role is necessary for:

1. Maintaining open lines of communication between the enrollee/family, the provider (individual or agency), the provider-based case manager, and the payer staff

2. Reduction of cost

3. Prevention of inappropriate access to health care services

4. Screening of enrollees and tracking of low-intensity patients and those who have improved and no longer require in-person case management services

J. Onsite case management is common when a large number of individuals from one insurance company (especially managed care) tend to seek care at the same provider agency (e.g., a hospital). In this context, the onsite case manager's role is necessary for:

1. Timely access to care by enrollees

2. Bridging the gaps, especially those related to communication, between the patient, payer, and the provider agency

3. Expediting the process of utilization review and management; that is, timely communication between the provider-based and payer-based case managers regarding treatment plans, treatment options, discharge plans and required services, and patients' progress

4. Coordination of discharge planning activities such as identifying the preferred provider of home care services, transportation services, or skilled nursing facility

5. Discussing post-hospital care, services, and options with the patient and family as needed

6. Providing health education services to patients and their families

7. Explaining the health plan and benefits to patients and their families

8. Solving problems and conflicts as they arise and in a timely manner

■ CASE MANAGEMENT IN THE COMMUNITY CARE SETTING

A. Designed to support and empower patients and their families in achieving or maintaining an optimal level of wellness and functioning by accessing and using community-based health care services and resources.

B. Programs focus on primary care and health promotion or prevention.

C. Target individuals who are healthy, but may be at risk for certain illnesses or needing to access health care services.

D. Work through outreach programs such as screening for illness (e.g., mammography, prostate cancer, cholesterol, and blood pressure screening). These programs identify individuals who are predisposed for illness and enroll them in specific care programs or refer them to other care providers.

E. Other examples of primary prevention include wellness programs such as yearly physical examinations, well-baby care, and immunizations.

F. Work closely with individuals to prevent illness or a sudden change in one's condition to a state that may require hospitalization.

G. In addition to screening, case managers offer health education services to those at risk and others who are interested. They also offer psychosocial and financial counseling and advice, especially to those who are poor or uninsured.

H. Programs also may focus on secondary prevention.

I. Case managers work closely with individuals who have already experienced certain illnesses, have been hospitalized in an acute care setting, and need to maintain optimal health and functioning.

J. Services offered may include health education, lifestyle changes and behavior modification (e.g., smoke cessation; diet and exercise counseling), psychosocial counseling, financial counseling, assessment and monitoring of health condition (e.g., home care services; laboratory testing such as blood sugar and coagulation profile), telephonic advice and counseling, and medication adherence.

K. A special focus here is on prevention of readmission to the acute care setting or ED, or exacerbation of one's health condition/disease state.

L. Case managers in the community care setting coordinate medical as well as social services, and provide care to patients in their homes, day care centers, or ambulatory clinics with the goal of enhancing self-care management skills and patient-directed decision making and empowerment.

M. Case managers assess the patient's condition (health, physical, psychosocial, and financial), plan and implement appropriate interventions, evaluate the patient's responses to treatment, provide patient and family education, and monitor the patient's use of necessary medical technologies, such as glucometers, scales, and blood pressure machines, for self-monitoring of health condition.

N. Case managers may incorporate health education and promotion activities into existing settings such as day care, youth and adult recreation programs, summer camps, schools, support groups, meals for elders, churches, charitable organizations/agencies, and other community development efforts.

■ CASE MANAGEMENT IN THE AMBULATORY OR CLINIC/OUTPATIENT CARE SETTING

A. Community-based case management services also can be provided in walk-in clinics (scheduled and unscheduled visits), home visits, day care centers, assisted living facilities, and telephonically.

B. Case management in the ambulatory or outpatient care setting may focus on the following:
   1. Patient access to care, scheduling appointments, documenting key information relevant to each visit, and answering patient/family questions
   2. Provision of care for specific populations with chronic illnesses and ensuring that treatment plans are oriented to the continuum of care; that is, including well care, acute care, chronic care, and terminal care. Case management in these cases is most beneficial if it encompasses the context of disease management

3. Reducing or preventing the demand for acute, complex, or expensive care. This is best accomplished by applying the strategy of demand management; for example, using nurse advice lines, call centers, telephone triage, health risk assessments, and outreach programs

4. Use of long-term plans of care that apply evidence-based guidelines and protocols

5. Reviewing results of laboratory and radiological tests and procedures, identifying any abnormalities, and intervening accordingly; for example, calling the patient about a change in dosage of a medication or frequency; asking a patient to come back for an early ambulatory care visit, or referring a patient to a specialist type care provider

6. Keeping a vital link between the patient/family, the medical team, and the payer company

7. Measuring outcomes of care (e.g., clinical and financial issues, and processes of care outcomes) and reporting on such to appropriate parties

8. Ensuring that the patient and family are satisfied with care delivery and service

9. Referring the patient for admission to the acute care setting when needed; securing transportation and bed availability

10. Obtaining authorizations for care as indicated and based on the payer's policies and procedures

11. Ensuring compliance with standards of regulatory and accreditation agencies

■ CASE MANAGEMENT IN THE ADMITTING DEPARTMENT

A. Case management in the admitting department has gained increased attention recently because of concerns regarding patient flow and throughput, particularly in the acute care setting. It has also become a necessary function due to the need for compliance with the utilization management standards of MCOs.

B. Case management in the admitting department takes the form of gatekeeping, including:
1. Management and control of who gets admitted to the acute care setting
2. Securing authorizations and precertifications for care from MCOs or other payers as needed
3. Communicating with the payer organization regarding patient conditions and the need for acute care stay (hospitalization)

C. The case manager in the admitting department may assume responsibility for the following functions:
1. Screening patients who are presented for admission to the acute care setting using specific criteria such as those described in InterQual or Milliman standards/guidelines

2. Evaluating the patient's condition to determine medical necessity for acute care; that is, examining the severity of illness and the intensity of needed resources or services. Based on these two factors the case manager determines whether the acute care setting is the best level of care needed by the patient.

3. Communicating with the admitting physician regarding medical necessity for acute care and negotiating the best level of care for the patient if hospitalization was not indicated based on the patient's presenting condition.

4. Providing the physician with an alternative level of care (e.g., ambulatory surgery, outpatient clinic, home care) is necessary when it is determined that admission to the inpatient/hospital care setting is not appropriate and is denied.

5. Timely communication with the physician, patient/family, and payer regarding the decision is important to prevent problems or delays in care.

6. An important factor in deciding the appropriateness of the admission to the acute care setting (hospital) is reimbursement, especially in the case of the MCO where preauthorization for hospital admission is expected. Timely communication with the payer is an important function of case managers in the admitting office.

7. Reviewing all surgical admissions to the hospital, especially those who are admitted a day or more prior to surgery. In this case, the case manager ensures that the admission is warranted based on the patient's condition. Some surgical patients may require hospitalization for medical management or further diagnostic testing prior to surgery.

8. The case manager determines appropriateness of the admission based on pre-established criteria and reimbursement for such. In this case, the case manager ensures that the admission is warranted based on the patient's condition. The intensity of service and the severity of condition are the main determining factors.

9. Under certain circumstances, the patient is still approved for admission to the hospital prior to the day of surgery regardless of lack of reimbursement (e.g., a patient who is unable to complete a bowel preparation for major abdominal surgery in the home setting prior to surgery).

10. Reviewing interhospital transfers for appropriateness and that the transfer meets the MCO's standards and Medicare guidelines; that is, to avoid noncompliance with the Emergency Medical Treatment and Active Labor Act (EMTALA).

    a. For the transfer to be appropriate and necessary the transferring organization must not be able to provide the level of care required by the patient and the receiving organization must have the capacity to provide the level of service needed.

11. Communicating with the admitting department staff the decisions made by the case manager regarding the potential admissions reviewed.

12. Reviewing the medical records of patients who are admitted to the hospital and released within 24 hours. This is an important function and assists in avoiding reimbursement denials. For example, if the case manager determines that the admission is not justified, he or she will convert the admission to an ambulatory encounter or observation status.

13. Preliminary assessment of the patient's condition focusing on the following:
    a. Appropriateness of the admission
    b. Appropriateness of the setting
    c. Type of patient—observation, outpatient, acute/admission
    d. Potential discharge planning needs
    e. Need for care facilitation/coordination
    f. Psychosocial situation

14. Notifying the inpatient case manager of the admission and the findings of the preliminary assessment, including the following:
    a. Coverage limitations; for example, sharing the outcome of conversations with the payer entity
    b. Special patient/family circumstances; for example, lack of family support, availability of next of kin/caregiver, health care proxy, or do not resuscitate status
    c. Potentially avoidable days; for example, pre-surgical days, pre-procedure days
    d. Other issues as appropriate; for example, recipient of home care services prior to admission, skilled nursing facility transfer

15. Keeping in touch with payer-based case managers and other staff

16. Consulting with other staff (e.g., finance, managed care office) and health care professionals (e.g., social worker, physician, patient representative) to eliminate barriers to care or delays in treatment

17. Documenting activities, interventions, assessment, and communications

18. Educating health care professionals and allied health staff about admitting office case management structure and functions

19. Providing patients and their families with health education, promotion, and prevention activities

20. Ensuring compliance with standards of regulatory and accreditation agencies

■ CASE MANAGEMENT IN THE PERI-OPERATIVE SERVICES

A. Peri-operative services case management have become more popular recently due to concern about patient flow and throughput in the acute care setting/hospital. It is also viewed as necessary because it represents a route of entry to an ambulatory or acute care setting, making it necessary for the case manager to ensure appropriateness of the admission, reimbursement, and that care will be provided at the relevant level or setting.

B. The main focus of case management here is the care of the surgical patient—pre-, intra-, and postsurgery. The process of case management is applied in the preadmission testing area, continues in the immediate preoperative and intraoperative periods, and terminates postoperatively in the post-anesthesia care unit (PACU) upon recovery and discharge of the patient to home or transfer to an inpatient care setting.

C. A major interest in case management in the peri-operative services setting is the provision of care for patients that is relevant to their needs and in compliance with regulatory and accreditation standards. Another is the focus on efficiency and efficacy of care and services.

D. Select case management functions in the preadmission testing area are sometimes assumed by the admitting department case manager, the dedicated preadmission testing area case manager, or the peri-operative services case manager. Regardless of who assumes responsibility, the preadmission case management role focuses on the following functions:

　1. Interviewing the patient and family to evaluate condition (medical, physical, psychosocial, and financial) and identify any preadmission or preoperative issues or concerns that might affect the postsurgical period including discharge to home

　2. Exploring discharge planning options and services. For example, determining the need for home care services if the patient or family is unable to assume responsibility for self-care management

　3. Educating the patient/family regarding the surgical procedure and course of treatment

　4. Referring for psychosocial counseling as necessary based on the patient's and family's situation; consulting with a social worker if needed

　5. Evaluating the patient's readiness for surgery; for example, reviewing results of laboratory and radiological tests and procedures; securing the availability of blood and blood products if required, medical and surgical clearance, and consent for surgery

　6. Confirming the date and time of surgery, and availability of the surgical team

　7. Keeping open communication with members of the health care team, especially the surgeon and the anesthesiologist, as well as inpatient case manager(s)

　8. Initiating the discharge planning process, especially in the case of a surgical procedure where it is clear in advance that the patient will require a transfer to a sub-acute or acute rehabilitation facility

　9. Communicating with the payer-based case manager to secure authorization for surgery and admission to the hospital

　10. Documenting in the patient's medical record all assessments, interventions, communication, outcomes, and services arranged for

E. Select case management functions in the immediate preoperative period may include the following:

　1. Assessing the patient's readiness for surgery

2. Reviewing the medical record, which entails the following:
   a. Evaluating results of laboratory and radiological tests and procedures;
   b. Securing the availability of blood and blood products if required;
   c. Ensuring that medical and surgical clearances have been obtained, including the history and physical and anesthesia evaluation; and
   d. Ensuring that the surgical and blood and blood products consents have been completed.
3. Communicating any abnormal results or other concerns to the physician (anesthesiologist and/or surgeon) in a timely manner. This task is important because abnormalities may delay surgery.
4. Confirming that certification for surgery by the payer (if needed) has been secured and documented.
5. Ensuring appropriateness of the level of care; that is, those scheduled for an ambulatory surgery meet the criteria for ambulatory surgery, and those who are to be admitted also meet the inpatient intensity of service and severity of illness criteria.

F. Select case management functions in the intraoperative period may include the following:
   1. Ensuring operating room efficiency; that is, maximizing the operating room utilization. This may entail specific activities such as:
      a. Tracking housekeeping turnaround time, first patient out–next patient in time, delays in surgery and reasons for delays, and so on;
      b. Communicating with the surgical team about any actual or potential delays and intervening as necessary;
      c. Ensuring availability of surgical equipment, trays, and supplies to maximize operating room readiness; and
      d. Changing operating room schedule to avoid waste, especially when the patient or surgical team is not ready.
   2. Addressing quality and risk management issues as they arise
   3. Maintaining a vital link between the patient/family, the surgical/medical team, and the peri-operative services staff
   4. Securing an inpatient or PACU bed for the patient
   5. Ensuring timely patient transfer to the next phase of care or next level of care/setting

G. Select case management functions during the post-anesthesia care period may include the following:
   1. Arranging for admission to an inpatient bed (regular and intensive care type bed); securing bed and medical/surgical care team availability; and expediting transfer out of the PACU
   2. Securing authorizations for care and treatment plans
   3. Identifying and addressing, or preventing, delays in care
   4. Reviewing appropriateness of level of care/setting and the involvement of relevant care providers

5. Obtaining authorizations for care from the payers (insurers) as needed to ensure reimbursement; also, providing them with progress reports and completing concurrent and retrospective review activities
6. Addressing quality and risk management issues as they arise
7. Maintaining a vital link between the patient/family, the surgical/medical team, the inpatient care team, the PACU team, and the perioperative services staff
8. Ensuring timely patient transfer to the next phase of care or next level of care/setting (i.e., the inpatient care unit)

■ INDEPENDENT/PRIVATE CASE MANAGEMENT

A. Independent or private case management is also known as *external* case management compared to the hospital-based case management, which is known as *internal* case management.

B. Defined as the provision of case management services by self-employed case managers or those who are employees of a privately owned company.

C. The term *independent* or *private* refers to the absence of oversight by an MCO or health care organization.

D. Independent and private case management services emerged as a cost-effective approach to the care of:
1. An increased number of the elderly population with complex and chronic illnesses
2. Disabled individuals who require coordination of expensive and intense services (medical, social, financial, and mental health) for an extended period of time—sometimes for a number of years
3. Workers' compensation or occupational health cases that have resulted in chronic or permanent injury and that are known to consume expensive and complex health care resources

E. Independent and private case management are similar in relation to the structure and type of services they provide to patients; however, subtle differences between the two do exist. They are usually used interchangeably; however as an expert, the case manager must be able to differentiate between these two terms and use them appropriately.
1. Private case management refers to the services provided by an independent case manager privately contracted or hired by a chronically ill individual or family member to manage the complex care and services needed.
2. Independent case management refers to services offered by a case manager who is hired by an independent case management firm and contracted by a health care organization (usually a managed care company, an employer, or a health care facility) to provide case management services on a long- or short-term basis to certain individuals, especially those who are disabled.

F. Case managers in the independent or private case management practice setting represent the health care organization or insurance company that hires them unless they are hired directly by the patient or family, in which case they represent the patient/family.

G. Independent and private case management focuses on the following:
1. Enabling the patient and family to transition along the health care continuum
2. Assisting the patient and family in successfully navigating the health care delivery system
3. Monitoring services and resource utilization
4. Evaluating outcomes
5. Managing cost of care and services and health benefits
6. Ensuring the provision of quality care and services which may include:
   a. Retirement planning
   b. Home health care; homemaker and companion services
   c. Respite care
   d. Transportation
   e. Family and legal counseling
   f. Physical and occupational therapy
   g. Psychosocial counseling and crisis intervention
   h. Referrals to specialty providers
7. Ensuring patient and family satisfaction
8. Advocating for the patient/family

H. The goals of independent and private case management are similar to those of other models or practice settings of case management. They may include, but are not limited to, the following:
1. Coordination and facilitation of complex medical, psychosocial, functional, and financial services
2. Provision of timely, quality, and appropriate services
3. Cost effectiveness
4. Provision of one-to-one individualized and personalized relationship between a health care provider and the patient/family
5. Integration of health care services and resources including mental health assessment and counseling and referrals to specialty providers

I. MCOs and employers are more likely to subcontract with an independent or private case management agency for services such as rehabilitation and disability case management.

J. Although hired by an insurance company, private and independent case managers are expected to comply with the utilization management procedures followed by the insurance company. They seek authorization for services, provide concurrent and ongoing utilization review and progress reports, and ensure the provision of services that are satisfactory to both the patient/family and the insurer.

K. Reimbursement for private and independent case management services is either on an hourly, daily, or case rate. Sometimes, sliding fee schedules are used.

L. Private and independent case management practice settings allow the case manager to function independently and autonomously, especially in decision making, achieve greater income, and attain professional satisfaction.

M. Private and independent case management practice settings provide the case manager with the opportunity to manage a personal/private business with all its aspects including hiring and firing staff, marketing, budgeting and financial management, accounting, public relations, purchasing, sales, and so on.

■ CASE MANAGEMENT IN THE EMERGENCY DEPARTMENT

A. The emergency department (ED) is a common route of entry to the acute care hospital setting. The recent issue of ED overcrowding has resulted in a dire need for case management services to ensure efficient, safe, and effective patient flow and throughput.

B. The benefits of ED case management are primarily (Tahan and Cesta, 2005):
   1. Cost effectiveness
   2. Provision of efficient, effective, timely, safe and quality care
   3. Patient and family satisfaction
   4. Reduction in diversion hours and frequency
   5. Elimination of unnecessary admissions to the hospital setting
   6. Expeditious admissions to inpatient beds/hospital setting
   7. Prevention of lost revenues due to diversions and inappropriate admissions

C. The ED case manager provides an important gatekeeping function for the hospital and ensures that patients are either appropriately admitted to the hospital or treated in and released from the ED.

D. The ED case manager facilitates care processes from the time of the patient's arrival in the ED, through registration and triage, assessment and treatment, until discharge from the ED or admission to the hospital setting (Tahan and Cesta, 2005). Activities may include the facilitation of:
   1. Timely triage and initiation of treatment according to urgency of the situation
   2. Diagnostic tests and procedures (e.g., laboratory, radiology)
   3. Therapeutic procedures (e.g., insertion of gastric tube for feeding)
   4. Discharge planning
   5. Patient and family education
   6. Transfers to inpatient beds or other facilities

E. ED case managers are active members of multidisciplinary teams that include physicians, nurses, social workers, patient representatives, admitting office staff, and other personnel.

F. Traditional admission and discharge planning responsibilities of the case manager in an acute care setting may be extended to the ED case manager.

This role allows for timely assessment of patients' needs and intervention accordingly. The case manager may:

1. Act as a liaison between the ED, hospital, and community case management programs and personnel, particularly to improve continuity and efficiency of care
2. Ensure and expedite appropriate patient disposition—hospital admission, transfer to another facility or level of care, discharge home with visiting nurse services, and alternative placements
3. Evaluate the decision to admit a patient to a hospital setting based on specific criteria (intensity of service and severity of illness)
4. Coordinate appropriate use of efficient services and resources
5. Evaluate outcomes and examine system efficiency and effectiveness
6. Arrange for post-discharge care such as visiting nurse services
7. Ensure compliance with standards of regulatory and accreditation agencies

G. Case managers in the ED make sure that patients who can be treated on an outpatient basis or in another level of care are not inappropriately admitted to an acute inpatient care setting. They work with physicians and others to avoid "social admissions."

H. Some of the other functions of ED case managers are:

1. Assisting indigent patients who need community services such as shelter and charity care
2. Engaging in financial screening activities and the necessary utilization management processes such as securing certifications for treatment and post-discharge services from MCOs
3. Coordinating the patient's admission to the hospital setting and facilitating the transfer of patients from the ED to the assigned inpatient beds
4. Securing medications and durable medical equipment for those in need
5. Ensuring provision of health education services to patients and families
6. Facilitating the patient's release after treatment and arranging for necessary transportation
7. Monitoring ED patient flow metrics and evaluating performance, especially those related to ED crowding. National indicators for ED crowding are (United States General Accounting Office, 2003):
   a. Diversion—number of hours the ED is unable to receive and care for patients who need transportation by the emergency medical services (EMS) personnel
   b. Boarding—number of patients remaining in the ED after a decision has been made to admit them to an inpatient bed
   c. Left before a medical evaluation—number of patients who leave the ED after triage but before receiving medical evaluation
8. Preventing unsafe discharges from the ED
9. Obtaining follow-up appointments for those discharged from the ED who require such care

10. Facilitating the exchange of information among physicians, social workers, nurses, other hospital staff, patient and family, and community providers

11. Ensuring compliance with EMTALA regulations (Wilson, Siegel, and Williams, 2005):

    a. All patients seen in the ED must receive:

        i. Appropriate medical screening examination within the capability of the ED;

        ii. No delay in care on account of insurance or reimbursement; and

        iii. Transfer to another facility should be because of the patient's request or due to inability of the ED to provide the needed service.

    b. It essentially established a universal federal right to ED care without earmarking payment for this care.

    c. EDs must provide open access to individuals who may not have real or perceived open choices for care.

■ PATIENT FLOW, THROUGHPUT, AND CASE MANAGEMENT

A. Patient flow focuses on the clinical and operational processes of care that facilitate the movement of the patient from point A to point B within the health care system (i.e., from one location/level of care to another). Usually these movements are necessary and required by the patient based on his or her condition, treatment plan, and related services.

B. Throughput encompasses the actual operations/activities of a care provision that are essential for effective delivery of care. Conceptually, throughput is "part and parcel" of patient flow; without it, a patient may not transition effectively and efficiently from one place to another.

C. For throughput to be efficient and effective, it must focus on the structure, processes, and expected outcomes of care delivery.

    1. Structure—Characteristics of the care setting and the patient population. Examples may include type of care setting (e.g., acute, ambulatory, ED), type and number of care providers (e.g., nurses, physicians, social workers), or services available (e.g., laboratory, pharmacy, physical therapy).

    2. Processes—The steps to be followed to ensure the completion of care activities. Examples may include the process of medications management, triage, insertion of an intravenous access, transfer of a patient from an ED to an inpatient unit.

    3. Outcomes—End results or outputs of a process. Examples are discharge of a patient to home, relief of symptoms.

D. Patient flow and throughput are terms that have often been used in reference to the hospital-based care setting as a result of ED crowding and inefficiency in moving patients from an ambulatory or procedural setting into inpatient beds.

E. Patient flow and throughput are terms that tend to be used interchangeably. In this section they will be addressed as if they are the same because both terms denote the way patients are transitioned across a set of locations (levels of care) within the hospital; however, implicit in that are the treatments they receive and the types of services they utilize.

F. Examining the hospital's efficiency in patient flow and throughput focuses on careful evaluation of the operations of areas known to experience bottlenecks, increased traffic, and process variations. These may include:
   1. EDs,
   2. PACUs,
   3. ICUs, and
   4. Procedure areas such as intervention cardiology laboratories, bronchoscopy and endoscopy suites, and operating rooms.

G. Case managers are professionals best prepared to assume an integral role in coordination, facilitation, or management of patient flow and throughput activities. With their leadership skills and knowledge of utilization management and patient care services/resources across the continuum of care, they are able to ensure the efficiency and effectiveness of the health care facility operations.

H. The 2005 patient flow standard from the Joint Commission on Accreditation of Healthcare Organizations (JCAHO) called for hospital leadership staff to have a process in place for managing patient flow and throughput, especially in the EDs and PACUs. This expectation is incorporated in the already-existing leadership standard, and requires hospitals to (JCAHO, 2006):
   1. Engage in an ongoing evaluation of patient flow practices;
   2. Develop and implement plans to identify and mitigate impediments to efficient patient flow throughout the hospital as a result of overcrowding;
      a. Patients who are admitted through the admitting office (elective admissions)
      b. Patients who are admitted post-surgery through the PACUs (elective and emergency admissions)
      c. Patients who are admitted through the ED (emergency admissions)
   3. Implement strategies for process improvement with a main focus on patient access to care (efficiency, effectiveness, and timeliness); and
   4. Manage overcrowding of patients in the ED, because this population is particularly vulnerable to experiencing negative effects of inefficiency.

I. Inefficient patient flow can affect patient safety and quality of care, as well as the hospital's bottom line. It may increase the number of denials and avoidable days, and therefore impacts negatively on reimbursement.

J. Patient flow can be viewed from two perspectives—clinical and operational.

   1. Clinically, patient flow represents the progression of a patient's health status as it relates to disease, treatment, and recovery progression.

   2. Operationally, patient flow means the transition of a patient through a set of locations in a health care facility or across facilities.

K. Patient flow is determined based on clinical needs (i.e., level of care needed, intensity of service, and severity of illness) of the patient and the best place that necessary health care services are available.

L. Patient flow is important today more than ever because of current reimbursement methods (e.g., managed care, capitation, federal prospective payment systems) that place the provider of care at financial risk or that place the patient at risk (e.g., risk for medical errors and unsafe experiences) as he or she transitions across the continuum of care.

M. Case managers may take the lead in their hospitals in ensuring efficient patient flow and throughput. They may collaborate with multidisciplinary health care teams, including administrators and staff from the admitting office, ED, medicine, surgery, nursing, social work, environmental services, information technology, and others, to:

   1. Oversee patient flow processes

   2. Measure outcomes of patient flow processes and practices. Examples of measures, according to JCAHO (2006) may include:

     a. Available supply of beds;

     b. Available supply of medical/surgical teams;

     c. Efficiency of patient care, treatment, and service areas;

     d. Safety of patient care, treatment, and service areas;

     e. Support service processes that impact patient flow; and

     f. Number of patients boarding in an area other than their destination.

   3. Examine relevant data that evaluate performance

   4. Execute actions for improvement

   5. Ensure compliance with regulatory and accreditation patient flow standards

N. The multidisciplinary patient flow team allows a better understanding of the issues of patient volume, demand for inpatient beds, bed capacity and supply, and necessary resources (staff and otherwise).

O. The patient flow standard requires that patients access services as soon as they are in the system (e.g., ED, admitting office, clinic, PACU, or other area of the hospital system) and that there is no delay in admission to an inpatient bed or in receiving diagnostic and therapeutic tests and treatments.

P. Case managers can facilitate timely patient flow and throughput by:

   1. Making sure that those in the ED are triaged in a timely manner and treated accordingly

   2. Expediting delivery of care

   3. Coordinating the completion of tests and procedures

   4. Ensuring that the results of tests and procedures are available to physicians and other clinicians/staff so they can make decisions about the plan of care

5. Securing inpatient beds for those who require admission to the hospital care setting
6. Facilitating a safe transfer process from one location to another, internal or external to a health care facility, especially as the patient's condition requires a transition from one level of care (or setting) to another
7. Evaluating the patient's health insurance plans or lack thereof

Q. Case managers not only check the appropriateness of admissions to the hospital setting, but also make sure that patients receive the care they need as well, in a timely manner and while in the ED awaiting admission or in the PACU awaiting transfer, as if they already were in an inpatient bed.

R. For any patient flow process, there always exists an entry point, an exit or checkout point, and a path connecting the two points together. The path is in essence what throughput is all about. Therefore, generally speaking, patient flow can be described as a model of "entry-path-exit."

S. Wilson, Siegel, and Williams (2005) applied a similar perspective to the ED and described their approach for improving the efficiency of ED operations as the "input-throughput-output" model. Although this model was specific to the ED, it has merits for other care settings across an organization or among organizations. Therefore, one can apply this model to managing and improving any patient flow and throughput issue in an organization.

T. The input-throughput-output model, for example as Wilson et al. (2005) described, provides a structure for examining the factors that impact on patient flow in the ED as follows:
   1. Examples of input factors are:
      a. The reasons why people present to the ED for care
      b. Patients' demographics
      c. Patients' health status
      d. Insurance status and type
      e. Availability of alternative sites of care such as "fast track," urgicare
      f. Perceptions of quality
      g. Skills and knowledge of clinicians
      h. ED space and capacity
      i. Patient's desire for immediate care
      j. Ambulance diversion
   2. Examples of throughput factors are:
      a. Actual processes of care in the ED
      b. Registration
      c. Triage
      d. Authorization for care (certification)
      e. Level of service
      f. Treatment

      g. Availability of staff

      h. Availability of specialists

      i. Diagnostic services

      j. Information systems and technology

      k. Communication channels

      l. Staff assignments and caseloads

      m. Case management services

      n. Physician's practice

      o. Equipment and therapeutic approaches

      p. Bed management and capacity

      q. Care rounds

      r. Boarding

  3. Examples of output factors are:

      a. The ability to move the patient to his or her next disposition

      b. Discharge decision/order

      c. Available care/services in the community

      d. Patient's discharge

      e. Transfer to other facilities

      f. Bed tracking and availability

      g. Availability of transportation services

      h. Availability of housekeeping/environmental services

      i. Access to follow-up care and follow-up appointments

U. For an organization attempting to improve the efficiency of its patient flow operations, it is important to evaluate the above factors to identify issues that result in undesirable performance and to address them accordingly.

V. Understanding the input-throughput-output model and the patient flow operations in a facility allow health care professionals, including case managers, to improve its performance. Case managers may assist in identifying the important metrics that must be used for measuring the system's efficiency and monitoring of these metrics.

■ TRANSITIONS OF CARE AND CASE MANAGEMENT

A. The provision of quality health care services to patients requires them to receive care in multiple settings and from varied providers. This is even more so in the case of individuals with chronic and complex illnesses, regardless of age.

B. Transitions from one care setting to the next or from one provider to the next often parallel changes (transitions or progression) in patients' health status. For example, patients who are transferred from a skilled nursing facility to an acute care hospital undergo such activity because of a change in condition that requires care (or the attention of a specialist health care provider) that is not available at the skilled nursing facility.

C. The health care system in the United States is not equipped with one single health care professional or team that assumes full responsibility for the coordination of care across settings or care providers during transitions of care.

D. Transitions of care occur during a time when patients journey the health care system. This journey may result in vulnerable situations, and require an increased need for coordination and continuity of care.

E. Case management is most important during transitions of care where inefficiencies may occur leaving the patient at risk for poor quality or negative and unexpected outcomes.

F. The National Quality Forum (NQF, 2006, p. D-9) describes care transition as a "change or interruption of patient care such as a discharge, a change in medications, a transfer among care units, a referral to services such as physical or occupational therapy, and the use of emergency services."

G. NQF also describes care coordination (a core aspect of case management) as the "synchronization of patient care and services during care transitions" (NQF, 2006, p. D-9). Care transitions may compromise patient safety and increase the likelihood for medical errors to occur primarily as a result of miscommunications.

H. Care transition is also described by the HMO Workgroup on Care Management (2004, p. 1) as "patient transfers from one care setting to another." This group focused its report on the improvement of the quality of care transitions for members of MCOs. However, the lessons to be learned from this report are beneficial to all other care settings.

I. The report describes a transition of care as occurring when there is a change in necessary care or services as follows:
   1. Transfer of responsibility of care from one health care professional to another such as from a primary care to a specialist physician or from one nurse to another
   2. Change in the environment of care (care setting or level of care) within a health care facility; that is, a transfer from an intensive care to a regular unit, or ED to an inpatient bed
   3. Change in care environment from one facility to another including hospitals, skilled nursing facilities, the patient's home, outpatient primary care and specialty clinics, and assisted living and other long-term care facilities

J. The HMO Workgroup on Care Management (2004) proposed six specific strategies for care of patients during transitions. These are:
   1. Ensuring that someone on the health care team assumes accountability for the patients' transitions;
   2. Facilitating the effective transfer of information;
   3. Enhancing health care practitioners' skills and support systems;
   4. Enabling patients and caregivers to play a more active role in their transitions;
   5. Aligning financial and structural incentives to improve patient flow across care settings, providers, and facilities; and

6. Initiating a quality improvement/management strategy for care transitions.

K. The Workgroup emphasized the importance of other aspects of care during the time when a patient transitions from one health care provider or care setting to another, including the following:
   1. Both entities assuming responsibilities in maintaining continuity of care and ensuring patient safety by controlling the risk for medical error.
   2. Keeping the patients informed about their plans of care, especially their transitional plans and what to expect during the transitions. Health care professionals must answer the patients' questions and alleviate their anxiety.
   3. Transfer of timely and accurate information, especially clinical. Such practice ensures effective and safe transitions. Information may include these described below.
      a. Goals and plan of care
      b. Patient's baseline functional status (physical and cognitive)
      c. Active medical and behavioral health problems
      d. Medications regimen
      e. Social support network and support resources
      f. Durable medical equipment needs and life-sustaining equipment use such as oxygen therapy
      g. Ability for self-care management
      h. Health care proxy and resuscitation status
      i. Financial status such as type of insurance and benefits
   4. Use of transfer note or summary that provides a comprehensive picture of the patient's status and the course of treatment followed prior to the transition.
   5. Making sure that enough time and attention are spent by health care professionals on patient transitions, similar amount compared to that exerted at the time of the patient's entry into the system.
   6. Making appropriate resources available—staff, equipment, space, etc.
   7. Shifting the perspective/framework of care provision from that of "discharge planning" to "transitions to continuous care".
   8. Collaboration in and integration of care provision across settings and disciplines.
   9. Using "transitional care managers".

L. The risk for suboptimal or unsafe care presented during transitions of care provides an excellent opportunity for case management.

M. In this regard, case managers may:
   1. Assume the role of the "single" professional on the health care team responsible and accountable for the essential activities that ought to occur during patients' transitions
   2. Speak up and act on behalf of the multidisciplinary team and the organization for which he or she works

3. Incorporate the "lessons learned" from the HMO Workgroup on Care Management report into their own practice in the care settings where they work

4. Focus on patient safety and error prevention (discussed in next section) as they assist patients, families, and other health care providers during care transitions

N. NQF (2006, p. D-9) identified transitions of care as one of four domains that constitute the framework for assessing the quality of care coordination in the hospital setting, a core aspect of case management. In fact, these four domains are integral to case management practice in any care setting:

1. Transitions of care, including transfer among units within a hospital as well as admission to and discharge from the hospital; discharge includes transfer to other facilities such as acute or sub-acute rehabilitation

2. Communications among providers

3. Information, including the availability of health information when needed and the provision of information to patients about their condition and plan of care

4. Capacity for services, including the availability of specialized services, waiting time for care, and the need for transfer to another facility or care setting when necessary services are unavailable

O. The above domains cover aspects of care coordination that occur within a facility or setting (internal) and those that require collaboration with other facilities or settings (external).

■ ROLE OF THE CASE MANAGER IN PATIENT SAFETY AND PREVENTION OF MEDICAL ERRORS

A. Across the health care continuum, patients are routinely transferred from one provider to another, one service to another specialty, or one practice/care setting to another. With such activity, risk for suboptimal (or poor) quality of care may exist.

B. At each juncture, there is a handoff and a necessary exchange of information that requires close attention to ensure safety, eliminate the likelihood of medical errors, and maintain continuity of care.

C. The case manager may assume responsibility for professional, legal, and ethical practices that extend beyond the patient's discharge from a practice/care setting.

D. If the transitions of care were not handled properly and with caution, the patient's health condition will be placed at risk for unsafe situation (e.g., deterioration), which may result in serious negative outcomes.

E. From assessment and planning to evaluation and outcomes, the case management process must provide a proactive approach to safety by ensuring access to quality, safe, effective, and timely care. Each step in the case management process provides an added and significant benefit; that is, the potential to reduce or prevent risk of medical errors.

F. The case management process provides numerous opportunities along the continuum of care and across providers to identify and address potential risks for errors and ensure patient safety. Tahan (2005a) described how essential activities of case management can enhance patient safety. For example,

1. An appropriate assessment of the patient's needs focusing on the "total patient," not just the medical condition at hand provides a step toward proactively preventing errors by being comprehensive in identifying the patient's concerns, interests, and health-related problems.

2. The design of a comprehensive plan of care that is patient- and family-centered, from the onset of the injury or illness through treatment and recovery or rehabilitation, and one that is based on the patient's individualized needs and desires will ensure safety.

3. Obtaining authorization for care from the payer (as needed) and advocating for the needs of patients and their families expedites access to care.

4. Understanding and communicating all facets of the patient's treatment plan to the patient/family and the members of the health care team and agreeing on the plan can also help prevent medical errors from occurring.

G. Through advocacy, the case manager is able to ensure that the care plan is closely followed by all health care providers. He or she ensures that specialty providers are consulted as indicated by the patient's condition and treatment plan including transitional planning. To avoid errors, this may involve open communication with all care providers, who may not necessarily have the same "global view" of the plan of care as the case manager.

H. Focusing on care across the continuum, the case manager can ensure that information is shared appropriately regarding such things as medications, diet, prior and future treatment, follow-up appointments, physical activity, and so on. Maintaining continuity of care through this sharing of information can reduce or prevent errors.

I. Monitoring of the delivery of care throughout the case management process, and adjustment of the treatment plan as needed enhances safety. For example, when there is a delay or variance in the provision of care (e.g., an important diagnostic test is delayed) the case manager identifies the cause of the delay and immediately institutes appropriate corrective actions.

J. Close monitoring and management of the patient's plan of care, progress, outcomes, as well as the behaviors of the care providers expedite patient's care and progression. Such actions can prevent undesirable events from occurring or delay in meeting the patient's interests and treatment goals.

K. Comprehensive view of the patient's plan of care and desired outcomes and evaluation of the overall plan for appropriateness, relevancy to the patient/family's interests, and timeliness of care activities identifies situations where the patient is not progressing according to expectations. This prompts the case manager to implement necessary actions and to ensure safety.

L. Collecting and analyzing outcomes data can help determine elements of the care plan that are not successful or have not been carried out according to plan. This may help determine whether a medical error did occur and provide for appropriate corrective action, and help prevent similar errors from reoccurring in the future.

M. The role of the case manager in ensuring patient safety during transitions of care has become integral to the health care system and essential in case management practice (Tahan, 2005b).

N. Individuals with chronic health conditions—and often more than one—frequently receive their care from a variety of health care professionals and across varied care settings across the continuum of care leaving the patient unsure of which primary provider is accountable for coordinating the plan of care and treatment options, and who possesses ultimate responsibility for outcomes.

O. Hospital stays have become shorter. Thus, more patients with serious and/or complicated chronic health conditions are being treated in non-acute (e.g., outpatient and home) care settings and perhaps by less-specialized providers.

P. There continues to be an element of increased fragmentation in the provision of health care services, ultimately leading to increased risk for medical errors.

Q. Case managers have a very clear role, regardless of practice settings, in improving patient safety whether in preventing, reporting, acknowledging, or correcting a situation. No matter where they work, they may:
   1. Advocate for patients and their families/caregivers;
   2. Promote education of individuals and their families or other caregivers;
   3. Improve communication and coordination among care providers; and
   4. Ensure continuity in patient care (Tahan, 2005b).

R. Case managers may assume a special focus on patient safety in their roles in five main areas. These are (Tahan, 2005b):
   1. Transitions or handoffs of care when a patient is transferred from one level of care or practice setting to another
   2. Medical regimen (including medications and other treatments) reconciliation. A special focus is on medications, including a complete listing of all medications—prescription drugs, over-the-counter drugs, and herbal treatments—that have been prescribed and/or a patient is taking.
   3. Patient/caregiver education, to empower and educate patients and their caregivers on self-care management skills and compliance with medical regimens
   4. Access to services through a plan of care that provides access to the right amount and type of care and treatment at the right time, with the right provider, and to achieve the right outcome

5. Communication among providers to make sure that all treating physicians, specialists and other care providers are aware of the latest treatment plan and to maintain timely communication and exchange of information

S. When medical errors occur, health care providers including case managers are ethically, morally, and legally obligated to disclose them.

T. The case manager might not be the right person to disclose a medical error, if one has occurred; however, he or she can be the right person to make sure the health care team is aware of its duty to disclose to the patient that an error has occurred, how it will be handled, what the patient can expect to do himself or herself, and what he or she can expect the team to do to rectify the error.

REFERENCES

Cesta, T., & Tahan, H. (2003). *The case manager's survival guide: Winning strategies for clinical practice,* 2nd ed. St Louis, MO: Mosby.

Cohen, E., & Cesta, T. (2005). *Nursing case management: From essentials to advanced practice applications,* 4th ed. St Louis, MO: Elsevier Mosby.

HMO Workgroup on Care Management (February 2004). *One patient, many places: Managing health care transitions.* Washington, DC: AAHP-HIAA Foundation.

Joint Commission on Accreditation of Healthcare Organizations (JCAHO). (2006). *Comprehensive accreditation manual for hospitals.* Chicago, IL: Author.

Mullahy, C. (2001). Case management and managed care. In P. Kongstvedt, *Essentials of managed health care,* 4th ed. (pp. 249–280). Gaithersburg, MD: Aspen.

National Quality Forum (NQF). (2006). *National voluntary consensus standards for hospital care: Additional priority areas—2005–2006: A consensus report.* Washington, DC: Author.

Tahan, H. (2005a). Identifying and reducing the risk for medical errors. *The Case Manager, 16*(3), 80–82.

Tahan, H. (2005b). Enhancing patient safety: The role of the case manager. *Care Management, 11*(5), 19–26.

Tahan, H., & Cesta, T. (2005). Managing emergency department overload. *Nurse Leader, 3*(6), 40–43.

United States General Accounting Office. (March, 2003). Hospital emergency departments: crowded conditions vary among hospitals and communities. Report to the Ranking Minority Member, Committee on Finance, US Senate, report number GAO-03-460. Website: *www.gao.gov/cgi-bin/getrpt?GAO-03-460.*

Wilson, M., Siegel, B., & Williams, M. (2005). *Perfecting patient flow: America's safety net hospitals and emergency department crowding.* Washington, DC: National Association of Public Hospitals and Health Systems.

SUGGESTED READING

Cesta, T.G. (2002). *Survival strategies for nurses in managed care.* St Louis, MO: Mosby.

Daniels, S., & Ramey, M. (2005). *The leader's guide to hospital case management.* Sudbury, MA: Jones and Bartlet.

Kongstvedt, P. (2003). *Essentials of managed healthcare,* 4th ed. Gaithersburg, MD: Aspen.

Mullahy, C. (2004). *The case manager's handbook,* 3rd ed. Sudbury, MA: Jones and Bartlet.

Powell, S. K. (2000). *Case management: A practical guide to success in managed* care. Philadelphia, Pa: Lippincott Williams & Wilkins.

Case Management in the Acute Care Setting

Stefani Daniels

Upon completion of this section, the reader will be able to:

1. Identify the prevalent models of hospital case management.
2. Distinguish functional case management models from clinical resource management models.
3. Discuss the dominant features of successful hospital case management programs.
4. Describe the primary purposes of a hospital case management program.
5. Outline essential knowledge to develop a framework for an acute care case management program.
6. Articulate the benefits of establishing a physician–case manager partnership.
7. Describe how the use of data is essential to produce measurable outcomes.

IMPORTANT TERMS AND CONCEPTS

Advocacy
Clinical Case Management
Congruency

Continuity
Dyad and Triad Models
Functional Models

Infrastructure	Resource Management
Leverage	Return on Investment
Measurable Outcomes	Visioning Process
Physician Partnerships	Workflow Operations

■ INTRODUCTION

It used to be that hospital case management (HCM) could succeed simply by providing solid utilization review and discharge planning activities. But as expectations for higher levels of service intensify and demands for value accelerate, those days have drawn to a close. Today, cutting-edge programs are identifying ways to meet or exceed the expectations of the baby boomers through assertive advocacy and a strong focus on access, cost, and outcomes (Wolfe, 2006).

A. According to industry observers, hospitals will succeed by establishing partnerships with their stakeholders and developing solutions that are tailored to their unique needs.

B. Case manager partnerships with physicians is a popular strategy to help the medical staff work through a morass of industry challenges that can, at times, be complex, frustrating, and intimidating.

C. Hospital case management continues on its evolutionary track and there is no single model of hospital case management, nor is there "one best way."

D. From the perspective of many progressive hospital executives, HCM should now achieve three major outcomes:
   1. Engage the physician in order to influence the quality of patient outcomes.
   2. Overcome process obstacles so that patients flow smoothly and efficiently through the acute care episode.
   3. Prevent or, at least, minimize the occurrence of unwanted clinical or operational events that add unnecessary risk.

E. The new generation of HCM programs are typically structured and operationalized to rapidly achieve these three goals. Within these programs, there are many features that should be integrated into every hospital's program no matter where they are on the evolutionary scale (Daniels and Ramey, 2005).

■ KEY DEFINITIONS

A. Advocacy—A process that promotes beneficence, justice, and autonomy for clients. Advocacy especially aims to foster the client's independence. It also involves educating clients about their rights, health care and human services, resources, and benefits. Advocacy facilitates appropriate and informed decision making, and includes considerations for the client's values, beliefs, and interests (Gilpin, 2005).

B. Congruency—The "fit" between HCM and its environment.

C. Continuity—In practical terms, continuity means that a single case manager will consistently serve as the patient's advocate, quality inspector, and information source in every geographic area in which the patient is placed.

D. Infrastructure—Relates to the alignment of HCM within the organizational structure; the nature of the team and the positions within the HCM program; and the assignment, staffing, and scheduling of case management team positions.

E. Resource management—Encompasses a diverse set of activities designed to influence the efficient and appropriate use of hospital resources; may be tangible or intangible; is a balance of patient advocacy and the organization's obligation to appropriately allocate resources; and is a prospective process to monitor the appropriate use of resources for the condition and to offer acceptable alternatives.

F. Visioning—A collective process of imagining the future.

■ BACKGROUND

A. Hospital case management has its roots in the expanded role of the clinical nurse at Massachusetts' New England Medical Center (Zander, 1988). It was originally conceived as a cost-containment strategy to help hospitals deal with the nursing shortage and the world of managed care, but has expanded as a means to decrease resource consumption, reduce costs, and improve the continuity and quality of patient care (Stonestreet, 1999).

B. Over the years, the influence of the New England Medical Center clinical model has led to a variety of similarly conceived programs, although no single model has surfaced.

C. As the U.S. hospital industry undergoes dramatic changes in the structure and processes of care delivery, the case manager has emerged as an important part of the workforce and a key driver of managing access to care, coordination of care, and cost/quality outcomes.

■ DISTINGUISHING THE HOSPITAL VENUE

The primary purposes of case management—to advocate on behalf of the patient, facilitate the delivery of quality and appropriate care in a cost-effective manner, while seeking to promote positive health care outcomes—remain constant regardless of the practice venue. However, the practice of case management in a hospital looks quite different from case management practiced in a community health program or an insurance company.

A. There are three key dimensions that distinguish case management in the hospital from those in other practice venues.
  1. Designation of the program
     a. HCM is often characterized in the literature as a clinical program despite the fact that case managers do not provide clinical, hands-on services.

    b. If described as a clinical service, careful thought must be given to what clinical services will be provided and whether those services are redundant to those provided by the patients' primary nurse or other clinicians.

    c. The role of the hospital case manager must be carefully aligned with the clinical team but should not be viewed as competitive with the patient's clinical nurse.

    d. Today's HCM programs are more often characterized as business programs to complement the clinical expertise present within the acute care setting.

2. Congruency

    a. HCM programs exist within the larger context of the political, economical, and cultural forces of the hospital.

    b. Congruency refers to the "fit" between HCM and its environment.

    c. There are three levels of congruency applicable to HCM to which successful programs give keen attention.

        i. Concept congruency refers to the translation of different perspectives or expectations into a single, harmonious frame of reference. Members of the executive team often have differing expectations from HCM. Successful programs use the planning phase as the time to get everyone on the same page with regard to purpose and outcome expectations.

        ii. Content congruency refers to the alignment between the model of case management used and the environment in which it is practiced. Successful programs make sure that its structure and activities are, to the extent feasible, congruent with the customs, preferences, experiences, and culture of the hospital.

        iii. Process congruency refers to the distinct cause-and-effect outcomes. Successful programs enlist support staff to conduct routine clerical and chart review activities so that the professional time of the case manager is focused on achieving expected outcomes.

3. Leverage

Hospital case managers have neither the positional authority nor the economic leverage to muster the support needed to overcome operational inertia or medical practice decisions. Leverage and influence must, therefore, be created.

    a. To create leverage and influence, HCM must consider its customer base and shift problem solving to the perspective of that customer.

        i. Providers—Other hospitals, skilled nursing facilities, home care agencies, long-term acute care hospitals, and clinical practitioners

        ii. Purchasers—Corporations, businesses, and other health care purchasers have become very vocal about the costs and quality of health care and are using their economic power to influence change.

        iii. Payers—The insurers caught between the demands of the purchasers and the expectations of their members

    iv. Physicians—Account for 80% of all clinical costs; direct 60% of all inpatient admissions; determine, through their practice behaviors, how nearly 15% of the gross domestic product is spent; are still considered "captain of the ship" in the hospital. Without physician buy-in, HCM will not achieve the level of success envisioned by planners.

    v. Patients—The ultimate HCM customer looking to the case manager to serve as advocate, educator, and advisor.

■ PHYSICIAN PARTNERSHIPS

Hospital case management operates within a supply-driven market. It is often the provider (the physician) rather than the consumer (the patient) who determines the type and extent of treatment, care, or services required. To a modest degree, the explosion of the baby-boomers, news media, the Internet, and direct-to-consumer advertising have eroded a portion of this market. Nevertheless, within the acute care environment, it is safe to say that, for the most part, the physicians' practice choices drive resource consumption, costs, and outcomes.

A. To influence the type and extent of practice choices and promote appropriate and cost-effective interventions, a collaborative partnership between the case manager and the physician must be nurtured and centered on the consumer (patient).

B. Case manager–physician partnerships are not forged overnight and often said partnership may be perceived as an infringement on partner prerogatives. Careful thought must be given to strategies meant to overcome the perceived static nature of the medical role.

C. While many HCMs might describe their relationship with the physicians as a "partnership," in reality, each provider works independently toward a common goal. An authentic collaborative partnership exists when the physician and the case manager work in tandem to achieve the desired goal.

D. Working in tandem may mean adopting new styles of communication or a new attitude. It means that the case manager will probably be: making rounds with the physician partner whenever feasible; questioning practice decisions and offering alternatives; and deciding together whether a patient's immediate needs require an acute care admission or whether the patients' continuing needs require an acute level of care. Optimal patient advocacy requires continual diligence to minimize the patient's exposure to unnecessary risk. Successful case managers work *with* the physician not *around* him/her.

E. Despite the case manager's level of clinical competence, the case manager's role is not to exercise clinical skills, but rather to apply critical thinking skills, knowledge of health care treatments, familiarity with evidence-based interventions, and erudition of the health care system to influence the physician's medical decision making. To promote a safe, cost-effective episode of acute care, working in tandem with the physician is key (Daniels and Ramey, 2005).

F. To influence a physician so that treatment decisions are made timely, appropriately, and in the patient's best interest, a conceptual shift to problem solving from the customer's perspective must occur and become second nature to the hospital case manager. If the case manager can recognize what is important to the physician, that insight can be used to offer a trade, or exchange, that brings value to the physician in practical terms.

G. Physicians want help in effectively managing their time while in the hospital. They are interested in having:
1. An advocate to make sure each patient receives prescribed treatments. The case manager is best suited to assume responsibility for this role.
2. Information to stay up to date and to make sound decisions that are in their patient's best interest.
3. Relief from the business transactions they see as obstacles to care.

H. Physicians are generally driven by professional commitment and a personal set of values. However, few are willing to commit to dramatic alterations in their practice, their routine, or their time unless it has personal value.

I. Physicians are typically driven by their own financial self-interest and will engage in a partnership with the case manager when they see that the exchange makes economic sense and brings value to him or her on a professional level ("The Performance Equation," 2003).

J. By and large, physicians will not buy into a case management program and acceptance will never occur if the physician perceives the role of the case manager as being simply to police his/her patients' charts, reduce length of stay, cut costs for the hospital, or challenge his/her medical judgment.

■ ACUTE CARE CASE MANAGEMENT MODELS

As programs continued to evolve, no single "reference model" of acute care case management has emerged. As a result, HCM today is often a reactive conglomeration of activities without a coherent vision or rational intent.

A. Envisioning the future—Given the chaos in the current hospital environment, coupled with the lack of a reference model for HCM, every successful program first creates a vision for the model.
1. Visioning is a collective process of imagining the future.
2. When a group of individuals get together to brainstorm about a case management model, creative juices start to flow and "why can't we . . ." ideas surface.
3. Through the visioning process, the purpose and intent of a program can be defined, along with its philosophy, core values, and principles.
4. When vision and intent are neglected, there is dissonance and confusion and the case managers feel the push and pull of multiple constituencies.

B. While determining the purpose and intent of the hospital's case management program, important and sensitive outcomes are articulated.

Knowledge at the outset on how HCM will be evaluated gives planners information to help design a relevant infrastructure and operations.

C. There are two overarching case management goals in the acute care setting.
   1. Quality care with boastful clinical outcomes
   2. Cost-effective care with the savings to prove it
   How each of these goals is translated into measurable objectives is a product of data accessibility, priorities, and manpower. With a clear understanding of the program's vision, purpose, goals, and objectives, a series of positive concepts or principles can be developed to serve as the framework for a model of HCM.

D. Some of the frequently encountered principles found in successful care delivery programs include activities related to the following domains:
   1. Accountability
   2. Responsibility
   3. Advocacy
   4. Collaboration
   5. Real-time communication
   6. Influence
   7. Customer-friendliness
   8. Teamwork
   9. Value
   10. Outcomes

E. Some elements of the original clinical New England model still exist. Clinical case management models or collaborative practice models are typically seen in larger, urban teaching centers. Although pure clinical care/case management models are rare, the collaborative model— known more popularly as a dyad or triad model—is frequently found in large, tertiary facilities where the high costs of these models can more easily be absorbed. The collaborative model typically features a team made up of a case manager, a utilization review specialist, and a social worker.

F. However, community hospitals overwhelmingly use a functional model created by either consolidating or integrating utilization review and discharge planning activities.
   1. Functional models are typically created when social work and utilization review departments are collapsed into a case management department.
   2. The job descriptions of the roles created in the functional model focus on the tasks associated with the two primary functions of social work/discharge planning and utilization review.
   3. A consolidation model is a subset of a functional model. In it, the activities of discharge planning and utilization review are performed by independent individuals.
      a. Separate roles are maintained under either a single director or a case management program director and a social work manager.

b. This model is fraught with challenges.
   i. Role definitions are often ill defined with overlapping or redundant activities.
   ii. Self-preservation turf battles are not uncommon, leading to tension and conflict (as is frequently documented in the literature).
4. In an integrated model, both functions—discharge planning and utilization review—are integrated into a *single* role.
   a. The social work and utilization review positions are eliminated or, in some cases, may convert to case manager positions.
   b. In this model, the responsibilities of the new case manager position are vaguely defined and the case manager ends up performing the same tasks related to discharge planning and utilization review.

G. Clinical resource management (CRM) models represent the next generation of case management programs in hospitals.
1. Clinical resource managers follow the patient through the phases of the acute care continuum.
2. Routine tasks are typically delegated to clerical support team members, thereby freeing up the case manager to help the patient navigate through the system in the safest, most cost-efficient manner.
3. In this model, case management activities focus on the process of access, the nature and appropriateness of treatment, and alternatives for timely transition to a post-acute venue.
4. This model capitalizes on the assets and skills of a well-rounded, business savvy case manager. They eschew task completion in favor of outcome achievement.
5. Two examples of CRM models
   a. Disease management models
      i. A case manager is aligned with a high-volume or high-risk patient population.
      ii. Though the case manager monitors resource utilization and offers possible post-acute services, the focus is more typically concerned with education, social intervention, and therapeutic compliance.
      iii. Disease management models are often launched to manage the chronic illnesses of patients who are repeatedly admitted to the hospital for acute care.
      iv. Patients with chronic illnesses such as heart failure, renal failure, asthma, diabetes, and others, are either followed by their case manager into the community, or a seamless handoff to a community/complex care case manager is effected.
      v. The growth of interactive tele-health connecting the case manager with the patient has yielded published success and has made this model a natural progression in acute care case management evolution (Roupe, 2004; Young, 2004).

    b. Outcome management models—Are heavily dependent on data to drive change, including:

       i. Change in medical practice decisions through the use of evidence-based protocols to protect the patient against non-contributory interventions that may add clinical or financial risk.

       ii. Change in delivery of care processes to remove barriers to the patient's swift and safe navigation through the acute care episode.

       iii. Change in the value proposition—Establishing benchmarks of HCM practice and demonstrating the impact of HCM interventions on both clinical and financial outcomes to prove value to the organization's multiple stakeholders.

H. Hybrid models incorporate multiple approaches.

    1. Experiments with disease management programs that coexist with integrated models are not uncommon.

    2. Likewise, an outcomes model to support the growing popularity of intensivists and hospitalists works very well while the rest of the organization is working from a CRM or functional model.

■ INFRASTRUCTURE

Infrastructure relates to the alignment of HCM within the organizational structure; the nature of the team and the positions within the HCM program; and the assignment, staffing and scheduling of case management team positions.

A. There is no one best way to structure HCM. Nevertheless, as mentioned previously, there are definite commonalities among successful programs, which are listed below.

B. One of the parameters of structure concerns the decision about the program's placement on the organizational chart.

    1. The organizational chart describes the hierarchical system of responsibility and supervision based on levels of authority.

    2. The organizational chart, also known as the table of organization (TO), represents the interconnectivity of the various components of the hospital organization and reflects the structure of relationships between people, positions, and departments.

    3. Although the TO is a static representation, it plays a role in setting the rules that guide behavior, promoting hospital culture, and changing or perpetuating mental models of behaviors.

       a. Mental models are a set of perceptions that color the images, assumptions, and stories that individuals carry in their minds about how things work.

       b. Where HCM is positioned on the TO will influence the image of the program, the rules of behavior governing the program, and the responsiveness of stakeholders to the program.

       c. Simply put, the accountability relationships and mental models of behavior that the TO represents will affect how people perceive case management (Daniels and Ramey, 2005).

    4. Vertical alignment refers to the line pattern of authority that supervises lower levels.

a. In the past, case management was typically positioned under the chief nursing officer. However, that trend has shifted and programs now report to the chief medical officer (CMO). (ACMA, 2003).

b. In smaller hospitals, or in the absence of a salaried CMO, programs generally report to the chief financial officer.

5. Horizontal alignment refers to the way hospital programs are separated or combined under a single administrator.

a. The richest path for information and ideas is often a lateral trail that includes social work, utilization review, and documentation specialists.

b. An expanded lateral alignment often includes risk management, infection control, and performance improvement (quality management/total quality management/core measures).

C. Assignment of responsibility and scope of accountability—The manner in which the case management workforce is distributed among patients—is important in HCM programs (Daniels and Ramey, 2005).

1. In geographic assignment, case managers are assigned to a physical unit and work with the staff and patients on that unit.

2. In service line assignment, case managers are assigned to a particular medical service line.

a. Assignment may be grouped by specialties (e.g., Department of Medicine, Department of Surgery, Division of Cardiology, Division of Orthopedics) or by Centers of Excellence (e.g., Center for Cancer Studies, Hypertension Management Program).

3. In physician assignment, case managers may be assigned to specific groups of physicians, generally sharing similar specialties, or employed hospitalists. Hospitals have seen the enhanced benefits of a hospitalist–case manager partnership as the trend keeps growing (Ramey and Daniels, 2004).

4. Case managers may be assigned to populations who share a common disease. This model is gaining support in small, community hospitals where case management is moving beyond the boundary of the hospital into the community.

5. There are pros and cons to each of these assignment models.

a. Geographic assignment is by far the most popular and, of course, the easiest for the case manager.

b. However, anecdotal evidence indicates that physician assignment models are preferred as case managers report that they have greater influence when they work with a consistent group of physicians.

c. Physician assignments in hospitals with more than 300 beds present unique challenges. Often these can be minimized by using a hybrid approach that uses both unit-based case managers and physician- or specialty-assigned case managers.

D. Staffing of HCM programs refers to the plan for how many case management personnel are needed and of what classification.

1. For several reasons, there is not a staffing "best practice."

      a. First, no two hospital case management programs are the same and every HCM program has a scope of practice and scope of service unique to its facility. Case management expectations in one hospital will not necessarily parallel the expectations in another hospital.

      b. Second, the degree of support staff is a major variable. In some hospitals, case managers are expected to perform clerical as well as professional activities, while others have "back room" support personnel.

      c. Third, the nature of the patient populations and the character of the case management assignment are additional variables that must be considered. Case managers working exclusively with physicians caring for orthopedic patients, for example, will be able to handle more patients than a colleague who is partnered with the internal medicine doctors caring for patients with multiple diagnoses.

      d. Fourth, staffing depends on the chosen model of practice, the relationships that the case manager is expected to nurture, the payer mix, managed care contractual obligations, and the availability of data (Daniels and Ramey, 2005).

  2. These four different issues are why there are no set staffing standards—nor should there be. However, for readers looking for more definitive numbers to justify or explain their staffing levels, the range of patient to case manager ratios have varied from a low of 12–15:1 (working with hospital-based intensivists or complex medical patients) to a high of 22–32:1 (working with low-risk maternity or orthopedic patients).

  3. Best advice—Look beyond caseload statistics and ask yourself what you are trying to achieve.

E. Scheduling refers to the most productive pattern of staff presence to achieve the best outcomes.

  1. Scheduling is most appropriate and meaningful when it is predicated on an aggregate of several factors.

      a. Needs of primary customers

      b. Pattern of presence based on scope of service (outpatient clinics may not require weekend case management, while emergency department case management may require 24/7 coverage)

      c. Payer accessibility

      d. Levels of intensity of the patient population

      e. Contextual issues including scope of responsibilities and available resources

      f. Level of preparation and experience of the case managers

F. Competency of the case management staff is a product of professional training, experience, mentorship, and exposure to new information. Critical thinking skills of any case manager are vital, but in the high-risk hospital environment where case managers lack any positional authority, failure to exercise critical thinking skills on behalf of the patient could be a matter of life or death.

1. Other basic skills of a successful hospital case manager include:
   a. Outstanding communication skills—Able to easily use language to present a position and build more productive relationships with key business partners
   b. Essential negotiation skills—Able to tackle difficult people situations effectively and improve collaboration with colleagues
   c. Self-confidence and assertiveness—Able to get message across in a secure manner
G. A mountain of anecdotal evidence suggests that a real-time, physician-centric partnership results in better outcomes for all stakeholders.
   1. Activities that diminish the case manager's role or removes her from the center of action and easy access to physicians will undermine the case manager's efforts to influence outcomes.
   2. Case manager–physician rounds represent a simple but highly effective strategy to begin the partnership building process.
H. Successful programs allocate a portion of available Full-time Employees (FTEs) to support staff, sometimes called case management associates. Commonplace tasks take up valuable time that would be better spent in dialog with clinical and business associates as well as patients and their families and community service representatives.
   1. Duties that are frequently delegated to case management support/associate staff
   a. Reception
   b. Data entry
   c. Phone calls triage
   d. Centralized post-acute placement activities
   e. Contractual utilization review
   f. Clerical processes
   g. Report generation and dissemination
   h. Maintaining and updating program resource manuals
I. The case management infrastructure typically includes a physician advisor (PA).
   1. Today's PA role differs significantly from the medical advisor of the past, an individual who was viewed as the "hatchet man" for utilization problems. Today, the PAs support the case managers both intellectually and emotionally.
   a. PAs serve as a resource to case managers who are dealing with specific challenging patient and care provider situations.
   b. PAs further the case managers' clinical knowledge, adding to their credibility when interacting with their physician partners.
   c. Effective PAs also coach case managers on approaches that will be best received by a physician colleague.
   d. Since case managers are typically functioning in a fast-paced and high-pressure environment, PAs can mitigate some of the daily

chaos associated with the role and provide a sense of organizational support (Smith, 2003).

2. Of all the structural issues that surface, the challenge of building a constructive relationship between the case manager and the social worker has proven the most tricky.

   a. Despite the industry's misguided attempt to eliminate social work positions, they are essential assets in a successful case management program. Nevertheless, tension between the social worker and the case manager exists often due to the social worker's feeling of vulnerability (Feuer, 2003).

   b. The issue is how to best align social work assets to minimize professional tension; eliminate redundant activities; avoid fragmentation, overlap, and competition; and keep personnel costs down.

   c. In small-to-medium-sized hospitals, social work departments have virtually disappeared and social work positions are incorporated under the case management umbrella. The relationship between the case manager and the social worker is reinforced through a referral process that recognizes the special expertise that the social worker brings to a situation. When the case manager determines that psychosocial issues could potentially obstruct the patient's swift and safe navigation through the acute episode of care, a referral to her social work colleague can save the day.

   d. In large teaching facilities, a social work department may continue to function and the growth of dyad or triad case management models has resulted in the reduction of functional silos.

   e. When case management programs include adequate support staff to implement the patient's discharge plan, the social work job description can be rewritten to refocus activities on the social worker's professional expertise in the field of psychosocial counseling, crisis management, and so on.

   f. Referrals by case managers and other professionals avoid the need for independent social work case finding, which only confuses patients, confounds physicians and other staff, and is often the root cause of case manager–social work tension (Daniels and Ramey, 2005).

   g. In a "best practice" environment, social workers are independent practitioners serving as professional consultants and are referred to patients and families according to predetermined criteria, patient needs, and care planning (including transitional planning) priorities.

■ OPERATIONS

A. There is a direct link between case management workflow activities and the purpose and objectives of the HCM program.

B. In an era where duplication of work and overlapping responsibilities are financially indefensible and coordination of services is highly desirable, the performance of the case manager includes activities that are meant to better integrate the level of care transition and the resource management processes.

1. Some aspects of these functions are best delegated to other personnel, such as case management support staff, to better leverage the time and skill of case managers.
   a. For example, once the determination is made that a patient requires durable medical equipment or transportation services at discharge, arranging for transportation or securing equipment does not require the involvement of a professional person such as the case manager (Smith, 2003). Rather, such activities can be delegated to support staff.
C. The workflow operations of a hospital case manager are best described in terms of two major categories: clinical management and resource management activities. Both represent the full scope of practice of a successful HCM.
D. Clinical case management
   1. Refers to activities that position the case manager as an advocate for quality and safe care and appropriate medical interventions.
   2. Is the equivalent of medical case management—a collaborative effort between the physician and the case manager (and other health care professionals as needed, such as clinical nutritionists and physical therapists) to promote interventions that are appropriate to the reason for the inpatient admission, the medical treatment plan, the patient's prognosis, the intended outcomes, and any continuing needs following the acute-care episode.
   3. There are several major components of clinical case management. With the current demand for quality, safety, and value, evidence-based protocols are the new generation of guidelines used for these purposes.
      a. A best-practice protocol ideally synthesizes research evidence, expert opinion, and local judgment and serves as a guide to enhance the physician's (as well as others') decision making in a clinical situation.
      b. Anecdotal evidence confirms that there must be a process in place so that practical case management advice can be made available at the time when the physician is making clinical decisions and writing orders for treatment.
      c. Because 80% of medical costs are initiated through physician orders, discussing alternative medical interventions before writing orders is an ideal strategy for cost containment.
         i. A real-time, point-of-care interaction is the single most effective activity where a combination of a case manager, physician, and the application of an evidence-based guideline could favorably affect the cost and quality of medical care.
         ii. In hospitals with a computerized physician order entry (CPOE) system, application of the guideline in concert with the automated order sets is highly effective. When guidelines are suggested as such—guidelines, not immutable mandates—it will be possible to gain the highest degree of physician compliance (Daniels and Ramey, 2005).

    iii. In hospitals without an electronic medical record or CPOE, the case management team must brainstorm ideas and strategies on how to bring the best of evidence-based medicine (EBM) to the point of care.

d. Physician profiling is another strategy to promote quality and curtail cost. It uses objective, physician-specific information to draw attention to the cost of rendering care and the wide variation in medical practice (Daniels and Ramey, 2005).

    i. Profiles are constructed using a collection of empirical data on demographics, diagnoses, procedures, and treatments. They are generated in the medical records department.

    ii. These data are linked to the resources that were consumed by the patient during the episode of care.

    iii. Resources include such items as medications (both oral and intravenous medications), diagnostic imaging, operating room time, use of an intensive care bed, minimally invasive procedures, the services of respiratory therapy, and other interventions that are a direct result of the physician's practice decisions.

    iv. Resources include those prescribed, not only by the attending physician of record, but by all of the consultants that are brought in on the case.

    v. Each intervention has an associated revenue code and each revenue code is converted to an associated cost. Thus, when a physician's order for a chest x-ray is entered into the order entry system, it is typically translated into a revenue code with a price tag attached to it for billing.

    vi. For the purposes of practice profile reporting, all the claims data are organized by either DRG or principle diagnosis and formatted so that the resources are categorized into major resource "buckets." For example, all DRG 89 patients (simple pneumonia with comorbidities) would be grouped together and all the resources reported under each attending physician caring for DRG 89 patients are listed in bucket columns such as respiratory services, medications, lab-hematology, lab-chemistry, IV meds, and so on. In this manner, comparisons of the resources used are made among different physicians caring for pneumonia patients. These reports come in many formats though the best practice is a simple spreadsheet format where physicians can see their profile in comparison with their peers and no interpretative explanation is required.

    vii. It can be anticipated that physicians whose profiles differ sharply from their colleagues will claim: "I use more resources because my patients are sicker."

    viii. The playing field must be leveled to make sure that apples are being measured against other apples. Leveling the playing field is done electronically by sophisticated software that considers many patient-specific demographic and clinical factors.

The results are known as *severity* or *risk-adjusted* data and are used widely by state, federal, and payer agencies to evaluate medical practice patterns.

   ix. Performance profiles are key resources to improve patient care outcomes, remove obstacles to care, and prevent unwanted events that add cost or present risk.

   x. Objective profiles help to connect the physician with the hospital's interests simply by sharing the relevant data with the physicians. These profiles serve as a resource to improve the case manager's efforts to motivate and influence physician decisions to achieve expected outcomes.

e. Crossing the continuum.

At a minimum, successful hospital case management programs encompass all three phases of the acute care continuum—access, throughput, and transition.

   i. Access is generally defined as the entry into the acute care environment.

   ii. Throughput or care management is often defined as all the people, processes, and systems that work independently or dependently to deliver care, treatment, or services to the patient.

   iii. Transition is the movement of the patient from one level of care to another, generally in diminishing order. Hospital case managers have traditionally focused on the exit phase—discharge planning. Progressive programs include access and care management as well.

f. Optimally, the case management process begins as soon as the patient crosses the hospital threshold. Whether the patient enters through the emergency department, as a direct admission, as a transfer, or through the preadmission ambulatory center, the case manager is on the scene.

g. Successful HCM programs have adequate resources to facilitate treatments and services and coordinate interventions with the clinical team. Such activities take place mostly in the throughput phase.

h. Coordination of care entails the provision of assistance to ensure the effective organization of, and access to, services and resources that are appropriate to the needs of the patients and their families.

i. Coordination can be categorized into five primary advocacy accountabilities.

   i. Advanced communication among clinical team members

   ii. Organization of the multidisciplinary discharge planning process

   iii. Liaison with payers and business team members

   iv. Initiation of referrals to internal and external resources

   v. Fueling the progress of the patient's transition to the next level of care

j. In practical terms, continuity means that a single case manager will consistently serve as the patient's advocate, quality inspector, and information source in every geographic area in which the patient is placed.

   i. This is not an easily obtainable goal in large hospitals where the physical distance between patient care areas can be considerable.

   ii. In those situations, case management designs mechanisms for a seamless handoff from one case manager to another to minimize communication gaps and to comply with new regulatory expectations.

k. Hospitals are required to develop an individualized plan for moving the patient from the acute care setting to a community setting prior to leaving the hospital. Patients and families, no matter how well adjusted, often need considerable consultation to help them explore and evaluate all the options regarding post-acute needs.

l. Ongoing evaluation of transition needs is the responsibility of the entire clinical team.

   i. Each member, including the patient and family, plays a role in planning for transition.

   ii. In most hospitals, it is the case manager who serves as the orchestra leader and pulls all the pieces together, often with the essential assistance of the patient's primary nurse and social worker.

m. Mature HCM programs have established a centralized position to serve as the transition planning coordinator.

   i. For those patients who are being followed by a case manager, the case manager is accountable for orchestrating the transition planning process. However, implementation of the plan—checking benefits, finding resources, completing forms, and so on—is delegated to the coordinator.

   ii. In addition, the coordinator is a resource for nurses caring for patients who are not being followed by a case manager. If the patient requires post-acute service or equipment, the nurse can access the centralized transition coordinator and receive the same support as the case manager.

E. Resource Management

   1. Resource management encompasses a diverse set of activities designed to influence the efficient and appropriate use of hospital resources. Resources may be tangible (like supplies, pharmaceuticals, a diagnostic test, or equipment) and intangible (like time).

   2. Resource management is a balance of patient advocacy and the organization's obligation to appropriately allocate resources.

   3. Resource management is a prospective process to monitor the appropriate use of resources for the condition presented and offer acceptable alternatives.

   4. The utilization review function practiced in most hospitals is a component of resource management.

    a. It is a compulsory obligation under the terms of the insurance contract.

    b. The process typically uses a method of chart review to evaluate the medical necessity and appropriateness of an admission and duration of stay, level of care, resources consumed, and readiness for discharge.

    c. Routine chart review for the purpose of gathering information for the payer can be delegated to a nonprofessional staff member such as a case management associate.

5. It is important to distinguish contractual obligations for utilization review from regulatory requirements for utilization review.

    a. For the most part, contracts are quite explicit about their procedures and policies regarding the review process. In contrast, regulatory agencies (e.g., Centers for Medicare and Medicaid Services, State Departments of Health) generally promulgate a set of guidelines but leave it to each hospital to determine its own procedures.

    b. The predominant chart review process of utilization review is a retrospective activity. The decision to admit, the intensity of services prescribed, and the level of care determinations *have all been done already* (Daniels and Ramey, 2005).

    c. Commercial contracts establish the utilization review and management arrangements.

        i. Since the insurer organization typically drafts the document, it is left to the health care provider to improve the agreement to achieve a mutually beneficial relationship.

        ii. While some provisions will inevitably favor one side or the other, overall balance is a key to more harmonious payer–provider relationships.

    d. Contracts are typically endorsed by the chief financial officer, managed care department, and chief executive officer once fees are negotiated.

    e. Boilerplate language dictating the terms of utilization review expectations should be reviewed by the director of case management to avoid placing the hospital in a defensive posture (Daniels and Ramey, 2005).

        i. The director should review the utilization language prior to each contract renewal. Once case management has succeeded in reducing denials (and factual data proves it), this information is used as a negotiating tool to reduce or eliminate contractual utilization review demands and allows case management to assume prospective resource management responsibility.

        ii. Every case manager should have knowledge of the payers' reimbursement methods. Case management activities and priorities may hinge on knowledge that reimbursement is per diem versus DRG versus discounted fee for service.

        iii. In addition, in an area with aggressively managed payer contracts, (e.g., Medicare Advantage), physician contracts may be capitated. Case manager knowledge of this information will prove beneficial in helping the physician efficiently manage the patient's treatment plan.

f. Physician practice behaviors (see physician profiles above) can be influenced through persistent point-of-care interactions and objective data quantifying practice habits.

g. Through real-time discussions about admissions, continued stays, or the value of practice decisions at the time the decision is being made, the case manager provides several value-added services:

   i. Provides the physician with immediate feedback

   ii. Avoids intrusive follow-up phone calls questioning the physician's decisions

   iii. Informs the physician of possible consequences both clinical and economical, for both the patient and the physician

   iv. Gives the physician the opportunity to modify his decision

   v. Reinforces new and desirable behaviors (Daniels and Ramey, 2005)

h. Timely delivery-of-care is a product of the processes in place.

   i. Processes are linked activities that produce outcomes.

   ii. Delays caused by these processes consume scarce resources and the ability of the hospital to provide care, treatment, and services in an efficient manner.

6. As part of resource management activities the hospital-based case managers capture and quantify information on the obstacles encountered that result in a potentially avoidable day (PAD).

a. Data on avoidable days must prevent pointing fingers or placing blame.

b. PAD is a cost issue to hospital administration but it is a quality issue for the hospital case manager and the patient. This distinction must be clearly understood.

c. The effectiveness of the case manager's efforts to reduce PAD and move the patient efficiently through the episode of care will suffer if the case manager connects PAD to the loss of revenue to the hospital.

d. The incentive for the physician to engage in resource management must be driven by quality of care or some personal, vested interest.

e. Best practice for the capture and quantification of PAD include:

   i. Identifying the full range of PAD variables

   ii. Categorizing the data by patient, physician, or system

   iii. Consistently capturing the necessary data

   iv. Focusing on capturing both delays and lost days

   v. Using a standard metric to quantify the issues

   vi. As trends begin to emerge, narrowing the list of variables to those necessary

   vii. Reporting and disseminating results to every department head as well as members of the executive team (Daniels and Ramey, 2005)

  f. If a process improvement is not forthcoming, the value of continuing to collect the data should be re-examined.

  g. Inpatient days for which payers deny payment and which may be influenced by a case manager result from five avoidable situations:

   i. Inappropriate admissions

   ii. Delay in discharge

   iii. Delay in treatment

   iv. Prescribed services not related to the reason for admission (not medically necessary)

   v. Tests performed just before a patient is discharged that could be performed in an outpatient setting

  h. These categories plus many other inefficient administrative processes are among the obstacles hospitals face in order to get paid for services rendered.

7. Denial management is typically a component of the hospital's revenue cycle.

  a. The revenue cycle is a series of financial processes that begin when the patient comes into the system and includes all of those activities that have to occur in order for the hospital to bill for services and collect revenue at the end of the process.

  b. The revenue cycle cuts across every area/department in the hospital from medical record face sheet completion, to charge capture by clinicians; from contract management to medical record documentation.

  c. Executives have only recently seen the revenue cycle as an enterprise-wide process rather than a series of department activities.

  d. Representatives from the HCM program are members of the revenue cycle team because of their participation in the episode of acute care and their knowledge of navigational breakdowns that may result in a PAD, and ultimately in a payer denial.

  e. Case managers are the front-line resources to respond to those categories of denial that are the result of medical decisions. All other denial appeals are delegated to the attributable source. For example, denials arising from a delay in treatment are referred to the department head for that treatment area. Similarly, denial due to the lack or delay of precertification is forwarded to the access management department (admissions and registration). However, a denial for a quality of care issue is followed up by the case manager.

  f. Hospitals with highly successful resource management programs have a low rate of clinical denials, as evidenced by an easily accessible system of financial record keeping that uses a separate posting code to capture and report denial information for every possible denial category.

8. Medical documentation drives reimbursement for both the physician and the hospital.

  a. Specifically, doctors complete their charting responsibilities, the chart flows to the health information management (HIM) department for the coder to abstract essential information and assign related codes.

b. The information captured as part of the abstracting and coding process is converted to the UB-92 format so that the patient accounting office can generate a bill.

c. Neither physicians nor case managers are knowledgeable about coding and would find it difficult to master the time-consuming and technically tricky coding function while also practicing clinical case management. Nevertheless, both would acknowledge that coding accuracy is a lynchpin for both regulatory compliance and the financial health of both the physician and the hospital (Daniels and Ramey, 2005).

d. In hospitals without documentation improvement specialists, the case managers and HIM coders collaborate at monthly "mapping" sessions to discuss problems about the capture of diagnoses and supporting medical necessity documentation.

e. The mapping sessions point out deficiencies in medical documentation and provide the case manager with some hints to reduce ambiguous or potentially incomplete charting related to a specific, high-volume, or high-risk diagnosis.

f. Documentation aids are often designed to reinforce the case manager's counsel by offering language to support the patient's severity of illness and the intensity of services prescribed.

F. Advocacy

1. Overarching both clinical management and resource management activities is the prime directive of advocacy.

2. The Commission for Case Manager Certification in its Code of Professional Conduct defines advocacy as: "A process that promotes beneficence, justice and autonomy for clients. Advocacy especially aims to foster the client's independence. It also involves educating clients about their rights, health care and human services, resources, and benefits, and facilitating appropriate and informed decision making, and includes considerations for the client's values, beliefs, and interests"(Gilpin, 2005).

3. In the hospital environment, the case manager's persuasive involvement in clinical and resource management activities reflects the supremacy of the advocacy role.

4. More than any other practice environment, the hospital represents the highest-risk setting for the patient and demands an assertive, self-confident case manager to guard the patient's exposure to unnecessary clinical, financial, and operational risks. In terms of day-to-day practice this means that the case manager must question any decision or delay that may negatively impact the patient.

G. Outcomes

1. The value of case management is a product of its contribution to the organization's clinical and financial bottom lines, therefore the case manager's performance in relationship to organizational goals is essential.

2. Case management activities must be congruent with the strategic results a hospital (including its HCM program) desires to achieve on behalf of its stakeholders.
3. There must be a cause and effect relationship between the work of the case manager and the desired results (Daniels and Ramey, 2005).
4. Outcomes measurement can be quite complicated especially if data is not easily accessible. Fortunately, the use of informatics has dramatically changed the face of the health care industry and has enabled case management to more easily demonstrate its influence.
5. HCM outcomes are the end results of the case managers' work activities that objectively measure the HCM program's effectiveness and demonstrate a positive correlation between its interventions and the outcomes being measured.
6. Case management outcome indicators are surrogate measures of the case manager's sphere of influence.
7. Outcomes generally fall into four major categories:
   a. Clinical outcomes reflect improvement in patient care. For example, data may show that more patients are getting beta-blockers as a result of point-of-care reminders by the case manager.
   b. Cost outcomes measure the cost of resources being consumed.
      i. Noncontributory medical practice decisions or delivery-of-care processes adds costs per patient day.
      ii. Lower costs per case through reductions in nonacute interventions exemplify an objective outcome that results from a case manager's influence.
   c. Revenue outcomes measure the resources gained as a result of the case manager's activities. An example would be an increase in case mix index (CMI) through the case manager's (or documentation improvement specialist's) point-of-service documentation advice or reductions in one- and two-day length of stay admissions.
   d. Value outcomes put a price tag on the achievement of outcomes. They make it easier to measure the relationship between the case management resources and the outcomes achieved. Often expressed as an equation: value = benefits − cost.
8. Building an outcomes framework often begins with the hospital's business objectives—economic, environmental, operational, and clinical.
   a. These objectives serve as a framework for developing department- or program-specific performance improvement initiatives.
   b. If one of the hospital's objectives is to improve physician relationships, then case management may identify objective indicators to demonstrate that as a result of their real-time physician partnerships, physician satisfaction has significantly increased. For example, an outcome may state that as a result of the case manager's presence to assist the physician, satisfaction with the case management program increased by 17% over a one-month period.
   c. If the hospital objective is operational excellence, then case management may identify a metric to show "avoidable days due to

untimely chemistry lab diagnostic testing and reporting were reduced by 11% over the last month."

9. A framework is often referred to as the dashboard or report card of case management outcomes. It provides a portal view into the state of achievement.

10. Outcomes require objective information, which is recorded and stored in department repositories.

    a. Case management leaders must work with information system or decision support specialists to set up systems that benchmark their performance and contributions.

    b. Integration of data and production of information from disparate systems is now possible because of the availability of interface engines, data-mining software, and decision support services.

    c. Case management access to information is essential to monitor program effectiveness.

11. Traditional discharge planning and utilization review models have a relatively clear return on investment (ROI) specifically in terms of length of stay (LOS). However, as case management programs continue to evolve, LOS reduction must be accompanied by aggressive demonstration of resource management outcomes.

12. For the purposes of case management, ROI is the profit or loss resulting from the hospital's investment in case management.

    a. Calculating the ROI requires a comparison of the costs of case management resources against the benefits it provides and is expressed in a formula: [(benefits − costs)/costs] × 100% = % ROI.

REFERENCES

American Case Management Association (ACMA). (2003). Survey provides objective view of case management profession. *Collaborative Case Management, 1*(2), 3.

Daniels, S., & Ramey, M. (2005). *The leader's guide to hospital case management.* Sudbury, MA: Jones and Bartlett.

Feuer, L. (2003). Ugly turf issues once again? *The Case Manager, 14*(3), 26–27.

Gilpin, S. (2005). Advocacy and case management. *Care Management, 11*(1), 28.

Ramey, M., & Daniels, S. (2004). Hospitalists and case managers. *Lippincott's Case Management, 9* (6), 280–286.

Roupe, M. Y. (2004). A vital component of disease management programs. *Lippincott's Case Management, 9*(1), 47–49.

Smith, A. P. (2003). Case management: Key to access, quality, and financial success. *Nursing Economics, 21*(5), 237–240, 244.

Stonestreet, J. A. (1999). *Acute care case management in US: A survey of structure, process and outcomes.* Unpublished PhD dissertation. Texas Woman's University, Denton, TX.

The Performance Equation. (2003). PriceWaterhouseCoopers Healthcare. Interview with Arthur T. Porter in *Modern Healthcare.*

Young, S. (2004). Outcomes and throughput. *Lippincott's Case Management, 9*(6), 300–302.

Wolfe, G. (2006). The cost of healthcare: Opportunities for case managers. *Care Management, 12*(3), 7.

Zander, K. (1988). Managed care within an acute care setting: Design and implementation via nursing case management. *Health Care Supervisor, 6*(2), 27–43.

Case Management in the Home Care Setting

Elizabeth Alvarado
Edward Sunderland

LEARNING OBJECTIVES

Upon completion of this chapter, the reader will be able to:

1. Discuss the different services available in the home care setting.
2. Describe reimbursement and insurance issues in relation to the home care setting.
3. Explain the importance of collaboration within the interdisciplinary team including durable medical equipment agencies and other representatives.
4. Explain the role of the case manager in the home care setting.

IMPORTANT TERMS AND CONCEPTS

Advance Request Payment
Certified Home Healthcare Agency (CHHA)
Custodial Care
Home Care
Home Health Aide
Home Health Resource Groups (HHRGs)
Homebound
Intermittent or Part-Time Care

Long-Term Care
Low Utilization Payment
Nonskilled Services
Occupational Therapy
Outcome and Assessment Information Set (OASIS)
Outlier Payment
Partial Episode Payment
Physical Therapy
Reasonable Care/Services

Significant Change in Condition	Skilled Services
Payment	Speech Therapy

■ INTRODUCTION

A. Throughout history, medical care was provided in the home by family members, with some guidance from outpatient or home visiting professionals.

B. During the second half of the twentieth century, medical practice shifted from this home-based model of care to the hospital-based care model, which allowed medical practice to expand its knowledge and improve individual outcomes and dramatically increase life expectancy.

C. Unfortunately, however, medical care costs also dramatically increased. These increases have brought about the necessity of controlling costs.

   1. In the private sector, insurance companies sought to control costs through utilization review/management and health maintenance organizations (HMOs).

   2. In the public sector, the Centers for Medicare and Medicaid Services (CMS), formerly the Health Care Financing Administration, have sought to control costs through the adoption of diagnosis related groups (DRGs) and the prospective payment system (PPS).

   3. The development of DRGs, HMOs, and the practice of utilization review has led to increased pressure on hospitals to control costs by limiting the number of days each patient spends in the hospital—that is, to reduce length of stay (LOS).

   4. The current pressure on hospitals has increased the need for home care services and therefore, case management.

D. Hospitals have found that utilizing interdisciplinary teams to develop post-hospital discharge plans can safely reduce length of stay without compromising patient safety. These teams are best facilitated by case managers to produce the most effective outcomes.

E. Home care, when appropriate, serves two vital functions in reducing costs by limiting length of stay in institutional settings.

   1. First, home care serves as a less expensive extension to hospital-based care.

      a. The average home care visit cost is significantly less than the cost of a day in the hospital. The visit can provide vital information to the physician that can confirm the plan of care or indicate the need for change.

      b. The assessment of a medical professional in the home can provide reassurance to patients and their families that the plan of care or health regimen is appropriate as well as provide important information to the interdisciplinary team about conditions in the home.

   2. Second, home care serves as a less expensive and more satisfying alternative to other types of institutional care.

a. The average cost of a home care visit is significantly less than the cost of a day in a skilled nursing care facility; and most, but by no means all, families would prefer to provide care in the home setting.

b. As an alternative to a hospital or skilled nursing facility, home care shifts the burden of round-the-clock institutional care from the insurer to the family. Therefore, across an effective continuum of care, one should expect to see increasing home care costs, not as a result of overutilization of home care services, but as a result of shifting utilization away from more costly settings into home care.

F. Case management in the home care setting is designed with similar goals in mind as those of case management in the acute care setting. These may include the following:

1. Optimization of the delivery of care across the continuum
2. Caring for patients in less costly care settings
3. Employing a proactive approach to patient care delivery by implementing strategies to keep patients out of acute care settings
4. Monitoring patients' conditions and preventing deterioration
5. Reducing patients' risks and need for acute care services
6. Improving quality of care and services
7. Maintaining patients' safety
8. Improving patients' quality of life

G. Patients who are eligible for home care services include those who were hospitalized in an acute care/hospital setting, those with chronic illnesses, or those with seriously complex medical conditions.

H. The demand for home care case management services has increased lately since the implementation of the federal home care PPS, the increase in managed care and capitation, the popularity of demand management programs, and the growth of integrated delivery systems.

■ KEY DEFINITIONS

A. Advance request payment—A home care services claim submitted at the completion of the initial assessment of the patient, upon admission into home care services, and at the completion of an initial OASIS score. This claim includes a partial payment amount that does not exceed 60% of the specific HHRG-designated reimbursement.

B. Certified home healthcare agency (CHHA)—A company that meets all the eligibility criteria required by CMS before it is permitted to provide home care services for Medicare beneficiaries.

C. Custodial care—Care provided primarily to assist a patient in meeting the activities of daily living, but not requiring the services of a licensed professional, such as bathing and eating.

D. Home care—Health care services that are provided to patients while in their own homes. These services may include professional (i.e., skilled) and paraprofessional (i.e., supportive) services.

E. Home health resource group (HHRG)—Groupings for prospective reimbursement under Medicare for home health agencies. Placement into an HHRG is based on the OASIS score. Reimbursement rates correspond to the level of home health services provided.

F. Homebound—Being confined to the home setting all (or almost all) the time. A patient who is considered homebound is only able to leave the home very infrequently and for short periods of time. Leaving the home requires a considerable or taxing effort with or without help. An example is a patient who experiences an unbearable and extreme effort to leave the home just for a clinic visit or to receive some sort of medical treatment.

G. Intermittent services—Care that is provided on a part-time basis; that is, for a portion of hours in a day and for few days of the week; for example, home care services provided by a nurse for 2 hours per day and 3 days per week.

H. Nonskilled services—Health care services that are provided by a paraprofessional or an unlicensed person. Examples of these services may include close observation, bathing, feeding, and transferring from bed to chair.

I. Outcome and Assessment Information Set (OASIS)—A uniform and standardized set of home care services–related outcomes data used by the CMS to examine the quality of home care services received by Medicare beneficiaries. The set includes clinical, financial, and administrative outcome indicators and is used by home health agencies for quality improvement.

J. Reasonable services—Services provided based on a patient's medical condition; acuity and severity of the disease, and the course of treatment meets what is described in national guidelines or standards.

K. Skilled services—Health care services that require delivery by a licensed professional such as a registered nurse; social worker; and physical, occupational, or speech therapists. Examples of these services may include wound care, vital signs assessment and monitoring, patient and family education, Foley catheter care, psychosocial counseling, physical rehabilitation, and intravenous medications administration.

■ THE ROLE OF THE HOSPITAL-BASED INTERDISCIPLINARY TEAM

A. The primary care physician, in cooperation with consulting physicians, has responsibility for discharging a patient. All those involved in the patient's treatment plan, including the nursing staff, the case manager, and the home care agency employees, share in the responsibility and liability for providing appropriate post-hospital discharge care (Mullahy and Jensen, 2004).

B. Hospital-based interdisciplinary teams include physicians, nurses, social workers, care coordinators, physical therapists, occupational therapists, chaplains, nutritionists, and others.

C. Daily interdisciplinary care rounds provide a forum to discuss the medical, financial, spiritual, and psychosocial issues that will impact the post-hospital discharge plan.

D. The role of the hospital-based case managers, whether they are called discharge planners or care coordinators, is to assess patient and family resources for post-hospital discharge planning and to assist with linkage to the appropriate community-based providers who can provide services determined to be necessary by the interdisciplinary team.

E. Before considering home care services, the interdisciplinary team must know that the patient and family would appreciate and agree to a home care referral. The case manager can facilitate such discussion and follow up on the referral with the patient, family, and one or more home care agencies.

1. Many people are reluctant to allow strangers into their homes and some homes may be too small to accommodate patients, families, and home care professionals.
2. Other families may not be willing, or able, to participate in a plan of care which includes home care.

F. The case manager, in collaboration with members of the health care team, conducts an assessment of needs. This should include, in addition to the clinical/medical condition of the patient, an evaluation of insurance benefits and restrictions placed by the patient's health plan on the number of hours of care to be provided per day, number of visits per week, the types of services, and which vendors have contracts with particular payers for provision of home care services.

1. For example, to be eligible for Medicare reimbursement of home care services, the patient must:
   a. Be homebound;
   b. Require intermittent or part time care;
   c. Require skilled care/services;
   d. Be under the supervision of a physician;
   e. Receive services that are reasonable and necessary; and
   f. In addition, the agency to provide the services must be a CHHA.

G. In addition to the assessment of needs, the case manager must use the findings of the clinical evaluation of the patient to determine the type of services needed such as nursing, both at the professional and paraprofessional levels, rehabilitation therapies, and social work/services such as counseling. The case manager makes such decisions by applying knowledge of the operations of home care services, its related rules and regulations, and policies and procedures. The case manager also works closely with the interdisciplinary team on these assessments and in decision making about what is best for the patient and family.

H. Patients who are eligible for home care services and are known to benefit from these services may include:

1. Those who may be recovering from a stroke, orthopedic or cardiac surgeries, or injuries; or those learning to live with other neurological or cardiac disorders, diabetes, and other chronic health problems
2. A number of high-risk populations that require special attention, such as the frail elderly who live alone, those with limited cognitive or

physical function, the severely mentally ill, the chemically dependent, the homeless, and people living with HIV/AIDS or other types of debilitating, chronic, and complex illnesses.

    a. Individuals in these high-risk groups merit special attention in discharge planning because of specific vulnerabilities that may make them eligible for additional community support or that may preclude a safe home care post-hospital discharge plan.

I. The case manager, on behalf of the health care team, works closely with health care professionals and support staff external to the hospital in coordinating the patient's discharge plan and home care services. These may include the case manager of the managed care organization, representatives from home care agencies such as the home care intake coordinator, staff from transportation agencies and laboratory services, and representatives of durable medical equipment.

■ HOME CARE VISITS

A. Home care professionals can be invaluable to patients and families in making a home visit prior to scheduled admissions or prior to discharge from the hospital, especially in the case of emergency admissions, to anticipate minor changes in ordinary family routines. Such a visit could make all the difference especially in understanding the family preferences and the dynamics of the home environment.

    1. For example, the extension cord carelessly connecting a television set to the closest electrical outlet is known not to be safe; but for someone returning home from the hospital with decreased vision, balance, strength, or unsteady gait, it could become a mortal hazard.

    2. Home visits provide invaluable information about the way the family functions, the neighborhood supports, and barriers to home care success.

B. Information gathered can be communicated to the hospital interdisciplinary care teams during subsequent inpatient hospital stays so that future discharge plans can be structured in light of the specific reality of the particular patient in his or her own environment.

C. The number, type, length, and frequency of home care visits are determined based on the patient's medical condition and treatment regimen, capacity for self-care, complexity of the types of services required, and health plan or insurance benefits.

D. Home care visits may include the provision of professional and/or paraprofessional services.

    1. Professional services are skilled in nature and require the involvement of licensed professionals such as a registered nurse; social worker; or physical, occupational, and speech therapists.

    2. Paraprofessional services are not skilled and do not require the involvement of licensed professionals. These may include the care provided by a home health attendant, homemaker, or housekeeper.

■ REIMBURSEMENT FOR HOME CARE SERVICES

A. Reimbursements for home care services vary based on the health plan. Some follow the managed care reimbursement methods; others apply the Medicare or Medicaid payment systems.

B. Managed care reimbursement is dependent on the contractual agreement between the provider and the managed care organization.

   1. Home care services are provided to enrollees in a managed care plan by an agency that is a contracted service provider.

   2. Authorization for home care services is usually expected prior to the delivery of these services.

   3. Patients' and family members' choice of provider is limited to those agencies that have a contractual agreement with the managed care organization.

C. In 2000, reimbursement by CMS for home care services and visits provided to Medicare beneficiaries was changed to a PPS.

   1. More visits no longer means higher reimbursement rates.

   2. Unlike the inpatient or hospital-based PPS, reimbursement for home care visits is determined based on a nursing assessment that is completed at the time a patient is admitted into home care services.

   3. Reimbursement is no longer based on the number and type of visits. Home care services are currently reimbursed based on an episode of care or 60 days.

   4. The dollar amount reimbursed is fixed regardless of the number of visits provided. It is determined based on the OASIS score a patient receives.

   5. OASIS scores are determined based on three categories: clinical, financial, and service utilization.

   6. The OASIS score results in the assignment of the patient into one of 80 HHRGs. Each HHRG has a predetermined dollar amount attached to it.

D. A CHHA may submit claims to Medicare for reimbursement on two occasions.

   1. An initial claim or a request for advance payment—completed upon admission of a patient into home care services and completion of the initial assessment of the patient (i.e., performing an initial OASIS assessment and score). The amount is limited to a maximum of 60% of the HHRG-designated rate.

   2. A final claim or request for payment—completed at the end of an episode of services; includes all line-item home care visit information or types of services rendered during the customary 60 days of service.

E. Special payment rates by Medicare occur in five occasions:

   1. If there is an interruption of service due to a patient's request for transfer from one home health agency to another before the conclusion of the 60 days of service. In this case, a partial-episode payment is deemed appropriate.

2. If a patient is discharged from home care and then returns to the same agency within the 60-day period. In this case, a partial-episode payment is considered appropriate—but only if the discharge from or return to service was not related to a significant change in the patient's condition.

3. If the patient experiences a change in condition that results in change in medical orders and course of treatment and ultimately leads to a change in the OASIS score or the HHRG assignment. In this case, a significant change in condition payment is deemed appropriate.

4. If a patient requires a minimal number of home care visits (e.g., five visits or fewer) during the 60-day period due to low acuity and resource utilization. In this case, a low-utilization payment is considered appropriate and the reimbursement is calculated based on the national standard per visit per discipline amount.

5. When unusual variations occur in the amount of medically necessary home health services. In this case, an outlier payment is considered appropriate.

■ HOME CARE NURSING SERVICES

A. When appropriate, home care services can extend the care of the hospital-based interdisciplinary team beyond the hospital boundaries and reduce length of stay or provide an alternative to institution-based custodial and skilled care.

B. As an extension of hospital-based care, short-term home care services are reimbursable under Medicare benefits and many health plans offered by private insurance companies.

C. Medicare and most health plans offered by private insurance companies may not provide long-term care or custodial care benefits; therefore, these services will not be reimbursed.

D. Medicaid, however, reimburses for long-term care and custodial care and therefore in some areas will reimburse for these same services at home.

E. To be reimbursable, short-term home care services must be medically necessary and for a limited period of time.

1. Medicare requires that the condition of the patient present a need for skilled services of a registered nurse, social worker, or therapist. In addition, services may include those provided by a registered nutritionist or a paraprofessional nursing aide.

a. In some states such as New York these aides are licensed as home health aides and follow a treatment plan performing tasks assigned by a registered nurse.

b. Home health aides are trained to measure and report vital signs and assist patients with the activities of daily living to enable them to remain safely at home.

F. Long-term home care services may involve the same services as short-term home care; however, they also may involve transportation and use of a less-skilled paraprofessional personal care assistant.

1. In some states such as New York, these assistants are licensed as home attendants.
2. Personal care assistants are only permitted to assist with the activities of daily living that will enable the patient to remain safely at home.
3. Over time, the CMS has permitted various demonstration projects in long-term home care, called "nursing homes without walls." Examples are the PACE program which started in San Francisco and New York, and the Lombardi programs in New York.

G. The third type of home care services widely available in the United States is hospice care.
   1. Initially started by Dame Cicely Saunders when she opened St. Christopher's Hospital in London, the hospice movement spread to the United States as a volunteer nurses program humanely caring for dying patients at home in the 1960s and 1970s. Hospice became a standard of care when Congress adopted the Medicare reimbursement for home hospice services in 1983.
   2. Hospice care as determined by the Medicare regulations includes nursing, pastoral care, social work, and volunteer services.
   3. Hospice care also includes reimbursement for bereavement services, most often provided by social workers or volunteers, to the survivors (e.g., family members) for 13 months following the death of the patient.
   4. Hospice care allows inpatient care for symptom control or respite care relief for caregivers of the terminally ill individual. Inpatient care is at a length of stay determined by the hospice. Hospice care also covers services that are related to the terminal illness.

■ HOME CARE REHABILITATION SERVICES

A. Rehabilitation therapy in the home is provided by a licensed physical therapist, occupational therapist, or speech therapist.

B. The goal of rehabilitation therapy is to maximize the patient's level of functioning to improve quality of life.

C. Physical therapy includes therapeutic exercises, balance activities, and ambulation training that will help the patient regain functional mobility and motor skills.

D. Occupational therapists use motor, cognitive perceptual, and sensory exercises and tasks to help improve the patient's ability to perform activities of daily living.

E. Speech/language therapists help patients improve their ability to produce and understand speech as well as help with communication skills. They also assist with swallowing disorders.

F. Professional therapists increase the value of home care services by providing therapy in the home where the patient lives. They can assess the patient, teach safety precautions and techniques, and provide exercise routines that work in the patient's home.

G. Case managers must be aware of these services and their purposes so that they can best incorporate them into the plans of care for their patients.

H. Case managers are effective in discussing the patient's need for these services with members of the interdisciplinary health care team and in incorporating such services into the patient's plan of care.

I. Case managers in the home care setting also follow up on the outcomes of these services for their specific patients and revise the home care plan of care accordingly to meet the patient's specific needs.

■ DURABLE MEDICAL EQUIPMENT AND OTHER SERVICES

A. Many homes are not equipped to provide short-term or long-term patient care. Such situations warrant the use of durable medical equipment (DME) such as a hospital bed, wheelchair, glucometer, etc. Case managers facilitate the acquisition of equipment as needed by patients.

B. An important role for the hospital-based interdisciplinary team is to help the patient and family obtain the equipment and supplies they will need to ensure the success of home-based care.

C. DME, including hospital bed, walker, cane, portable oxygen, wheelchair, commode, tub chair, transfer bench, grab bars, oxygen canisters, and concentrators can be ordered and delivered to the patient's home prior to the patient's discharge from the hospital to ensure continuity of care and comfort when the patient arrives home. Sometimes the DME is delivered to the patient while in the hospital, at the time of discharge in order for the case manager to ensure a safe transition to home.

D. Supplies such as diapers, chucks, diabetic, wound and ostomy supplies, nebulizers, intravenous tubing, syringes, and even medications can be ordered prior to the patient's discharge for home delivery as a way to ensure continuity of care and comfort. This is especially true of newer medications, expensive medications, or less-often-used medications.

E. Case managers may alert patients and their families as well as the health care team that particular doses of pain medication or blood thinners, such as Lovenox, may not be available in all strengths at all pharmacies. In such situations, they negotiate the ordering of appropriate dosages or types of medications.

F. Case managers may educate patients and families and members of the health care teams about the variety of services provided in the varied patients' communities and provide them with lists of these services and contact information.

G. Case managers may teach patients not only about the choices available but also empower them to seek additional services and equipment as the patient's condition changes and new needs arise.

■ HOME CARE SOCIAL WORK SERVICES

A. Although hospital social workers are responsible for the completion of psychosocial assessments and the development of appropriate post-hospital discharge plans, many times in the current health care environment length of stay has shortened to the point that it is difficult to find time to educate patients and families about the range of social services available to them, let alone make appropriate referrals and have time to follow up.

B. Social workers who come to the patient's home in the context of home care services not only have additional time, they have additional important information about the patients' conditions including their home environment, social network, and caregivers. Such information is made available to them as they walk through the door, and most of the time is not as apparent to the hospital-based colleagues.

C. Home visiting social workers can assist the patient in completing the patient's portion of the referral processes and follow up. The fact that the patient is at home and has access to important documents and files facilitates this work.

D. Home visiting social workers also are able to assess why a particular referral may not have worked and assist the client in obtaining needed services through subsequent referrals.

E. Home care social workers can help families to identify strengths, overcome obstacles, and provide better care, which may result in improved outcomes for patients and their families.

F. As short-term home care services are about to be terminated, community-based social workers reassess patients and assist them, the interdisciplinary team, and family in developing the next plan of care. They may find it necessary to expand services or to adjust the type of services needed based on the patient's condition.

G. Plans of care may include transitioning the patient to long-term home care services, hospice services, or institutionalized care.

H. Adequate home care discharge plans not only prevent the need for hospital readmissions, but also can optimize the patients' quality of life by helping them and their families to transition easily to new care plans.

■ THE ROLE OF THE HOSPITAL-BASED CASE MANAGER

A. The role of the hospital-based case manager varies from hospital to hospital depending on the ways the hospital, the case management program directors, and the individual case managers have divided the work.

B. When the case manager or any member of the interdisciplinary team has identified a patient who would benefit from home care services, and the patient and family have agreed to a discharge plan that includes home care, the patient/family must be educated about the agencies that offer the services recommended by the team so that they can identify the preferred agency. Next, the case manager facilitates the referral and the service brokerage process.

C. The Balanced Budget Act of 1996 requires that all patients be provided with written information, such as a list of agencies providing services in their area. The case manager may:
   1. Make the list available to patients

2. Use the list to educate patients and their families about the role of the insurance company/health plan in authorizing and managing the home care services

3. Inform patients of the procedures applied by managed care organizations in securing home care services, such as the use of preferred contracts and limits on the number of visits per calendar year

D. When a home care agency has been selected and permission for the release of medical information has been obtained, it is important for the case manager to consult with the indicated home care provider to confirm that the agency has a contract with the insurer and to discover whether the requested services are available through the agency.

E. In these times of growing shortages of professional nurses and therapists, case managers not only must check to see whether services are offered by the selected agency, but also need to clarify that the agency has adequate personnel to deliver the needed services in a timely fashion.

F. Rehabilitation therapies following joint replacement, laboratory tests for coumadin levels, and patient education about new medications or reinforcement of hospital-based diabetic education are three examples of services that must be delivered in a timely fashion; otherwise serious complications in the patient's health condition may occur, which in turn may warrant the patient's return to the hospital setting.

G. The case manager can facilitate the communication between the patient, family members, and the home care agency. This communication is essential so that the patient and family know what is expected of them and the agency knows what the family expects.

H. It is also important for the case manager to ask the agency and the insurer whether the patient is responsible for any costs associated with home care services and promptly relay the information to the patient and the family.

I. It is also important to review with patients what home care is *not* about. Go over their expectations.

1. One type of cost is insurance policy deductible. If, for example, patients have Medicare benefits and have been hospitalized under the Medicare benefits, they will have already met their Medicare deductible.

2. However, if a patient is hospitalized under the insurance policy of a spouse but the insurance company has refused to authorize home care services, then the astute case manager would use the patient's Medicare benefit.

3. Many private insurance policies utilize per visit co-payments to discourage overuse of benefits. This strategy to reduce home care costs has been suggested but not approved for Medicare at this time.

J. The case manager should communicate with the community doctor responsible for the patient's follow-up and be sure that the community doctor is in agreement with the plan of care developed by the hospital-based interdisciplinary team, the patient, the family, and the home care agency.

K. The handoff of information is not only a courtesy but also provides continuity of care for the patient and provides the agency with ongoing physician orders for medical treatment that allows for a safe transition of care for the patient.

■ THE ROLE OF THE COMMUNITY-BASED CASE MANAGER

A. Community-based case management programs have evolved in response to changes in the health care delivery system and to mainly meet the needs of the disabled and noninstitutionalized elderly.

B. Community-based case management is intended to improve the lives of high-risk patients through outreach, screening, and risk-reduction programs.

C. The main purposes of community-based case management programs are care planning, continuity of care and services, and follow-up care.

D. Home care–based nurses and social workers work closely with community-based case managers who monitor the patient's medical and psychosocial progress, referrals, and interventions.

E. No one profession can be responsible to provide all the services. Both social workers and nurses have different professional skills and talents. When working collaboratively, each brings a unique perspective within his/her discipline and then reaches across to improve patient care—"when the focus is on the client and not on professional self-image, the combination of the two worlds is dynamite" (Hawkins, Veeder, & Pearce, 1998, p. 44).

■ CONCLUSION: SAVINGS, SAFETY, AND SATISFACTION

A. Home care can provide savings to the health care system in two ways:
1. By reducing the length of stay in the acute inpatient settings
2. By reducing the length of stay in custodial or other institutional inpatient settings such as skilled nursing facilities

B. As private and public insurance and institutional costs are controlled it should never be forgotten that these reductions are possible not by eliminating costs but by shifting the burden of care from the health care system to the family.

C. Most families are ready, willing, and able to shoulder this burden but case managers must never take their contribution for granted.

D. The most important issue of home care today is patient safety.
1. When people have spent time in the acute care hospital setting, the inpatient acute rehabilitation unit, or the skilled nursing facility, they have been cared for by professional and paraprofessional staff around the clock. During such times, they develop, even after a short while, a type of dependency on the health care professional.

2. No matter what pressures might exist to reduce patient stay and no matter how much patients may wish to return to the home setting, the only successful home care plan is a safe plan.

3. Individuals who cannot ambulate, readily speak or understand the speech of others, or are demented, cannot be safely left alone. If family members are not ready, willing, and able to stay with these individuals 24 hours a day, 7 days a week (or hire help), they cannot be safely discharged home.

E. Most patients are safer in their own homes surrounded by the loving care of their family and friends than in unfamiliar institutional settings.

F. If the patient, the family, the community physician, home care agency, and the interdisciplinary team have communicated effectively and developed a safe plan there can be no more satisfying plan than home care.

G. Home care may reduce the risk of nosocomial illnesses—illnesses developed from a hospital-born infection (Mullahy and Jensen, 2004).

H. Home care encourages greater independence and promotes recovery by allowing patients to resume some parts of their ordinary life before they are completely healed.

I. Home care also encourages loving care by family and friends rather than limiting care to visiting hours.

J. Home care can help reduce Medicare and Medicaid expenditures by caring for people in their homes and by reducing the number of far more costly days in skilled nursing facilities or hospitals.

REFERENCES

Hawkins, J., Veeder, N., & Pearce, C. (1998). *Nurse social work collaboration in managed care: A model of community case management.* New York: Springer.

Mullahy, C., & Jensen, D. (2004). *The case manager's handbook,* 3rd edition. Sudbury, MA: Jones and Bartlett.

SUGGESTED READING

American Geriatrics Society. (2000). *Care management position statement.* NewYork, NY.

Birmingham, J. (2004). Discharge planning: A collaboration between provider and payer case manager's using Medicare's conditions of participation. *Lippincott's Case Management, 9*(3):147–151.

Lane, N. Senate Fiscal Year (SFY) (2005–06). Executive Budget Joint Budget Hearing: New York State Office for the Aging.

Watt, H. (2001). Community-based case management: A model for outcome-based research for non-institutional elderly. *Home Health Care Services Quarterly, 20*(1):39–65.

chapter

6

Case Management in the Long-Term Care and Rehabilitation Settings

Linda N. Schoenbeck
Hussein A. Tahan
Suzanne K. Powell

LEARNING OBJECTIVES

Upon completion of this chapter, the reader will be able to:

1. Identify levels of care available for the elderly person, including rehabilitation, skilled nursing facility, long-term care, and non-medical levels of care.
2. Determine criteria for placement of the elderly in various levels of care.
3. Distinguish between custodial care, assisted living, and "aging in place."
4. Identify the nonmedical care settings or options, especially those available for the elderly patient.
5. Describe the use of respite care.
6. Determine critical questions to ask when completing a financial assessment.
7. Describe the role of the case manager in rehabilitation and long-term care settings.

IMPORTANT TERMS AND CONCEPTS

Activities of Daily Living (ADLs)	Long-Term Care Insurance
Aging in Place	Occupational Therapy (OT)
Assisted Living	Reasonable and Necessary Care
Comprehensive Outpatient Rehabilitation Facility (CORF)	Personal Care Services
	Physical Therapy (PT)
Custodial Care	Rehabilitation
Inpatient Rehabilitation Facility (IRF)	Respite Care
Instrumental Activities of Daily Living (IADLs)	Restorative Nursing Services (NRS)
	Skilled Nursing Care
Limitation of Activity	Skilled Nursing Facility (SNF)
Long-Term Care	Speech and Language Pathology (SLP)

■ INTRODUCTION

A. This chapter discusses post-acute levels of care, from acute rehabilitation hospitals, to nursing homes, to "aging in place" (Fig. 6-1).

B. Most of the frail elderly in the United States require at some point or another long-term care or rehabilitation services in acute or sub-acute care facilities. This is mostly due to deconditioning post-acute care hospitalization.

C. Today's elderly patients who seek health care services encounter a variety of providers and organizations, including primary care physicians, specialists, acute care hospitals, skilled nursing facilities (SNFs), nursing homes, rehabilitation facilities, and home health care.

D. Assessment for placement of the client/patient in a specific level of care should:
   1. Yield the *least* restrictive level of care possible for safe care;
   2. Be financially feasible and sustainable for the patient/client/family;
   3. Meet the conditions stipulated in either laws and regulations or insurance policies; and
   4. Ensure a reimbursable episode of care.

E. Health insurance plans usually pay for "medically reasonable and necessary" care. However, each insurance company has its own rules and definitions of "medical necessity" and "skilled" versus "unskilled" services that play an integral role in deciding whether to reimburse for care or not.

F. The prospective payment system (PPS) has resulted in patients' early discharge from the acute care/hospital setting. This has increased the need for follow-up care in settings such as the home, but most commonly in the long-term care and rehabilitation settings.

G. As integrated care delivery systems have become more common, new approaches to care, especially for the elderly, disabled, or functionally impaired, have been created. A common approach is sub-acute care,

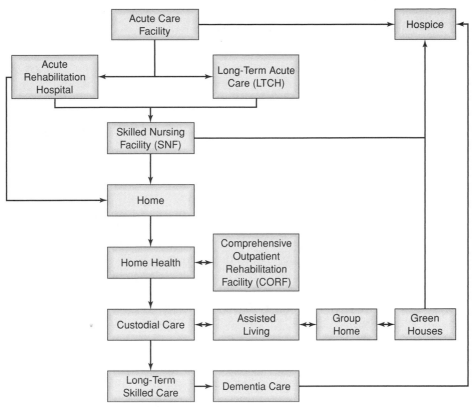

FIGURE 6–1   Post-acute levels of care.

which is a level of care that blends acute and long-term care skills and philosophies (Carr, 2000).

H. Recent changes in health care delivery systems have resulted in an increased demand for case management and the role of the case manager in settings beyond the acute care/hospital; i.e., long-term care and rehabilitation.

I. Care of the elderly requires the services of a multidisciplinary team of health care professionals including geriatricians, nurses, social workers, dieticians, physical therapists, occupational therapists, speech and language therapists, and pharmacists, but especially case managers.

J. To ensure effective care of the elderly, the multidisciplinary team must focus on the following:
   1. Functional and medical assessments to develop a full understanding of the elderly patient's needs
   2. Physical and mental status examination
   3. Balance and gait test
   4. Dietary assessment
   5. Psychosocial history and support system

    6. Home safety

    7. Battery of laboratory and x-ray (radiologic) tests as necessary

    8. Other tests as indicated by the elderly patient's condition

K. Care for the aged, chronically sick, and mentally ill has been affected by specific milestones in laws and regulations in the United States.

    1. Almshouses: institutions to house the poor, aged, and mentally ill; regulation in 1873.

    2. County homes: result of regulation; historically, terrible conditions for the older adult.

    3. 1935—Social Security Act: provided catalyst for privately funded institutions for the aged.

    4. 1965—Medicare and Medicaid reimbursement: allowed expansion of this industry.

    5. 1965—Older Americans Act: created primary vehicle for organizing, coordinating, and providing community-based services and opportunities for older Americans and their families.

    6. Office of Nursing Home Affairs of 1971 and Nursing Reform Act of 1987: established minimum requirements for nursing assistants, created a resident rights statement, and implemented a single standard for 24-hour care for all residents in nursing homes.

■ KEY DEFINITIONS

A. Activities of daily living (ADLs)—Activities related to personal care and include bathing or showering, dressing, getting in or out of bed or a chair, using the toilet, and eating. If a person has any difficulty performing an activity by himself or herself and without special equipment, or did not perform the activity at all because of health problems (physical, mental, or emotional), the person is categorized as having a limitation in that activity. The limitation may be temporary or chronic.

B. Aging in place—Process by which a person chooses to remain in his or her living environment (home) and to remain as independent as possible despite the physical or mental decline.

C. Assisted living—A type of living arrangement in which personal care services such as meals, housekeeping, transportation, and assistance with activities of daily living are available as needed to people who still live on their own in a residential facility. In most cases, the assisted living residents pay a regular monthly rent and an additional fee for the services they receive.

D. Comprehensive outpatient rehabilitation facility (CORF)—A facility that provides coordinated outpatient diagnostic, therapeutic, and restorative services, at a single fixed location, to outpatients for the rehabilitation of injured, disabled, or sick individuals.

E. Continuing care retirement community (CCRC)—A housing community that provides different levels of care based on what each resident needs over time. This is sometimes called *life care* and can range from independent living in an apartment, to assisted living, to full-time care in a nursing home. Residents move from one setting to another based on their needs but continue to live as part of the community. Care in CCRCs is usually expensive. Generally, CCRCs require a large payment before an individual moves in, and then a certain monthly fee.

F. Custodial care—The provision of services that can be safely and reasonably given by individuals who are neither skilled nor licensed medical personnel. These may include personal care, such as help with activities of daily living (bathing, dressing, eating, getting in or out of a bed or chair, moving around, and toileting). It may also include care that most people do themselves, like administering eye drops. In most cases, Medicare does not pay for custodial care.

G. Custodial care facility—A facility that provides room, board, and other personal assistance services, generally on a long-term basis, which does not include a medical component.

H. Independent living—A service delivery concept that encourages the maintenance of control over one's life based on the choice of acceptable options that minimize reliance on others performing everyday activities.

I. Inpatient rehabilitation facility (IRF)—A free-standing rehabilitation hospital or rehabilitation unit(s) in an acute care hospital that provides intensive rehabilitation programs; patients who are admitted to such facilities must be able to tolerate 3 hours of intense rehabilitation services per day.

J. Instrumental activities of daily living (IADLs)—Activities related to independent living, including preparing meals, managing money, shopping for groceries or personal items, performing light or heavy housework, and using a telephone. If a person has any difficulty performing an activity by himself or herself and without special equipment, or does not perform the activity at all because of health problems, the person is categorized as having a limitation in that activity. The limitation may be temporary or chronic.

K. Limitation of activity—Refers to a long-term reduction in a person's capacity to perform the usual kind or amount of activities associated with his or her age group due to a chronic condition. This may include a limitation in activities of daily living, instrumental activities of daily living, play, school, work, difficulty in walking or remembering, or any other.

L. Long-term care—A variety of services that help people with health or personal needs and activities of daily living over a period of time. Long-term care can be provided at home, in the community, or in various types of facilities, including nursing homes and assisted living facilities. Most long-term care is custodial care, which few (if any) insurance companies will pay for if skilled care is also not required.

M. Long-term care insurance—A private insurance policy to help pay for some long-term medical and nonmedical care. Some long-term care insurance policies offer tax benefits; these are called *tax-qualified policies.*

N. Non-covered services—These services are not considered skilled and do not meet the requirements of a Medicare benefit category, are statutorily excluded from coverage on grounds other than 1862(a)(1), or are not considered reasonable and necessary under 1862(a)(1).

O. Nursing facility—See skilled nursing facility (SNF).

P. Nursing home—A residence that provides individuals with a room and meals, and assists with activities of daily living and recreation. Generally, nursing home residents have physical or mental problems that keep them from living on their own. They usually require daily assistance.

Q. Occupational therapy (OT)—Structured activity focused on activities of daily living skills (feeding, dressing, bathing, grooming), arm flexibility and strengthening, neck control and posture, perceptual and cognitive skills, and using adaptive equipment to facilitate activities of daily living.

R. Outpatient care—Medical or surgical care that is provided in a clinic/ambulatory setting and does not include an overnight hospital stay.

S. Personal care services—Nonskilled assistance (bathing, dressing, light housework) provided to individuals in their homes.

T. Physical therapy (PT)—Structured activity focused on mobility skills (bed and chair transfers, wheelchair use, walking), leg flexibility and strengthening, trunk or gait control and balance, endurance training, and use of adaptive equipment to facilitate mobility and physical functioning.

U. Reasonable and necessary care—Health care or services that are required by Medicare recipients and that is considered important for their medical condition. The Medicare program generally covers only items or services that are "reasonable and necessary" for the diagnosis or treatment of illness or injury, or "to improve the functioning of a malformed body member." This "reasonable and necessary" language is the basis for most Medicare coverage policies, but its meaning remains ill defined and controversial.

V. Rehabilitation—A restorative process through which an individual with a complex, chronic, or terminal illness develops and maintains self-sufficient functioning consistent with his/her capability. Usually provided by licensed health care professionals such as nurses and physical, occupational, and speech therapists.

W. Respite care—Temporary or periodic care provided in a nursing home, assisted living residence, or other type of long-term care program so that the usual caregiver can rest or take some time off.

X. Restorative nursing services (NRS)—Replication of activities initiated by a physical therapist (PT), occupational therapist (OT), or a speech-language pathologist (SLP) and then performed and maintained by the nursing staff. These may include services such as range of motion exercises, dressing, personal hygiene, walking, and feeding.

Y. Skilled care—The provision of services that can be given only by or under the supervision of skilled and licensed medical personnel/health care professionals; that is, skilled and competent staff such as registered nurses; social workers; physical, occupational, and speech therapists; rehabilitation counselors; and registered dietitians/nutritionists. These staff are required to manage, observe, and evaluate the skilled care activities.

Z. Skilled nursing care—A level of care that includes services that can only be performed safely and correctly by a licensed nurse (either a registered nurse or a licensed practical nurse).

AA. Skilled nursing facility (SNF)—A facility (which meets specific regulatory certification requirements) that primarily provides inpatient skilled nursing care and related services to patients who require medical, nursing, or rehabilitative services but does not provide the level of care or treatment available in a hospital.

BB. Skilled nursing facility care—A level of care that requires the daily involvement of skilled nursing or rehabilitation staff. Examples of skilled nursing facility care include intravenous injections, wound care, and physical therapy. The need for custodial care (for example, assistance with activities of daily living, like bathing and dressing) cannot, in itself, qualify for Medicare coverage in a skilled nursing facility.

CC. SNF Co-insurance—For day 21 through 100 of extended care services in a benefit period, a daily amount for which the beneficiary is responsible, equal to one-eighth of the inpatient hospital deductible.

DD. Speech and language pathology (SLP)—Structured activity focused on communication skills, perceptual and cognitive skills, and swallowing.

■ LONG-TERM CARE

A. Long-term care is necessary when individuals require someone else to help them with their physical and/or emotional needs. This help may be required for many of the activities or needs healthy and active people take for granted.

B. Long-term care and assistance may be necessary as a result of a terminal condition, disability, illness, injury, or merely old age.

C. The need for long-term care may last for a few weeks, months, or years. The length of time needed depends on the underlying reasons and medical/health condition.

D. Long-term care may take the form of temporary or ongoing care.
   1. Temporary long-term care—Need for care for a limited period of time, usually for only a few weeks or months. This may take place to address the following conditions:
      a. Rehabilitation from a hospital stay

      b. Recovery from illness

      c. Recovery from injury

      d. Recovery from surgery

      e. Terminal medical condition

   2. Ongoing long-term care—Need for care for an extended period of time, usually many months or years. This may take place to address the following conditions:

      a. Chronic medical illness

      b. Chronic severe pain

      c. Permanent disability

      d. Dementia

      e. Ongoing need for help with ADLs

      f. Need for supervision

E. Long-term services are provided in varied care settings such as:

   1. Home (either the patient's or that of a family member)

   2. Adult day care center

   3. Assisted living facility

   4. Board-and-care home

   5. Hospice facility

   6. Nursing home

F. Case management in the home care setting is discussed in Chapter 5 and case management in the palliative care and hospice settings is discussed in Chapter 7. Other settings are discussed in this chapter.

G. Health care services provided in the long-term care settings are of two types: custodial and skilled (Day, 2006).

   1. Custodial services

      a. The provision of services that can be safely and reasonably given by individuals who are neither skilled nor licensed medical personnel.

      b. Services may include personal care such as help with ADLs (bathing, dressing, eating, getting in or out of a bed or chair, moving around, and toileting). It may also include care that most people do themselves, like administering eye drops.

      c. In most cases, Medicare does not pay for custodial care, unless it is provided in combination with skilled services and as part of a skilled plan of care.

      d. Custodial care may include any or all of the following:

         i. Walking

         ii. Bathing, personal hygiene, and grooming

         iii. Dressing

         iv. Feeding and providing meals

         v. Toileting and helping with incontinence

         vi. Managing pain

      vii. Preventing unsafe behavior such as wandering around aimlessly

     viii. Providing comfort and assurance

      ix. Providing physical or occupational therapy

       x. Attending to medical needs

      xi. Counseling

     xii. Answering the phone

    xiii. Meeting doctors' appointments

    xiv. Maintaining the household

     xv. Shopping and running errands

    xvi. Providing transportation

   xvii. Administering medications

  xviii. Managing money

    xix. Paying bills

     xx. Doing the laundry

    xxi. Writing letters or notes

   xxii. Maintaining a yard

  xxiii. Removing snow

e. The individual who requires custodial services is someone who:
   i. Can no longer perform daily tasks necessary to maintain health and safety
   ii. Cannot safely perform ADLs or preserve health from further decline
   iii. By choice or circumstance has decided to reside in the nursing home as primary residence
   iv. Receives nonskilled physical therapy services (restorative nursing by nursing assistants) to maintain function

2. Skilled services
   a. The provision of services that can be given only by or under the supervision of skilled and licensed medical personnel/health care professionals; that is, skilled and competent staff such as registered nurses, social workers, physical, occupational, and speech therapists, rehabilitation counselors, and registered dietitians/nutritionists.
   b. Members of the professional staff are required to manage, observe, supervise, and evaluate the skilled care activities.
   c. Skilled care activities may include the following:
      i. Monitoring vital signs
      ii. Ordering medical tests
      iii. Diagnosing problems
      iv. Administering intravenous medications
      v. Administering intravenous fluids/nutritional support
      vi. Dispensing medications, including injections
      vii. Drawing blood

        viii. Wound care and dressing changes

        ix. Psychosocial counseling and therapy

        x. Physical therapy and exercise

        xi. Occupational therapy

        xii. Speech therapy

    d. The individual who requires skilled services is someone who:

        i. May have exhausted Medicare Part A benefit period or is not eligible for benefits

        ii. Can no longer care for himself or herself

        iii. Requires assistance in ADLs, IADLs, taking medication, or skilled treatments

H. Skilled and custodial services do not refer to a specific type of long-term care services; rather, they are referred to based on the people who deliver/provide the care—not the actual care given. The main differentiating factor between these two terms is the employment of 1) skilled versus nonskilled, and 2) licensed versus unlicensed providers (Day, 2006).

I. Generally, skilled care is available only for a short period of time after a hospitalization. Custodial care is for a much longer period of time. Sometimes both levels of care are provided in the same facility (e.g., nursing home) and the patients (usually called *residents*) may transfer between levels of care within the facility without having to move from one room or unit into another.

J. A skilled and licensed care provider can provide custodial services; however, a nonskilled and unlicensed provider cannot provide skilled services. In rare situations, skilled services such as blood pressure monitoring, administering medications, or changing wound dressings may be given by a custodial care provider.

K. A long-term care treatment plan usually includes skilled and custodial services (care activities), goals, and expected outcomes. It addresses the following:

    1. Applied therapies

    2. Frequency of the therapies consistent with goals and expected outcomes

    3. Potential for patient's restoration and prognosis

    4. Time frame in which the physician/provider prescribing the treatment will review the plan and evaluate medical necessity and progress

    5. Maintenance, palliative relief, or measures to be implemented to prevent deterioration in the patient's status

L. Medicare pays for skilled care. Custodial care is covered under Medicare if it is provided in a skilled care setting and under a skilled plan of care.

M. Medicare and other health insurance plans pay for the care of patients with certain acute medical needs where recovery is anticipated. Patients with chronic medical problems are usually covered under Medicaid.

■ REHABILITATION LEVELS OF CARE (TABLE 6-1)

A. Rehabilitation is "the restoration of the handicapped [individuals] to the fullest physical, mental, social, vocational, and economic usefulness of which they are capable" (Wright, 1983, p. 3).

B. The Commission on Accreditation of Rehabilitation Facilities (CARF) defines rehabilitation as, "the process of providing, in a coordinated manner, those comprehensive services deemed appropriate to the needs of a person with a disability in a program designed to achieve objectives of improved health, welfare and the realization of the person's maximal physical, social, psychological and vocational potential for useful and productive activity" (CARF, 1991, p. 138).

C. Rehabilitation services are provided in many different settings, including the following:
   1. Acute care and rehabilitation hospitals
   2. Sub-acute facilities
   3. Intermediate rehabilitation facilities (IRFs)
   4. Long-term care facilities
   5. Comprehensive outpatient rehabilitation facilities (CORFs)
   6. Day rehabilitation services (DRSs)
   7. Home rehabilitation through home health agencies

D. Regardless of setting, rehabilitation services are provided through a multidisciplinary rehabilitation team that revolves around the patient and family. The team helps set short- and long-term treatment goals for recovery and is made up of many skilled professionals, including the following:
   1. Physicians such as a physiatrist—a physician who specializes in physical medicine and rehabilitation
   2. An internist or a specialist physician depending on the medical condition of the patient (e.g., a neurologist, in the case of a stroke patient)
   3. Rehabilitation nurses
   4. Physical therapists
   5. Occupational therapists
   6. Speech and language pathologists
   7. Dietitians
   8. Social workers
   9. Chaplains
   10. Psychologists, neuropsychologists, and psychiatrists
   11. Case managers

E. There are two fundamental requirements (criteria) for insurance coverage that must be met for inpatient hospital stays for rehabilitation care (CMS Medicare Benefit Policy Manual, 2003). The care/services must be:
   1. Reasonable and necessary (in terms of efficacy, duration, frequency, and amount) for the treatment of the patient's condition; and

TABLE 6-1

Summary of Rehabilitation Options and Criteria

Type of Rehab Services	Hours/Day Services Needed	Days/Week Services Needed	Approval Criteria	Funding Services	Target Turnaround Time
Acute Care Rehab	0.5/1.5	5–7	New or exacerbated disability	Billed as part of acute hospital stay	12 hr
Outpatient Rehab	0.5–2	3	Acute disability At home, but can be transported Ability to progress	Precertification Medicare Part B cap $1,500/yr Charges $75–$100/hr	24 hr
Day Rehab	3	5	Acute disability that does not prevent return home Medically stable Participate in therapy 1 hr 2× day Ability to progress Home support available	Precertification except for Medicare Charges $400–$600/day	12 hr
Home Health Rehab	0.5–1	3	Homebound Acute disability Medically stable Ability to progress	Precertification Cap on total visits Charges $75–$150/hr	48 hr
Inpatient Rehab	3	5–7	Acute disability prevents return home Medically stable Participate in therapy 1 hr 2× day Ability to progress Home support available	Precertification Coverage varies Charges $50–$1500/day	24 hr
Skilled Nursing Facility (SNF)	0.5–2	5–7	Acute disability Medically stable Participate in therapy 1 hr 2× day	Precertification Coverage varies Charges $120–$750/day	48 hr

Source: www.rrc.pmr.vcu.edu/misc/guide_to.htm (Virginia Commonwealth University, The Rehabilitation & Research Center).

    2. Reasonable and necessary to furnish the care on an inpatient hospital basis, rather than in a less-intensive facility such as an SNF, or on an outpatient basis (Carr, 2005).

F. Determinations of whether inpatient rehabilitation hospital stays are reasonable and necessary are made through a preadmission screening process. These determinations are based on an assessment of each beneficiary's individual care needs. The screening involves a preliminary review of the patient's condition, medical record(s), and health history to determine if the patient is likely to benefit significantly from an intensive inpatient rehabilitation program (Carr, 2005).

G. Rehabilitation may occur in specialized centers that:
    1. Are dedicated to the provision of such services
    2. Are staffed by the full gamut of rehabilitation professionals
    3. Include 24-hour physician coverage
    4. Develop an individualized program of intense rehabilitation that usually involves a minimum of 3 hours of therapy per day
    5. Include a team of professionals that meets at least once a week to evaluate the patient's progress and to amend the care plan

H. The main goal of rehabilitation:
    1. A reduction in or reversal of impairment, disability, or handicap caused by disease, enabling individuals (patients) to achieve their fullest possible physical, mental, and social capability.

I. The range of goals varies according to the individual. Different goals and prognoses place patients into different levels of rehabilitation.
    1. Full activity after a severe illness
    2. Maximum achievable activity after a damaging illness
    3. As much independence as possible when continuing impairment is unavoidable

J. The process of rehabilitation includes full patient and family assessment, goal setting, action planning and implementation, and evaluation/feedback.

K. Rehabilitation care and services are designed to meet each person's specific needs; thus, each program is different. Some general treatment components for rehabilitation programs include the following:
    1. Treating the basic disease and preventing complications
    2. Treating the disability and improving function
    3. Providing adaptive tools and altering the environment
    4. Teaching the patient and family and helping them adapt to lifestyle changes as caused by the disease and limitation in functioning

L. The success of rehabilitation treatments depend on many variables, including the following:
    1. The cause, location, and severity of physical functioning
    2. The type and degree of any impairments and disabilities from the medical condition

3. The overall health of the patient
4. Family and community support
5. The multidisciplinary health care team

M. Rehabilitation services in a hospital/acute care setting (i.e., inpatient rehabilitation) is:

1. Considered to be reasonable and necessary for a patient who requires a more coordinated, intensive program of multiple services than is generally found outside of a hospital.
2. Appropriate for patients who have either one or more conditions requiring intensive and multidisciplinary rehabilitation services, or a medical complication/comorbidity in addition to their primary condition, so that the continuing availability of a physician is required to ensure safe and effective treatment (Carr, 2005).
3. Necessary if an individual requires and is able to tolerate an intensive level of rehabilitation; that is, at least 3 hours per day, 5 to 7 days per week, and of at least two different types of therapy and interdisciplinary services.

N. Areas of treatment targeted in rehabilitation programs may include the following:

1. Self-care skills—ADLs such as feeding, grooming, bathing, dressing, and toileting
2. Mobility skills—Walking, transferring from bed to chair and vice versa, and self-propelling a wheelchair
3. Communication skills—Speech, writing, and alternative methods of communication
4. Cognitive skills—Memory, concentration, judgment, problem solving, and organizational skills
5. Socialization skills—Interacting with others at home and within the community
6. Vocational training—Work-related skills
7. Pain management—Medicines and alternative methods of managing pain
8. Psychological testing—Identifying problems and solutions with thinking, behavioral, and emotional issues
9. Family support—Assistance with adapting to lifestyle changes, physical limitations, financial concerns, and discharge planning
10. Education—Patient and family education and training about coping with illness (e.g., coping with stroke, amputation), medical care, and adaptive techniques

O. Any acutely hospitalized individual who has a new disability (or an exacerbation of an existing one) is often an appropriate candidate for acute rehabilitation services.

P. Individuals who meet the following criteria are appropriate for inpatient rehabilitation:

1. Have an acute disability that prevents them from returning home with family care

2. Have medical or surgical conditions that are sufficiently stable to allow participation in therapies
3. Have the ability to participate in at least 1 hour of therapy two times a day
4. Are able to make progress in acute care therapies
5. Have a social support system that will allow them to return home after reasonable improvement of function
6. Receive financial clearance from their insurer

Q. Most insurers will pay for acute care therapy-based rehabilitation.

R. The Centers for Medicare and Medicaid Services (CMS) has identified the specific evidence-based criteria to be used when evaluating potential candidates for placement in the inpatient rehabilitation setting (Table 6-2) (Carr, 2005).

■ REHABILITATION SERVICES IN VARIOUS SETTINGS

A. Intermediate rehabilitation facilities (IRFs)
1. IRFs are free-standing rehabilitation hospitals or rehabilitation unit(s) within acute care hospitals.
2. IRFs provide an intensive rehabilitation program. Patients who are admitted to these facilities must be able to tolerate 3 hours of intense rehabilitation services per day, 5 to 7 days per week.
3. IRFs are exempt from the Medicare Hospital PPS and are paid under the IRF PPS that went into effect on 1/1/2002. However, CMS collects patient assessment data only on Medicare Part A fee-for-service patients who are cared for in these facilities.
4. In order to be paid under the IRF PPS structure, such facilities must submit specific data based on the IRF patient assessment instrument (PAI).

B. Comprehensive outpatient rehabilitation facilities (CORFs)
1. CORFs are highly specialized outpatient facilities that provide services to individuals who require complex rehabilitative services.
2. CORFs provide coordinated outpatient diagnostic, therapeutic, and restorative services, at a single fixed location. These services are geared toward rehabilitation of injured, disabled, or sick individuals.
3. CORFs are designed to deliver physical therapy, occupational therapy, and speech-language pathology services. Other services available in these facilities may include:
    a. Prosthetic and orthotic devices, including testing, fitting, or proper training in the use of such devices.
    b. Supplies, appliances, and equipment, including the purchase or rental of durable medical equipment (DME).
4. CORFs tend to care for the mobile, more active patient.
5. Individuals who meet the following criteria are appropriate for outpatient rehabilitation in a CORF facility:
    a. Having an acute disability or physical complaint (e.g., back pain),
    b. Having a medical or surgical condition that allows the individual to return home and be transported to and from therapy,

TABLE 6–2
Rehabilitation Hospital Screening Criteria

Criteria	Explanation
1. Close medical supervision by a physician with specialized training or experience in rehabilitation	• A patient's condition must require the 24-hr availability of a physician with special training or experience in the field of rehabilitation. The medical record should reflect frequent, direct, and medically necessary physician involvement in the patient's care, that is, at least every day for moderately stable patients to every 2 to 3 days for stable patients throughout the patient's stay (CMS Medicare Benefit Policy Manual, 2003).
2. Twenty-four-hour rehabilitation nursing	• The patient requires the 24-hr availability of a registered nurse with specialized training or experience in rehabilitation. This degree of availability represents a higher level of care than is normally found in a skilled nursing facility (SNF) patient (CMS Medicare Benefit Policy Manual, 2003).
3. Relatively intense level of rehabilitation services	• The general threshold of establishing the need for inpatient rehabilitation facility (IRF) services is that the patient must require and receive at least 3 hr a day of physical and/or occupational therapy. In some cases the 3 hr a day requirement can be met by a combination of therapeutic services instead of, or in addition to, physical therapy and/or occupational therapy. Furnishing services no less than 5 days a week satisfies the requirement for "daily" services (CMS Medicare Benefit Policy Manual, 2003).
4. Multidisciplinary team approach to delivery of program	• A multidisciplinary team usually includes a physician, a rehabilitation nurse, a social worker, and/or a psychologist, and those therapists involved in the patient's care, that is, speech—language pathologist, recreation therapist (CMS Medicare Benefit Policy Manual, 2003).
5. Coordinated program of care	• The patient's records must reflect evidence of a coordinated program, that is, documentation that periodic team conferences are held at least every 2 weeks to • assess the individual's progress or the problems impeding progress; • consider possible resolutions to such problems; and • reassess the validity of the rehabilitation goals initially established. A team conference may be formal or informal. The decisions made during such conferences, and any changes to the care plan and/or treatment goals, and/or discharge planning must be recorded in the clinical record (CMS Medicare Benefit Policy Manual, 2003).
6. Significant practical improvement	• Hospitalization is covered only in those cases where a significant practical improvement can be expected in a reasonable period of time. The expectation of improvement must be of practical value to the patient, measured against the patient's condition at the start of the rehabilitation program (CMS Medicare Benefit Policy Manual, 2003).
7. Realistic goals	• The most realistic rehabilitation goal for most beneficiaries is self-care or independence in the activities of daily living, or sufficient improvement to allow the individual to live at home with assistance, rather than in an institution. The aim of treatment is to achieve the maximum level of function possible (CMS Medicare Benefit Policy Manual, 2003).

Note. From "The Case Manager's Role in Optimizing Acute Rehabilitation Services," by D.D. Carr, 2005, *Lippincott's Case Management, 10*(4), pp. 190–200. (Reprinted with permission. Carr, 2005.)

      c. Ability to participate in therapy and to demonstrate progress toward agreed-upon goals, and

      d. Acceptance of fiscal responsibility by the insurer and/or patient.

  6. Individuals who are not homebound must receive this type of therapy after hospital discharge.

  7. Most insurers provide for outpatient therapy services; however precertification is usually required and there are specific limits on the duration of services.

  8. Medicare Part B has a $1,500 per year cap on outpatient PT/OT services. Charges are typically $75 per hour to $150 per hour.

C. Day rehabilitation services (DRSs)

  1. Patients must be able to participate in at least a 3-hour rehabilitation program per day, 5 days per week, and use at least two different types of therapy.

  2. Interdisciplinary services are performed in a discrete location, often adjacent to an inpatient rehabilitation unit.

  3. Transportation to and from the services is provided.

  4. Some advantages of DRSs

      a. Patients spend from 3 to 5 days per week in a facility that provides skilled nursing care and rehabilitation services.

      b. Patients may continue to live at home.

D. Skilled nursing facilities—Short-term sub-acute services

  1. Sub-acute rehabilitation care is comprehensive and cost effective for patients who have been hospitalized for treatment of an injury or illness. This type of care is not limited to the elderly patient.

  2. The candidate for sub-acute care no longer requires the intensive procedures of an acute care hospital, but does require the diagnostic or invasive procedures of an inpatient health care facility.

  3. The patient's care still requires active physician direction, professional nursing care, significant ancillary services, an outcomes-focused interdisciplinary approach to care, and complex medical and/or rehabilitative care.

  4. Sub-acute rehabilitation care assists patients in regaining lost or diminished abilities and restoring independence and confidence by focusing on realistic, attainable goals.

  5. Sub-acute care usually requires that the patient is hospitalized for a short period of time and focuses on continuing the treatment plan initiated in the hospital/acute care setting while providing needed rehabilitation support to facilitate the patient's return to his or her prior living arrangement.

  6. Sub-acute care facilities or units provide rehabilitative care through a multidisciplinary team of professionals including:

      a. Nurses

      b. Physical therapists

      c. Occupational therapists

   d. Speech pathologists

   e. Case managers

   f. Physicians

   g. Social workers

7. Sub-acute care facilities provide 4 or more hours of daily direct nursing care, plus 24-hour nursing supervision. Direct skilled nursing assessment is completed once per day.

8. Care is led by a physician—internist, family practitioner, geriatric specialist, or physiatrist (a specialist in physical and rehabilitation medicine). Physicians are also available on call at all times to respond to emergency situations.

9. Sub-acute care facilities see patients who have a variety of diagnoses requiring rehabilitation. Some of these are:

   a. Orthopedic conditions such as hip and knee replacements, amputations, and multiple traumas

   b. Neurological conditions, such as stroke, Parkinson disease and Guillain-Barré, brain injury, and spinal cord injury

   c. Other conditions such as post-cardiac surgery, post–major abdominal surgery, infections requiring extended intravenous antibiotic treatment

   d. Complicated wounds and pressure ulcer/skin breakdown

10. Rehabilitation services in sub-acute care facilities focus on restoring function. Eligible patients are those who:

   a. Require skilled nursing services on a daily basis

   b. Have a potential for improvement or ability to return to prior level of functioning in a reasonable amount of time

   c. Have an acute disability

   d. Have medical or surgical conditions that may not be sufficiently stable to allow full participation in therapies, but do not require acute inpatient hospitalization

   e. Demonstrate the ability to participate in at least 1 hour of therapy per day

11. Sub-acute care is not intended for chronic illnesses or disabilities. It is paid for by Medicare, following a qualifying hospitalization.

12. Sub-acute rehabilitation may take place in an SNF or a free-standing rehabilitation facility.

13. Sub-acute rehabilitation services can be divided into three broad categories (Carr, 2000):

   a. Short-term/rehabilitative:

      i. Patients with significant medical and nursing needs and who are too ill to tolerate rigorous rehabilitation therapy in an acute care rehabilitation facility

      ii. Require 4.5 to 5.5 daily direct nursing care hours

      iii. High use of PT, OT, and SPT

        iv. Common medical problems include orthopedics (amputation, total hip or knee replacements) and neurology (stroke, brain or spinal injury)

        v. Length of stay/treatment ranges between 7 and 21 days

    b. Short-term complex medical:

        i. Patients who are post-surgical or medically stable but require intense medical and nursing management

        ii. Require 4.5 to 8.0 daily direct nursing care hours

        iii. High use of respiratory, laboratory, pharmacy, and medical supplies

        iv. Common medical problems include cardiology, oncology, pulmonary, renal disease, post-surgical, complex wounds, intravenous therapy, parenteral nutrition, and dialysis

        v. Length of stay/treatment ranges between 7 and 21 days

    c. Long-term/chronic:

        i. Patients who have experienced extended acute care stays and are medically stable but still have relatively high need for nursing and/or ancillary services

        ii. Require 4.5 to 8.0 daily direct nursing care hours

        iii. Common medical problems include head injury, coma, multiple trauma, and ventilator dependence

        iv. Length of stay/treatment is 25 days or longer

14. Most insurers have sub-acute rehabilitation benefits, including non–managed care Medicaid.

    a. No limit on length of stay as long as progress occurs every 2 to 3 weeks

    b. Non–managed care Medicare Part A (100 days coverage for each new disability as long as progress occurs every 2 to 3 weeks) and most private insurers

    c. Sub-acute rehabilitation in an acute rehabilitation unit or acute hospital is only occasionally covered by insurers.

    d. Medicaid reimbursement for SNF-level care specifically directed at rehabilitation as opposed to medical needs is poor. Charges range from $120 to $400 per day (non–hospital-based SNF) to $450 to 750 per day (hospital or rehabilitation unit-based services)

E. Long-term acute care in specialty acute care hospitals

  1. Long-term acute care hospitals are facilities specializing in the treatment and rehabilitation of medically complicated, chronically ill, and critically ill patients.

  2. Areas of specialization may include pulmonary, ventilator dependency and weaning, cardiac, trauma, wound, and neurology.

  3. Average length of stay is 25 days or longer.

  4. Usually the patient cannot tolerate more than 3 hours of therapy per day.

5. Typically, patients are admitted to these facilities after illness such as stroke or severe infections.

6. Care is directed by internal medicine and may include:
   a. Ventilator management, intravenous therapy, or other high-technology treatment available
   b. Daily physician assessments
   c. Complicated wound care
   d. Management of multi-system organ failure

7. Care provided in these facilities is usually covered by Medicare.

F. Long-term care—skilled nursing facilities

1. SNFs are considered cost-effective ways to enable patients with injuries, acute illnesses, or postoperative care needs to recover in an environment outside the acute care hospital setting.

2. Individuals who require placement in SNFs are covered under Medicare Part A.

3. Medicare coverage is only up to 100 days of skilled care during a benefit period, and only if strict skilled criteria are met.

4. SNFs are not intended for the care of patients with chronic illness or disabilities.

5. All skilled services needed by patients must be "reasonable and necessary." Refer to the long-term care section above for more details.
   a. The individual must have potential for improvement or ability to return to prior level of function in a reasonable amount of time.
   b. Skilled service does not mean that the individual cannot care for himself or herself.
   c. Not intended to provide maintenance therapies to maintain function (e.g., restorative nursing).

G. Long-term care—nursing homes

1. Nursing homes primarily exist to serve a small portion of the elderly population—those with severe medical and/or disability problems that require 24-hour care.

2. This population cannot stay in the home for many reasons, including:
   a. Financial resources are limited
   b. Caregivers are unavailable
   c. Personal choice
   d. The intensity of the required home services is no longer possible
   e. The elderly is no longer safe in a home environment
   f. The elderly may require skilled care but has exhausted Medicare Part A benefits or is not eligible for Medicare Part A benefits

3. Long-term care in the nursing home setting may provide rehabilitation services (restorative nursing) to maintain function in the geriatric patient:
   a. Walking the patient on a daily basis
   b. Passive range-of-motion exercises
   c. Help with feeding activities
4. Functional characteristics may contribute to the decision to place a patient in a nursing home for long-term care. Examples may include:
   a. Difficulty with toileting and incontinence
   b. Memory or orientation problems
   c. Behavior problems
   d. Sensory and communication problems
   e. Speech therapy; does not include restorative speech programs

◼ NONMEDICAL LEVELS OF CARE

A. Assisted living facilities (ALFs):
   1. A type of living arrangement in which personal care services are provided as needed. These may include, but are not limited to, the following:
      a. Meals
      b. Housekeeping services
      c. Transportation services
      d. Assistance with activities of daily living
      e. 24-hour security and staff availability
      f. Emergency call systems
      g. Health care services such as visiting nurse
      h. Wellness and exercise programs
      i. Medications management
      j. Laundry services
      k. Social and recreational activities
   2. ALFs are also called *residential care facilities* and tend to fill a gap between home care and nursing homes.
   3. The physical environment of ALFs is set up with the geriatric/elderly patient in mind. They look more like apartment buildings with private rooms or suites. Some of the environmental characteristics include:
      a. Higher toilets
      b. Wheelchair accessibility
      c. Showers
      d. Electric outlets at hip level
      e. Communication devices
      f. Commodes
   4. Residents in ALFs can receive medication reminders and have access to health care professionals such as registered nurses, social workers, and nurse aides.

5. ALFs are not covered by Medicare.

6. Each state has its own licensing regulations or requirements for ALFs. Allowable services also vary among the states.

7. ALFs are known by various names in different states—*personal care, adult congregate living care, board and care, adult homes, adult living facilities, sheltered housing,* and *community-based retirement facilities.*

B. Group homes

1. Often patients, known as *residents*, live in a facility with 4 to 10 other individuals.

2. Meals, recreation, and other housekeeping assistance are provided.

3. Residents must be able to ambulate to the bathroom and not require any skilled care.

4. Group homes are not covered by Medicare.

5. Used by state Medicaid systems to care for residents who have no other means of care or support.

C. Dementia care, adult day care, or 24-hour living units

1. Adult day care facilities (ADCFs) have been in use for more than 30 years. They are designed especially for the care of patients with Alzheimer disease or other types of dementia.

2. ADCFs may also be called *adult day centers, adult day health, adult day services, adult day residential care,* or *medical adult day care centers.*

3. ADCFs offer an alternative to caregivers by providing a daytime care environment outside the home setting.

4. ADCFs offer simple daily activities, supervision, and routine daily caregiving. They decrease stimulation and confusion.

5. ADCFs maintain the individual's dignity and highest potential of functioning.

6. ADCFs employ a family-centered approach to care and services and offer special training for caregivers and involved families.

7. ADCFs focus on planned activities that fit the needs of elderly patients and help them to function as comfortably and independently as possible, for as long as possible.

8. There are three types or models of ADCFs.

   a. The traditional model includes social services, activities, crafts, and individual attention from ADCF staff.

   b. The medical model includes, in addition to the services offered in the traditional model, skilled services by nurses, therapists, social workers, psychiatrists, and geriatricians.

   c. The Alzheimer model includes specialized services designed specifically for the care of the Alzheimer patient.

9. ADCFs aim to keep patients active and to teach them skills that will prevent them from needing to be in institutions such as nursing homes.

10. Some ADCFs may be eligible for Medicaid reimbursement or other public funds; however, most caregivers incur significant out-of-pocket

payments for these services. Some are reimbursed under long-term insurance plans.

D. Green houses
   1. Group homes, with a focus on elders' quality of life.
   2. Focus on providing an environment that includes more "home" features and less of the clinical coldness of other care facilities.
   3. Residents eat together like a family (communal dining).
   4. Focus is not on care, rather on the dignity of the elder.
   5. Built on a residential scale, not large scale like other facilities.
   6. Residents are able to choose interior design of their own space.
   7. Depending on their functional abilities, residents may help in the cooking of meals or daily routines, as if they were living in their own homes.
   8. Caregivers have higher job satisfaction.
   9. Less cost overall.

E. Aging in place
   1. Occurs when a person chooses to remain in his or her living environment (home) and to remain as independent as possible, despite the physical or mental decline that may occur with chronic disabilities or the aging process (Callahan, 1992).
   2. This independence can be maintained by contracting with providers of any health services that are needed, including skilled care such as nursing care or skilled rehabilitative therapy services.
   3. Independence may also be maintained by contracting with providers for other needs, such as:
      a. Assistance with ADLs
      b. Incontinence care
      c. Assistance with IADLs
      d. Assistance with personal and legal affairs
   4. Barriers to aging in place may include:
      a. Financial barriers
         i. The individual may lack ability to pay for services.
         ii. The individual may not want to pay for services.
      b. Lack of community services
         i. This may be an issue mainly in rural areas with no access to services.
         ii. There may not be enough community services to meet needs.
         iii. Frailness of the individual may require more assistance than possible or available from the community.
      c. Quality of care concerns
         i. Caregivers may not be properly trained.
         ii. Caregivers may not be licensed or supervised adequately.
         iii. Possible abuse and neglect
         iv. Lack of quality care

      d. Individual barriers
         i. Owing to physical or psychological factors
         ii. Danger to self and/or others may exist
    5. Programs for aging in place
      a. Federal—Older Americans Act of 1965
         i. Administration on Aging
         ii. Administers key programs to help vulnerable older Americans
         iii. Works closely with state, regional, and Areas of Aging agencies
      b. State and community programs
         i. Provide supportive in-home and community-based services
           (a) Nutrition
           (b) Transportation
           (c) Senior center
           (d) Homemaker services
         ii. Emphasis on elder rights programs
           (a) Nursing Home Ombudsmen programs
           (b) Legal and insurance counseling services
           (c) Elder abuse prevention efforts
         iii. Contracts with public or private groups
           (a) Referral, outreach, case management, escort, and transportation
           (b) In-home services for homemakers, personal care, home repair, and rehabilitation
           (c) Educational programs

F. Custodial care
    1. A level of care that is available mainly for the purpose of performing ADLs and IADLs
    2. May be provided by persons without professional skills or training
    3. This level of care is intended to:
      a. Maintain and support the patient's existing level of health
      b. Preserve health from further decline
      c. May be provided in a long-term care (nursing home) setting

■ RESPITE CARE

A. Family members provide approximately 80% of the care needed by older relatives.

B. When caring for a loved one, it is easy for caregivers to overlook their own personal needs. They often juggle the demands of a family and career along with their responsibility to a sick or disabled family member or friend. Therefore, many caregivers often find themselves victims of stress and depression.

C. In order to maintain both their own and a loved one's quality of life it is important for caregivers to take a rest.

D. A respite care program can offer temporary relief for a caregiver from the day-to-day demands of caring for an aging or disabled patient.

E. The idea of respite care emerged in the early 1970s when home care became a trend in the field of human services. It is typically defined as any type of "relief" care provided to families who care for a loved one having a chronic illness or disability.

F. Respite care may include temporary relief ranging from a few hours to a few weeks or periodic care up to a few months. This temporary relief may be provided on an emergency or regular basis.

G. Ideally, respite care should be preventive, rather than the result of a crisis. Planning ahead by seeking outside help will ensure that good care will be provided.

H. Respite care services are provided in many ways, depending on the needs of the family/caregiver. In general there are three types of respite care services:
  1. Adult day programs
  2. In-home health aide or companion services
  3. Overnight care in a residential facility

I. Respite care services are part of an overall support system necessary for families or caregivers to provide care for a loved one at home.

J. One of the most important purposes of respite care is to give caregivers temporary relief from the stress they experience while providing care to an ill or disabled patient.

K. Respite care enables caregivers to take extended vacations or just a few hours off to spend time with friends or family, or the opportunity to discuss a loved one's health status with a health care professional.

L. Most respite care programs are provided by health care organizations/agencies such as hospitals, nursing homes, assisted living facilities, and private agencies. In some cases, families with an ill or disabled individual arrange for respite care with neighbors, family members, or friends.

M. Many caregivers are reluctant to rely on a respite care program. They may question the need for this type of service.

N. Respite care not only gives caregivers time to concentrate on themselves but it provides an ill or disabled loved one with a change in their daily routine. It encourages the development of new relationships and friendships, boosts self-esteem and confidence, and inspires a move toward independence.

O. Case managers may engage in the following activities in relation to respite care:
  1. Educate family members and caregivers of patients about respite care, its goals/purpose, its availability, and how to access it
  2. Encourage families and caregivers to take advantage of respite care programs

3. Arrange for respite care and coordinate its services
4. Counsel families and caregivers regarding their need for respite care
5. Support the actions of families and caregivers in obtaining respite care and assure them that this does not mean abandonment of their loved one

■ FINANCIAL ASPECTS OF LONG-TERM AND REHABILITATION CARE SETTINGS

A. Prior to 1997, Medicare reimbursement for nursing homes was based on actual costs submitted on each patient. The Balanced Budget Act of 1996 forced Medicare to phase in a PPS of reimbursement that is currently fully implemented. Medicaid also reimburses for care based on the PPS.
   1. Reimbursement is determined based on intensity of care needed and the length of stay.

B. Nursing homes that only take Medicaid residents might offer longer term but less intensive levels of care. Nursing homes that do not accept Medicaid payment may make a resident move when Medicare coverage or the resident's own money runs out.

C. Medicare pays for 20 days of a SNF at full cost and the difference between $114 per day and the actual cost for another 80 days.

D. To qualify for Medicare nursing home coverage, a patient must stay in an acute care hospital setting for at least 3 full days and must have a skilled nursing care need that is ordered by a physician.

E. Medicaid covers skilled nursing care services when an individual spends-down his/her liquid assets to $2000.

F. Long-term care recipients of Medicaid come almost exclusively from the aged, blind, and disabled group of eligible beneficiaries but very few of those are actually receiving Supplemental Security Income (SSI).

G. SSI is a welfare payment for certain disabled or handicapped individuals who are unable to work, have no assets, and have no extended family financial support.

H. Reimbursement in the rehabilitation care setting employs a PPS, similar to that of acute care/hospital-based care (i.e., the DRG system).
   1. This system includes a Patient Assesment Instrument (PAI) that captures a score that is used to place a patient in a case mix group (CMG) and to establish the reimbursement rate.
   2. In the CMG system, rehabilitation patients are classified into groups based on clinical/medical characteristics and expected resource consumption.

I. SNFs also employ a PPS for reimbursement, similar to that of the acute care/hospital-based care (i.e., the DRG system); this system is called resource utilization groups (RUGs).
   1. The system classifies SNF patients into 7 major hierarchies and 44 RUGs based on information from the minimum data set (MDS).

2. The MDS includes data that reflects the patient's medical/clinical condition and resources/services required for care.

3. Reimbursement is based on the assigned hierarchy and RUG.

J. Inquiries regarding finances are often difficult to initiate. In general, individuals are not comfortable providing information about their finances. This is especially true if the inquiries are over the telephone.

K. Economic issues can have a direct impact on the health of an elderly individual.

L. The Older Americans Resources and Services Multidimensional Functional Assessment Questionnaire (OARS) contains an assessment of financial resources case managers may use for the financial assessment of the elderly individual.

M. Case managers can arrange for this type of in-depth assessment of finances via the help of a social worker or, depending on the practice setting, may complete the assessment themselves.

N. Even without the complete assessment, the case manager should identify whether finances may be the root cause of other issues:

1. Does the person fail to follow his or her special diet because of lack of funds?

2. Does he or she ever alter the medication schedule to prolong the interval between refills to save money, or not take the medication at all?

3. Does the patient miss his/her doctor's appointments for health maintenance or chronic illness management owing to insufficient funds?

4. Does the patient's housing substandard or unsafe environment occur due to a lack of funding for a more suitable living situation?

O. Case managers may intervene in any of the above situations (or others) to limit the impact of financial issues on the health and well-being of all patients including older adults.

P. Case managers must understand the various care settings, eligibility criteria for admission into these settings, and the financial reimbursement methods associated with them so that they can best be able to assist their patients and ensure positive outcomes.

■ CASE MANAGEMENT ROLES IN LONG-TERM AND ACUTE REHABILITATION CARE SETTINGS

A. Case managers in the long-term and acute rehabilitation care settings balance the clinical and financial considerations of treatments.

B. Use of evidence-based criteria in the inpatient rehabilitation setting provides an excellent framework by which case managers are able to ensure that patients are admitted to the most appropriate level of care (Fig. 6-2).

C. Registered nurse (RN) case managers in the long-term and rehabilitation care settings act as gatekeepers for health services, advocates for

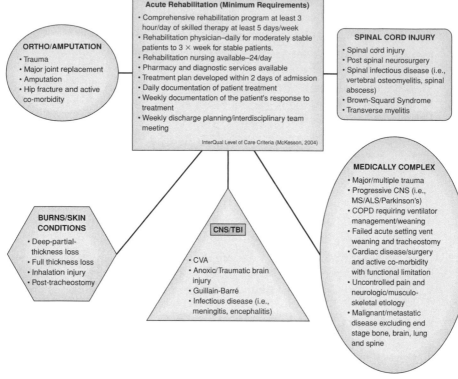

FIGURE 6–2   Adult rehabilitation criteria (Carr, 2005).

rehabilitation services and other treatment plans, and experts on case management issues.

D. Rehabilitation case managers are able to organize complex treatment plans and establish clear and attainable goals for the patient and family. They use creativity, adaptability, and flexibility to enhance resources, maximize health care benefits, and seek solutions to short- or long-term problems.

E. The case managers in the long-term and rehabilitation care settings must possess specialized knowledge related to the client population served; that is, they must act as clinical experts, insurance experts, and health care delivery systems and management experts.

F. The accomplishment of case management interventions depends largely on the case manager's ability to move effectively between the multidimensional aspects of their role. These dimensions are clinical, managerial, and financial/business as described by Carr (2005) and summarized in Table 6-3.

G. The case management process in the long-term or rehabilitation care setting begins with a referral from health care professionals in the acute care settings, including the acute care case managers. Case managers then initiate contact with the referring professionals and arrange for an

TABLE 6–3

The Case Manager's Role Dimensions in the Acute Rehabilitation Setting

The Clinical Role Dimension	The Managerial Role Dimension	The Financial/Business Role Dimension
• Conducts the initial and ongoing clinical assessment	• Coordinates interdisciplinary team activities	• Monitors financial margins
• Manages and coordinates the treatment plan toward favorable outcomes	• Collaborates with managed care case managers as indicated	• Verifies benefits and authorization of services
• Ensures the timeliness of clinical and rehabilitation interventions	• Identifies preferred providers and evaluates the availability/appropriateness of goods and services	• Negotiates rates and services
• Facilitates patient and family education	• Determines appropriate care settings and discharge planning needs	• Confers with third-party payers regarding the availability and scope of continued care services
• Identifies and facilitates referrals for patient-related issues that require intervention	• Identifies utilization limits and outliers	• Conducts cost-benefit analysis as indicated (Cohen and Cesta, 1996)
• Does early identification of potential problems that might adversely impact the plan of care (Cohen and Cesta, 1996)	• Establishes and facilitates ongoing lines of communication with the team	• Maintains open lines of communication with third-party payers and facility business office
• Maintains open lines of communication with the team and the patient	• Ensures documentation supports the plan of care and treatment (Cohen and Cesta, 1996)	• Acts as a liaison to the business office to facilitate services for the underinsured

Note. From "The Case Manager's Role in Optimizing Acute Rehabilitation Services," by D.D. Carr, 2005, *Lippincott's Case Management, 10*(4), pp. 190–200. Reprinted with permission.

onsite visit to assess the patient's condition and potential treatment needed.

H. Whenever possible, the case manager may meet with members of the acute care multidisciplinary team and discuss the patient's condition and treatment plan before a decision is made to accept the patient into long-term or rehabilitation care setting.

I. As part of the patient assessment, the case manager:

1. Completes a patient's history

2. Gathers relevant data about hospital length of stay and treatment plan

3. Meets with the patient and family to discuss the transfer to the rehabilitation or long-term care setting

J. The role of the case manager in the rehabilitation or long-term care setting may include the following activities:
  1. Coordination of the flow of patients through the facility
  2. Collaboration with members of the multidisciplinary care team
  3. Optimization of care outcomes, including safety, cost effectiveness, and quality of life
  4. Liaison between the referral sources, patient and family, managed care/insurance company, and community-based physicians
  5. Negotiating services and resources, and obtaining authorizations for such services
  6. Advocating for patients and families

■ RESOURCES FOR THE CARE OF THE ELDERLY

A. The American Association of Retired Persons (AARP) has information on virtually every aspect of successful aging and serves as a resource for case managers and patients.

B. The American Society on Aging has an extensive library of educational materials aimed at case managers and patients. In addition, it sponsors numerous conferences throughout the year for those working with older adults.

C. The Area Agency on Aging (AAA) offers a variety of programs, from information and referral to hands-on support programs. This is a number that should be in every case manager's telephone book. Both new and seasoned case managers should contact the AAA in their area and familiarize themselves with the services available.

D. Local public health departments often provide for in-home visits by public health nurses for health promotion activities. This is especially valuable for low-income elderly.

E. Service organizations such as the Salvation Army or St. Vincent DePaul Society often offer a variety of programs for the elderly population, such as:
  1. Adult day health programs
  2. Friendly visitor programs (on the phone or in person)
  3. Equipment loan programs
  4. Free or low-cost transportation

F. Churches and religious groups often offer services to their members or the community at large.

REFERENCES

Callahan, J. (1992). *Aging in Place*. Generations, 16(2), 5–7.
Carr, D. D. (2000). Case management for the subacute patient in a skilled nursing facility. *Lippincott's Case Management*, 5(2), 83–92.

Carr, D. D. (2005). The case manager's role in optimizing acute rehabilitation services. *Lippincott's Case Management, 10*(4), 190–200.
Centers for Medicare and Medicaid Services (CMS) Medicare Benefit Policy Manual. (2003). Conditions of participation for hospitals: Inpatient hospital stays for rehabilitation 110.0–110.5. Revised October 1, 2003. Website: *www.cms.hhs.gov/manuals/102_policy/bp102c01.pdf* [Context Link]. Retrieved October 20, 2004.
Commission on Accreditation of Rehabilitation Facilities (CARF). (1991). *Standards manual for organizations serving people with disabilities.* Tucson, AZ: Author.
Day, T. (2006). About long-term care. Guide to long-term care planning. Website: *www.longtermcarelink.net/eldercare_long_term_care.htm.* Accessed August 19, 2006.
Wright, B. (1983). *Physical disability: A psychosocial approach,* 2nd ed. New York: Harper & Row.

SUGGESTED READING

Clinical Practice Guidelines. *Guidelines abstracted from the American Academy of Neurology's dementia guidelines for early detection, diagnosis and management of dementia.* The American Geriatrics Society. Website: *http://americangeriatrics.org/products/positionpapaers/aan_dementiashtml.* Accessed August 13, 2006.
Gallo, J., Reichel, W., & Andersen, L. (1988). *Handbook of geriatric assessment.* Gaithersburg, MD: Aspen.
Hamilton, G. A. (1999). Council for Case Management Accountability. Patient adherence outcome indicators and measurement in case management and health care. A state of the science paper. 8.
HIAA guide to long-term care insurance. (1999). *Consumer Information,* December, 1–13. Website: *www.hiaa.org/cons/guideltc.html.*
HMO Work Group on Care Management. (1996). *Identifying high-risk Medicare HMO members: A report from the HMO Work Group on Care Management: Chronic care initiatives in HMOs.* Washington, DC: Group Health Foundation.
Hoenig, H., et al. (1994). Adult rehabilitation: What do physicians know about it and how should they use it? *Journal of American Geriatrics, 42,* 341–347.
Lawler, K. (2001). *Aging in place, coordinating housing and health care provision for America's growing elderly population.* Joint Center for Housing. Studies of Harvard University, Cambridge, MA.
Miller, K. E., Zylstra, R. G., & Standbridge, J. B. (2001). The geriatric patient: A systematic approach to maintaining health. *American Family Physician, 61*(4), 1089–1104.
Miller, C. A. (1999). *Nursing care of older adults: Theory and practice,* 3rd ed. Philadelphia: Lippincott Williams & Wilkins.
National Center for Injury Prevention and Control. A tool kit to prevent senior falls. Website: *www.cdc.gov.*
NebGuide. (1999). Nursing home insights. December, 1–7. Website: *www.unl.edu/pubs/homemgt/g1013.htm.*
Studenski, S., Rigler, S. (1999). Rehabilitation of geriatric patients. *Scientific American, 3rd ed.* Vol. 2 DC (Dale, Feldennan, Eds). *Scientific American, 8*(10), 1–6.
Senior Resource for Aging. (2006). Aging in place. Website: *www.seniorresource.com/ageinpl.htm.*
The Merck manual of geriatrics, Chapter 2: U.S. Demographics. Website: *www.merck.com/mrkshared/mmg/sec1/ch2/ch2b.jsp.*
U.S. Care. (1999). *Glossary of long-term care terms.* Website: *www.uscare.com/glossary.html.* Accessed April, 2006.
Wieland, D., & Hirth, V. (2003). Comprehensive geriatric assessment. *Cancer Control, 10*(6), 454–462.

Case Management in the Palliative Care and Hospice Settings

Lyla J. Correoso
Linda Santiago

LEARNING OBJECTIVES

Upon completion of this chapter, the reader will be able to:

1. Understand the difference between palliative care and hospice care.
2. Recognize how case management practice applies to palliative and hospice end-of-life care issues.
3. Describe patient identification and criteria for palliative versus hospice care services.
4. Explain the main principles and scope of services for palliative and hospice care programs.
5. Describe the role of the case manager in the palliative and hospice care settings.

IMPORTANT TERMS AND CONCEPTS

Advance Directives
Collaboration
Coordination
End-of-Life Care
Good Death
Health Care Proxy

Hospice Care
Interdisciplinary Team
Palliative Care
Primary Palliative Care Level
Self-Determination
Specialty Palliative Care Level

■ INTRODUCTION

A. Studies have consistently demonstrated that when patients are asked about their desires for end-of-life care, they indicate that they wish to die free of physical symptoms; they do not want to die alone; and they want to receive care in accordance with personal (especially spiritual) preferences, and in ways that honor the individual's life and do not present a burden to the family.

B. For more than 30 years, the venue for end-of-life care has been the hospice setting. However, due to multiple barriers, hospice has been underutilized in the United States.

C. Over the past few years, demand for palliative and hospice care has grown tremendously. Palliative and hospice care are provided across a variety of health care settings and professional disciplines. These areas of health care will continue to grow as the American population continues to age and seek desired alternatives to having their health care services met.

D. With the advent of Education on Palliative and End-of-life Care (EPEC) (EPEC, 2006) and End-of-life Nursing Education Consortium (ELNEC) (ELNEC, 2006), there has been a slow but increasing understanding of the importance of symptom control, advanced care planning, hospice care and patient's preferences, quality of life, and end-of-life care.

E. One long-standing barrier has been the lack of understanding by patients and health care providers, including physicians, about Medicare benefits for hospice.

F. With the explosive growth of palliative care in hospitals and fledgling growth in the community, there has been further confusion with respect to the two levels of care (i.e., primary and specialty care levels).

G. The impact of increased cost to consumers and decreased insurance coverage for service delivery including Medicare capitation for end-stage illness has increased the need for palliative and hospice services in the community.

   1. Capitation has led to the need for utilization of cost-containment strategies to improve the efficiency and quality of services to those clients with end-stage illnesses.

   2. An example of such strategies is the coordination and management of service through palliative care and hospice programs.

H. The number of palliative care and hospice programs have grown in recent years in response to the growth in the population living with chronic, debilitating, and life-threatening illnesses (NHPCO, 2005).

I. Studies suggest that a referral to palliative care programs and hospice results in beneficial effects on patients' symptoms, reduced hospital costs, a greater likelihood of death at home rather than at an institutionalized facility, and a higher level of patient and family satisfaction than does conventional care (Morrison and Meier, 2004).

■ KEY DEFINITIONS

A. Advance directive—Legally executed document that explains the patient's health care–related wishes and decisions. It is drawn up while the patient is still competent and is used if the patient becomes incapacitated or incompetent.

B. End-of-life care—Care provided by the health care team during the last few months of a person's life and when experiencing an end-stage illness that is life threatening or steadily progressing toward death. It is an integrated, patient/family-centered, and compassionate approach to care that is guided by a sense of respect for one's dignity and comfort. It also addresses the unique needs of patients and their families at a time when life-prolonging interventions are no longer considered appropriate or effective.

C. Good death—Death that is free from avoidable distress and suffering for patients and their families, and in accordance with the patient's and family's wishes. It is care that is considered reasonable and consistent with clinical, cultural, and ethical standards of care.

D. Health care proxy—A legal document that directs whom the health care provider/agency should contact for approval/consent of treatment decisions or options when the patient is no longer deemed competent to decide for himself or herself.

E. Hospice care—A model of quality and compassionate care at the end of life. It focuses on caring not curing, and the belief that each person has the right to die pain free and with dignity.

F. Palliative care—A health care approach that seeks to provide the best possible quality of life for people with chronically progressive or life-threatening illnesses and in accordance with their particular values, beliefs, needs, and preferences.

G. Patient self-determination—Making treatment decisions, such as designating a health care proxy, establishing advance directives, deciding to refuse or discontinue care, and choosing to not be resuscitated or to withdraw nutritional support.

H. Primary palliative and hospice care level—Palliative and hospice care provided by the same health care team responsible for routine care of the patient's life-threatening illness.

I. Specialty palliative and hospice care level—Palliative and hospice care provided by a health care team of appropriately trained and credentialed professionals, such as physicians, nurses, social workers, chaplains, and others.

■ PALLIATIVE CARE

A. Palliative care is both a philosophy of care and an organized, highly structured care delivery system.

B. Palliative care can be delivered by a multidisciplinary team concurrently with life-prolonging measures or as the main focus of care. It may begin

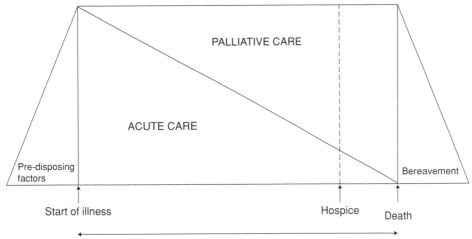

PALLIATIVE CARE

ACUTE CARE

Pre-disposing
factors

Bereavement

Start of illness

Hospice

Death

ILLNESS TRAJECTORY

FIGURE 7–1   Palliative and hospice care across the continuum of health and illness.

at the time a life-threatening or debilitating illness or injury is diagnosed, and continues through care or until after the patient's death—that is, into the family's bereavement period.

C. Palliative care is best defined as an interdisciplinary care that aims to relieve suffering and improve quality of life for patients with advanced illness and their families. It is offered *simultaneously with all other appropriate medical treatment* (see Fig. 7-1) (Meier, 2006).

D. Palliative care involves addressing the physical, intellectual, emotional, social, and spiritual needs of patients and their families. It facilitates the patient's autonomy, self-determination, access to critical information, and right to choice of care and treatment options.

E. Palliative care programs aim to improve or optimize the quality of life for patients with advanced illness in collaboration with their families and caregivers. This is achieved by anticipating, preventing, and treating suffering.

F. The delivery of palliative care may occur in the setting of the administration of life-prolonging therapy or in a setting where the sole aim is amelioration of suffering.

G. Palliative care may require end-of-life care and services. The delivery of such services requires the involvement of health care professionals who possess specialized skills, knowledge, and competencies in caring for the terminally ill at the end stage of illness or when nearing death.

■ **HOSPICE CARE**

A. Hospice care is a service delivery system that provides comprehensive care for patients suffering from a terminal illness and who have a limited life expectancy—generally 6 months or less if the disease follows its usual course.

1. The hospice population includes a subset of palliative care patients who have entered the end-of-life stage of their illness.
2. The care is patient centered and extends to the care of the family unit as well.
3. Family is defined by the patient.
4. Care requires comprehensive biomedical, psychosocial, and spiritual support, especially during the final stage of illness.
5. Hospice care supports family members coping with the complex consequences of illness as death nears, as well as post-death during the bereavement phase.

B. The hospice benefit is designed to cover the needs of a patient with respect to physician services, medications, durable medical equipment, nursing services, home health aid, social services, and spiritual care. Essentially, costs are related to the services required to care for the terminal diagnosis for which a patient is on hospice care.

C. Home is considered the patient's residence and is not necessarily limited to a "typical" home setting. Home could also be a nursing home, jail or prison, hospice residence, or assisted living facility.

D. Hospice statistics continue to demonstrate that one of the barriers to receiving good hospice care is late referrals.
1. Patients are often not referred until the last few days or weeks of life as opposed to earlier when they would be able to benefit more fully from the services that are offered to them and their family.
2. The reasons for late referrals are multifactorial and include but are not limited to:
   a. Physicians' overly optimistic views of their patients' prognoses
   b. Inability of physicians to provide bad news to patients and their families/caregivers
   c. Inability of physicians to discuss hospice as an option for care at the end of life (Hakim, Teno, Harrell et al., 1996; Hofmann, Wenger, Davis et al., 1997).

E. Studies that have looked at the quality of life of patients on hospice care have continuously demonstrated improvement in their overall condition.

F. With the improvement in the level of education of case management staff, including case managers, about the barriers to hospice care, it is hoped that better communication, collaboration, and coordination of care will move patients upstream early for palliative and hospice referrals.

G. The barrier most commonly encountered by health care providers, including case managers, is identifying patients with chronic illnesses that have entered into the end-stage phase of the disease trajectory.
1. Patients with cancer are more easily identifiable.
2. Patients with end-stage illnesses other than cancer are not easily recognized.

TABLE 7–1
Karnofsky Performance Status Scale

Definitions Rating (%) Criteria

The Karnofsky Performance Scale Index allows patients to be classified as to their funtional impairment. This can be used to compare effectiveness of different therapies and to assess the prognosis in individual patients. The lower the Karnofsky score, the worse the survival for most serious illnesses.

Able to carry on normal activity and work; no special care needed

100	Normal, no complaints; no evidence of disease
90	Able to carry on normal activity or do active work; minimal signs or symptoms of disease
80	Normal activity with effort; some signs or symptoms of disease

Unable to work; able to live at home and care for most personal needs; varying amount of assistance needed

70	Cares for self; unable to carry on normal activity or do active work
60	Requires occasional assistance, but is able to care for most personal needs
50	Requires considerable assistance and frequent medical care

Unable to care for self; requires equivalent of institutional or hospital care; disease may be progressing rapidly

40	Disabled; requires special care and assistance
30	Severely disabled; hospital admission is indicated although death is not imminent
20	Very sick; hospital admission necessary; active supportive treatment necessary
10	Moribund; fatal processes progressing rapidly
0	Dead

From *Oxford Textbook of Palliative Medicine*, by Doyle, D., Hanks, G., Cherny, N., & Calman, K. (eds). (1993). (p.109). Oxford United Kingdom: Oxford University Press. Adapted with permission.

H. The National Hospice and Palliative Care Organization has printed guidelines that are used to select patients that are hospice appropriate. (These are available at www.nhpco.org.)

I. Recent educational efforts have tried to simplify for health care providers the identification of appropriate patients for hospice or palliative care. As a rule of thumb, health care providers have been encouraged to ask themselves "Would you be surprised if this patient died within the next 6 months to a year?" If you would not be surprised, then the patient could be receiving palliative care measures or hospice benefits.

J. For more detailed information refer to Tables 7-1 and 7-2. Once the patient has been identified, plans for case management of this patient can be developed.

K. Many studies suggest that medical care for patients with serious and advanced illnesses is characterized by the undertreatment of symptoms,

TABLE 7–2
Common Indicators of End-Stage Disease

The patient may exhibit one or more of the following core and disease-specific indicators.

Core Indicators
- Physical decline
- Weight loss
- Multiple comorbidities
- Serum albumin <2.5 g/dl
- Dependence in most ADLs
- Karnofsky score ≤50%
- Desire/will to die

Amyotrophic Lateral Sclerosis
Unable to walk, needs assistance with ADLs
Barely intelligible speech
Difficulty swallowing
Nutritional status down
Declines feeding tube
Significant dyspnea, on O_2 at rest
Declines assisted ventilation
Medical complications—pneumonia, upper respiratory infection, sepsis

Cerebrovascular Accident and Coma
Level of consciousness down; coma
Persistent vegetative state
Dysphagia age >70
Paralysis post-stroke dementia
Nutritional status down (despite feeding tube if present)
Medical complications up
Family wants palliative care

Debility Unspecified
Multiple comorbidities with no primary diagnosis
Emphasis on core indicators

Dementia
Unable to walk without assistance
Urinary and fecal incontinence
Speech limited to ≤6 words/day
Unable to dress without assistance
Unable to sit up or hold head up
Complications—aspiration pneumonia, urinary tract infection, sepsis, decubitus ulcers
Difficulty swallowing/eating
Nutritional status down
Weight loss

Failure to Thrive
Body Mass Index ≤22kg/m^2
Declining enteral/parenteral support
Not responding to nutritional support
Karnofsky score ≤40%

TABLE 7–2
Common Indicators of End-Stage Disease (*continued*)

Heart Disease/Congestive Heart Failure
NYHA Class IV
Ejection fraction ≤20%
Discomfort with physical activity
Symptomatic despite maximal medical management with diuretics and vasodilators
Arrhythmias resistant to treatment
History of cardiac arrest
Cardiogenic embolic CVA

Liver Disease
No liver transplant
PT >5 sec above control
Ascites despite maximum diuretics
Peritonitis
Hepatorenal syndrome
Encephalopathy with asterixis, somnolence, coma
Recurrent variceal bleeding

Pulmonary Disease/Chronic Obstructive Pulmonary Disease
Dyspnea at rest
FEV1 <30% after bronchodilators
Recurrent pulmonary infections
Cor pulmonale/right heart failure
pO_2 ≤55mm Hg; O_2 sat ≤88% (on O_2)
Weight loss >10% in past 6 mos
Resting tachycardia >100/min
pCO_2 >55

Renal Disease
Creatinine clear <10cc/min (<15cc/min in diabetics)
No dialysis, no renal transplant
Signs of uremia (confusion, nausea, pruritus, restlessness, pericarditis)
Intractable fluid overload
Oliguria <40cc/24 hr
Hyperkalemia >7.0 mEq/L

Note. Visiting Nurse Services of New York. (VNSNY) End Stage Disease Indicators for Non-Cancer Diagnoses: Common Indicators of End-Stage Disease. Published with permission.

conflicts about decision making regarding care, inadequate support for patients/families, and inadequate utilization of resources.

L. Deficits in care provider's support for palliative care services including palliation of symptoms, rehabilitation, combination of life-prolonging treatments (when possible and appropriate), support for families, and advanced care planning.

M. Several studies have demonstrated that the personal and practical care needs of patients who are seriously ill and their families are not adequately addressed by routine office visits or hospital and nursing home stays, and that this failure results in substantial burdens—medical, psychological, and financial—on patients and their caregivers. (Meier, 2006)

N. Communication is an essential core skill for palliative care. Clear communication leads to the successful assessment and management of pain and other associated symptoms. This starts with the identification of each individual patient's/family's needs, such as:

1. Pain
2. Symptom control
3. Treatment decision making
4. Financial burdens
5. Psychological support
6. Caregiver burdens

■ GENERAL PRINCIPLES AND GOALS OF PALLIATIVE AND HOSPICE CARE PROGRAMS

A. There are general principles that guide palliative and hospice care programs. These may include the following:

1. Provision of information to support care decisions
2. Treating the patient's and family's values, beliefs (cultural and social), and preferences with respect
3. Addressing the total needs of the patient and family—symptom control, especially pain and suffering; psychosocial distress; spiritual issues; social, practical, financial, and legal ramifications of the patient's condition; patient/family education; and bereavement services
4. Care and services are delivered by a multidisciplinary team and coordinated by a designated health care professional such as a case manager. Members of the core team are competent and knowledgeable in palliative and hospice care and practices.
5. Care and services are administered across all settings of the continuum of care.
6. Access to palliative and hospice care is available across care settings and patient populations regardless of ethnicity, race, age, ability to pay, and so on.
7. Palliative and hospice care professionals, including case managers, act as advocates for patients and their families.

B. The goals of palliative and hospice care programs are several. They focus on enhancing the patient's quality of life and quality of death. They include the following:

1. Addressing and controlling pain and symptoms
2. Promoting advance care planning, especially incorporating the principles of palliative and hospice care in the plan and by all members of the health care team, regardless of the care setting
3. Providing patients and their families with the needed information that may be crucial for decision making, especially regarding treatment options

4. Coordination and facilitation of care activities, especially as patients transition from one level of care/setting into another or from one health care provider to another

5. Preparing both the patient and the family for dignified death when it is anticipated

6. Providing bereavement support to the family after the patient's death.

7. Providing palliative and hospice care that is patient and family centered.

■ ADVANCE DIRECTIVES AND HEALTH CARE PROXIES

A. The patient Self-Determination Act has set the tone for health care providers to ensure patients' and families' education about the need for the designation of a health care proxy and the completion of an advance directive. It is necessary for patients to choose a person, or an advocate, to speak on their behalf in the event that they are unresponsive or incompetent. This designation is a necessity whether a person is healthy or has an advanced disease state (Perry, Churchill, and Kirshner, 2005).

B. An advance directive (AD) is a set of written instructions that when completed, outlines what types of treatment the patient would or would not desire when faced with a terminal illness.

1. Examples of ADs include a living will, health care proxy, or a health care power of attorney.

2. The legal acceptance of these documents varies from state to state. Case managers should become familiar with their individual state's legislation with respect to these items.

3. NHPCO has an excellent website resource for ADs (www.nhpco.org).

C. A health care proxy (HCP) is a person, an advocate, who has been selected by the patient to speak for the patient in the event that he or she is unable to speak for himself or herself.

1. The HCP can be anyone that the patient trusts. It does not necessarily have to be a family member.

2. The HCP should have a sense of what the person would desire since they will be providing substituted judgment for the patient.

3. The patient should have discussions with the HCP about wishes and desires for care. This dialogue is crucial for the HCP to be able to adequately represent the person's wishes.

4. Details that should be covered with an HCP include but are not limited to:

   a. Resuscitation

   b. Feeding tubes and nutritional support

   c. Dialysis

   d. Mechanical respirator/ventilator support

   e. Transfusions of blood and blood products

   f. Antibiotics

D. In developing an AD and selecting an HCP, patients and families should be aware of the importance of these documents and the role they play in decision making regarding health care options.

E. Copies of ADs should be given to the HCP and the primary care physician. Should the dynamics of a family change and a new AD needs to be created, this can be done at any time as long as the process and the documents conform to state regulations.

F. ADs do not need to be completed by a lawyer. Proper witnessing and signatures are required but do not entail the use of a notary.

G. Case managers may find it difficult to explain to patients the need for ADs and HCPs.
   1. In communicating this to a family and patient, it is best to use simplified concepts that patients/families may comprehend.
   2. Equating the AD to a road map of life and the HCP as the designated driver may assist families and patients in better understanding the concepts.

H. When traumatic events do occur and the HCP and AD are needed and followed, these documents can be empowering and comforting to the family because they feel confident that they are following their loved one's wishes.

■ SCOPE OF PALLIATIVE AND HOSPICE CARE AND SERVICES

A. A primary principle in palliative and hospice care is that services are provided seamlessly across all care settings and phases of illness.

B. Palliative and hospice services are provided to patients who are entering the terminal stages of their illness as a result of a life-threatening or debilitating illness or injury. Such a patient population encompasses individuals of all ages and those with a broad range of diagnostic categories that reduce their life expectancy.

C. Palliative and hospice care is provided in all care settings including the following:
   1. Inpatient
      a. Acute care hospitals
      b. Acute and sub-acute rehabilitation facilities
      c. Dedicated hospice and/or palliative care units within a facility
      d. Free-standing hospice and palliative care facilities
   2. Outpatient clinics
   3. Chronic care facilities
   4. Nursing homes or other skilled nursing facilities
   5. Assisted living facilities
   6. Boarding care and residential care facilities
   7. Home

D. Palliative and hospice care and services are provided at two levels—primary and specialty.
   1. The primary level is care provided by the same multidisciplinary team responsible for routine care of the terminal illness.

2. The specialty level is care provided by a specialized palliative and hospice care team of "core" health care professionals who are trained and credentialed in such specialties. This team may include:
   a. Physicians
   b. Nurses
   c. Social workers
   d. Case managers
   e. Therapists (physical, occupational)
   f. Chaplains
   g. Counselors
   h. Pharmacists
   i. Nutritionists

■ CASE MANAGEMENT SERVICES IN PALLIATIVE AND HOSPICE CARE PROGRAMS

A. Utilizing case management strategies in palliative and hospice care involves:
   1. Assessment
   2. Treatment planning
   3. Treatment decision making
   4. Collaboration with other disciplines and care providers
   5. Implementation of the plan of care
   6. Evaluation of outcomes
   7. Ensuring that the patient's/family's needs are met
   8. Provision of bereavement services for the family
   9. Patient and family education
   10. Managing the practical burdens of illness
   11. Conferencing with the patient and family and health care team to facilitate communication and decision making regarding the plan of care

B. Palliative care acts as a bridge for the hospice referral and services. The case manager can play a major role in ensuring that timely and appropriate referrals are made.

C. Hospice service coverage includes physician and nursing care, durable medical equipment, medications for pain and symptom management, home health aide (HHA) services, social work, physical therapy, occupational therapy, short hospitalization stay, crisis care, and respite services as they relate to the terminal illness. The case manager oversees these services and ensures patients' access to these services.

D. Palliative and hospice care include end-of-life care that is focused on symptom management, pain management and control, and assisting patients and families in providing care at home while assisting with advanced care planning.

   E. Once an initial assessment for palliative and/or hospice care is made by the coordinator of care (COC), the initial plan of care is set and agreed upon by the core team. The interdisciplinary team meets every 2 weeks (14 days) and collaborates regarding each individual patient's plan of care, evaluates the effectiveness of the plan, and revises the plan as indicated. The patient and family are actively involved in the care planning process.

   F. The COC is the case manager (most of the time an RN) responsible for overseeing and facilitating the care of each patient.

   G. Ensuring reimbursement is a primary role for the case manager in hospice and palliative care programs. Utilization management practices, principles and concepts, and roles and responsibilities of case managers are similar to those applied in other care settings.

      1. Hospice services provided under Medicare are a capitated service. Once the Medicare benefit is signed over to hospice, the hospice receives (national average) $126 daily for management of the patient's certified terminal illness.

   H. In addition to the goals of palliative and hospice care described above, the goals/outcomes of case management are:

      1. Efficient utilization of services, decreased emergent care and emergency department utilization

      2. Improved patient outcomes and quality of life (especially in end-of-life issues)

      3. Increased knowledge and confidence for care provision regarding end-stage diagnosis and symptom management

      4. Increased consistency of care delivery

      5. Increased patient/family satisfaction

      6. Honoring patient/family wishes regarding whether care is to be at home or inpatient placement

   I. The COC plays a significant role as a case manager in hospice to help facilitate the patient's care through advanced care planning and bereavement psychosocial support services. The COC as a case manager facilitates communication and care provision with the patient, family, physician, and interdisciplinary team to achieve outcomes/goals mutually set in a collaborative fashion.

   J. The expected patient/case management program outcomes utilizing palliative care and hospice services include:

      1. Efficient utilization of services

      2. Cost effectiveness through the coordination and management of health care services

      3. Improved patient outcomes such as satisfaction with care and symptom management

      4. Resolution of identified issues while maintaining the patient at home with support of the caregiver

   K. The achievement of these goals results in decreased use of emergent care, better symptom control, provision of quality and cost-efficient care, and interdisciplinary team concept and approach to care while meeting the terminally ill patient's/family's wishes to care for their loved ones in their own home or facility.

L. Palliative and hospice services and the role of the case manager in the provision of these services are crucial in helping patients/caregivers navigate the difficult terrain of end-of-life issues.

REFERENCES

Education on Palliative and End-of-life Care (EPEC). (2006). Website: *www.epec.net*. Accessed July 26, 2006.

End of Life Nursing Education Consortium (ELNEC). (2006). Website: *www.aacn.nche.edu/elnec*. Accessed July 26, 2006.

Hakim, R. B., Teno, J. M., Harrell, F. E., et al. (1996). Factors associated with Do-Not Resuscitate Orders: Patients' preferences, prognoses, and physicians judgements. *Annals of Internal Medicine, 125,* 284–293.

Hofmann, J. C., Wenger, N. S., Davis, R. B., Teno, J., et al. (1997). Patient preferences for communication with physicians about End-of-life decisions. *Annals of Internal Medicine, 127,* 1–12.

Meier, D. (2006). The case for palliative care. Website: *www.capc.org*. Accessed July 26, 2006.

Morrison, S., & Meier, D. (2004). Palliative care: Clinical practice. *New England Journal of Medicine, 350,* 2582–2590.

National Hospice and Palliative Care Organization (NHPCO). (2005). NHPCO's 2004 facts and figures. Website: *www.nhpco.org/files/public/Facts_ Figures_for2004data.pdf*. Accessed July 26, 2006.

Perry, J. E., Churchill, L. R., & Kirshner, H. S. (2005). The Terri Schiavo case: Legal, ethical, and medical Perspectives. *Annals of Internal Med, 143,* 744–748.

SUGGESTED READING

Case Management Society of America: *www.cmsa.org*

Centers for Medicare and Medicaid Services, Health and Human Services: *www.cms.hhs.gov/providers/hospiceps/end_of_life.asp*

Education in Palliative and End-of-Life Care: *www.epec.net*

Hospice and Palliative Nurses Association: *www.hpna.org*

Medical guidelines for determining prognosis in selected non-cancer diseases, 2nd ed. National Hospice Organization. Available at *www.nhpco.org*. Accessed July 26, 2006.

National Guideline Clearing House: *www.guideline.gov*

National Hospice and Palliative Care Organization: *www.nhpco.org*

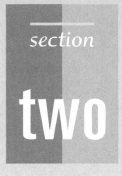

Roles and Functions of Case Managers

The Case Manager

Elizabeth Bodie Gross
Hussein A. Tahan

LEARNING OBJECTIVES

Upon completion of this chapter, the reader will be able to:

1. Differentiate between a role and function, and how they apply to the case manager.
2. Understand how the practice of the case manager has changed and expanded over time in the United States.
3. Identify how and why clients/patients have embraced and accepted case management services.
4. Understand why the case manager's role continues to change and be dynamic in practice.
5. List the various functions case managers perform across the various venues of practice.

IMPORTANT TERMS AND CONCEPTS

Activity
Care Management
Case Management
Case Manager
Context

Domain
Function
Job Description
Role
Venue

■ INTRODUCTION

A. Roles and functions of case managers are defined by professional organizations/societies (e.g., Case Management Society of America, American Nurses Association, and Commission for Case Manager Certification), based on scientific evidence, literature published by organizations that have implemented case management programs, and educational materials used in training and education of case managers.

B. Roles and functions of case managers are usually written in an organization in the form of job descriptions. However, the research literature that addresses what case managers do tends to report a taxonomy (or a list) of activities and tasks of case management based on which job descriptions can be delineated.

C. The role of the case manager has been implemented in every setting of the health care continuum (pre-acute, acute, post-acute, and rehabilitative) and is assumed by a variety of professionals such as nurses, social workers, rehabilitation counselors, disability specialists, workers' compensation specialists, and others.

D. There is no standard job description for case managers. However, the literature shares common or core aspects of case management practice: clinical/patient care, managerial/leadership, financial/business, and information management.

■ KEY DEFINITIONS

A. According to the *Merriam-Webster Dictionary* (2000), key case manager role-related terms are defined as follows:
   1. Domain— A sphere of knowledge, influence, or activity. In case management, it refers to an area or category of practice and/or knowledge.
   2. Function—Any of a group of related actions contributing to a larger action. In case management, it is the activities a case manager performs in his or her job.
   3. Role—A function or part performed especially in a particular operation or process; the proper function of a person or thing. In case management, it refers to the case manager's job title or position.
   4. Venue—The scene or locale of any action or event. In case management, it refers to the type of agency/organization a case manager works in and what population he or she serves.

B. Tahan, Huber, and Downey (2006) defined the terms *activity, function,* and *role* as described below and used these conceptualizations to guide their research on roles and functions of case managers.
   1. Activity—A discrete action, task, or behavior performed by the person in the role to meet the goals of the role; for example, "list the medications a patient takes while at home."
   2. Function—A grouping or composite of specific activities within the role. These activities are interrelated and share a common goal; for example "coordination of care activities."

3. Role—A general and abstract term that refers to a set of behaviors and expected results that is associated with one's position in a social structure. A proxy usually used for the role is the individual's title; for example, the "case manager."

C. Other case management–related terms are as follows:
1. Case manager—A health care professional who works with the patient and family as well as the health care team in the coordination of care activities and treatment or plan of care. He or she may be engaged in many activities such as patient and family education, counseling, outcomes monitoring, utilization management, and others. The case manager may be a registered nurse, a social worker, a physical therapist, a vocational rehabilitation counselor, or some other licensed health care professional.
2. Context—The environment or work structure in which a case manager functions; for example, managed care organization or payer-based case manager, hospital or acute care.
3. Job description—A document that describes roles and responsibilities, which when executed produces intended results. It also describes general tasks, responsibilities, and functions; identifies the individual/position to whom the case manager reports; and specifies the required qualifications for the job such as educational background, years of experience, and certification.

■ BACKGROUND

A. Over the past 25 years, the field of case management has evolved to meet the changing nature of the health, social, and medical care systems. Although the process of case management remains the same, the roles, functions, and venues continue to change and evolve.
1. The process of case management (discussed in Chapter 9) permeates every aspect of the health and medical care systems, and now this process is beginning to be used in other industries as well (e.g., legal and business).
2. This chapter focuses on how the roles and functions of a case manager are executed via the case management process.

B. Chapter 1 provides a great summary of the practice of case management over the past 100 years.

C. In 1982, when the U.S. Congress passed the Tax Equity and Fiscal Responsibility Act (TEFRA), it pushed third-party payers to integrate case management services across all lines of health, social, financial, and medical services to control costs and manage limited resources.

D. The case management community established several professional case management associations and organizations that were focused on advancing the practice of case management and its value in the United States. For example,
1. Case Management Society of America (CSMA)—established in 1990

2. National Association of Professional Geriatric Care Managers (NAPGCM)—established in 1985

3. Commission for Case Manager Certification (CCMC)—established in 1992

E. In the 1980s, the difference between *case* and *care* management was established.

1. *Case management* is a term used to refer to the management of acute and rehabilitative health care services. Services are delivered under a medical model, primarily by nurses.

2. *Care management* is a term used to refer to the management of long-term health care, legal, and financial services by professionals serving social welfare, aging, and nonprofit care delivery systems. Services are delivered under a psychosocial model.

3. In the mid-1980s, case and care management entrepreneurs emerged and started independent, for-profit companies or private practices that focused on selling case management services as a niche product for the care of a specific population (e.g., the disabled, the work-related severely injured, and most recently the chronically ill).

F. By the 1990s, other health care–related professionals (e.g., physical, occupational, and speech therapists; gerontologists; etc.) began to offer case and care management services on a fee-for-service basis in different practice venues.

G. In 1997, the Foundation for Rehabilitation Education Research (FRER) and NAPGCM co-sponsored a case/care management summit to discuss the future of case and care management in the United States.

1. The summit was held in Chicago in October, 1997. Sixteen (16) professional associations/organizations attended to discuss their vested interest in case/care management and its future in the United States. Participants included the following:

a. American Association of Occupational Health Nurses

b. American Nurses Credentialing Center

c. American Society on Aging

d. Case Management Society of America

e. Certification of Disability Management Specialist Commission

f. Commission for Case Manager Certification

g. Commission on Rehabilitation Counselor Certification

h. Foundation for Rehabilitation Education and Research

i. Health Insurance Association of America

j. Institute of Case Management

k. National Academy of Certified Care Managers

l. National Association of Case Management

m. National Association of Professional Geriatric Care Managers

n. National Association of Social Workers

o. National Guardianship Association

p. National Guardianship Foundation

2. The goal of the 1997 Case and Care Management Summit was to: "foster cost-efficient, collaborative professional interactions that effectively integrate the medical, psychological, and social elements of each client/provider relationship in a manner that includes the essential activities of case management in order to provide timely, appropriate and beneficial service delivery to the client. These activities include, but are not limited to, assessment, planning, coordination, implementation, monitoring, education, evaluation, and advocacy. Such integration would encompass, but not be limited to, clients and their families, health care providers, community agencies, legal and financial resources, third-party payers and employers" (Gross and Holt, 1998, p. 4).

3. The 1998 summit also recommended that a second summit be organized to:
   a. Examine and establish minimum standards for qualified case management practitioners and how case managers demonstrate ongoing competency (includes reviewing the different levels of education required for existing credentials and determining the need to standardize the entry level criteria)
   b. Document successful case management outcomes in order to demonstrate the value of the case manager credential
   c. Develop educational materials to answer basic questions and inform consumers about the qualifications of various providers, as well as the types of services care and case managers offer their clients.
   d. Use market research to identify the information needs of specific stakeholders.
   e. Review organizational codes of ethics in order to establish a common code of conduct that all care and case managers could endorse (in addition to their existing codes). Overall code would include, at a minimum, individual scope of practice, requirements for professional disclosure, clarity on conflicts in interests, cultural competency of practitioners, and client confidentiality.
   f. Identify minimum requirements for a qualified practice, develop a mechanism to standardize existing credentials, conduct periodic review of professional development criteria, and determine the need for advanced credentials for care and case managers

4. The Second Case and Care Management Summit (1999) was held in Chicago to discuss the topics outlined in the 1998 Summit I Discussion Paper. Participants remained the same, except that the Institute on Case Management did not attend. At the conclusion of this summit, the Coalition for Consumer-Centered Care and Case Management was established. The Coalition was dissolved in 2001 due to a lack of funding.

H. In 1999, Michaels and Cohen (Cohen and Cesta, 2005) redefined care and case management as follows:
   1. *Care* management establishes a system of care for a particular condition, across the continuum of care to ensure seamless transition to the right services, right providers, and at the right time and encourages

patients and their family/caregiver to manage their own health. Such care is facilitated by a case manager.

2. *Case* management is a way of managing unique and high-risk situations often associated with costly acute care and hospital stay. Typically, those who require case management are individuals whose self-care capacity is diminished at a time when their health condition is most complex or even life threatening. Such care is facilitated by a case manager.

■ CASE MANAGEMENT ROLES

A. Since the 1980s, the case manager's role has evolved, transforming itself from being an evaluator of health care services to a procurer and negotiator of health, medical, social, legal, and financial services. The role of a case manager has become more sophisticated and active in the care of an individual. Case managers are required to professionally and legally provide state-of-the-art and ethical services.

B. The changes that have catapulted case managers into the forefront of the health and medical care delivery systems include the following:

1. Increased complexity of coordinating and financing health/medical care services

2. More than 50 million Americans do not have medical/health insurance and need a case manager to help them navigate and procure needed health/medical care services with limited financial resources.

3. Due to the economy, many health, medical, and social care agencies and institutions are reducing their list of services because they are deemed to be unprofitable or a "losing asset."

4. Many social service agencies have reduced or eliminated services and subsidies (e.g., sliding scales) due to a lack of government funding and grants.

5. Nonprofit and federally/state-funded social service agencies and organizations are closing down due to a lack of overall funding. This situation is referred to as the "dissolution of the U.S. social service infrastructure."

C. Most important case management roles as identified by Tahan (2005) include the following:

1. Educator—Given the complexities of our health, medical, and long-term care systems, case managers are able to:

a. Assess the educational needs of their clients/patients and their family members and educate them in the areas identified, which may include medications, treatments, healthy lifestyles, and illness risk-reduction strategies

b. Educate health/medical/social service clinicians about the services they offer and how to obtain these needed services. Case managers also educate clinicians about health insurance benefits, reimbursement, and other appropriate aspects of care delivery.

2. Coordinator—Case managers are coordinators of complex service patterns. Through multidisciplinary collaboration efforts, they are able to:

    a. Organize service providers so that they meet the needs of their clients/patients and their families.

    b. Facilitate the delivery of care, such as the completion of tests and procedures, transition planning, and teaching activities.

3. Communicator—Case managers are effective communicators. They articulate, and clearly communicate, the needs of their clients/ patients to family members, health/medical clinicians, and other service providers so that clients can reach their highest level of functioning.

4. Collaborator—Case managers are able to collaborate with numerous health, medical, and social service providers about the needs of their clients/patients. Some health care professionals case managers collaborate with are internal to the organization where they work such as physicians, pharmacists, and physical therapists; others are external to the organization such as representatives from durable medical equipment agencies, employers, and providers of transportation services.

5. Clinician—Case managers are expert clinicians as well. They posses a level of expertise in a particular specialty such as cardiac, oncology, or disability care. Some of them, however, are general practitioners. They use their knowledge to identify the client's problems and develop an effective plan of care.

6. Utilization manager—Case managers ensure cost-effective care delivery and use of services as well as reimbursement. They focus on the continuum of care and the transition of patients from one level of care to another. In addition, they conduct specific reviews for the purpose of securing certification/authorization of care from the managed care/insurance company.

7. Transition planner—Case managers facilitate the movement of patients from one level of care to another across the continuum of care and settings. They accomplish this by examining the patient's condition, necessary treatment options, and where the relevant services are available, and by developing a plan of care that includes a discharge or transition plan; for example, a plan that addresses the transition of a patient from most to least acute care setting.

8. Leader—Case managers assume leadership responsibilities in their role especially in the areas of allocation and utilization of resources, gatekeeping of services, reimbursement review and revenue management, changing the care delivery systems, and performance review and management.

9. Quality manager—Case managers are responsible for ensuring patient safety and improving the quality of the care provided. They identify variances or delays in care (system-, practitioner-, and patient/family-related variances) and institute action. They also participate in activities of a quality improvement team and function as team leaders, facilitators, or members. In addition, they evaluate the

effectiveness of case management services through monitoring organizational and client-oriented outcomes.

10. Negotiator—Case managers assume an important role in negotiating the plan of care and services. They are skilled in coordinating the scheduling of tests and procedures and the communication of results. They also are effective in negotiating with managed care organizations the services required for patients, length of hospital stay, community-based services, and reimbursement for care provided.

11. Advocate—Case managers ensure that the needs of patients and their families are met and place their interests above all others. In addition, they educate patients about their treatment options and facilitate the making of informed decisions.

12. Researcher—Case managers evaluate case management services and outcomes via research and recommend the utilization of research outcomes in their practice, changes in standards of care, policies, procedures, and treatment protocols; that is, ensure evidence-based practice.

13. Risk manager—Case managers identify areas of risk in the care environment and processes while they review patient care and services and recommend, if not execute, an action plan. They are first to identify significant events that warrant immediate attention and resolution. They also ensure that the organization and other professionals adhere to regulatory and accreditation standards at all times.

■ CASE MANAGEMENT FUNCTIONS

A. In 1998 when the Case and Care Management Summit I Paper was distributed, for the first time it was publicly stated that the function of a case manager was dependent upon his or her job title (role) and setting (venue).

B. Often a case manager's role does not correlate with or reflect his or her job function, so it is important to know where the case manager works and whom he or she serves.

C. Regardless of work setting or clinical specialty, case managers perform the essential activities of case management (assessment, planning, goal setting, coordinating, managing, monitoring, advocating, and evaluating), but these activities are greatly influenced or directed by a case manager's venue of practice.

D. Case management functions are also influenced by the expectations a client/patient, family member, health/medical/social service provider, or employer has of the role. Case managers must always weigh the functions of their job against what is realistic to expect in a given situation or case.

E. Every 5 years, the CCMC conducts a formal role and function study to identify those changes that have taken place in the case management industry. The most recent study was concluded in 2005 and the results were published by Tahan, Huber, and Downey (2006) and Tahan, Downey, and Huber (2006). This study identified the six essential activity domains of the case manager's practice based on the opinion of more than 4,000 practicing case managers. The domains are described below.

1. The Case Finding and Intake domain focuses on:
   a. Identifying clients requiring case management services
   b. Obtaining client consent for services
   c. Communicating the client's needs to other health care providers including the physician
   d. Identifying clients who would benefit from alternate levels of care, such as sub-acute or skilled nursing services
   e. Reviewing the client's insurance coverage, negotiating rates to maximize the funding available for an individual's health care needs, and appealing service denials such as admission to an acute care setting

2. The Provision of Case Management Services domain addresses:
   a. The client's health condition, needs, and case management plans
   b. The role of the case manager as facilitator and coordinator of care activities and the person accountable for keeping communication open among care providers
   c. Monitoring care and client's progress toward expected/desired goals
   d. Reviewing and modifying the delivery of health care services as needed
   e. Reviewing the health history of the patient
   f. Communicating case management assessment findings to providers, payers, employers, family, and other key stakeholders
   g. Collaborating with the stakeholders in establishing comprehensive goals, objectives, and expected outcomes of care
   h. Organizing resources and integrating the delivery of health care services
   i. Serving as an advocate for an individual's health care needs
   j. Adhering to ethical, as well as legal, regulatory, and accreditation standards

3. The Outcomes Evaluation and Case Closure domain focuses on:
   a. Collection, analysis, and reporting of outcomes data (e.g., clinical, financial, variance, quality of life, patient satisfaction)
   b. Evaluation of the quality of case management services and the effectiveness of the case management plan
   c. Ensuring client's access to timely and necessary services
   d. Using evidence-based practice guidelines in the development of the case management plan
   e. Educating and/or facilitating the education of clients about wellness and illness prevention
   f. Monitoring disease management activities

    g. Preparing reports in compliance with regulatory requirements

    h. Communicating termination of service notification to stakeholders

    i. Bringing the case manager–client relationship to closure

4. The Utilization Management Activities domain focuses on:

    a. Appropriateness of the level of care

    b. Utilization review

    c. Ongoing communication with payers and insurance companies

    d. Resource allocation and matching resources with client's needs

    e. Reimbursement denials and appeals management

    f. Reviewing the completeness of the care providers' documentation in the client's record

    g. Reviewing information about the client's condition that necessitates hospitalization

    h. Identifying cases at high risk for complications and those that would benefit from additional types of services (e.g., disease management, physical therapy, durable medical equipment, vocational services, diagnostic testing, counseling, and assistive technology)

    i. Assessing the client's readiness, willingness, and ability to participate in case management services or self-care activities

    j. Determining the client's baseline and ongoing levels of physical, emotional, psychological, and spiritual functioning

    k. Performing appropriate assessments of situations using established case management processes and standards

5. The Psychosocial and Economic Issues domain describes the case manager's activities relative to:

    a. Integrating the knowledge of specific interventions, family dynamics, cultural issues, and resources into case management practice

    b. Reviewing information about a client's social and financial resources

    c. Assessing the social support system and relationships, multicultural issues, and health behaviors that may impact the client's health status

    d. Evaluating the ability and availability of the designated caregiver to deliver the needed services

    e. Referring clients to formal and informal community resources and support programs

    f. Determining eligibility for private- and public-sector funding sources for health care services

6. The Vocational Concepts and Strategies domain focuses on case management activities in the areas of:

    a. Disability, workplace issues, and strategies for work as a life activity

    b. Identifying the need for modifications in the client's home environment to eliminate accessibility barriers

  c. Determining the need for specialized services (e.g., rehabilitative services) to facilitate achievement of an optimal level of wellness, functioning, and productivity

  d. Arranging for vocational assessment and services

  e. Coordinating client's job analysis for job modifications and accommodation

  f. Recommending job modifications and accommodations to employers

F. Another recent study sponsored by the CCMC (Tahan and Huber, 2006) reported the use of more than 75 case management activities by case managers working in a variety of settings and specialties throughout the United States. The researchers identified these activities based on a qualitative analysis of more than 1,000 case manager job descriptions obtained from different health care organizations during the time of application for the Certified Case Manager (CCM) examination/credential. These activities are listed below—not in any order of priority or frequency.

  1. Evaluating case management outcomes
  2. Monitoring patient care and progress
  3. Assuming the role of patient advocate
  4. Assessing patient's progress
  5. Writing summary reports
  6. Engaging in quality assurance activities
  7. Determining patient needs and resources, including insurance/financial
  8. Acting as liaison between payers and health care team
  9. Determining medical necessity of admissions and services
  10. Assessing patient's level of impairment
  11. Identifying patients using a high level of services
  12. Preventing overutilization/underutilization of resources
  13. Analyzing data
  14. Communicating with health care team
  15. Collecting medical history information
  16. Acting as a professional role model
  17. Collaborating in the development of treatment plan/care plan
  18. Identifying gaps in treatment plan/care plan
  19. Communicating with patients and their family/caregivers
  20. Avoiding the use of high-cost services
  21. Developing quality assessment methods
  22. Determining patient compliance with the treatment plan
  23. Ensuring care is provided in the most appropriate setting
  24. Meeting time management and quality assurance standards
  25. Completing necessary documentation
  26. Monitoring the appropriateness of test procedures and care settings

27. Communicating with payers
28. Completing admission reviews
29. Analyzing medical files for effectiveness of case management
30. Reviewing active cases with employers
31. Attending or holding case conferences
32. Maintaining confidentiality
33. Educating patients in health promotion
34. Implementing cost-management strategies
35. Engaging in discharge planning activities
36. Identifying community resources
37. Analyzing utilization patterns and denied cases
38. Processing appeal requests
39. Developing and documenting policies and procedures
40. Establishing new client files
41. Implementing treatment plans
42. Maintaining Utilization Review Accreditation Commission (URAC) accreditation standards
43. Reporting inappropriate utilization of resources
44. Identifying gaps in general treatment
45. Monitoring medical progress
46. Scheduling medical evaluations
47. Collecting data on utilization patterns and denied cases
48. Meeting billing requirements
49. Coordinating transfers to appropriate facilities, home care, or alternative settings
50. Fostering professional development of personnel
51. Traveling to patients' homes, job sites, or other health care facilities
52. Collecting general data
53. Ascertaining the reasons for high service use
54. Obtaining approval for contacts
55. Educating and training other staff
56. Training case managers on computer systems
57. Initiating vocational service referrals
58. Coaching case managers on time management
59. Training case managers on philosophy, systems, and departmental guidelines
60. Assessing staff competencies
61. Reviewing files for claims adjusters
62. Supervising staff
63. Facilitating Return to Work (RTW)
64. Monitoring physical care and therapy
65. Completing clerical functions
66. Obtaining claims records

67. Planning for resolution of audit issues
68. Completing quality audits
69. Engaging in budget activities
70. Overseeing consultant work for thoroughness
71. Completing referral activities to other services
72. Assessing need for follow up
73. Coordinating discharge planning activities and services
74. Developing short- and long-term care goals
75. Performing job site evaluations
76. Initiating discharge planning
77. Engaging in marketing activities
78. Planning medical rehabilitation processes
79. Coordinating patient care

G. The care settings case managers work in usually determine how many and what type of these functions/activities are required and necessary to succeed in a specific case management role.

H. The case manager's roles, responsibilities, and functions are impacted by the type of health care organization, purpose of the role, the specific practice setting, and the patient population served.

I. Case managers are found to function in variety of settings such as the following:
   1. Acute and medical case management
   2. Insurance companies
   3. Traditional group or individual medical insurance plans
   4. Managed care organizations (e.g., HMOs, PPOs, EPOs, etc.)
   5. Long-term care insurance plans
   6. Hospital-based
   7. Home health care companies
   8. Government (e.g., Medicaid, Medicare, etc.)
   9. Long-term care facility (e.g., skilled nursing facility, assisted living, acute and sub-acute rehabilitation, etc.)
   10. Community-based organizations
   11. Hospice and palliative care
   12. Social service agencies
   13. Not-for-profit and religious organizations
   14. Agencies on Aging
   15. Workers' compensation companies
   16. Disability management companies
   17. Independent case management companies
   18. Life care planning
   19. Law firms
   20. Day care centers

■ CASE MANAGEMENT KNOWLEDGE FOR PRACTICE AND QUALIFICATIONS

A. In addition to the case manager's essential activities, the role and functions study completed by CCMC in 2005 also identified six main knowledge domains for effective case management practice (Tahan, Huber, and Downey [2006]; Tahan, Downey, and Huber [2006]). These are described below:

1. The Case Management Concepts domain addresses:
   a. Processes of case management practice
   b. Methods of establishing quality measures and parameters of practice
   c. Quality and performance improvement concepts
   d. Program evaluation and research methods
   e. Cost–benefit analyses, and cost-containment principles

2. The Case Management Principles and Strategies domain focuses on:
   a. Professional practice behaviors of case managers and the impact of external influences upon these behaviors
   b. Roles and functions of case managers and other health care providers
   c. Health care delivery systems
   d. Continuum of care and services
   e. Assistive technology
   f. Community resources
   g. Clinical pathways and practice guidelines

3. The Psychosocial and Support Systems domain discusses:
   a. Specific case management interventions
   b. Family and cultural issues and resources that must be integrated into case management practice
   c. Disability concepts
   d. Psychosocial aspects of chronic illness
   e. Wellness promotion and illness prevention
   f. Family dynamics and multicultural issues
   g. Crisis intervention strategies
   h. Complimentary and alternative medicine practices

4. The Health Care Management and Delivery domain describes:
   a. Health care delivery systems
   b. Collaboration with other providers
   c. Case management across practice settings
   d. Case management models, processes, and tools
   e. Confidentiality
   f. Risk management
   g. Standards of practice
   h. Legal and regulatory requirements

      i. Legislation

      j. Ethics and client advocacy

  5. The Health Care Reimbursement domain addresses:

     a. Responsibilities in relation to health care insurance and payers

     b. Managed care concepts

     c. Third-party payers

     d. Prospective payment systems

     e. Private and public benefit programs

     f. Utilization management and resource allocation

  6. The Vocational Concepts and Strategies domain

     a. Disability management

     b. Workplace issues

     c. Return-to-work strategies

     d. Disability compensation systems

     e. Job analysis, modification, and accommodation

     f. Job development

     g. Work adjustment and hardening

     h. Workers' compensation principles

     i. Life care planning

B. Tahan and Huber (2006), in their job description analysis study, also reported on the qualifications considered by employers in hiring case managers. These qualifications were identified based on the qualitative analysis of more than 1,000 job descriptions of case managers working in variety of health care practice settings. These qualifications are listed below—not in any order of priority or frequency.

    1. Clinical experience in a specific specialty

    2. Independent decision making

    3. Teamwork

    4. Professional licensure such as Registered Nurse, Social Worker, Rehabilitation Counselor

    5. Computer literacy such as skills in word processing, spreadsheets, and presentation software

    6. Customer service

    7. Critical thinking and creativity

    8. Education—Bachelor or Master's degree

    9. Initiative

  10. Knowledge or experience in Workers' Compensation

  11. Multitasking abilities

  12. Utilization management experience

  13. Knowledge or experience in disability management

  14. Knowledge of medical technology and vocabulary

  15. Knowledge of medical management

  16. Flexibility

17. Negotiation
18. Knowledge of age-related differences in care needs
19. Licensure and/or specialty certification, such as Case Management Certification
20. Mentoring
21. Knowledge of Americans with Disabilities Act/Law
22. Supervisory/managerial experience
23. Knowledge of specialized services, including referrals to other providers or services
24. Knowledge of cost analysis, cost–benefit analysis, cost-effectiveness analysis methods
25. Knowledge of labor laws and benefits
26. Knowledge of reimbursement and benefit systems—prospective payment systems, managed care, etc.
27. Communication
28. Long-term care experience
29. Data analysis and management
30. Past experience in case management

C. To be successful in their roles, case managers must possess specific skills that allow them to carry out their roles, functions, and activities and apply their knowledge into practice. Below is a list of skills described by Tahan (2005).
   1. Clinical and patient care
      a. Direct and indirect care provision
      b. Expertise in a clinical area/specialty
      c. Patient and family teaching
      d. Transitional planning
      e. Coordination, facilitation, and expedition of care activities
      f. Holistic and pastoral care
      g. Crisis intervention and counseling
      h. Development and implementation of plans of care
   2. Managerial and leadership
      a. Problem solving and conflict resolution
      b. Critical thinking and clinical judgment
      c. Project management
      d. Conducting meetings
      e. Goals setting
      f. Management of change
      g. Management of ethical and legal issues
      h. Time management and priority setting
      i. Delegation
      j. Negotiation
      k. Cultural competence

  l. Consensus building

  m. Integration

  n. Advocacy

  o. Variance and delay management

  p. Outcomes management

  q. Quality and patient safety

 3. Business and financial

  a. Resource allocation

  b. Utilization management

  c. Certification of services

  d. Financial analysis/cost–benefit (and cost-effectiveness) analysis

  e. Financial reimbursement procedures

  f. Claims and denials management

  g. Gatekeeping

  h. Health benefits and entitlements

 4. Information management and communication

  a. Customer relations

  b. Cultural sensitivity

  c. Writing reports

  d. Information sharing

  e. Communication

  f. Documentation

  g. Dealing with challenging people

  h. Active listening

  i. Collaboration

 5. Professional

  a. Research and evidence-based practice

  b. Specialty certification

  c. Writing for publication

  d. Consulting

  e. Networking

  f. Membership in professional organizations

■ CONCLUSION

A. The case management industry will continue to expand and evolve in response to the dynamic health care environment so that it can meet the challenges of tomorrow. By 2012, approximately 10,000 "baby boomers" will turn 65 years old everyday, changing how we look at and deliver long-term case management services in the future.

B. Case management services will continue to be integrated into exciting new models; thus challenging how we will educate and train future case managers.

C. The above descriptions of the roles, functions, activities, knowledge, and skills of case managers and case management practice are a guide for designing job descriptions for the case managers of today and the future. These lists should be taken into consideration carefully and applied in a way specific to the practice setting of case management. They are not to be applied in totality in any setting; rather, health care and case management executives should incorporate in the case manager's job description what is considered applicable to their organization, the specialty or service, and the practice setting.

REFERENCES

Bodie-Gross, E., & Holt, E. (July 1998). Care and Case Management Summit, October 19–20, 1997, The White Paper, Chicago, IL. Sponsered by the National Association of Professional Geriatric Case Managers, Tucson, AZ and the Fondation for Rehabilitation, Education and Research, Rolling Meadows, IL. FRER, IL.

Merriam-Webster Dictionary. (2000). New York: Random House.

Michaels, C., & Cohen, E. (2005). Two strategies for managing care: Care management and case management. In E. Cohen and T. Cesta, *Nursing case management: From essentials to advanced practice applications,* 4th ed. (pp. 33–37). St Louis, MO: Elsevier Mosby.

Tahan, H. (2005). The role of the nurse case manager. In E. Cohen and T. Cesta, *Nursing case management: From essentials to advanced practice applications,* 4th ed. (pp. 277–295). St Louis, MO: Elsevier Mosby.

Tahan, H., Downey, W., & Huber, D. (2006). Case managers' roles and functions: Commission for Case Manager Certification's 2004 research, Part II. *Lippincott's Case Management, 11*(2), 71–87.

Tahan, H., & Huber, D. (2006). The CCMC's national study of case manager job descriptions: An understanding of the activities, role relationships, knowledge, skills, and abilities. *Lippincott's Case Management, 11*(3), 127–144.

Tahan, H., Huber, D., & Downey, W. (2006). Case managers' roles and functions: Commission for Case Manager Certification's 2004 research, Part I. *Lippincott's Case Management, 11*(1), 4–22.

SUGGESTED READING

Alliance for Aging Research. (2002). *Medical never-never land: Ten reasons why America is not ready for the coming aging boom.* New York: New York.

Case Management Society of America (CMSA). (2002). *Standards of practice for case management.* Little Rock, AR: CMSA.

Commission for Case Manager Certification. (2005). *CCM certification guide.* Rolling Meadows, IL: Author.

Fitzpatrick, J., Glasgow, A., & Young, J. (Eds.). (2003). *Managing your practice: A guide for advanced practice nurses.* New York: Springer.

Mullahy, C. M. (2004). *The case manager's handbook,* 3rd ed. Gaithersburg, MD: Aspen.

National Association of Professional Geriatric Care Managers (NAPGCM). (2002). *Standards of practice.* Tucson, AZ: NAPGCM.

The Case Management Process

Hussein A. Tahan

Upon completion of this chapter, the reader will be able to:

1. List the six steps of the case management process.
2. Describe the process of patient identification and selection for case management services.
3. Discuss the difference between the case selection process and the assessment/problem identification process.
3. Explain the steps in the development and coordination of the case management plan and care activities.
4. Discuss the importance of the "evaluation and follow-up" step of the case management process and how it relates to the achievement of outcomes.
5. Explain the roles and benefits of continuous monitoring, re-assessment, and re-evaluation activities and how they are related to the evaluation and follow-up step.

IMPORTANT TERMS AND CONCEPTS

Advocacy	Client Selection
Assessment	Collaboration
Client Identification	Continuum of Care

Coordination	Monitoring
Evaluation	Outcomes
Implementation	Planning
Intervention	Problem Identification

■ INTRODUCTION

A. Case management is an interdisciplinary practice that focuses on the coordination of the care activities and the allocation of resources required by a patient during an acute or non-acute episode of illness.

B. A case manager manages, facilitates, and coordinates the necessary care activities and treatments, applying an approach to care delivery that is called the *case management process.*

C. The case manager also manages communication among the varied care providers and other essential parties internal and external to the health care organization.

D. The case management process focuses on the identification of patients who would benefit from case management services, and the activities of assessment, problem identification, care planning, care delivery, monitoring, and evaluation of the care provided, specifically for its relevance to the needs of the patient/family, and for the health care team's ability to meet the desired outcomes and established goals.

E. Each patient is unique, and the case management process takes into consideration the individual needs of the patient, family, and caregiver. This is not only limited to the patients' medical condition and treatment; rather, it includes their financial and psychosocial state, as well as their culture, values, and belief system.

F. Each case manager has her or his own unique style of case management based on one's own experience, education, skills, knowledge, ability, creativity, specialization (e.g., critical care, organ transplantation, rehabilitation, home care), professional discipline (e.g., nursing, social work, rehabilitation counselors, workers' compensation specialists), and professional networks.

G. The case management process is a set of steps applied by case managers in their approach to patient care management. It is similar to the nursing process (and other processes used by other disciplines such as social work and medicine).

   1. The nursing process is applied to the care of patients in a particular setting by all nurses in that setting.

   2. The case management process is used by case managers only in settings where case management is the delivery system in use (Cesta and Tahan, 2003).

This chapter is a revised version of what was previously published in the first edition of *CMSA Core Curriculum for Case Management*. The contributor wishes to acknowledge Patricia M. Pecqueux, as some of the timeless material was retained from the previous version.

3. The process of case management is much broader than the nursing process.
    a. The nursing process assesses the patient for changes in the physical, medical, psychosocial, cultural, and safety needs; plans how to meet these needs; implements these plans; and evaluates the results of these plans.
    b. The case management process entails—in addition to the activities assumed in the nursing process—collecting assessment data, including those before the onset of the current illness; assessing the environmental, financial, and support systems available to meet the identified needs; planning future care; and evaluating the impact of case management care delivery on both patient- and organization-based outcomes.

H. The case management process has been applied in the care of a select group of patients based on certain criteria determined by the health care organization. These criteria are the necessary factors that indicate the patient's need for case management services.
    1. In some organizations, the case managers screen all patients for case management services, identify their needs, and implement the case management process accordingly.

I. Some activities of the case management process may vary significantly based on the case management setting (preventive, pre-acute, acute, post-acute or managed care, ambulatory, hospital, community, home, skilled facilities, and so on) and the population served (pediatric, geriatric, behavioral health, and so on).
    1. Activities that may vary based on the above variables are case selection/identification, implementation of the case management plan of care, utilization management, transitional planning, and the necessary evaluation and follow up.
    2. Other activities of the case management process may apply to case management practice in many of the care settings. These activities are assessment/problem identification; development and coordination of the case management plan; and continuous monitoring, reassessing and re-evaluation.

J. Through the case management process, case managers eliminate fragmentation and/or duplication in care delivery. They also maintain open and timely communication with all parties involved in care in an effort to ensure continuity, safety, quality, and cost-effective outcomes.

K. The case management plan designed by the case manager in collaboration with the patient, family, and other health care providers identifies immediate, short-term, and ongoing needs, as well as where and how these care needs can be met.
    1. The plan sets goals and time frames for achieved goals that are appropriate to the individual and his or her family, and are agreed to by the patient or family and treatment team.

2. The case manager ensures that funding or community resources, or both, are available to support the implementation of the case management plan.

■ KEY DEFINITIONS

A. Advocacy—According to the Commission for Case Manager Certification (CCMC), advocacy is "acting on behalf of those who are not able to speak for or represent themselves. It is also defending others and acting in their best interest. A person or group involved in such activities is called an advocate" (CCMC, 2005a, p. 18).

B. Assessment—The collection of "in-depth information about a client's situation and functioning to identify individual needs and in order to develop a comprehensive case management plan that will address those needs. In addition to direct client contact, information should be gathered from other relevant sources (patient/client, professional caregivers, non-professional caregivers, employers, health records, education/military records, etc.) (CCMC, 2005b, p. 5).

C. Collaboration—Working together with the client/family, care providers, and other agents who are both internal and external to the health care organization for the purpose of achieving consensus on the case management plan and to maximize care outcomes (CMSA, 2002).

D. Continuum of care—"The continuum of care matches ongoing needs of the individuals being served by the case management process with the appropriate level and type of health, medical, financial, legal and psychosocial care for services within a setting or across multiple settings" (CCMC, 2005a, p. 3).

E. Coordination—"Organizing, securing, integrating, modifying, and documenting the resources necessary to accomplish the goals set forth in the case management plan" (CCMC, 2005b, p. 6).

F. Discharge planning—"The process of assessing the patient's needs of care after discharge from a health care facility and ensuring that the necessary services are in place before discharge. This process ensures a patient's timely, appropriate, and safe discharge to the next level of care or setting, including appropriate use of resources necessary for ongoing care" (CCMC, 2005a, p. 4).

G. Evaluation—"Determining and documenting the case management plan's effectiveness in reaching desired outcomes and goals. This might lead to a modification or change in the case management plan in its entirety or in any of its component parts" (CCMC, 2005b, p. 6). This activity is repeated at appropriate intervals and is adjusted or changed as necessary based on the plan and the client's condition.

H. Facilitation—An activity assumed by the case manager to promote communication among the client/family and the health care team members including the insurer. Facilitation also focuses on collaboration among all parties to achieve the case management goals and to ensure informed decisions (CMSA, 2002).

I. Implementation of the final plan—Linking the patient's assessed needs with private and community services, filling the gaps in care and services, avoiding duplication of services, and obtaining agreement on the plan of care from the patient and his or her support systems. The main goal in these activities is maximizing the safety and total well-being of the patient (Powell, 2000).

J. Implementation—"Executing and documenting specific case management activities and/or interventions that will lead to accomplishing the goals set forth in the case management plan" (CCMC, 2005b, p. 6).

K. Intervention—"Planned strategies and activities that [are employed to] modify a maladaptive behavior or state of being and facilitate growth and change. Intervention is analogous to the medical term *treatment*. Intervention may include activities such as advocacy, psychotherapy, or speech language therapy" (CCMC, 2005a, p. 5).

L. Monitoring—"Reviewing and gathering sufficient information from all relevant sources and its documentation regarding the case management plan, and its activities and/or services to enable the case manager to determine the plan's effectiveness" (CCMC, 2005b, p. 6).

M. Outcomes—"Measuring the [effectiveness of case management] interventions to determine the [impact] of case management (e.g., clinical, financial, variance, quality/quality of life, client satisfaction)" (CCMC, 2005b, p. 6).

N. Planning—"Determining and documenting specific [case management] objectives, goals, and actions designed to meet the client's needs as identified through the assessment process" (CCMC, 2005b, p. 5).

O. Problem identification—"Utilizing objective data gathered through careful assessment and examination of the potential for effective intervention, the case manager identifies problems requiring case management interventions, reflecting practice patterns and trends wherein client outcomes can be positively influenced" (CMSA, 2002, p. 14).

■ STEPS OF THE CASE MANAGEMENT PROCESS

A. The case management process is a systematic approach to patient care delivery and management.
  1. The process identifies what the case manager should do, and at what time intervals during the patient's course of treatment.
  2. The case manager works closely with the interdisciplinary team in implementing the case management process.
  3. The process consists of six steps that are executed as necessary and as indicated by the patient's condition or the demands of the health care delivery system.

B. Step 1: Client identification/selection—Focuses on identifying clients who would benefit from case management services.
  1. In some health care organizations, it is considered the first step in the case management process. In some others, it is viewed as being unnecessary due to the fact that case managers may follow all types

of patients regardless of acuity levels, intensity of services and resources required, or needs.

2. In organizations where selection is necessary, the case manager identifies the clients who will most benefit from case management services based on certain criteria specific to the organization.

3. According to the Case Management Society of America (CMSA), identification of clients for case management services is accomplished through the use of methods and tools that include, but are not limited to:
   a. Health-risk screening;
   b. Evidence-based criteria;
   c. Risk stratification through data management; and
   d. Referrals from other health care providers such as physicians and clinical nurses (CMSA, 2002).

4. Client identification/selection may be applied in the evaluation of individuals who are referred by other health care providers to the case manager for the purpose of providing case management services.
   a. The case manager decides whether to accept the individual based on an established set of criteria developed by the health care organization where she or he works.
   b. The criteria applied enable the case manager to determine whether the patient needs case management services and the type of services that will be needed.

5. Criteria for case management services are not limited to a single condition or diagnosis. For example, sentinel or significant/reportable events may be considered by some organizations as automatic situations that necessitate full case management services and follow up by case managers.

6. Through client identification and selection, the case manager is able to systematically review all patients' situations and select those individuals who absolutely need case management services and would benefit from them the most. This activity is essential for streamlining the case managers' workloads and to allow them to spend their time and efforts where they are needed the most.

7. During the client identification/selection step, case managers determine the necessity for case management services using a rapid and brief assessment or a special screening tool. Not all patients need a case manager. Case management may *not* be necessary if:
   a. The patient meets intensity of services and severity of illness criteria;
   b. No major discharge barriers are identified;
   c. If readmission to the hospital or service is not a concern; and
   d. There are no financial or psychosocial barriers present.

8. Case management may be necessary when there are:
   a. Complex medical issues or comorbidities;
   b. Needs for complex and costly services/resources;
   c. Complex discharge needs;
   d. Complex psychosocial issues;

    e. Risks for untoward events including legal/ethical concerns; or

    f. Compromised financial situations or absence of health insurance.

9. Selection criteria can be generic and applicable across care settings and levels of care or specific to a population or setting. Regardless, they must be based on issues that may affect length of stay or service, quality, safety, and cost of care. Their use by case managers should be based on the condition and anticipated needs of the patient (Cesta and Tahan, 2003).

10. Selection criteria must be prospectively identified by an organization and communicated to all staff in a case management policy or procedure format.

11. Avoid exclusively using length-of-stay and claims data as selection criteria. These criteria are late indicators of case management needs. By the time the patient has exceeded the established length of stay and maximum dollar expenditure for the diagnosis, much case management intervention could have already taken place.

12. The selection criteria are to be used with caution or in conjunction with other factors. They may include, but are not limited to, the following:

    a. Lives alone or with someone with a disability

    b. Age over 65 years

    c. Payer source; for example, managed care type insurance/health plans

    d. Readmission, or readmissions within 15 days

    e. Multiple physician involvement including specialists

    f. Overdose (unintentional/intentional)

    g. Chemical dependency (alcohol and drugs)

    h. Eating disorder (e.g., bulimia, anorexia nervosa, failure to thrive)

    i. Chronic mental illness

    j. Alzheimer/dementia

    k. Noncompliance

    l. Uncooperative, manipulative, or aggressive behavior

    m. Coexisting behavioral and physical conditions

    n. Miscellaneous conditions (Munchausen syndrome)

    o. Socioeconomic indicators

    p. Suspected child or elder abuse and neglect

    q. Victim of violent crime

    r. Homelessness

    s. Poor living environment

    t. No known social or family support system

    u. Admission from an extended care facility (ECF) or sheltered living arrangement

    v. Need for transitional care in an ECF or sheltered living arrangement

    w. Out-of-state or out-of-country residence, undocumented immigrants

    x. Residence in rural community with limited or nonexistent services

    y. Limited or no financial resources

  z. Absence of or inadequate health insurance

 aa. Single or first-time parent

 bb. Dependent in activities of daily living; inability to shop for groceries, drive, or cook for self

 cc. Repeated admissions to acute care

 dd. Frequent visits to the emergency room (ER), family physician, or clinic

 ee. Disruptive or obstructive family member or significant other

C. Step 2: Assessment and problem identification—This step of the process begins after the completion of the case selection and intake into case management.

 1. A thorough assessment must be done at this point in order to determine the needs of the patients, particularly as they relate to the treatment and transitional/discharge plans.

 2. An inaccurate or poor assessment can lead to an unsafe discharge plan.

 3. Sources of assessment data are:

  a. Patient and family/caregiver

  b. Family physician or primary care provider

  c. Office and hospital medical records, including old and current emergency department records

  d. Ancillary staff

  e. Employers

  f. Other external agencies such as extended/skilled care facilities and home care services.

 4. The assessment must be comprehensive and address the following:

  a. Patient's health demographics and history

  b. Appropriateness for admission to the level of care or setting the patient is in

  c. Current medical status, including the chief complaint that prompted the patient to seek medical care

  d. Nutritional status

  e. Adjustment to illness

  f. Health education needs

  g. Medication assessment

  h. Financial assessment including health insurance, certification/authorization status

  i. Functional assessment and environmental factors

   i. Home environment assessment

   ii. Activities of daily living (ADLs and IADLs) assessment

  j. Psychosocial assessment, including family and support systems

  k. Cultural, spiritual, and religious characteristics

 5. Based on the assessment data and findings, case managers are able to:

  a. Identify the actual and potential problems to be addressed;

   b. Set the goals of the treatment;

   c. Identify the necessary interventions and strategies that will need to be incorporated in the case management plan of care in order to achieve the goals; and

   d. Determine the resources needed for addressing these problems.

D. Step 3: Development of the case management plan—The case management plan is necessary to establish goals of the treatment and to prioritize the patient's needs as well as determine the types of services and resources required to meet the established goals/desired outcomes.

   1. The case management plan is multidisciplinary in nature and requires input from those involved in the care of the patient as well as the patient and family.

   2. A well-developed case management plan helps decrease the risk for incomplete tasks or inappropriate care. It also provides a seamless approach to care that supports the standards of accreditation and regulatory agencies.

   3. Case managers may answer the following questions to ensure the appropriateness of the case management plan:

      a. What are the patient's and family's problems that need to be addressed in this episode of care? Are the patient and family in agreement with these problems?

      b. What are the treatment goals and desired outcomes the health care team must accomplish?

      c. What are the necessary interventions (both diagnostic and therapeutic) that would address these problems and goals?

      d. What timeframe should be established for meeting the goals and outcomes?

      e. What are the barriers to meeting the goals and the desired outcomes?

   4. The case management plan is used by all disciplines and providers when caring for the patient. The case manager facilitates the development of the plan and the revision of plan as she or he engages in ongoing assessment and reassessment of the patient's condition and the goals of treatment.

E. Step 4: Implementation and coordination of care activities—In this step the case manager puts the case management plan into action.

F. Step 4 also encompasses all the interventions indicated in the plan that are meant to meet the treatment goals and resolve the patient's problems or presenting chief complaint.

   1. Implementation and coordination requires case managers to reassess the patient's condition on an ongoing basis looking for:

      a. Resolution of the identified problems;

      b. Status of the treatment goals and the transitional plan; and

      c. Whether new needs have arisen that require modification in the plan.

   2. In this step, case managers continue to obtain certifications/authorizations for care and services from managed care organizations as

needed. They engage in concurrent reviews as well as follow up on any outstanding issues with the insurer or members of the health care team.

3. Case managers facilitate and coordinate the work of the health care team in an effort to promote cost-effective, safe, and efficient care. This may include:

   a. The required tests and procedures;

   b. Patient and family education;

   c. Discharge/transitional planning;

   d. Brokerage of services such as specialty consultations, physical therapy, and home care services; and

   e. Completion of all required paperwork such as those needed for the placement of patients in skilled nursing or rehabilitation facilities.

4. For effective implementation and coordination of the case management plan, case managers work closely with:

   a. Health care providers internal to the organizations that employ them, such as physicians, social workers, and physical therapists

   b. Key health care providers and agents external to the organizations, including staff from transportation agencies, durable medical equipment companies, home care agencies, charitable organizations, and skilled nursing facilities

5. Case managers address the family's needs to help members of the patient's family cope with illness and sometimes hospitalization. These may include:

   a. The need for hope and the need for information about their family member's condition (seen by the patient's family as the most important of all the needs identified)

   b. Communicating accurate information to the family to enable them to make informed decisions, thereby assisting them to gain understanding and a feeling of control over a difficult situation (Powell, 2000)

6. For effective implementation of the case management plan and for ensuring that it is patient- and family-centered, case managers may answer the following questions:

   a. Does the patient/family have any new needs that must be incorporated into the case management plan?

   b. Are the patient, family, and health care team in agreement with the plan?

   c. What is the appropriate timeframe for implementing the treatments and interventions? Is this timeframe appropriate for resolving the identified problems?

   d. Does the transitional/discharge plan meet the patient's condition and needs?

   e. Have all the necessary authorizations for treatment and services been obtained?

   f. Have the barriers to meeting the plan been addressed or resolved?

G. Step 5: Evaluation of the case management plan and follow up—This step involves the evaluation of the patient care activities and treatments, and the associated outcomes.

H. Case managers complete this evaluation by examining the patient's condition and the status of the goals and desired outcomes. During these activities, case managers may answer the following questions:

1. Are the activities and outcomes on target?
2. Is care progressing according to the case management plan?
3. Are treatments occurring as per the established timeline?
4. Is the patient ready for discharge?
5. Is the patient being cared for in the appropriate level of care or setting?
6. Are there any issues with reimbursement? Have all required authorizations been obtained?
7. Does the case management plan meet the needs and interests of the patient and family?
8. Are there any legal or ethical risks present?
9. What modifications in the case management plan are necessary?

I. Case managers continuously monitor and reassess the patient's condition, responses to interventions, and progress toward recovery. Such activities are necessary for ensuring timely care delivery and patient-focused modifications of the plan.

J. Case managers also ensure that the discharge/transition plan is safe and that the patient and family are satisfied with care.

K. During the evaluation and follow-up step, case managers are able to identify any variances or delays in the care and address them immediately as indicated. These activities ensure that care is efficient, safe, and cost effective.

L. Step 6: Termination of the case management process—This step brings closure to the care and the episode of illness. It focuses on discontinuing the case management services and the transition of the patient to a community-based level of care including the patient's home.

1. Case managers determine the need for terminating the case management services based on the patient's and family's condition or choice, the health care team, or the payer/insurer.
2. Situations that require termination of case management services may include, but are not limited to, the following:
   a. Achievement of targeted goals and outcomes;
   b. Required change in health care setting or level of care;
   c. Loss of or change in the benefits;
   d. Patient/family wishes;
   e. Case manager is no longer able to provide case management services;
   f. Patient and family met maximum benefit from case management services; and

g. Patient and/or family exhibit nonadherent behaviors to the case management plan of care (CMSA, 2002).

3. When terminating the case management process and/or services, case managers must provide ample notice and explanation to the patient, family, and health care team members. Such decisions should be discussed with all involved in the care and must be made based on the situations shared above.

M. Throughout the case management process, case managers engage in other necessary activities. These activities are applicable to almost all of the steps of the case management process. They are: advocacy, continuous monitoring, re-assessment, and re-evaluation.

1. Advocacy focuses on being patient- and family-centered in the case management activities; that is, meeting the patient and family needs, interests, and wishes, and ensuring that care activities and decisions focus on what is in the best interest of the patient and family.

2. Continuous monitoring where the case manager uses a method of checking, regulating, and documenting the quality of care, services, and products delivered to the patient to determine whether the goals of the case management plan are being achieved, or whether the goals remain appropriate and realistic.

3. Re-assessment is similar to continuous monitoring and focuses on frequently examining the patient's and family's condition and the status of the plan of care looking for data that allows the case manager to decide whether the case management plan is on target or if it requires any modifications.

4. Re-evaluation is an activity case managers engage in especially after they institute action such as examining whether their attempts to expedite the reporting of test results or to counteract the effects of a delay in care have been successful, and if not, to determine the next necessary steps.

5. The frequency of these activities depends on the care setting or level of care where case management services are provided. For example, case management services in a hospital setting may require more frequent follow up (e.g., hourly) than for an individual in a private home (e.g., few times a week), clinic (e.g., quarterly), or extended care facility (e.g., weekly).

6. Re-assessment, monitoring, and re-evaluation may be necessary if there is:
   a. Change in the patient's medical condition;
   b. Change in the patient's social stability and network;
   c. Quality of care issue;
   d. Risk management issue;
   e. Concern regarding the transitional/discharge plan;
   f. Change in the patient's functional capacity and mobility;
   g. Evolving educational need; or
   h. Issues in the availability of community resources/services.

N. Case managers may decide to repeat the case management process at any time during the episode of care or they may revisit any of the six steps.

1. Engaging in activities such as continuous monitoring, re-assessment, and re-evaluation requires the case managers to go through every step of the case management process. This is important to assess whether a goal has been met or an outcome needs to be revisited.
2. Repeating the process is one way of ensuring that care activities are being completed as predetermined, the transitional/discharge plan is safe, and care is of utmost quality, efficient, and cost effective.

O. Throughout the case management process, case managers:
1. Document their observations, decisions, actions/interventions, and outcomes in the patients' records
2. Keep a record of their assessment, monitoring, and evaluation findings
3. Keep a record of the modifications they make to the case management plan, including the rationale
4. Document their interactions with the patient/family, the insurer/payer, and other health care providers/agents internal and external to their organization

REFERENCES

Case Management Society of America (CMSA). (2002). *Standards of practice for case management.* Little Rock, AR: CMSA.

Cesta, T. G., & Tahan, H. A. (2003). *The case manager's survival guide: Winning strategies for clinical practice,* 2nd ed. St Louis, MO: Mosby.

Commission for Case Manager Certification (CCMC). (2005a). *CCM glossary of terms.* Rolling Meadows, IL: Author. Website: *www.ccmcertification.org/pages/22frame_set.html.* Accessed March 23, 2006.

Commission for Case Manager Certification (CCMC). (2005b). *CCM certification guide.* Rolling Meadows, IL: Author.

Powell, S. K. (2000). *Case management: A practical guide to success in managed care.* Philadelphia: Lippincott Williams & Wilkins.

SUGGESTED READING

Daniels, S., and Ramey, M. (2005). *The leader's guide to hospital case management.* Sudbury, MA: Jones and Bartlet.

Kongstvedt, P. R. (2003). *Essentials of managed health care,* 4th ed. Gaithersburg, MD: Aspen.

Mullahy, C. M. (2004). *The case manager's handbook,* 3rd ed. Gaithersburg, MD: Aspen.

Todd, W., & Nash, D. (1996). *Disease management: A systems approach to improving patient outcomes.* Chicago: American Hospital Publishing.

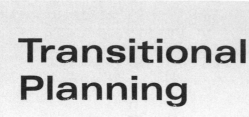

chapter 10

Transitional Planning

Jackie Birmingham

LEARNING OBJECTIVES

Upon completion of this chapter, the reader will be able to:

1. Define transitional planning.
2. Differentiate between transitional planning and discharge planning.
3. List the key federal Conditions of Participation that influence transitional and discharge planning in an acute care setting.
4. Discuss the role of the case manager in the process of transitional planning.
   a. Role of provider-based case manager
   b. Role of payer-based case manager
   c. Role of case manager in post-acute settings such as nursing facilities, home health agencies, and inpatient rehabilitation facilities
5. List and describe selected levels of care that make up the continuum of care.
   a. Conditions of Participation for all levels of care
6. Discuss transitional planning resources for case managers.
   a. Joint Commission on Accreditation of Health Care Organizations (JCAHO)
   b. American Osteopathic Association (AOA)
   c. Case Management Adherence Guidelines (CMAG)

d. National Guidelines Clearinghouse (AHRQ—Agency for Healthcare Research and Quality, Department of Health and Human Services)

IMPORTANT TERMS AND CONCEPTS

Appropriateness: Continued Stay
Assessment of Continuing Care
  Needs Status
At Risk for Adverse Outcome
Care Fragmentation
Conditions of Participation (CoPs)
Continuity of Care
Decision-Making Capacity
Discharge Planning
Discharge Status

Functional Status
Handoff
Levels of Care
Nondiscrimination in Referral Selection
Prospective Payment System (PPS)
Readmission
Referral
Transfers
Transitional Care Unit (TCU)
Transitional Planning

■ INTRODUCTION

The concept of transitional planning is based on "continuity of care." Case management and the process of transitional planning are relatively new concepts in health care delivery. Prior to the implementation of payment methods that influenced where and when health care services were delivered, the primary setting of health care delivery for persons with active health problems was in a hospital, and those with chronic diagnoses depended on physician office visits. As the post-acute health care delivery system developed into a viable alternative to acute care, the movement of patients between levels increased. Navigating through the acute to post-acute and chronic-acute to post-acute system was, and is, very complex. Case management grew out of this phenomenon as a way to help transition patients from one level of care to another while maintaining quality of and access to needed services, while simultaneously managing costs.

■ KEY DEFINITIONS

A. Conditions of Participation— The Centers for Medicare and Medicaid Services (CMS) develops Conditions of Participation (CoPs) that health care organizations must meet to participate in the Medicare and Medicaid programs. These standards are used to improve quality and protect the health and safety of beneficiaries. The CMS also ensures that the standards of accrediting organizations recognized by the CMS, such as the Joint Commission on the Accreditation of Healthcare Organizations (JCAHO) or the American Osteopathic Association (AOA), through a process called *deeming*, meet or exceed Medicare standards as stated in the CoP. The standards apply to anyone receiving services, regardless of payment source.

1. Discharge planning—CoPs are associated directly with the hospital's responsibility for discharge planning.
2. Patients' rights—CoPs are associated with assuring that patients' rights to freedom of choice and other issues are followed.

3. Medical records—CoPs are associated with the patient's inpatient medical record and the need to ensure that the closed record contains information related to the course of the hospital stay and plans for follow-up care.

B. Continuity of care—The coordination of care received by a patient over time and across multiple health care providers and settings.

C. Discharge—The formal release, or signing out by a physician, of a patient from an episode of care. The episode of care can be from hospital inpatient status, observation status, or emergency room stay. A discharge can also be applied to an inpatient skilled nursing facility, acute and subacute rehabilitation facility, or a home health episode of care.

   1. Discharge status—Disposition of the patient at discharge indicating to what level of care a patient has been transferred or discharged. Discharge status, particularly from acute care, has significance in how a hospital is paid, and in how health care organizations track care. Because of this, there are specific codes that are assigned to the various types of dispositions (Table 10-1).

   2. Leaving Against Medical Advice (LAMA) or Against Medical Advice (AMA)—A term used to describe a patient who is discharged from the hospital against the advice of his or her attending physician. The person signing out is usually asked to sign a form stating his or her awareness that the discharge is against medical advice.

   3. Patient elopement—A term used to describe a situation in which a patient leaves without the knowledge of the hospital staff. The patient is then determined to be "missing."

D. Discharge planning—The process of assessing the patient's needs of care after discharge from a health care facility and ensuring that the necessary services are in place before discharge. This process ensures a patient's timely, appropriate, and safe discharge to the next level of care or setting, including appropriate use of resources necessary for ongoing care (CCMC, 2005).

E. Functional status—The assessment of an individual's ability to manage his or her own care needs.

   1. Activities of daily living (ADL)—Activities that are considered an everyday part of normal life. These include dressing, bathing, toileting, transferring (e.g., moving from and into a chair), and eating. The functional levels of ADLs are used to measure the degree of impairment and can affect eligibility for certain types of insurance benefits.

   2. Instrumental activities of daily living (IADL)—Regularly necessary home management activities, including meal preparation, housework, grocery shopping, and other similar activities.

   3. Executive function—An integrated set of cognitive abilities that allow an individual to process available information in planning, prioritizing, sequencing, self-monitoring, self-correcting, inhibiting, initiating, controlling, or altering behavior. It includes evaluation of such parameters as "capacity" and "competency." Evaluating a patient's executive function is a multidisciplinary process involving physicians,

TABLE 10–1
Disposition Codes Used at the Time of Discharge

Code	Description
01	**Discharged to home or self-care (routine discharge).** Includes: discharged on home oxygen or home DME services (without home health), court/law enforcement, residential care, foster care.
02*	**Discharged/transferred to a short-term general hospital for inpatient care.** Use this code to bill a same-day transfer claim for an inpatient claim. The "from" and "through" dates in the statement coverage period (FL6) must be the same. Use condition code 40—same-day transfer (FLs 24–30), and show the one day as noncovered in FL 8 with the noncovered charges reported in FL 48.
03†	**Discharged/transferred to SNF with Medicare certification in anticipation of covered skilled care** *(effective 2/23/05)*. Indicates that the patient is discharged/transferred to a Medicare-certified skilled nursing bed and qualifies for skilled care (regardless of whether the patient has skilled benefit days). For hospitals with an approved swing bed arrangement, use Code 61—swing bed. For reporting transfers to nursing facilities see 04 and 64.
04	**Discharged/transferred to an intermediate care facility (ICF).** Typically defined at the state level for specifically designated intermediate care facilities. Also used to designate patients who are discharged/transferred to a nursing facility with neither Medicare nor Medicaid certification and for discharges/transfers to state-designated assisted living facilities. For transfers to dual-certified facilities, confirm level of care with physician/discharge planner, i.e., skilled (03), hospice (50/51), or intermediate care (04).
05†	**Discharged/transferred to another type of institution not defined elsewhere in this code list** *(effective 2/23/05)*. Cancer hospitals excluded from Medicare PPS and children's hospitals are examples of such other types of institutions. Includes: chemical dependency treatment facility that is not part of a hospital; patient transferred from hospital-based SNF to observation; discharge from acute care to another acute care facility for outpatient procedure with intention that patient will not be returning to the first acute care facility following the procedure.
06†	**Discharged/transferred to home under care of organized home health service organization in anticipation of covered skilled care** *(effective 2/23/05)*. Report this code when the patient is discharged/transferred to home with a written plan of care for home care services.
07	**Left against medical advice or discontinued care.** Effective April 1, 2004, these claims are treated as transfers if the patient is subsequently admitted to another inpatient PPS hospital on the same day. Medicare PM A-03-073, August 22, 2003.
20	**Expired.** (Or did not recover—Christian Science patient.)
43	**Discharged/transferred to a federal hospital (VA hospital).** Use whenever the destination at discharge is a federal hospital, whether or not the patient lives there.
50	**Discharged to hospice—home**
51	**Discharged to hospice—medical facility**
61	**Discharged/transferred to a hospital-based Medicare-approved swing bed**
62†	**Discharged/transferred to a rehab facility, including rehabilitation unit as distinct part of a hospital**

TABLE 10-1
Disposition Codes Used at the Time of Discharge (*continued*)

Code	Description
63[†]	**Discharged/transferred to a long-term care hospital** (Long-term hospitals provide acute inpatient care with an average LOS >25 days, provider numbers include XX2000–XX2299.)
64	**Discharged/transferred to a nursing facility certified under Medicaid but not certified under Medicare.** Acute care hospitals, SNFs, outpatient hospital providers are required to report this code, if appropriate, although the use of this code does not impact payment.
65[†]	**Discharged/transferred to a psychiatric hospital or psychiatric unit as distinct part of a hospital**
66	**Discharged/transferred to a critical access hospital** (*effective for discharges after 1/1/06*).

*Each transferring hospital is paid a per diem rate, not to exceed the full DRG payment that would have been made if the patient had been discharged without being transferred.
†Affects reimbursement if assigned to one of 182 select DRGs.
From Centers for Medicare & Medicaid Services (CMS) (2005). Completing and processing the form CMS-150 data set. In Medicare claims and processing manual (Chap. 25). Retrieved from *http://www.cms.hhs.gov/manuals/downloads/clm104c25.pdf*

nurses, social workers, and other health care professionals and can, in some situations, involve the court system (Cooney et al., 2004).

F. Handoff—The exchange of a patient's care between incoming and outgoing caregivers; any transfer of role and responsibility from one person to another or one setting to another. Successful handoffs overcome barriers such as physical setting, social setting, language and communication barriers, and time and convenience (Solet et al., 2005).

G. Level of care—Different kinds and locations of care provided to patients, based on a scale of intensity or amount of care/services provided.
   1. Acute level of care—The most intense level of care related to necessity for medical (physician) services.
   2. Sub-acute level of care—The level of care that combines a high need for nursing, therapy, and physician services. Intermediate between acute and chronic, this level of care can be provided in acute care facilities or other facilities as determined by licensing in each state.
   3. Transitional care unit (TCU)—A unit of care, usually in a hospital, that is dedicated to supporting a patient's transition of care from acute to a lesser level of care. The level of care is similar to sub-acute.
   4. Skilled nursing facility (SNF)—A facility offering 24-hour skilled nursing care along with rehabilitation services, such as physical, speech, and occupational therapy; assistance with personal care activities, such as eating, walking, toileting, and bathing; coordinated management of patient care; social services; and activities. Some nursing facilities offer specialized care programs for Alzheimer disease or other illnesses, or short-term respite care for frail or disabled persons

when a family member requires a break from providing care in the home. Payment for a stay in an SNF varies depending on the payer criteria, whether the patient was an inpatient in a hospital for 3 consecutive days, and the reason for admission.

5. Home health care services—Care provided to individuals and families in their place of residence for the purpose of promoting, maintaining, or restoring health; or for minimizing the effects of disability and illness, including terminal illness. Patients must meet the definition of homebound status, and require intermittent professional services, including nursing, physical therapy, occupational and speech language services, or social work services. Eligibility criteria for insurance coverage for home care services vary between payer groups.

6. Hospice—A program that provides special care for people who are near the end of life and for their families, either at home, in freestanding facilities, or within hospitals.

H. Prospective payment system (PPS)—A method of reimbursement used by CMS that bases Medicare payments on a predetermined, fixed amount. The payment amount derived for a particular episode of care is based on a classification system of a specific level of care and an episode of care, e.g., *diagnosis related groups* (DRGs) classification for inpatient hospital services, *resource utilization groups* (RUGs) classification for nursing facilities; *home health resource groups* (HHRGs) classification for home health agencies.

1. Diagnosis related groups (DRGs)—The system used to pay for acute inpatient care that is based primarily on the patient's principal diagnosis.

2. Resource utilization groups (RUGs)—The system used to pay for care provided in a nursing facility that is based on the amount, intensity, and type of "resources used," including nursing care and therapies.

3. Home health resource groups (HHRGs): The system used to pay home health agencies for services based on the resources used and the duration of the services.

I. Readmission—The admission of a patient back into the hospital, for the same disease or condition as the previous admission. Some payers review both admissions if they occur within a specified number of days, e.g., 72 hours or 15 or 30 days. Readmission is the focus of a great deal of attention by health professionals and regulators (Phillips et al., 2004).

J. Referral—The process of sending a patient from one practitioner to another for health care services; in the case of transitional planning, usually for services related to the current episode of care (e.g., rehabilitation consultation).

K. Transfer—The planned action of sending a patient from one place of care to another. It can be to the same level of care (acute to acute) or to a lower level of care (acute to post-acute), or vice versa. The planning of the transfer involves notification of the next level of care and the transfer of necessary medical information.

L. Transfer/Qualified DRG—A situation in which a patient's care is coded as being within a predetermined list of DRGs, the patient is discharged to either a skilled nursing facility or home health agency for services related to the reason for hospitalization, and the patient is transferred before the national geometric length of stay for that DRG. Because the patient is determined to be leaving prior to the number of days in that DRG, and because the patient is receiving continuing care for which Medicare is paying, the hospital is paid only for the days of care provided, and not the full DRG.

M. Transitional planning—The process that case managers apply to ensure that appropriate resources and services are provided to patients and that these services are provided in the most appropriate setting or level of care, as delineated in the standards and guidelines of regulatory and accreditation agencies. It focuses on moving a patient from the most complex to less complex care settings (CCMC, 2005).

■ TRANSITIONAL PLANNING

A. Transitional planning generally refers to care and services that promote the safe and timely transfer of patients from one level of care to another (e.g., acute to sub-acute, intensive/critical care unit in a hospital to a regular patient care unit), or from one type of setting to another (e.g., hospital to home). It focuses on moving a patient from the most complex to less complex care settings, or in some cases the reverse, should the patient require more intense services.

B. Case managers apply their special care-related functions and responsibilities to ensure that appropriate resources and services are available to patients in the most appropriate setting or level of care.

C. Case managers in all settings participate in the transitional care process. Case managers work for payers; providers, including hospitals, nursing homes, and home health agencies; workers' compensation; and community-based programs for the elderly.

D. Transitional planning is a set of actions designed to ensure the coordination and continuity of health care services and resources as patients transfer between different locations or different levels of care in the same location.
    1. The time frame for transitional planning primarily concerns the relatively brief time interval that begins with preparing a patient to leave one setting and concludes when the patient is received in the next setting.
    2. Transitions may be unplanned, result from unanticipated medical problems, occur during off hours such as at night and on weekends, involve clinicians who may not have an ongoing relationship with the patient, and happen so quickly that formal and informal support mechanisms cannot respond in a timely manner.
        During transitions between settings or levels of care, patients are particularly vulnerable to care fragmentation and risk for medical errors.

■ DIFFERENTIATING BETWEEN TRANSITIONAL CARE PLANNING AND DISCHARGE PLANNING

A. Transitional care planning is a general term that is used to describe the focused planning for patients who are moving through the health care system.

B. Discharge planning is a term generally applied to the process in which patients in an acute care setting are assessed for continuing care needs required after discharge from an acute setting.

1. Discharge planning is a specialty process within transitional planning.
2. Discharge planning is mandated by federal regulations.
3. The process involves identifying patients who are at risk for adverse outcomes after discharge without specific interventions.
   a. All patients are required to have a discharge plan, but not all patients require the detailed interventions required by regulations.
   b. Determining whether the patient's ongoing needs are related to the reason for admission to an acute care setting, or if the ongoing needs are related to a chronic health condition or non-acute health problem, is involved. Reimbursement for post-acute services depends on the origin of the need (acute vs. chronic).
   c. Assessment of the patient's post-acute care needs is based on the patient's predicted functional status and the capacity for self-care and management.
   d. Level of care determinations are based on the patient's assessed functional needs at or near the time of discharge. Functional assessment is a more reliable predictor of level of care than is the patient's principal diagnosis.
   e. The focus of discharge planning is moving the patient from the complex-acute care health system to the next appropriate level of care, which is usually less complex. Patients may need to move through two or three levels before they are in the least complex setting.
   f. The least complex setting can be described as the level of care where the patient is stabilized from a functional point of view and has reached his or her maximum capacity for self-care.
   g. Although case managers participate in discharge planning activities, it is the physician who determines the patient's readiness for discharge and appropriateness of the next level of care based on the patient's health condition and needs.

■ PROFESSIONAL STANDARDS FOR TRANSITIONAL AND DISCHARGE PLANNING

A. Transitional planning has been mandated by federal agencies in the form of legislation, by accreditation agencies in the form of accreditation or professional performance standards, and by professional organizations and societies in the form of policies or practice guidelines.

B. Currently, there are specific case management standards and guidelines available that explain the roles and responsibilities of case managers in both transitional and discharge planning. These standards are advocated for by case management professional organizations such as the Commission for Case Manager Certification (CCMC) and the Case Management Society of America (CMSA), and others that promote case management practice such as the American Nurses Association (ANA) and the National Association of Social Workers (NASW).

C. Transitional or discharge planning is one of the core knowledge areas covered in the CCMC's case manager certification examination. This topic addresses specific knowledge that pertains to case management practice, including the continuum of care, levels of care and services, care planning and goal setting, community services and resources, rehabilitation services and support programs, assistive technologies and durable medical equipment, continuity of care, and benefit programs.

D. Transitional and discharge planning standards are also addressed in the CMSA's Case Management Standards of Practice. In this regard, the standards discuss the roles and responsibilities of the case manager in care planning, including identification of needs and development of short- and long-term goals; planning with the patient and family and obtaining their consent to the transitional plan; working with other professionals internal and external to the organization to meet the patient's and family's needs; brokering of services and procurement of health care resources as needed by the patient; and working in concert within payer demands and expectations.

■ REGULATIONS AFFECTING TRANSITIONAL AND DISCHARGE PLANNING

A. Hospitals—Discharge planning (Box 10-1).

B. Clinical records—The requirement that a discharge summary be completed and available to the next care provider(s) is included in health care regulations for providers of services (e.g., hospitals, home health agencies, critical access hospitals, and specialty care hospitals, including psychiatric facilities).
   1. All patient medical records must contain a discharge summary. A discharge summary discusses the primary plan of care as received by the patient during the acute phase of illness and treatment, the outcomes of the hospitalization, the disposition of the patient, and the relevant provisions for follow-up care.
   2. Follow-up care provisions include any post-hospital appointments, how post-hospital patient care needs are to be met, and any plans for post-hospital care by providers such as home health services, hospice care, nursing homes, or assisted living facilities.

C. Patient rights—Throughout the Medicare program literature, reference is made to patients' rights to participate in planning for their own care.

BOX 10–1
Conditions of Participation for Discharge Planning
• •

TITLE 42—PUBLIC HEALTH/CHAPTER IV—CENTERS FOR MEDICARE & MEDICAID SERVICES, DEPARTMENT OF HEALTH AND HUMAN SERVICES

PART 482—CONDITIONS OF PARTICIPATION FOR HOSPITALS— Subpart C: Basic Hospital Functions/Sec. 482.43: Conditions of participation: Discharge planning.

The hospital must have in effect a discharge planning process that applies to all patients. The hospital's policies and procedures must be specified in writing.

(a) *Standard: Identification of patients in need of discharge planning.* The hospital must identify at an early stage of hospitalization all patients who are likely to suffer adverse health consequences upon discharge if there is no adequate discharge planning.

(b) *Standard: Discharge planning evaluation.*

(1) The hospital must provide a discharge planning evaluation to the patients identified in paragraph (a) of this section, and to other patients upon the patient's request, the request of a person acting on the patient's behalf, or the request of the physician.

(2) A registered nurse, social worker, or other appropriately qualified personnel must develop, or supervise the development of the evaluation.

(3) The discharge planning evaluation must include an evaluation of the likelihood of a patient needing post-hospital services and of the availability of the services.

(4) The discharge planning evaluation must include an evaluation of the likelihood of a patient's capacity for self-care or of the possibility of the patient being cared for in the environment from which he or she entered the hospital.

(5) The hospital personnel must complete the evaluation on a timely basis so that appropriate arrangements for post-hospital care are made before discharge, and to avoid unnecessary delays in discharge.

(6) The hospital must include the discharge planning evaluation in the patient's medical record for use in establishing an appropriate discharge plan and must discuss the results of the evaluation with the patient or individual acting on his or her behalf.

(c) *Standard: Discharge plan.*

(1) A registered nurse, social worker, or other appropriately qualified personnel must develop, or supervise the development of, a discharge plan if the discharge planning evaluation indicates a need for a discharge plan.

(2) In the absence of a finding by the hospital that a patient needs a discharge plan, the patient's physician may request a discharge plan. In such a case, the hospital must develop a discharge plan for the patient.

BOX 10–1

Conditions of Participation for Discharge Planning (*continued*)
• •

(3) The hospital must arrange for the initial implementation of the patient's discharge plan.

(4) The hospital must reassess the patient's discharge plan if there are factors that may affect continuing care needs or the appropriateness of the discharge plan.

(5) As needed, the patient and family members or interested persons must be counseled to prepare them for post-hospital care.

(6) The hospital must include in the discharge plan a list of HHAs or SNFs that are available to the patient, that are participating in the Medicare program, and that serve the geographic area (as defined by the HHA) in which the patient resides, or in the case of a SNF, in the geographic area requested by the patient. HHAs must request to be listed by the hospital as available.

(i) This list must only be presented to patients for whom home health care or post-hospital extended care services are indicated and appropriate as determined by the discharge planning evaluation.

(ii) For patients enrolled in managed care organizations, the hospital must indicate the availability of home health and post-hospital extended care services through individuals and entities that have a contract with the managed care organizations.

(iii) The hospital must document in the patient's medical record that the list was presented to the patient or to the individual acting on the patient's behalf.

(7) The hospital, as part of the discharge planning process, must inform the patient or the patient's family of their freedom to choose among participating Medicare providers of post-hospital care services and must, when possible, respect patient and family preferences when they are expressed. The hospital must not specify or otherwise limit the qualified providers that are available to the patient.

(8) The discharge plan must identify any HHA or SNF to which the patient is referred in which the hospital has a disclosable financial interest, as specified by the Secretary, and any HHA or SNF that has a disclosable financial interest in a hospital under Medicare. Financial interests that are disclosable under Medicare are determined in accordance with the provisions of Part 420, Subpart C, of this chapter.

(d) *Standard: Transfer or referral.* The hospital must transfer or refer patients, along with necessary medical information, to appropriate facilities, agencies, or outpatient services, as needed, for follow-up or ancillary care.

(e) *Standard: Reassessment.* The hospital must reassess its discharge planning process on an ongoing basis. The reassessment must include

---

BOX 10–1

Conditions of Participation for Discharge Planning (*continued*)

• •

a review of discharge plans to ensure that they are responsive to discharge needs.

> [Code of Federal Regulations]
> [Title 42, Volume 3]
> [Revised as of October 1, 2004]
> From the U.S. Government Printing Office via GPO Access
> [CITE: 42CFR482.43]
> [Page 494–495]

Source: Centers for Medicare and Medicaid Services (CMS) Conditions of Participation. [59 FR 64152, Dec. 13, 1994, as amended at 69 FR 49268, Aug. 11, 2004]. Retrieved on July 15, 2006 at *http://a257.g.akamaitech.net/7/257/2422/12feb20041500/edocket. access.gpo.gov/cfr_2004/octqtr/pdf/42cfr482.43.pdf*

Patients have the right to make their own decisions regarding current and future care.

1. The patient's capacity for decision-making influences the extent of his or her rights.
2. Determining the capacity for decision-making can be the function of the physician, the health care team, or in some cases a court of law.
3. Determining the patient's executive function is critical when planning the transition to a lesser level of care (Cooney et al., 2004).

D. Nondiscrimination in referral selection—Patients and their responsible parties have the right to choose among providers for care, including post-acute care providers such as home health care agencies, skilled nursing facilities, ambulance providers, durable medical equipment providers, or other providers of products or services necessary for self-care management.

1. Patients must be given a choice among providers.
2. The choice should be among appropriate providers that are deemed capable of meeting the patient's assessed needs.
3. Where possible, the request of a patient, or responsible person, for selection of specific level of care or provider should be honored. When it is not possible, the reason the preferred level of care or service provider is not being used should be documented in the patient's medical record (e.g., "no available bed at preferred skilled nursing facility").

■ THE ROLE OF THE CASE MANAGER IN THE PROCESS OF TRANSITIONAL PLANNING

A. Role of the provider-based case manager
   1. Providers with responsibility for transitional planning or discharge planning include any organization that is providing or managing care for a patient receiving medical or nursing services. Examples include:
      a. Hospitals
      b. Nursing facilities
      c. Inpatient rehabilitation facilities
      d. Psychiatric facilities
      e. Home health care agencies
      f. Hospice
      g. Others in specific markets (e.g., Indian Health Service, Critical Access Hospital)
   2. Functions within provider-based case management
      a. Identification of individuals who are at risk for adverse outcomes during the transition or discharge from one level of care or setting to another
      b. Evaluation of the patient's continuing care needs
      c. Assessment of resources appropriate and available to the patient/family
      d. Planning for transition to the next level of care
      e. Implementation of the plan
      f. Monitoring and ongoing reassessment of the plan
      g. Use of evidence-based guidelines for patients with specific care needs and where applicable
      h. Documentation of all pertinent information related to the planning for discharge or transition
      i. Knowledge of the admission criteria for various levels of care (e.g., home health care with the requirement that patient be homebound)
      j. Advocacy for patients' rights, needs, and values; ensuring that patients' ethnic, cultural, or religious values, beliefs, preferences, and needs are considered during the transition or discharge phase
      k. Collaboration with the multidisciplinary health care team, and in particular with the patient's attending physician   ·
      l. Coordination of the plan of care and discharge plan with other providers and payer-based case managers, where applicable
      m. Communication of relevant information across the continuum
      n. Knowledge of the roles and responsibilities of other members of the health care team, including nurses, social workers, therapists, pharmacists, dietitians, utilization review staff, and other case managers within the organization
      o. Validation that the services ordered or arranged for at the next level of care are reasonably assured

p. Education and counseling of patients and their families regarding the transition or discharge phase of care

q. Education of the patients and their families about their roles and responsibilities in care, especially after discharge from an acute care setting

r. Protection of the privacy of health care information during the referral process (Health Information Privacy and Accountability Act—HIPAA).

s. Participation in coordination of benefits for patients with more than one interested payer (e.g., Medicare and workers' compensation)

t. Reporting of abuse, neglect, abandonment, or exploitation as mandated by the individual state laws and regulations

u. Participation in the evaluation of the patient's capacity for decision-making

v. Engaging in quality assurance and quality improvement initiates and activities

w. Reporting any complaints or concerns about other providers to administration for appropriate follow up

x. Participation in follow-up contact with patients per the organization's policy and protocol

y. Education of other health care professionals in the transition and discharge planning process and other relevant information (e.g., community resources)

z. Compliance with all related regulations as applicable to one's own organization

aa. Assurance of patient safety throughout the care process, especially during the handoff period

bb. Assurance of open communication between health care providers at all levels during the handoff phase

cc. Collection of data as required by the department for reporting purposes and completion of related reports as required by own organization or by law (e.g., referral patterns)

B. Role of the payer-based case manager

1. Identification of at-risk members or populations within their membership (i.e., health plan members), with emphasis on risks associated with transition or discharge to a new level of care

2. Acting as a resource to provider-based staff during the evaluation of a member's transition or discharge planning needs

3. Advocating for patient's rights, needs, values, and for the patient's ethnic, cultural or religious needs and preferences to be considered during the transition or discharge phase

4. Collaboration with the health care team, and in particular with the patient's attending physician, and when possible, with the member's/patient's community-based primary care physician

5. Assessment of resources within the member's health care plan

    a. Assessment of other public or private programs that can supplement the member's continuing care needs, for example the American Cancer Society

6. Planning for the transition of the member to the next level of care

    a. Determining the patient's health insurance benefits. Participation in the coordination of benefits for members with more than one payer source. For example, HMO and workers' compensation claim

    b. Determining providers that are contracted with the payer and that can meet the next level of care needs for the patient

    c. Assuring availability of the contracted provider and communicating that information to the provider based staff

    d. Assisting the current provider in implementing the transition or discharge plan, keeping in mind that the responsibility for the implementation belongs to the direct care provider

    e. Monitoring the progress of the transition or discharge plan with a focus on expected outcomes and relevancy to the patient's condition

    f. Utilization of evidence-based protocols in working with members or populations

    g. Use of established certain criteria, such as discharge criteria, as a guide during the transition or discharge phase

    h. Collaboration with provider staff during the transition or discharge phase

    i. Knowing the roles and responsibilities of provider-based members of the health care team including nurses, social workers, therapists, pharmacists, dietitians, utilization review staff, other case managers within the organization. Collaborating with these staff

    j. Knowing the roles and responsibilities of other members of the payer-based health care team including nurses, social workers, therapists, pharmacists, dietitians, utilization review staff, and other case managers within the organization, such as disease management case managers, oncology case managers

    k. Utilization of resources within the payer organization as needed

      i. Understanding the role of the medical director

      ii. Understanding the coverage determination procedures

    l. Advocacy for members within the payer system and when requested outside the payer system

    m. Discontinuing case management services when appropriate

    n. Educating members on their benefits

    o. Educating members on their responsibilities in participating in the transition or discharge phase of care

    p. Assuring that there is opportunity for questions and responses between health care providers and payers at all levels during the handoff phase

q. Collecting data as required by the case management department or the organization for reporting purposes

r. Documenting according to the policies and procedures of the organization including the policy on transitional/discharge planning or continuity of care

s. Following mandatory reporting of abuse, neglect, abandonment, exploitation if and when applicable

t. Conforming to the HIPAA and privacy rules as applicable

■ THE CASE MANAGEMENT/TRANSITIONAL PLANNING CONNECTION

A. Transitional and discharge planning activities include those that aim to address patients' needs at every phase of care—preadmission to a hospital or episode of care, the admission process, the hospital stay or care provision, before discharge from the hospital or episode of care, and time of discharge (JCAHO, 2006).

1. Before admission to the hospital or episode of care, the case manager must collect all pertinent information about the patient's condition and family's situation to identify the patient's and family's needs and communicate such information to other care providers as necessary.

2. During the admission process, the case manager ensures the provision of care and services that are consistent with the patient's condition and makes appropriate referrals to other care providers as indicated by the patient's condition and treatment plan. The case manager also facilitates the transfer of the patient to the appropriate level of care and setting or to other facilities based on the patient's acuity and needs.

3. While in the hospital or in other specific care settings (e.g., a clinic), the case manager maintains continuity of services through the phases of assessment, treatment, and reassessment of the patient's condition. The case manager also ensures that care is well coordinated among all care providers involved, including the post-discharge services and resources.

4. Before discharge from the hospital or an episode of care, the case manager evaluates the patient's and family's post-discharge needs and arranges for their availability to maintain continuity of care and prevent disruption of treatment. These activities also include referrals to other care providers and teaching the patient and family in self-care management and the treatment regimen.

5. At the time of discharge from a hospital or other episode of care, the case manager reassesses the patient's condition and the patient's and family's ability to manage self-care, as well as ensures that the arranged post-discharge resources and services continue to be appropriate for the patient. In addition, the case manager communicates pertinent information about the patient's condition and treatment plan to other agencies to be involved in the care of the patient post-discharge, such as skilled nursing facilities and home care

agencies. In the end, the case manager ensures a safe discharge or transition to another level of care.

B. Relationship between the transitional planning process and the case management process

1. The transitional and discharge planning process is part and parcel of the case management process. In fact, transitional planning activities take place at every step of the case management process to a point that such activities may appear seamless.

2. Upon the patient's admission to a hospital or an episode of care, the case manager screens the patient for post-discharge needs and arranges for such services after obtaining agreement from the patient, the patient's family, and the health care team.

3. The case manager identifies the patient's actual and potential problems and incorporates them in the transitional or discharge plan.

4. The case manager engages in interdisciplinary planning, implementation, and coordination activities that not only focus on the necessary treatment plan but also on the transitional plan as well. These activities include brokerage of services and referrals to other specialty care providers, such as rehabilitation medicine (physical and occupational therapy), and home care agencies.

5. The case manager also incorporates patient and family education in the transitional plan as well as engages in ongoing assessments and reassessments of the patient and family to ensure that the plan is appropriate.

6. The case manager prepares the patient and family for discharge or transfer to another facility when expected outcomes and goals of care specific to the hospital stay or to the episode of care are met.

7. Throughout the episode of care, the case manager repeats the transitional planning process (i.e., the case management process) as indicated by the patient's condition, such as in the case of deterioration in the patient's condition that requires a drastic change in the plan of care.

REFERENCES

Centers for Medicare and Medicaid Services (CMS) Conditions of Participation. [59 FR 64152, Dec. 13, 1994, as amended at 69 FR 49268, Aug. 11, 2004]. Website: *http://a257.g.akamaitech. net/7/257/2422/12feb20041500/edocket.access.gpo.gov/cfr_2004/octqtr/pdf/42cfr482.43.pdf.* Retrieved July 15, 2006.

Commission for Case Manager Certification (CCMC). (2005). *Glossary of terms.* Website: *www. ccmcertification.org.*

Cooney, L., Kennedy, G., Hawkins, K., & Hurme, S. B. (2004). Who can stay at home? Assessing the capacity to choose to live in the community. *Archives of Internal Medicine, 164,* 357–360.

JCAHO Patient Safety Standards, 2nd ed. (2006). Implement a standardized approach to "hand off" communications, including an opportunity to ask and respond to questions. *Critical Access Hospital and Hospital National Patient Safety Goals.*

Phillips, C. O., Wright, S. M., Kern, D. E., et al. (2004). Comprehensive discharge planning with postdischarge support for older patients with congestive heart failure: A meta-analysis. *Journal of the American Medical Association, 291*(11), 1358–1367.

Solet, D. J., Norvell, J. M., Rutan, G. H., & Frankel, R. M. (2005). Lost in translation: Challenges and opportunities in physician-to-physician communication during patient handoffs. *Academic Medicine*, 1094–1099. Website: *http://psnet.ahrq.gov/resource.aspx?resourceID=3032.*

SUGGESTED READING

Birmingham, J. (2004). Discharge planning: A collaboration between provider and payer case managers using Medicare Conditions of Participation. *Lippincott's Case Management, 9*(3), 147–151.

Birmingham, J. (2004). Documentation guide for case managers: Inside case management, Parts 1–2. *Lippincott's Case Management, 9,* 2–3.

Birmingham, J. (2002). The science of collaboration. *The Case Manager, 13*(2), 67–70.

Birmingham, J., & Anctil, B. (2002). Managing the dynamics of collaboration. *The Case Manager, 13*(3), 73–77.

Bowles, K. H., Foust, J. B., & Naylor, M. D. (2003). Hospital discharge referral decision making: A multidisciplinary perspective. *Applied Nursing Research 16*(3), 134–143.

Medicare Conditions of Participation for Discharge Planning. (Revised 1986, 1994, 2004). Social Security Act § 1861 (ee). Website: *http://www.ssa.gov/OP_Home/ssact/title18/1861.htm.*

Robbins, C. L., & Birmingham, J. (2005). The social worker and nurse roles in case management: Applying the three R's. *Lippincott's Case Management, 10*(3), 120–127.

Solet, D. J., Norvell, J. M., Rutan, G. H., & Frankel, R. M. (2005). Lost in translation: Challenges and opportunities in physician-to-physician communication during patient handoffs. *Academic Medicine, 80,* 1094–1099. Website: *http://psnet.ahrq.gov/resource.aspx?resourceID=3032.*

Stewart, K. (2003). Seven ways to help your hospital stay in business. *Family Practice Management, 10*(3), 27–30.

Utilization Management and Resource Management

Cheri Lattimer

Michael B. Garrett

LEARNING OBJECTIVES

Upon completion of this chapter, the reader will be able to:

1. Identify terms and concepts associated with utilization management.
2. Understand the utilization management process.
3. Describe the various criteria used in utilization management.
4. Identify the areas of focused or targeted utilization management.
5. Review the outcomes and reporting of utilization management programs.

IMPORTANT TERMS AND CONCEPTS

Admission Certification
Alternative Level of Care
Appeal
Appropriateness of Setting
Case Management
Case Manager

Case Rates
Continued Stay Review
Continuum of Care
Denials
Diagnostic Related Groups (DRGs)
Discharge Outcomes

Discharge Planning
Fee-for-Service (FFS)
Focused/Targeted Utilization
    Management
InterQual Clinical Decision Support
    Tools
Length of Stay (LOS)
Milliman Care Guidelines
National Committee for Quality
    Assurance (NCQA)

Overutilization
Preadmission Certification
Prospective Payment System (PPS)
Quality Improvement Organization (QIO)
Resource Management (RM)
Retrospective Review
Utilization Management (UM)
Utilization Review (UR)
Utilization Review Accreditation
    Commission (URAC)

■ INTRODUCTION

A. Utilization management (UM) as a program or process has existed for more than 30 years. UM functions began in the early 1970s with the creation of professional standards review organizations (now called quality improvement organizations or QIOs), which evaluated health care services provided to Medicare and Medicaid beneficiaries. The initial focus of UM was on reviewing hospital care, but gradually included outpatient services as well. By the 1980s, health maintenance organizations (HMOs) used the UM process to control referrals to specialists and gradually to health care services across the continuum of the delivery system. UM programs may be all-inclusive or focused on one or more areas of precertification, admission and concurrent review, outpatient and ancillary services, imaging and x-ray, pharmacy management, or ambulatory surgery centers.

B. In the commercial sector, UM traditionally was conducted by insurance companies, HMOs, or third-party utilization review vendors. The industry is now seeing physician organizations and hospital facilities developing UM programs and information systems to conduct UM reviews and coordination within a risk contract and/or pay-for-performance (Managed Care Resources, 2006).

C. The validated clinical and outcome impact of UM is still unclear. Supporters cite a positive shift from inpatient to outpatient care, reduction of inpatient days, and an enhanced referral process for identifying patients for discharge planning and disease and case management programs. Critics of the program identify significant administrative costs with unclear cost benefit, access barriers and delays for patients to care, and increasing patient and physician dissatisfaction with an unfriendly system (Managed Care Resources, 2006).

■ KEY DEFINITIONS[1]

A. Admission certification—A form of utilization review in which an assessment is made of the medical necessity of a patient's admission to a hospital

---

[1]From *Glossary of Terms*, published by the Commission for Case Manager Certification (2005).

or other inpatient facility. Admission certification ensures that patients requiring a hospital-based level of care and length of stay appropriate for the admission diagnosis are usually assigned and certified as medically necessary according to care guidelines; but this is not necessarily a guarantee of payment for such services (payment is a benefit and/or claims determination).

B. Alternative level of care—A level of care that can safely be used in place of the current level and is determined based on the acuity and complexity of the patient's condition and the type of needed services and resources.

C. Appeal—The formal process or request to reconsider a decision made not to approve an admission or health care services, reimbursement for services rendered, or a patient's request for postponing the discharge date and extending the length of stay.

D. Case rate—Rate of reimbursement that packages pricing for a certain category of services. Typically combines facility and professional practitioner fees for care and services.

E. Continued stay review (also known as *concurrent review*)—A type of review used to determine whether each day of the hospital stay is necessary and that care is being rendered at the appropriate level. It takes place during a patient's hospitalization for care.

F. Continuum of care—The continuum of care matches ongoing needs of individuals being served by the case management process with the appropriate level and type of health, medical, financial, legal, and psychosocial care for services within a setting or across multiple settings.

G. Denials (also called *noncertifications*)—Issuance of a notice of noncertification decision within the utilization management process for health care services.

H. Diagnostic related groups (DRGs)—A patient classification scheme that provides a means of relating the type of patient a hospital treats to the costs incurred by the hospital. DRGs include groups of patients using similar resource consumption and length of stay. Use of DRGs also is known as a statistical system of classifying any inpatient stay into groups for the purposes of payment. DRGs may be primary or secondary; an outlier classification also exists. This is the form of reimbursement that the Centers for Medicare and Medicaid Services (CMS) uses to pay hospitals for Medicare and Medicaid recipients. Also used by a few states for all payers and by many private health plans (usually non-HMO) for contracting purposes.

I. Discharge outcomes (criteria)—Clinical criteria to be met before or at the time of the patient's discharge. They are the expected or projected outcomes of care that indicate a safe discharge.

J. Discharge planning—The process of assessing the patient's needs of care after discharge from a health care facility and ensuring that the necessary services are in place before discharge. This process ensures a patient's timely, appropriate, and safe discharge to the next level of care or setting including appropriate use of resources necessary for ongoing care.

K. Evidence-based medicine—Involves the practice of medicine by use of nationally accepted clinical practice guidelines for a disease/disorder, including screening, diagnosis, and treatment of patients, based on what is referred to as the current "best evidence." Best evidence comes from medical studies or clinical trials (Hayes OnHealth, 2006).

L. InterQual clinical decision support tools—Evidence-based criteria sets that support care planning and level-of-care decisions across the continuum of care.

M. Length of stay (LOS)—The number of days that a health plan member/patient stays in an inpatient facility, home health, or hospice.

N. Level of care (LOC)—The intensity of effort required to diagnose, treat, preserve, or maintain an individual's physical or emotional status.

O. Milliman Care Guidelines—Span the continuum of care providing access to evidence-based clinical practice guidelines, clinical/medical knowledge, and best medical practice relevant to patients in a broad range of care settings.

P. National Committee for Quality Assurance (NCQA)—An independent nonprofit organization dedicated to improving health care quality through review and accreditation to the managed care industry.

Q. Overutilization review—Using established criteria as a guide, determination is made as to whether the patient is receiving services that are redundant, unnecessary, or in excess.

R. Preadmission certification (also known as *prospective review*)—An element of utilization review that examines the need for proposed services before admission to an institution to determine the appropriateness of the setting, procedures, treatments, and length of stay.

S. Precertification/prospective review—The process of obtaining and documenting advanced approval from the health plan by the provider before delivering the medical services needed. This is required when services are of a nonemergent nature.

T. Prospective payment system (PPS)—A health care payment system used by the federal government since 1983 for reimbursing health care providers/agencies for medical care provided to Medicare and Medicaid participants. The payment is fixed and based on the operating costs of the patient's diagnosis.

U. Quality Improvement Organization (QIO)—A federal program established by the Tax Equity and Fiscal Responsibility Act of 1982 that monitors the medical necessity and quality of services provided to Medicare and Medicaid beneficiaries under the prospective payment system.

V. Resource management (RM)—A quality improvement activity that analyzes resources used in patient care processes to improve quality, efficiency, and value (Brown, 2005).

W. Retrospective review—A form of medical records review that is conducted after the patient's discharge to track appropriateness of care and consumption of resources.

X. Utilization management (UM)—Review of services to ensure that they are medically necessary, provided in the most appropriate care setting, and at or above quality standards.

Y. Utilization review (UR)—A mechanism used by some insurers and employers to evaluate health care on the basis of appropriateness, necessity, and quality.

Z. Utilization Review Accreditation Commission (URAC)—A not-for-profit organization that provides reviews and accreditation for UR services/ programs provided by freestanding agencies.

■ UM PROGRAM AND PROCESS

A. A UM program is a comprehensive, systematic, and ongoing effort. UM review activities are conducted through telephonic, fax, and web services, and onsite interfaces with members and their contracted provider or designee. Review activities encompass the utilization of clinical care and services, including inpatient and outpatient services.

B. UM program goals
1. To ensure effective utilization of health care resources through ongoing monitoring
2. To determine medical necessity and appropriateness of care
3. To identify patterns of overutilization, underutilization, and inefficient scheduling of resources
4. To promote quality patient care and optimal outcomes
5. To assist in the identification of coordination of care options for members and providers
6. To facilitate appropriate, safe, timely, and effective discharge to the most appropriate level of care (LOC)
7. To provide education concerning the UM program to providers and department staff
8. To identify potential participants in disease management and case management programs

C. UM review process
1. Verification of the patient's eligibility for services—this can be accomplished by a nonclinical customer service representative who can access the eligibility database of the health plan
2. Determination of whether the requested service is a covered benefit and requires a review—this can also be done by a nonclinical customer service representative by accessing the benefit plan for covered services and the UM review requirements description
3. Collection of demographic and clinical information necessary to certify a requested service or length of stay, including history of prior health care services, current medical situation, and anticipated treatment plan (including surgeries, therapies, and other treatment modalities)

4. Documentation of gathered information within an information system or medical record-keeping process (e.g., chart, logbook, etc.)
5. Selection of the applicable criteria or guidelines to evaluate the requested services
6. Clinical information is reviewed against evidence-based decision support criteria or guidelines for a review determination. The UM clinical reviewer evaluates, based on the information provided, whether the case meets criteria or guidelines.
7. If the criteria or guidelines are met, the requesting provider will be notified of the request approval. If the criteria or guidelines are not met, then the review will be sent for peer review by an appropriate physician advisor or medical director.
8. The physician advisor reviews the clinical information, and may choose to approve the case based on medical judgment. If the physician advisor believes the request should not be approved, then an offer is made to communicate with the attending physician about the case (sometimes called a *peer-to-peer conversation* or *reconsideration*). At the end of the discussion with the attending physician (or at the end of the timeframe available for the discussion), the physician advisor makes a determination as to whether the request is approved or denied. If the request is denied, the provider or member can initiate the appeal process.

D. UM review types
 1. Prospective review/precertification admissions[2]
 2. Continued stay/concurrent review
 3. Retrospective review
 4. Second surgical opinion
 5. Discharge planning review
 6. Pharmacy therapy management
 7. Referral review to case management

■ UM CLINICAL REVIEWERS

A. The UM staff who perform URs should be appropriately educated, trained, and licensed (if applicable) according to their job responsibilities.
B. Personnel who obtain information and evaluate medical necessity regarding a patient's specific medical condition, diagnosis, and treatment options are usually registered nurses or other health care providers (such as social workers for behavioral health) who are qualified to review the service requested by providers.
C. A UM team may consist of:
 1. Initial clinical reviewers, including nurses, nurse case managers, behavioral health professionals (e.g., social workers), or other qualified health care professionals and/or paraprofessionals (in a support role)
 2. Medical director and physician advisors/peer reviewers

---

[2]Prospective and concurrent reviews can be either nonurgent or urgent in nature.

    3. Physician specialist panel

    4. Administrative staff/nonclinical staff

■ UM CRITERIA AND STRATEGIES

A. Clinical decision support tools such as guidelines, protocols, algorithms, and pathways are used by health plans and providers in managing the utilization, quality, and cost of health care services.

B. The application of these tools assists the initial clinical reviewer in determining whether proposed services are clinically indicated and provided at the appropriate LOC.

C. Criteria may be developed by organizations that specialize in the development of clinical criteria, specialty providers through the coordination of their associations, or internally by a health plan or health care organization.

D. Criteria need to be up to date, clinically sound, objective, and based on either evidence-based medicine or consensus-based processes.

E. Health plans will provide access to the criteria tools for both providers and patients and encourage shared decision making between them.

■ INTERQUAL CLINICAL DECISION SUPPORT TOOLS

A. InterQual (McKesson Health Solutions, 2005c) has provided UM tools for almost 30 years. An offering within the CareEnhance products of McKesson Corporation, InterQual provides evidence-based and clinically validated content to hospitals, health plans, government services, and other care management providers. InterQual clinical decision support tools are available in book format, PC software, browser-based application, and CD-ROM.

B. InterQual criteria began as a UR tool, evolved to support of UM, and today has become a care management tool that focuses on:

    1. Proactive care management

    2. Improvement of patient care and safety

    3. Resource management

    4. Improving clinical decision making based upon the best available evidence for care management decisions

    5. Fostering collaborative relationships

    6. Enhancing quality for organizations in helping to identify the need for quality improvement processes

C. InterQual offers a range of clinical decision support products. They can be used prospectively, concurrently, and retrospectively.

    1. *Level-of-Care Criteria*—include acute, long-term acute, rehabilitation, sub-acute, skilled nursing facility, home care, and outpatient rehabilitation and chiropractic care

    2. *Care Planning Criteria*—tools that provide support to evaluate the appropriateness and optimal sequencing of care-related interventions

3. *Behavioral Health Level-of-Care Continuum*—a criteria suite that aids in making initial and concurrent level-of-care decisions for psychiatric conditions, chemical dependency, and dual diagnoses for specific age groups
4. *Retrospective Monitoring*—a tool that helps provider organizations analyze the appropriateness of surgical and invasive procedures after they have been performed
5. *Workers' Compensation and Disability Management Products*—help guide decisions about appropriate medical utilization and return-to-work strategies
6. *Clinical Evidence Summaries*—address diagnosis-specific topics to support second-level medical review recommendations and promote evidence-based standards of care among providers

D. InterQual uses a five-stage development cycle in providing their tools to the health care industry.
   1. The development cycle begins with a comprehensive search of current evidence-based medical literature supported by a diverse panel of clinical consultants.
   2. The development team selects new topics and content for revisions.
   3. The development team performs a comprehensive research of evidence-based literature.
   4. Clinical consultants review the criteria and provide suggested revisions.
   5. In areas where no agreement is reached, the development team includes a rationale for the clinical stance chosen with supporting notes and literature references in the criteria.

E. Consultants who have not been part of the development process assess and validate the criteria sets for clinical accuracy.

F. Criteria sets are prepared for software and book versions and reviewed for clinical consistency.

■ CERTIFICATION PROGRAMS IN UR AND UM

A. Two certification programs are offered by McKesson in UM and UR. Both programs were developed in response to the industry's request for education and evidence of a basic level of competency for staff performing UR and UM.

B. The Certified Professional Utilization Review (CPUR) program can be likened to managed care or medical management 101. It examines why we manage health care services with a specific focus on UR. The program covers the history of health care from a quality, access, and cost perspective; examines integrating UR and case management; and explores legal issues related to managing health care services (McKesson Health Solutions, 2005a).

C. The Certified Profession Utilization Management (CPUM) program is an advanced course comparable to a 301 level class. It focuses on how to manage services and develop strategies from a medical management perspective, and covers developing a quality management program, working with outcomes, and managing legal issues and ethical concerns (McKesson Health Solutions, 2005b).

■ MILLIMAN CARE GUIDELINES

A. Milliman (2005) is an international consulting firm. The Milliman Care Guidelines division develops updates and publishes the Milliman Care Guidelines series providing evidence-based clinical tools for hospitals, health plans, and other professionals in the health care industry.

B. The Milliman Care Guidelines span the continuum of care, providing access to evidence-based knowledge and best practices relevant to patients in a broad range of care settings:
1. Ambulatory care
2. Inpatient and surgical care
3. General recovery guidelines
4. Recovery facility care
5. Home care
6. Chronic care guidelines

C. Hierarchy of evidence—information for the care guidelines is drawn from analysis of abstracts, articles, databases, textbooks, nationally-recognized guidelines, and practice observations. This data is embedded into the guideline products web version for users to access. In weighing and grading the evidence, the following generally accepted hierarchy of evidence is used (in order of importance)
1. Evidence Grade 1—Randomized controlled trials
2. Evidence Grade 2—Other published sources
3. Evidence Grade 3—Unpublished data

D. Milliman Care Guidelines
1. *Ambulatory care*—a care management tool for reviewing outpatient referrals, imaging, diagnostic testing, rehabilitative services, injectables, and pharmacy utilization
2. *Inpatient and surgical care*—a resource providing goals and care templates for patients facing hospitalization and/or surgery
3. *General recovery guidelines*—a resource for when a guideline does not exist for the diagnosis or when the clinical situation is so complex that a guideline is not easily applied
4. *Recovery facility care*—a comprehensive tool to help develop well-coordinated plans for recovery facility admission, care, and discharge
5. *Home care*—a comprehensive planning resource for home health care, enabling case managers and other health care professionals to transfer patients smoothly to home care, while managing quality and efficiency
6. *Chronic care guidelines*—a tool to facilitate outpatient care for chronic and complex patients covering 20 conditions

E. The Milliman Care Guidelines are available in several formats:
   1. Web
   2. PC
   3. Intranet
   4. Care Guide QI
   5. QI Care Web

■ OTHER UM CRITERIA SETS

A. Managed Care Appropriateness Program (MCAP)—criteria scientifically developed through consensus and evidence-based medicine to comprehensively reflect a best-practice approach to patient care. The criteria are updated at least annually in order to maintain clinical relevance (MCAP, 2005). Criteria sets are offered in:
   1. Acute care
   2. Alternative care
   3. Rehabilitation
   4. Pre-procedure
   5. Psychiatry—inpatient
   6. Psychiatry—outpatient
   7. Substance use disorder

B. American Society of Addiction Medicine (ASAM)

C. American College of Obstetric and Gynecology (ACOG)

D. The American Academy of Pediatrics (AAP)

E. The Department of Health and Human Services (DHHS) Health Care Guidelines

■ FOCUSED UM

A. Many UM programs and organizations have restructured their traditional UM services to target special populations or key areas of medical services where focusing with early UM interventions provides enhanced coordination of resources, timely interventions, improved patient safety, and appropriate referrals to ongoing outpatient disease and case management services.
   1. Elder care management
   2. Chronic care management
   3. Specialty management
   4. Targeted ICD-9 conditions for hospital management
   5. Pharmacy benefit management
   6. Pharmacy therapy management
   7. High-risk population management

B. Data indicate that this type of focused intervention reduces the overall administrative cost of a traditional UM program and improves the overall organizational management of patient care.

C. UM organizations employ primarily licensed RNs and LPNs as first-level reviewers for medical and surgical services, and social workers for behavioral health services, and are faced with the reality of the nursing shortage in their workforce. They are constantly faced with how to deploy staffing resources for the most positive support and impact of patient care. The business implications have pushed the questions of how to provide UM in more efficient, cost-effective, and customer service–friendly models. This has included some new methods for the UM review process, such as using technology for web-based UM in which only those cases that do not meet criteria/guidelines are reviewed by a health care professional. Also, some contracts and jurisdictions allow for LPNs to be initial clinical reviewers. Some health plans conduct scripted clinical reviews in which nonclinical customer service representatives strictly follow scripts in collecting demographic and clinical information (also known as *pre-review screening*). The evolution of UM will continue with a focus on how to use interventions not as isolated functions but as collaborative practice interventions with triage, disease management, and case management to coordinate patient care throughout the continuum of care options.

1. An example of this restructuring within the health care industry is case managers who are assigned the responsibility of UM, disease management, and pharmacy management interventions within their overall case work.

2. If a case manager is not providing UM, then the case manager must access this information so that UM decisions are taken into account during the care planning process.

3. It is just as important that the UM nurse provide timely referrals to case management and disease management to ensure optimum care coordination.

4. UM is one component of patient care and as such must be managed as a collaborative practice intervention with the total health care team.

■ APPEAL PROCESS

A. The appeal process is the formal mechanism by which a service provider or a member, or both, can request reconsideration of an initial determination or decision, with the goal being to find a mutually acceptable solution. The appeal process consists of the following four levels:

1. *Reconsideration* (peer-to-peer discussion)—a request by telephone for additional review of an impending UM determination to not certify (usually done prior to the issuance of noncertification determination). It is performed by the peer reviewer who performed the original review and is based on the need for additional information from the requesting provider. For example, a provider can discuss the potential denial with the initial clinical reviewer/medical director or advisor for possible reversal of an impending decision based on additional verbal clinical information.

2. *Appeal* (first-level appeal)—a request (in writing, by telephone, by email, etc.) for additional review of a decision to not certify imminent

or ongoing services, requiring a review conducted by a clinical peer who was not involved in the original decision to not certify. The appeal may be done, according to request, on an expedited/urgent basis or a standard/nonurgent basis. The member or provider can request an expedited decision (no longer than 24 to 72 hours, depending on the type of review). A standard appeal must be done within 30 days. The appeal must be performed by a physician advisor who was not involved in the original denial (URAC, 2005).

3. *Standard appeal*—a request to review a denial of an admission, extension of stay, or other health care service. It is conducted by a peer reviewer who was not involved in any of the previous determinations pertaining to the same episode of care. Standard appeals are completed, and written notification of the appeal decision issued, within 30 calendar days of the receipt of the request for appeal (URAC, 2005).

4. *Arbitration* (final level)—mediation is usually handled by objective outside parties.

B. An appeals process is generally in place for reconsideration of the denial.

C. Poor communication and/or documentation are often factors that contribute to a denial.

D. Quality improvement organizations (QIOs) contract with CMS to review the quality and appropriateness of care being rendered to hospitalized patients receiving Medicare benefits. Processes are developed for review and referral when a denial is issued.

E. Notice of noncoverage (NONC)—a generic term for a notification of noncoverage, usually due to the request being for a noncovered service or benefit

F. Hospital-issued notice of noncoverage (HINN)—a notice of noncoverage for fee-for-service Medicare beneficiaries

G. Notice of discharge and Medicare appeal rights (NODMAR)—a notice of noncoverage for Medicare beneficiaries in managed care plans (Powell, 2000)

■ DENIALS OF ADMISSIONS AND SERVICES

A. A denial notice, also known as a *lack of certification* or an *adverse determination,* may be issued when admission to, or continued stay in, the facility cannot be justified as medically necessary, or for procedures or ancillary services.

B. There are different types of denials and specific regulations that govern their use for Medicare and Medicaid patients.

C. Private review agencies may have specific policies and procedures for denials according to their specific payor groups. The U.S. Department of Labor (USDOL) has issued "claims regulations" that also govern UM review decisions that all fully insured and self-funded health plans must follow.

D. Those UM review organizations that are accredited by URAC or NCQA must adhere to and remain compliant with their standards and processes.

■ ADVERSE REVIEW DETERMINATION

A. Adverse review determination is defined as the nonauthorization (denial) of payment for a request for care or services.

B. URAC and NCQA consider nonauthorization decisions that are based on either medical appropriateness or benefit coverage or experimental treatments to be denials.

C. Partial approvals and care terminations are also considered denials.

D. If the UM review does not meet clinical decision support criteria (InterQual, Milliman, etc.) or there are no criteria for that diagnosis, procedure, or imaging procedure, then
  1. There could be a supervisor review, and then the initial nurse reviewer would refer the request to a physician for medical review.
  2. The medical reviewer might also refer to a second-level medical review, particularly if the request or review is outside the scope of the initial medical reviewer's scope of expertise.

E. Non-physician reviewers cannot deny certification for any care or procedure.

■ MEDICAL REVIEW OUTCOMES

A. Medical review determinations are based on the medical reviewer's judgment and expertise after reviewing the case for medical appropriateness. The health plan might also deny a service because it is not covered in the plan benefit coverage or is considered to be experimental. Types of medical review outcomes include:
  1. Closed for lack of information
  2. Approval or partial approval/certification
  3. Awaiting more information after request (time restricted)
  4. Denial (adverse determination or lack of certification)

■ UM PERFORMANCE REPORTING

A. Admission reported by LOC (inpatient, rehabilitation, hospice, psychiatric, substance abuse, deliveries)

B. Readmission reported by LOC

C. Average length of stay (ALOS) reported by LOC

D. Procedures per thousand

E. Alternative LOC transition (cost per day, savings per day)

F. Delays in services (days delayed, cost per day delayed) (Brown, 2005)

G. Emergency department visits

H. Number and type of denials (inpatient days, procedures, services)

I. Reconsiderations

J. Appeals of denials based on a statistic, such as percentage of denied cases brought to appeal

K. Denials based on a statistic, such as percentage of all reviews that result in a denial

L. Peer reviews based on a statistic, such as percentage of all reviews that are referred to a physician advisor for clinical peer review

M. Case referrals to disease management and case management services

N. UM statistics may be reported by facility, provider and/or type of insurance (Medicare, Medicaid, commercial, etc.)

■ **KEY REGULATORY AND ACCREDITATION BODIES ASSOCIATED WITH THE UM PROCESS**

A. Centers for Medicare and Medicaid Services (CMS)—a federal regulatory agency that oversees the Medicare program and oversees the states' administration of Medicaid programs

B. Joint Commission on Accreditation of Healthcare Organizations (JCAHO)—a private not-for-profit organization developed to improve the quality of care provided to the public; provides standards and evaluates for a variety of settings (e.g., hospitals, long-term care, home health)

C. Utilization Review Accreditation Commission (URAC)—an independent non-profit organization that promotes quality and efficiency of health care delivery among purchasers, providers, and patients by establishing standards, education programs, and communication (URAC, 2005)

D. National Committee for Quality Assurance (NCQA)—an independent non-profit organization that develops quality standards and performance measures for a broad range of health care entities (NCQA, 2005)

■ **UM REGULATORY AND ACCREDITATION PROCESSES**

A. It is desirable for UM service companies to obtain accreditation for services. Accreditation demonstrates:

1. Accountability to external customers
2. Compliance with regulations, including state regulatory processes
3. Objective and transparent review processes
4. Process consistency
5. Process efficiencies
6. Due processes and procedures
7. Designated timeframes for completion of review activities

REFERENCES

Brown, Janet, A. (2005). *The health care quality handbook: A professional resource and study guide.* Pasadena: JB Quality Solutions.

Commission for Case Manager Certification (CCMC). (2005). *Glossary of terms.* Website: *www.ccm-certification.org.*

Hayes OnHealth. (January 2006). *Evidence based medicine: Best evidence.* Website: *www.hayeson-health.com/factsheet/.*

Managed Care Appropriateness Program (MCAP). (2005). Oak Group Website: *www.oakgroup.com.*

Managed Care Resources, Inc. (January 2006). *Signature series*. Website: *www.mcres.com/,crless.htm#S2*.

McKesson Health Solutions. (2005a). *Certified professional utilization management*. InterQual Website: *www.interqual.com/iqsite/services/cpum.aspx*.

McKesson Health Solutions. (2005b). *Certified professional utilization review*. InterQual Website: *www.interqual.com/iqsite/services/cpur.aspx*.

McKesson Health Solutions. (2005c). *InterQual® clinical decision support tools*. Newton, MA: McKesson.

Milliman Care Guidelines. (2005). *Evidence-based medicine defined*. Seattle: Milliman Care Guidelines LLC.

National Committee for Quality Assurance (NCQA). (January 2006). Website: *www.NCQA.org/about/about.htm*.

Powell, S. K. (2000). *Case management: A practical guide to success in managed care*. Philadelphia: Lippincott Williams & Wilkins.

Utilization Review Accreditation Commission (URAC). (December 2005). Website: *www.urac.org*.

12 Leadership Skills and Concepts

Suzanne K. Powell

LEARNING OBJECTIVES

Upon completion of this chapter, the reader will be able to:

1. Define important terms and concepts relative to leadership, including styles of leadership.
2. List the essential components of effective leadership.
3. Differentiate between aggressive and cooperative negotiation.
4. Describe components of emotional intelligence.
5. Identify key critical thinking strategies and skills for case managers.
6. Describe the role of the case manager in delegation and supervision.
7. Compare and contrast hard and soft savings.
8. Discuss the role of the case manager as an agent of change.
9. Identify key communication skills.

IMPORTANT TERMS AND CONCEPTS

Change Agent

Communication

Conflict Management

Cost–Benefit Analysis

Critical Thinking

Delegation

Emotional Intelligence

Empowerment

Hard Savings

Leadership

Negotiation

Soft Savings

■ INTRODUCTION

A. Case management requires a wide array of management skills: delegation, conflict resolution, crisis intervention, collaboration, consultation, coordination, identification, communication, and documentation. However, case managers are no longer just managers of care; they are leaders, and there is a difference. *Managers manage systems; leaders lead people.* Case managers do both; they manage cases and lead, or guide, people. Leadership is one step up the ladder of professional growth. As case management responsibilities continue to grow, leadership qualities will necessarily be presumed (Powell, 2000a).

B. Management and leadership are *not* the same thing; they are not synonyms.
   1. A *manager* is an individual who holds an office—attached to which are multiple roles.
   2. *Leadership* is one of those roles (Shortell and Kaluzny, 2000).

C. Leadership is about the ability to influence people to accomplish goals. Leaders can be *formal* (by their position in the organization or society) or *informal* (by the amount of influence they have on others). Case managers are constantly in a position to influence people to accomplish health care goals.

D. Leadership is defined as a "process by which an individual exerts influence over other people and inspires, motivates, and directs their activities to help achieve group or organization goals" (Jones, George, and Hill, 1998, p. 403).

E. Six core components within the definition of leadership expound on the description (Shortell and Kaluzny, 2000):
   1. Leading is a *process,* an action word, a verb.
   2. The *locus* of leadership is a person; only individuals (as opposed to corporations or inanimate objects) can lead.
   3. The *focus* of leadership is other people or groups. This connection must exist for leadership to take place.
   4. Leadership necessitates *influencing.* It is the leader's ability to influence others that sets apart an effective leader from an ineffective one. This may be the most critical of the leadership components.

This chapter is a revised version of what was previously published in the first edition of *CMSA Core Curriculum for Case Management.* The contributor wishes to acknowledge Donna Ignatavicius, as some of the timeless material was retained from the previous version.

5. The object of leadership is *goal accomplishment.*

6. Leadership is *intentional,* not accidental.

F. How the above definition and criteria relate to case management roles and responsibilities:

1. Case management is a process where the case manager (the leader) must assess multiple variables that relate to the patient, the family, the disease process, the treatment, the insurance, the psychosocial situation, and the multidisciplinary health care team.

2. The goals chosen are the roadmap for the creation of best outcomes; the case manager must intentionally influence the situation to bring about the best outcomes for the patient and family.

3. The ability to influence others may be the case manager's "center of gravity" and most critical skill. Influence is a multipronged concept, and, on a daily basis, case managers intentionally influence patients/families to take appropriate medications, to think carefully about possible treatment choices, or to eat a diet that is best for their disease state (for examples). Case managers influence insurance companies, and other important health care team members.

■ KEY DEFINITIONS

A. Critical thinking—purposeful, outcome-directed thinking that aims to make judgments based on facts and is based on scientific principles (Alfaro-LeFevre, 1999).

B. Delegation—the process of assigning tasks to a qualified person and supervising that individual as needed.

C. Emotional intelligence—also called EI or EQ; describes an ability, capacity, or skill to perceive, assess, and manage the emotions of one's self, of others, and of groups.

D. Empowerment—allowing employees or subordinates to make decisions with support from the leader or manager.

E. Hard savings—occur when costs can be measurably saved or avoided.

F. Leadership—a process by which an individual exerts influence over other people and inspires, motivates, and directs their activities to help achieve group or organization goals.

G. Negotiation—essentially a communication exchange for the purpose of reaching agreement.

H. Soft savings—also called potential savings (or potential costs or charges); are less tangibly measurable than are hard savings (see hard savings, above).

■ LEADERSHIP STYLES

A. A leader's style is often based on a combination of beliefs, values, and preferences, in addition to the leader's organization's culture and norms, which will encourage some styles and discourage others. There are several styles of leadership. Case managers use these styles differently,

TABLE 12–1

Participative Leadership Styles

Not Participative			Highly Participative	
Autocratic decision by leader	Leader proposes decision, listens to feedback, then decides	Team proposes decision, leader has final decision	Joint decision with team as equals	Full delegation of decision to team

Note. *http://changingminds.org/disciplines/leadership/styles/leadership_styles.htm.*

depending on the situation and the role at the time. However, personality traits may make one or two styles predominant (or nonexistent).

1. Charismatic leadership—The word *charisma* is derived from a Greek word meaning "divinely inspired gift." Charismatic leaders feel that charm and grace are all that is needed to create followers and that people follow others that they personally admire. Charismatic leaders pay a great deal of attention in scanning and reading their environment, and are good at picking up the moods and concerns of both individuals and larger audiences. They then will hone their actions and words to suit the situation ("Leadership Styles," 2006).

2. Participative leadership—Participative leaders believe that involvement in decision making improves the understanding of the issues concerned by those who must carry out the decisions. Further, people are more committed to actions when they have been involved in the relevant decision making, and are less competitive and more collaborative when they are working on joint goals ("Leadership Styles," 2006) (see Table 12-1).

3. Situational leadership—Situational leaders use a range of actions and styles that depend on the situation. This style may be *transactional* or *transformational* (see below) or any of the leadership styles discussed.[1]

4. Transactional leadership—Transactional leaders believe that people are motivated by reward and punishment. Social systems work best with a clear chain of command. When people have agreed to do a job (the transaction), a part of the deal is that they cede all authority to their manager. The prime purpose of a subordinate is to do what their manager tells them to do ("Leadership Styles," 2006).

5. Transformational leadership—While transactional leadership attempts to preserve and work within the constraints of the status quo, transformational leadership seeks to subvert and replace it and looks at the greater good (Shortell and Kaluzny, 2000). Transformational leaders believe people will follow a person who inspires them, has vision and passion, and can achieve great things. The way to get things done is by injecting enthusiasm and energy. Transformational leadership starts with the development of a vision (by the leader or by the

---

[1]One caution of situational leadership: The leader's *perception* of the follower and the situation will affect what they do rather than the *truth* of the situation. The leader's perception of themselves and other factors such as stress and mood will also modify the leader's behavior ("Leadership Styles," 2006).

team)—a view of the future that will excite and convert potential followers ("Leadership Styles," 2006).

6. Quiet leader—The quiet leader believes that the actions of a leader speak louder than his or her words. People are motivated when you give them credit rather than take it yourself. Ego and aggression are neither necessary nor constructive ("Leadership Styles," 2006).

7. Servant leadership—The servant leader believes the leader has responsibility for the followers and toward society and those who are disadvantaged. The servant leader serves others, rather than others serving the leader ("Leadership Styles," 2006).

■ LEADERSHIP SKILLS

A. The jury is still out about whether leaders are born or made. However, experts have noticed specific actions that successful leaders share, regardless of the type of organization they lead.

B. Qualities of effective leaders are listed below. Note the similarities between effectively working with patients/clients, and leaders working within their organizations. Effective leaders:

1. *Promote empowerment.* They emphasize the strengths and utilize the talents of others in the organization. Leaders share decision making with others, allowing those people at the point of care or service to be the key decision makers. Then they share in the success and give credit where it is due.

2. *Promote a vision.* People need a vision of where they are going. Leaders provide that vision (*Manager's Intelligence Report*, 1997).

3. *Follow the golden rule.* Anyone who has been demeaned or treated with disrespect knows what effect that treatment has on the work (*Manager's Intelligence Report*, 1997).

4. *Admit mistakes.*

5. *Praise others in public.* And criticize others only in private.

6. *Stay close to the action.* In case management, this is the administrator who goes to the "front lines" occasionally to stay in touch with the reality of the working situation. This also means that the leader is visible and accessible.

7. Say, "*I don't know*" when confronted with a case management problem, then assist with a solution.

8. Focus on *what* is right, not *who* is right.

9. *Motivate others* by:
   a. Establishing credibility
   b. Improving communication skills
   c. Being a role model
   d. Taking an interest in others
   e. Rewarding positive behaviors
   f. Sharing decision making
   g. Offering constructive criticism (Ellis and Hartley, 1995)

10. *Hold their staff accountable*, but also let them do their jobs.

   C. Conflict management is an important skill for leaders. Five strategies can be employed, from less desirable to most desirable.
1. Avoidance
2. Competition ("I win, you lose")
3. Accommodation ("You win, I lose")
4. Negotiation (also known as compromise) (see next section)
5. Collaboration ("You win, I win") (the best strategy)
   a. Takes more time to use
   b. Saved for complex or emotional issues

■ NEGOTIATION SKILLS

   A. In the current health care environment of scarce resource availability and declining benefits, the art of negotiation is extremely important.

   B. Negotiation serves several important purposes (Powell, 2000a):
1. It has the capacity to control costs. This is one of the primary reasons case managers negotiate.
2. It has the capacity to gain medically necessary benefits for the patient that the patient would otherwise not receive. This is the other primary reason case managers negotiate.
3. It can avoid chaos (Jones, Skelton, and Hochuli, 1998). Many case managers have lived through the frustration and chaos that results when a patient's condition deteriorates, at least partly because the negotiation for the requested service or equipment was denied.
4. Negotiation can be a learning experience. Case managers may learn why the request is denied (sometimes there is a valid reason). They may also reveal weaknesses in the "No!" argument that could lead to further strengths in the case manager's negotiation stance.

   C. Successful negotiation steps include:
1. Be optimally prepared. Before negotiation begins, it is wise to do some research; understand the other side before negotiation. For example, if you are negotiating the price of a resource or service, research current prices of the same service offered by competitors.
2. Negotiation starts by stating the problem or problems and the goal, and stating what is needed to solve the problem. State the request in a positive and thorough way. Areas in which there is agreement can be put aside; then begin to search for a mutual compromise where there is disagreement (Rehberg and Sullivan, 1997).
3. Use the three Cs—communicate, communicate, communicate. Common mistakes can create a defensive environment that is not conducive to negotiation. Some behaviors that may be problematic include poor listening skills, poor use of questions, improper disclosure of ideas, mismanagement of issues, inappropriate stress reactions, rejecting alternatives too quickly, misusing a negotiating team member, not disclosing true feelings, improper timing, and being aggressive rather than assertive (Hein and Nicholson, 1994).

4. Be realistic. Attempting to negotiate for a service or a price that absolutely will not be covered or met, wastes everyone's time and energy.

5. Put it in writing. Once an agreement has been reached, write it down and have all parties sign it.

D. There are two types of negotiators: aggressive and cooperative. Aggressive negotiators use psychological maneuvers such as intimidation and threats to make their "opponent" feel disparaged. Cooperative negotiators try to establish trust.

1. The aggressive negotiator (Jones, Skelton, and Hochuli, 1998):

   a. Moves psychologically against his or her opponent. Note the key word *psychologically*. If the case manager feels that something is amiss—that is, that he or she is being toyed with—he or she should bring the case back to facts.

   b. Common tactics include intimidation, accusation, threats, sarcasm, and ridicule.

   c. There is an overt or covert claim that the aggressive negotiator is superior.

   d. The aggressive negotiator will make extreme demands and few concessions.

   e. There will be frequent threats to terminate negotiations.

   f. False issues will be brought up time and again. This is another opportunity to bring the case back to facts.

2. Weaknesses of the aggressive method (Jones, Skelton, and Hochuli, 1998):

   a. It is more difficult to be a successful aggressive.

   b. Tension and mistrust that develop may increase the likelihood of misunderstandings.

   c. Deadlock over one trivial issue may escalate other issues.

   d. The opponent may develop righteous indignation and pursue the case with more vengeance.

   e. The reputation as an aggressive hurts future negotiations.

   f. Aggressive tactics increase the number of failed negotiations.

   g. The trial rate for aggressive negotiators is more than double.

3. The cooperative negotiator (Jones, Skelton, and Hochuli, 1998):

   a. Moves psychologically toward his or her opponent.

   b. This negotiator establishes a common ground. For case managers, the common ground is the patient.

   c. This negotiator is trustworthy, fair, objective, and reasonable. This is very important. Respect and trustworthiness are critical for negotiations and for self-respect as a case management professional.

   d. This negotiator works to establish credibility and unilateral concessions. The attitude is one of "win-win."

   e. This negotiator seeks to obtain the best joint outcome for everyone. This requires respect, empathy, and active listening, as described in other sections of this text.

4. Strengths of the cooperative method (Jones, Skelton, and Hochuli, 1998):
   a. Promotes mutual understanding.
   b. Generally produces agreement in less time than the aggressive approach.
   c. Produces agreements in a larger percentage of cases than aggressiveness.
   d. Often produces a better outcome than aggressive strategies.
   e. There is a much higher percentage of "successful" negotiations.
   f. Future negotiations are made easier.
5. Weaknesses of the cooperative method (Jones, Skelton, and Hochuli, 1998):
   a. Aggressive negotiators view cooperative negotiators as weak, so they push harder.
   b. Cooperative negotiators risk being manipulative or exploitive because of the assumption that, "if I am fair and trustworthy and make decisions with all parties in mind, then the other side will feel an irresistible moral obligation to reciprocate."

E. A critical trait to possess when negotiating (or dealing with humanity) is *emotional intelligence.*

F. Emotional intelligence, also called EI or EQ, describes an ability, capacity, or skill to perceive, assess, and manage the emotions of one's self, of others, and of groups. However, being a relatively new area, the definition of emotional intelligence is still in a state of flux (Wikipedia, 2006).

G. The Mayer-Salovey model defines emotional intelligence as the capacity to understand emotional information and to reason with emotions. More specifically, in their four-branch model, they divide emotional intelligence abilities into four areas (Wikipedia, 2006):
   a. The capacity to accurately perceive emotions
   b. The capacity to use emotions to facilitate thinking
   c. The capacity to understand emotional meanings
   d. The capacity to manage emotions

H. Goleman divides emotional intelligence into the following five emotional competencies, all essential in case management work (Wikipedia, 2006):
   a. The ability to identify and name one's emotional states and to understand the links among emotions, thought, and action
   b. The capacity to manage one's emotional states—to control emotions or to shift undesirable emotional states to more adequate ones
   c. The ability to enter into emotional states (at will) associated with a drive to achieve and be successful
   d. The capacity to read, be sensitive to, and influence other people's emotions
   e. The ability to enter and sustain satisfactory interpersonal relationships

■ DELEGATION SKILLS

A. Some case managers see delegation as a loss of power and control.

B. Some case managers simply do not trust others to do the job correctly. They live by the credo, if you want something done correctly, do it yourself.

C. Some case managers feel a legal liability when delegating responsibility.

D. Delegation standards that will minimize risk are (Powell, 2000a):
1. Always act in a reasonable and prudent manner.
2. Ensure that the delegate is qualified to perform the tasks.
3. Assign tasks that are within the person's scope of practice.
4. Provide proper supervision (guidance and monitoring) to the person to whom the task was delegated. However, let the delegate put their "spin" on the task (it may be better than your idea).
5. Assign a due date.

E. Effective delegation recommendations:
1. Stress results, not details. Make it clear that you are more concerned with the final outcome than with all of the day-to-day details. This provides autonomy to the one who is responsible for the results.
2. Do not always become the solution to everyone's problems. Teach others how to solve problems, rather than just providing the answers. Again, this builds confidence and independence and provides autonomy.
3. When an employee or coworker comes to you with a problem and a question, ask him or her for possible solutions. Be there to brainstorm when needed.
4. Establish measurable and concrete objectives. Make them clear and specific. This is the road map that others can follow.
5. Develop reporting systems. Obtain feedback from written reports, statistical data, and planned face-to-face meetings. This does not always work in case management if a particularly tough problem arises; teach employees when to come to you with details, and when to come to you after exhausting other avenues.
6. When appropriate, give strict but realistic deadlines. This gives the task credibility and gives the person accountability.
7. Keep a delegation log. This is especially important for very busy people or those with many employees.
8. Recognize and use the talents and personalities of the people you work with. Being a good delegator is very much like being a good coach.

■ COMMUNICATION SKILLS FOR PATIENT SAFETY

A. Poor communication skills can have ramifications that range from stressful working environments to unsafe patient environments.

B. Unsafe patient environments can have many causes, and take many forms. Clearly, communication plays a large role, and communicating clearly and completely is essential.

1. The transfer of timely and accurate information across settings (transitions of care) is critical to the execution of effective care transitions.
2. One definition of care transfers includes transfers to or from an acute hospital, skilled nursing or rehabilitation facility, or home with or without home health care (HMO Workgroup, 2004).
3. Not all patients undergoing transitions are at high risk for adverse events; however, those with poor transitional care plans are particularly likely to "fall through the cracks" (HMO Workgroup, 2004).
4. Processes for accurate and complete transitions of care must be developed by health care organizations. However, at this time, there is often a lack of agreement about what comprises the core clinical information that all practitioners require irrespective of setting.
5. The Care Transitions Measure (CTM) was developed by researchers at University of Colorado Health Sciences Center to assess the quality of care transitions from the perspective of the patient or his or her proxy. CTM scores have been shown to be significantly associated with a patient's return to a hospital or emergency department after discharge (HMO Workgroup, 2004).

C. Stressful working environments are often a result of poor communication skills that lead one to "act out," rather than "talk it out" when the topic is one of high stress/high stakes (Patterson et al., 2002).
1. In the "Silence Kills" study, it was found that the ability to hold crucial conversations is key to creating a culture of safety in health care; conversely, the prevalent culture of poor communication and faulty collaboration among health professionals relates significantly to continued medical errors and patient complaints.
2. Crucial conversations occur when (Patterson et al., 2002):
   a. Opinions vary (e.g., What is the *best* course of treatment or discharge plan for this case?)
   b. The stakes are high (e.g., there is an imminent danger to patient safety)
   c. Emotions are strong (e.g., adrenalin is already flowing, so thought processes are impaired)
3. Dialogue skills are learnable and can be used in nearly every case management encounter. For positive dialogue (Patterson et al., 2002):
   a. Figure out what you really want: for yourself and for others.
   b. People often act out (go to "silence or violence") when they do not feel *safe*. Learn to notice when the other party does this.
   c. Make it safe. Conditions/dialogue that promotes *mutual respect* is one place to start.
   d. Apologize when appropriate. Agree when appropriate.
   e. Consider that what YOU think is happening, may not be exactly correct (i.e., What "story" are you telling yourself?). If you are telling a negative "story" about the other person, go back to "just the facts." And ask what part you play in the scene.
   f. *Ask* others questions, and consider that they have good information to add to the pool of knowledge.

■ CRITICAL THINKING AND DECISION MAKING

A. Critical thinking is broader than problem solving. It is more than finding a single solution to a problem (Alfaro-LeFevre, 1999).

B. In health care, critical thinking may be referred to as clinical reasoning; in nursing, it is sometimes equated to the nursing process. In case management, critical thinking equates with the global thinking necessary to appropriately put all the pieces of the client/patient puzzle together.

C. Critical thinking is being creative and/or "connecting the dots." In general, it is the ability to:
1. Put together the known components of the problem or situation
2. Research all possible solutions
3. Find a way to improve the condition (Powell, 2000a)

D. Critical thinking is focused on outcomes, not tasks. It is purposeful, outcome-directed thinking that aims to make judgments based on facts. It is reflective and reasonable thinking about client problems and is focused on deciding what to do.

E. Good critical thinkers are:
1. Flexible
2. Creative
3. Communicators, especially listening
4. Open minded
5. Willing to change
6. Outcome focused
7. Able to see "the big picture"
8. Caring

F. Variables that affect critical thinking (Ignatavicius, 1999):
1. Thinking styles
2. Personal factors, such as age, gender, and education
3. Situational factors, such as available time, resources, peer support, and administrative support

G. Levels of critical thinking
1. Basic level—knowing right from wrong
2. Complex level—identifying all possible alternatives or solutions (e.g., "It depends.")
3. Committed level: selecting the most reasonable alternative ("Plan A") and having one or more backup plans in case Plan A is unsuccessful

H. Critical thinking strategies and cognitive skills based on an American Philosophical Association (APA) study (Facione and Facione, 1996)
1. Interpretation (clarifying meaning)
2. Analysis (examining ideas, data)
3. Evaluation (assessing outcomes)
4. Inference (drawing conclusions)

     5. Explanation (justifying actions)

     6. Self-regulation (self-examination and correction)

I. Critical thinking process

     1. Analyze all of the problems.

     2. Determine the expected outcomes.

     3. List all possible alternatives and solutions to the problems.

     4. Select the best or highest-priority alternative.

     5. Determine if the plan worked (i.e., Were the outcomes met?).

■ THE ETHICS OF DECISION MAKING

A. The ethics of decision making includes how to recognize ethical issues, make ethical judgments, and then convert them into *action.*

B. Consider the following:

     1. Identify which stakeholders will be affected by the decision(s).

     2. Identify costs/benefits of the decision(s) *alternatives* for these stakeholders.

     3. Consider any moral expectations of the decision(s) (look at norms, regulatory issues, laws, organizational ethics, codes of conduct, principles related to honest communication and fair treatment).

     4. Be familiar with ethical dilemmas that leaders in your organization/profession commonly face.

     5. Discuss ethical matters with those affected.

     6. Convert your ethical judgments into appropriate action (Jones, 1996).

■ FINANCIAL/COST–BENEFIT ANALYSIS

A. Not only is a solid knowledge of financial methodologies important to case management, but the above leadership skills will help the case manager discuss the financial issues that follow when the stakes are high and the potential conflicts may be intensified. Case managers *and especially* case management supervisors must thoroughly understand—and judiciously manage—individual cases, staff resources, departmental resources, and organizational resources.

B. Case management leaders must understand and be savvy about budgetary issues.

C. Many case managers will be asked to conduct a cost analysis of a case or of parts of a case. For example:

     1. Occasionally, family members need comparative financial information.

     2. Insurance companies who are inclined to refuse payment for a requested plan if they believe that a less cost-intensive solution is available may request prices.

     3. Many case managers are required to make a formal documentation of savings per case for accounting purposes.

     4. Disease management case managers may be required to contribute to the savings information for an entire population of disease-specific patients.

D. Some case managers shun this responsibility. There may be several reasons for the dislike (Powell, 2000b), such as the following:
   1. We did not go into the helping professions to do accounting work. We are case managers to improve the quality of a patient's life.
   2. We already know that we improve quality and decrease costs per case; justifying our existence is another's responsibility.
   3. It is difficult to understand accounting and budgeting concepts.
   4. It is often tedious and time consuming to address and report financial details.
E. Case managers are as real an expense to the payers and facilities who hire us as are physician services, hospital costs, and medications. Cost analysis is one method used to prove our worth in the business world.
F. Hard savings or avoided costs are costs that can be measurably saved or avoided. Examples of hard savings facilitated by the case manager include (Powell, 2000b):
   1. Change in the level of care
   2. Change in the patient's length of stay
   3. Change to a contracted PPO provider
   4. Negotiation of price of services, supplies, equipment, or per diem rates
   5. Negotiation of frequency of services
   6. Negotiation of duration of services
   7. Prevention of unnecessary bed days, supplies, equipment, services, or charges
   8. Finding nonauthorized charges that are not warranted
G. Soft savings or potential savings (or potential costs or charges) are less tangibly measurable than are hard savings. If no case manager is assigned to a particular patient, the potential costs incurred could be much higher than with case management; soft savings represent costs that are avoided most likely because of case management intervention.
H. Examples of soft savings include avoidance of potential (Powell, 2000b):
   1. Hospital readmissions
   2. Emergency department visits
   3. Medical complications
   4. Legal exposure
   5. Costs, equipment, and supplies
   6. Acute care days
   7. Home health visits
I. Other soft savings relate to quality and satisfaction. It is difficult to put a dollar amount on improved:
   1. Quality of care
   2. Patient and family satisfaction with case management
   3. Patient compliance
   4. Quality of life

■ CASE MANAGEMENT OUTCOMES IN THE SUPERVISORY ROLE

A. Leaders/supervisors must look at outcomes in their department, staff, or organization. Well-chosen outcomes give case management leaders knowledge of *where* they currently are, and act as a compass for future improvement.

B. First attempts at measuring outcomes should be easily and concretely measurable.

1. Begin by looking at only one or two outcomes.

2. Traditionally, cost savings have been one of the most common measurements used for case management outcomes. Hard savings are more tangible and easily measured; soft savings are more obscure.

3. Quality of life issues are also more nebulous and require careful consideration when turning them into something that is measurable (Powell, 2000b).

C. Defining an "outcomes" budget when beginning an outcomes management program is important.

1. Measuring outcomes is an important marketing tool, but the process requires resources of time, money, and personnel.

2. It is important to assess what resources will be needed and to define a budget for the project that is acceptable to the organization. Consider the following (Powell, 2000b):

a. What resources are *available* to plan, select, modify or develop, and implement an effective case management intervention?

b. What resources are *required* to plan, select, modify or develop, and implement a case management intervention?

c. In some projects, other people or organizations are asked to commit resources to the project. In those instances, determine what resources will be required of others. Are they willing and able to provide the resources? Some resources to consider are provider staffing, physician time, and beneficiary co-payments or deductibles.

d. Can the improved outcome be translated into projected cost savings? If the cost of the case management intervention exceeds the amount of projected cost savings, is this still acceptable to the organization?

e. Data collection and analysis is complex and costly. Does the case management organization have the necessary resources and information systems to execute these tasks, or can the organization secure appropriate data elements from other avenues that will provide the information necessary to record outcome measurements? Put a dollar amount on this and assess whether it is feasible.

■ CASE MANAGERS AS CHANGE AGENTS

A. Although some people embrace change, most find it intimidating. Because of the unpredictable nature of change, some people respond to it with fear. Change is often at the core of stress.

B. New and fast-changing managed care and financial constraints must be managed.

C. Case management is more important than ever before in managing these changes in the best interests of the patients; case managers are essentially change agents.

D. The three components of the change process are:
1. Unfreezing the current behavior or situation
   a. Determine driving forces (supportive forces for the change).
   b. Determine restraining forces (opposing forces for the change).
   c. Develop a plan to overcome resistance to change.
2. Implementing the change
   a. Enable the change
   b. Monitor the change
3. Freezing the new change
   a. Sustain and support the change
   b. Evaluate the change

E. Attitudes to help agents of change cope:
1. Sometimes these methods fail. You have worked hard with the case and used the clinical pathways. Then it seems the case is falling off the path at every turn, and variances are winning. There is no shortage of problems.
   a. First, assess whether you could have done anything differently for a better outcome.
   b. If so, learn from it.
   c. If not, realize that sometimes these methods fail.
2. Choose your battles carefully. Many aspects of case management are completely out of the case manager's realm of control. Assess whether the problem is really something over which you have influence.
3. Consider that one approach to change includes a resistance to change (as though the ones who need to change are donkeys sitting down instead of moving where we want them to be). Instead, create attractors to promote change (Plsek and Kilo, 1999).
4. Remember this wise adage—Robert Eliot, a cardiologist at the University of Nebraska, has developed two rules for keeping things in perspective (Charlesworth and Nathan, 1984):
   a. Don't sweat the small stuff.
   b. It's all small stuff.
5. Remember that change is risk.
6. It is OK to disagree. Not everyone has to be in agreement to move forward. Use the continuous quality improvement (CQI) tool of "consensus".
7. Anticipate changes. Do not wait for changes to happen. Be proactive with other possibilities.

F. The Eight-Stage Change Process—Successful transformations are neither easy nor linear. Still, some change experts believe that a general sequence of change *does* occur, that no steps should be missed, and that—at times—multiple phases occur at once. The Eight-Stage Change Process (Kotter,

1996) includes timeless concepts that can help case managers in many aspects of their work (both at the patient level and at the corporate level).

1. *Establish a sense of urgency.* This can be accomplished by examining the market and competitive realities or the patient's clinical trajectory, identifying crises or potential crises, and/or identifying major opportunities.

2. *Create a guiding coalition.* Put together a group with enough power to lead the change; then, get the group to work together like a team (leadership is needed here). In case management, this may be the essential patient care team.

3. *Develop a vision and strategy.* The vision created will direct the change effort. Then, develop strategies to achieve the vision. What does the team want? More importantly, what does the patient/family want?

4. *Communicate the change.* Use all vehicles to communicate the vision and strategies. Have the guiding coalition to role model the behavior.

5. *Empower broad-based action.* Remove obstacles (from the team, the patient, the case, if possible). Change systems or structures that undermine the change vision. Encourage risk taking and nontraditional ideas.

6. *Generate short-term wins.* Plan for visible improvements early in the process. Visibly recognize and reward the people who made the "win" possible. From a patient perspective, this may help the patient/family become more autonomous.

7. *Consolidate the gains and produce more change.* As the patient/family becomes more knowledgeable or independent, use this progress to instill more sense of autonomy and produce more results.

8. Last—and perhaps most important for a department/organization— *anchor the new approaches in the culture.* Create better performance through customer service and excellent leadership. Articulate the connection between new behaviors and organization success. And develop ways to ensure leadership development and succession.

REFERENCES

Alfaro-LeFevre, R. (1999). *Critical thinking in nursing.* Philadelphia: W.B. Saunders.

Charlesworth, E., & Nathan, R. (1984). *Stress management: A comprehensive guide to wellness.* New York: Atheneum.

Ellis, J. R., & Hartley, C. L. (1995). *Managing and coordinating nursing care.* Philadelphia: J.B. Lippincott.

Facione, N. C., & Facione, P. A. (1996). Externalizing the critical thinking in knowledge development and clinical judgment. *Nursing Outlook, 44*(3), 129–136.

Hein, E. C., & Nicholson, M. J. (1994). *Contemporary leadership behavior.* Philadelphia: J.B. Lippincott.

HMO Workgroup on Care Management. (2004). *One patient, many places: Managing health care transitions.* Washington, DC: AAHP-HIAA Foundation.

Ignatavicius, D. D. (1999). Critical thinking workshops.

Jones, G. (1996). *Organizational behavior: Understanding and managing life at work,* 4th ed. New York: HarperCollins College Publishers.

Jones, G. R., George, J. M., & Hill, C. W. L. (1998). *Contemporary management.* Jones, Skelton, & Hochuli. (1998). Seminar in Phoenix, AZ.

Kotter, J. P. (1996). *Leading change.* Boston: Harvard Business School Press.

Leadership styles. (2006). Website: *http://changingminds.org/disciplines/leadership/styles/leadership_styles.htm.* Retrieved March 19, 2006.

Manager's intelligence report. (1997). Chicago: Lawrence Ragan Communications, Inc.

Patterson, K., Grenny, J., McMillan, R., & Switzler, A. (2002). *Crucial conversations: Tools for talking when the stakes are high.* McGraw-Hill Publishers: New York.

Plsek, P. E., & Kilo, C. M. (1999). From resistance to attraction: A different approach to change. *The Physician Executive,* Nov/Dec, 40–42.

Powell, S. K. (2000a). *Case management: A practical guide to success in managed care.* Philadelphia: Lippincott Williams & Wilkins.

Powell, S. K. (2000b). *Advanced case management: Outcomes and beyond.* Philadelphia: Lippincott Williams & Wilkins.

Rehberg, C., & Sullivan, G. (1997). The art of negotiation: A delicate balance. *Nursing Case Management,* 2(4), 177–179.

Shortell, S. M., & Kaluzny, A. D. (2000). *Health care management: Organization design and behavior,* 4th ed. Albany: Delmar.

Wikipedia (2006). Emotional intelligence. Website: *http://en.wikipedia.org/wiki/Emotional_intelligence.* Retrieved March 19.

chapter

13 Education, Training, and Certification of Case Managers

Marietta P. Stanton
Hussein A. Tahan

LEARNING OBJECTIVES

Upon completion of this chapter, the reader will be able to:

1. Identify those organizations and standards that exert an influence over case management education, training, and certification.
2. Describe key components of the case manager's initial education and clinical preparation, including life experience.
3. Describe competency-based approaches to case management education and training.
4. Examine the relationship between various certifying agencies in case management and case management education and training curriculum development.
5. Delineate topics appropriate for continuing education and staff development in case management.
6. Determine the differences in academic preparation and how these relate to basic and advanced levels of case management practice.
7. Define credentialing, certification, and accreditation.
8. List the components of the credentialing process employed for accreditation of case management organizations, programs, or services.
9. List essential criteria for certification.

240

IMPORTANT TERMS AND CONCEPTS

Accreditation
Accreditation of Case Management
  Organizations
Accreditation Standards
American Nurses Credentialing
  Center
Case Management
Case Management Philosophy
Case Management Society of America's
  Standards of Practice

Center for Case Management
Certificate
Certification
Commission for Case Manager
  Certification
Core Components of Case
  Management
Credentialing
Licensure

■ INTRODUCTION

A. Essential information related to the education, clinical preparation, and work life experience of case management practice comes from several important sources.

  1. Professional organizations, case management certification organizations, and accrediting agencies provide an overview of the knowledge required for case management education and training.

  2. Certification in and accreditation of case management are valued and therefore are powerful forces in shaping educational requirements for case management preparation.

B. Educational preparation of case managers is critical to the success of the case management role in the health care system. Consensus information about core areas of knowledge needed by case managers for basic, intermediate, and advanced levels of practice have been delineated in the literature.

C. Because case management preparation is dependent on both experience and educational preparation, using competency standards for case management in the clinical area is an effective mechanism for training, continuing education, and staff development.

D. Academic preparation and clinical experience are determinants of knowledge and skill levels of the case manager. There are case management skills that appear to be at the basic entry level of practice and there are other skills that appear to be at the advanced practice or master's-degree level of academic preparation.

E. Necessary training and education in specialty areas vary according to the specialty area and related certifications.

F. Certifications in case management have been in existence since the early 1990s. Currently, there are more than 30 different certifications in case management or its related practices, which presents a challenge for the interested case manager in deciding which one best fits her or his specialty practice or professional discipline.

G. *Certification, accreditation,* and *credentialing* are three terms that tend to be confused and used interchangeably. These terms are different and professionals in the case management field should be clear on their definitions and should use these terms appropriately.

■ KEY DEFINITIONS

A. Accreditation—A process in which a nationally recognized agency (other than a health care provider organization), usually nongovernmental, assesses a health care organization's operations and performance to determine whether it meets a set of nationally recognized and accepted standards, mainly designed to demonstrate quality and safe care.

B. Case manager—A health care professional who is responsible for coordinating the care delivered to a group of patients based on diagnosis or need. Other responsibilities may include patient and family education, advocacy, management of delays in care, utilization management, transitional planning, and outcomes monitoring and management. Case managers work with people to get the health care and other community services they need, when they need them, and for the best value (quality and cost).

C. Certificate—A document awarded to affirm that an individual participated or attended a given educational program. It can be provided by any professional agency (private or public, for-profit and not-for-profit), university, or college. Usually a certificate is not nationally recognized in any form other than an educational credit.

D. Certification (individual)—An official form of credential that is provided by a nationally recognized governmental or nongovernmental certifying agency to a professional who meets the eligibility criteria and requirement of a particular field, practice, or specialty. It usually signifies the achievement of a passing score on an examination prepared by the certifying agency for that purpose. It also denotes an advanced degree of competence.

E. Certification (organization or program)—An official form of accreditation that is provided by a nationally recognized governmental or nongovernmental agency to an organization or a program within an organization (e.g., center of excellence) that meets nationally recognized requirements or standards of quality and safe performance.

F. Consensus—Agreement in opinion of experts. Building consensus is a method used when developing case management plans.

G. Credentialing (individual)—The process used to protect the consumer and to ensure that individuals hired to practice case management are providing quality case management services. This involves a review of the provider's licensure, certification, insurance, evidence of malpractice insurance (if applicable), performance, knowledge, skills, and competencies, and history of lawsuits/malpractices.

H. Credentialing (organization or program/service)—The process used in the review of a case management program or organization to ensure that it meets nationally recognized industry standards of quality. This is necessary for the provision of quality case management services and to protect the consumer.

I. Credentials—Evidence of competence, current and relevant licensure, certification, education, and experience.

J. Licensure—A mandatory and official form of validation provided by a state governmental agency affirming that an individual has acquired the basic knowledge and skill, and minimum degree of competence required for safe practice in one's profession such as nursing, medicine, and social work. This is usually conducted in compliance with a statute for a given occupation and carries the expectation that the licensed individual act in an unsupervised way.

K. Standard (individual)—An authoritative statement by which a profession defines the responsibilities for which its practitioners are accountable.

L. Standard (organization)—An authoritative statement that defines the performance expectations, structures, or processes that must be substantially in place in an organization to enhance the quality of care.

M. Standards of care—Statements that delineate care that is expected to be provided to all clients. They include predefined outcomes of care that clients can expect from providers and that are accepted within the community of professionals, based on the best scientific knowledge, current outcomes data, and clinical expertise.

N. Standards of practice—Statements of acceptable level of performance or expectation for professional intervention or behavior associated with one's professional practice. They are generally formulated by practitioner organizations based on clinical expertise and the most current research findings.

O. Utilization Review Accreditation Commission (URAC)—A not-for-profit organization that provides reviews and accreditation for utilization review services/programs provided by freestanding agencies. It is also known as the American Accreditation Health Care Commission.

■ EDUCATION AND TRAINING OF CASE MANAGERS

A. Education and training programs of case managers are developed based on the standards of practice, evidence-based outcomes, accreditation and credentialing criteria, and certification examination content.

B. Key elements for case management education and training are specified in the URAC Case Management Accreditation Standards. These standards specify that case managers must be educated in:
   1. Current case management principles and practices, and
   2. Procedures and knowledge of case management based on nationally recognized standards.

C. Education should include knowledge of the organization's policies and procedures, case management process, state requirements, professional roles, organizational ethics and confidentiality, health care requirements of specific populations, URAC standards, and Case Management Society of America (CMSA) standards of practice.

D. URAC requires annual training and recognizes major case management certifications.[1]

E. The Commission for Case Management Certification (CCMC, 2005) has identified eight essential activities of case management:
   1. Assessment
   2. Planning
   3. Implementation
   4. Coordination
   5. Monitoring
   6. Evaluation
   7. Outcomes
   8. General (across all activities)

F. CCMC has also delineated six core components of case management knowledge necessary for effective performance.[2] These core components provide a basic foundation for case management education, training and continuing education, and competencies:
   1. Case management concepts
   2. Case management principles and strategies
   3. Psychosocial and support systems
   4. Health care management and delivery
   5. Health care reimbursement
   6. Vocational concepts and strategies

G. Similarly, the Center for Case Management (CFCM) delineates specific content for the Case Management Administrators Certification (CMAC).[3] Topics covered in the exam include:
   1. Identification of at-risk populations
   2. Assessment of clinical systems' components
   3. Development strategies to manage at-risk populations
   4. Leadership for change
   5. Market assessment and strategic planning
   6. Human resource management
   7. Program evaluation through outcomes management

H. CMSA provides a foundation for education of case managers with the specification of their standards of practice (2002). The standards for care

---

[1] *www.urac.org/prog_accred_CM*
[2] Detailed descriptions of these core components and subtopics are available at the CCMC Website (*www.ccmcertification.org*).
[3] *http://cfcm.com/resources/certification.asp*

and the related "performance indicators" are essential elements in case management education and training.

1. Educational components include client identification and selection for case management services, problem identification, planning, monitoring, evaluating, and outcomes.
2. Each step in the case management process provides measurement guidelines that give direction for education and training.
3. Performance indicators prescribed by CMSA in the area of quality of care, qualifications of case managers, collaboration with patients and providers, as well as legal, ethical, and advocacy considerations for case management practice also provide direction for education and training.
4. CMSA's standards of practice also address resource management and stewardship, as well as provide measurement guidelines for each of the performance indicators, resulting in a comprehensive overview of the requirements for the training, education, and ongoing continuing development of case managers.
5. The standards specify educational preparation and certification qualifications for case managers, including professional licensure, specific training related to case management and a minimum of 2 years' experience related to the health needs of the target population, appropriate continuing education, and maintaining certifications. These specifications regarding preparation have laid the groundwork for consideration of case management as advanced practice in nursing (CMSA, 2002).

I. The American Nurses Association (ANA), through its credentialing arm (the American Nurses Credentialing Center, ANCC) has identified five components of case management practice—assessment, planning, implementation, evaluation, and interaction (ANCC, 2005).

J. The CCMC also specifies criteria for validating practice for certification as a certified case manager (CCM). For example, an individual can practice under the auspices of a CCM for 12 months, or 24 months under the supervision of a case manager. There is a mechanism for validating experience as a self-employed case manager.

1. Persons supervising case managers for 12 months may be able to sit for the certification exam. Similarly, the CMAC exam acknowledges length of experience as a master's-degree–prepared case manager and case management administrator as a criterion for application to sit for the examination.

K. The education and training for case management has included extensive experience as a licensed professional and extensive practice as a case manager. The practice element in case management should be coupled with education and training.

L. Areas of specialization, like workers' compensation, disability case management, or maternal child case management, also provide additional foundational areas for case management education and training. Many of these are similar to the CCM in terms of content and focus.

■ CONSENSUS AREAS FOR CASE MANAGEMENT EDUCATION: CORE COMPONENTS

A. The literature in case management provides an indication of what needs to be included in case management education and training.

B. Reviewing previous research studies and articles on case management education and training provides insight into topics that should be included. This also promotes the development of evidence-based training and education programs.

C. A large survey of case managers provided an in-depth description of their services in a variety of work settings (Leahy et al., 1997). Foundational elements were abstracted from this data and five core areas were identified:

   1. Coordination and service delivery
   2. Physical and psychosocial issues
   3. Benefit systems/cost–benefit analysis
   4. Case management concepts
   5. Community re-entry

D. In a survey of nurse educators, content areas for case management were grouped into four levels of complexity as well as by content (Kulbok and Utz, 1999). These were:

   1. Background in history and trends
   2. Case management process (basic levels)
   3. Ethical and legal issues (intermediate level)
   4. Case management research (advanced)

E. Benner and colleagues (Kulbok and Utz, 1999) categorized the stages of skill development as novice, advanced beginner, competent, proficient, and expert.

   1. Applying these levels to case managers, a new graduate would be an advanced beginner.
   2. Through experience, maturity, and formal and informal learning, the case manager would progress through the experience levels to expert level within the role of the case manager.
   3. For some expert-level case managers with advanced education, a natural progression into a leadership position as a case management director responsible for educating and mentoring other beginning or intermediate case managers may occur.
   4. Based on this notion, much of the content that is appropriate for nursing administrators is also appropriate for case management administrators.

F. In social work, graduate courses in case management assist social workers in preparing for advanced practice. Core elements that have been integral to graduate coursework for social workers include five content areas that give case management a transdisciplinary character (Moxley, 1996). These five content areas are:

   1. Policy environment and problem formulation
   2. Diverse purposes, aims, and models of case management
   3. Context of case management practice

4. Role definitions and staffing implications

5. Ethical challenges to practice

G. Not all case management is advanced practice, nor does it require graduate education. However, it is becoming abundantly clear that in the past several years, case managers are performing more complex duties that appear to match the competencies and skill levels of other advanced practice roles.

H. Case managers perform their roles at individual, group, and system levels. Case management at the system level requires advanced practice skills that are traditionally not found in entry-level professional education (Stanton Swanson, Sherwood, and Packa, 2005).

I. The differences between basic and advanced case management skills are depicted in Tables 13-1 and 13-2 (Stanton and Dunkin, 2002).

1. Basically, case management at the baccalaureate level involves individual case management or care coordination.

2. Case management at the graduate level focuses not only on individuals, but on cohorts, population aggregates, and disease management groups.

3. Outcomes at the basic level focus on clinical, satisfaction, cost, and functional outcomes for the individual client.

4. Outcomes at the systems level focus on a roll up and analysis of these individual outcomes for the entire group of patients.

■ APPROACHES TO CASE MANAGEMENT EDUCATION AND TRAINING

A. Professional licensure is the basic mechanism for credentialing of case managers (Kulbok and Utz, 1999). Certification in case management has become increasingly available.

B. There is a growing list of distinct certification examinations. Some of the better known and well regarded have been influential in determining content for case manager education and training. They also provide entry level for case management clinical skills acquisition.

C. Competency in case management is paramount. Individual competence is the foundation or backbone for the case management process.

1. A variety of methods can be used to assess, develop, and evaluate competency, including self-assessment tools, orientation curricula, skills checklists, and/or onsite/online education (Stanton, Swanson, and Baker, 2005).

2. Assessing competence can be used to determine beginning competence or increasing knowledge and skills, and as a mechanism for performance appraisal on an ongoing basis.

D. There are continuing education and certificate programs that are available as preparation courses in case management. The better educational programs have core accreditation from URAC and/or continuing education approval by the CCMC.

E. There are an increasing number of graduate-level programs in nursing and social work that include case management in their preparation of

TABLE 13-1

Case Management at the Basic Practice Level: An Overview of the Role of the Nurse Case Manager

Aspect	Content
Practice	• Uses basic knowledge of physiology and pathophysiology • Uses basic health assessment skills • Designs, implements, and evaluates health promotion and disease prevention programs for selected individuals • Uses knowledge and understanding of ethical standards of practice according to ANA • Coordinates case management services for individual clients/family • Participates in disease management programs • Fulfills practice standards outlined by AACN, CMSA and CCM • Collects outcomes data • Participates in the development of evidence-based practice guidelines • Collaborates with utilization and resource management in the coordination of patient case management services • Screens patients for case management • Collaborates with discharge planners, social workers, and other internal and external resources to coordinate case management services
Research	• Participates in research studies under the direction of an advanced practice nurse or other professionals • Uses published research to apply to case management practice • Participates on multidisciplinary teams in the provision of case management services
Administration	• Uses basic knowledge in the policy, organization, and financing of health care and case management systems • Uses tools under the supervision of a graduate level to collect data for assessing clinical, financial, humanistic/satisfaction, quality, and functional outcomes for patients, families, disease management populations, and communities • Participates in case or disease management systems • Participates in Continuous Quality Improvement (CQI) programs
Education	• Participates in professional organizations and staff development programs related to case management • Maintains certification as case manager

clinical specialists and nurse practitioners. Some schools also include case management courses in their undergraduate curriculum.

F. Several graduate programs in nursing focus on case management as a specialty at the graduate level of nursing practice. There are also programs that combine nursing and social work with a focus on case management.

TABLE 13–2 ————————————————————————————
Case Management at the Advanced Practice Level: An Overview of the Role of the Case Manager

Aspect	Content
Practice	• Uses advanced knowledge of pathophysiology
	• Uses advanced health assessment skills
	• Synthesizes theories from natural, behavioral, social, and applied sciences to support advanced practice and role development for case management
	• Uses community development and intervention processes to design, implement, and evaluate health promotion and disease prevention programs for patient populations and communities
	• Collaborates with providers and consumers in designing, implementing, and evaluating innovative health programs and community services for patient populations
	• Assumes accountability of ethical values, principles, and personal beliefs that acknowledge human diversity and influence professional practice decisions and nursing interventions
	• Designs and administers quality case management services at the individual, disease management, and/or community level
	• Designs case management systems that address human diversity and social issues
	• Becomes "expert" generalist in terms of dealing with health care issues
	• Provides leadership in coordinating, managing, and improving health programs and health services to culturally diverse individuals and populations
	• Develops and/or accesses evidenced-based practice guidelines
Research	• Initiates research to address case management issues and practices in rural areas
	• Acts as a consultant to other researchers and providers regarding case management
	• Provides research consultation to members of multidisciplinary team on all aspects of case management for patient populations
	• Supervises interdisciplinary research on case management requirements for patient populations
	• Develops research proposals for external funding
	• Assesses and accesses preexisting data bases to facilitate case management processes at all levels
	• Contributes through research to elaboration of case management conceptual frameworks
Administration	• Uses advanced knowledge in health policy, organization, and financing of health care and case management systems to design, coordinate, and evaluate case management systems
	• Designs cost-effective intervention/strategies collaboratively with multiple disciplines to provide quality health care for patient populations

(continued)

TABLE 13–2 —————————————————————————

Case Management at the Advanced Practice Level: An Overview of the Role of the Case Manager (*continued*)

Aspect	Content
	• Assumes leadership in professional role definition and development for case managers
	• Develops informational and organizational systems for assessing clinical, financial, humanistic/satisfaction, quality, and functional outcomes for all levels of case management within patient populations
	• Designs, implements, and evaluates methods for efficient and effective use of human and material resources to support case management services
	• Organizes and evaluates case management systems
	• Organizes CQI programs that address unique characteristics of case management
	• Advocates for patient populations in policy formulation, organization, and financing of health care
Education	• Acts as a facilitator and mentor to advanced practice case management students
	• Serves as case management expert for staff development processes in area of rural case management
	• Provides leadership in professional organizations
	• Educates consumers and health care professionals about the role of case manager
	• Provides leadership in the design, implementation, and evaluation of education for patient populations
	• Disseminates research findings at professional meetings

G. The case management literature describes a variety of training and education programs for preparing case managers for their roles:
   1. Degree- or non–degree-granting programs
   2. Programs offered by health care organizations in the practice sector, independent continuing education agencies, or colleges and universities.

H. The case management training and education programs are classified by Cesta and Tahan (2003) into five types or levels as follows:
   1. Non-certificate programs offered by health care organizations as part of orientation or inservice education sessions.
   2. Certificate programs offered by independent agencies through conferences conducted for the purpose of continuing education in case management, such as those offered by Contemporary Forum, CMSA, and American Health Consultants.
   3. Multiple-credit certificate courses offered by colleges and universities.

    4. Post-baccalaureate certificate programs also offered by universities and colleges.

    5. Master's degree–granting programs; that is, graduate-level educational programs offered by universities or colleges.

I. Case management training programs that are offered by health care organizations may include topics such as:

    1. Leadership

    2. The change process

    3. Communication and interpersonal skills

    4. Case management concepts and models

    5. The case management process

    6. The role of the case manager

    7. Utilization management

    8. Transitional planning

    9. Case management plans and tools

    10. Legal and ethical considerations

    11. Patient and family education and patients' rights

J. Case management educational programs offered by colleges and universities include courses in the areas of:

    1. Health care delivery systems and models

    2. The continuum of care and settings including community resources and the transitional planning process

    3. Integrated health care delivery systems

    4. Health care finance and reimbursement concepts including utilization management

    5. Implementation of case management systems and the role of the case manager

    6. Research and program evaluation including outcomes management

    7. Ethical and legal issues of health care delivery and case management practice

    8. Leadership concepts including systems theory, change theory, multidisciplinary collaboration, negotiation, conflict resolution, and delegation

    9. Client advocacy

    10. Case management tools and plans

    11. Health care policy and legislation

    12. Quality and performance improvement including working in teams

K. Educational programs that grant academic degrees usually include clinical courses or practicum.

    1. Clinical courses consist of the case manager student spending a few hundred hours in a clinical setting practicing with a case manager mentor.

    2. Examples of colleges or universities that offer academic degrees in case management are University of San Francisco, CA; University of Tucson, AZ; University of Washington, Seattle, WA.

L. Case management training and education programs that are offered by professional organizations or continuing education agencies include specific topics that are related to case management practice, especially those that are based on practical experiences, tell the success stories or learned lessons of some health care organizations, research findings, and innovations/advances.

1. Generally, each topic is addressed over a 45-minute to 3-hour period.

2. Topics addressed in these sessions are geared toward building the knowledge, skills, and competencies of case managers, administrators of case management programs, and health care professionals associated with case management practice.

■ CREDENTIALING IN CASE MANAGEMENT

A. Credentialing is an essential activity in case management and aims to protect the consumer of health care services—to ensure that the individuals hired to practice case management are qualified, knowledgeable, and competent, as well as able to provide quality services.

B. Certification is but one aspect of credentialing. Others may include a review of knowledge, skills, performance, competence, licensure, work history, and experience.

C. Credentialing is the process of evaluating a person's education and experience against a standard to determine whether he or she is qualified to perform the job, taking into consideration community standards; national standards; and state practice acts, statutes, and liability.

D. Credentialing also is a dynamic process in determining the qualifications of a person compared with standards to perform a given responsibility safely, effectively, and legally.

E. URAC has developed accreditation standards for case management organizations and programs.

F. Standards of Practice for Case Management, adopted by CMSA in 1995 and revised in 2002, are authoritative statements defining the behaviors expected of case managers; that is, roles, functions, and responsibilities.

G. Components of credentialing

1. Definition of case management—"A collaborative process that accesses, plans, implements, coordinates, monitors, and evaluates the options and services required to meet an individual's health and human services needs. It is characterized by advocacy, communication, and resource management and promotes quality and cost-effective outcomes and interventions" (CCMC, 2005, p. iv).

2. Philosophy of case management

a. A philosophy is a statement of belief, setting forth principles that guide case management programs and the case manager in his or her practice.

b. Philosophy of case management as developed by the CCMC (2005, p. iv) indicates that case management:

    i. Is an area of specialty practice within one's health and human services profession. Its underlying premise is that everyone benefits when clients (e.g., patients, employees) reach their optimum level of wellness, self-management, and functional capability—the clients being served; their support systems; the health care delivery systems; and the various payer sources.

    ii. Facilitates the achievement of client wellness and autonomy through advocacy, assessment, planning, communication, education, resource management, and service facilitation. Based on the needs and values of the client, and in collaboration with all service providers, the case manager links clients with appropriate providers and resources throughout the continuum of health and human services and care settings, while ensuring that the care provided is safe, effective, client centered, timely, efficient, and equitable. This approach achieves optimum value and desirable outcomes for all—the clients, their support systems, the providers, and the payers.

    iii. Provides services that are optimized best when offered in a climate that allows direct communication among the case manager, the client, the payer, the primary care provider, and other service delivery professionals. The case manager is able to enhance these services by maintaining the client's privacy, confidentiality, health, and safety through advocacy and adherence to ethical, legal, accreditation, certification, and regulatory standards or guidelines.

3. Certification, which determines that the case manager possesses the education, skills, knowledge, and experience required to render appropriate services according to sound principles of practice.

4. The case manager's job description is an important part of credentialing. It is used as the day-to-day working document delineating the roles and responsibilities of the case manager (activities and role relationships) and requirements for practice (knowledge, skills, abilities, educational degrees, licensure, and certification).

5. The components of the case manager's job description are:
   a. Job title
   b. Reports to whom
   c. Summary of position
   d. Duties and responsibilities
   e. Required knowledge
   f. Functions
   g. Qualifications, including education, experience, licenses, and certifications

6. The employment application or contract, which sets forth in writing the education, work experience, and skills of the individual.

7. The applicant (candidate for the case manager job) interview conducted by a supervisor, peers, and subordinates, if any.

8. Verification of licenses or certifications, or both.

H. Credentialing occurs usually annually and includes a competency-based performance appraisal. This process focuses on the ability of the case manager to perform his or her roles and responsibilities as described in the job description. It is a measure of maintaining continued competence especially for the protection of the consumer and to ensure the provision of quality care.

I. Recredentialing ensures that case managers continue to meet professional standards in their performance. It is also a process for identifying the areas of knowledge or performance case managers need to improve in and therefore, identifies continuing training and education needs.

■ OVERVIEW OF CERTIFICATION IN CASE MANAGEMENT

A. Certification is a process of validation of knowledge, skills, and abilities of individual practitioners. It is usually provided by a nationally recognized agency such as the CCMC or the ANCC.

B. Certification is based on predetermined standards, including licensure, education, acceptable past experience, and examination. It builds on an existing and defined health license such as registered nurse (RN), medical doctor (MD), or licensed clinical social worker (LCSW).

C. The CCMC has developed a certification process for case managers since 1992. CCMC is the first multidisciplinary and largest organization to certify case managers in the practice of case management. The credential used by CCMC is called the *certified case manager* (CCM). Today, however, there are more than 30 different certifications in case management offered by varying professional organizations and agencies.

D. Certification is governed by independent bodies created to define and set standards for certification and administer the certification and the recertification process.

E. Certification-governing bodies are composed of individuals certified by that body and a variety of other individuals who represent the broad spectrum of individuals served, including consumers (public members), academicians, researchers, and other experts in the field.

F. Certification is for an initial period, which is typically 3 to 5 years on average, at which time recertification is required to maintain the certification or credential.

G. Recertification is completed in either of two ways:
1. Based on continued acceptable employment in the field and a predetermined number of continuing education requirements.
2. By retaking the certification examination itself.

H. Individuals who are certified have a specific credential (designation) they are allowed to use after their name, such as CCM or Care Manager Certified (CMC), for as long as their certification is active.

I. Certification is voluntary. However, some accreditation standards recommend certification.

J. Certifying bodies/agencies have a code of professional conduct for the individuals they certify. CCMs are expected to abide by the codes of professional conduct of their own professional specialty (e.g., nursing, social work, rehabilitation counseling) and that of case management.

1. A code of professional conduct protects the public interest and delineates the behavioral expectations of case managers.

2. Codes of professional conduct contain

   a. Principles;

   b. Rules of conduct; and

   c. Guidelines for professional conduct.

3. Individuals may have more than one code of professional conduct if they are licensed or a member of a profession.

K. Certification examinations should be free of bias and nondiscriminatory. There should be validity of the examination established through a job analysis survey and ongoing scientific research that helps maintain the currency of the examination and its representation of the case management field and practice.

L. There are many certifications in case management; however, credible ones employ research in the development of the examination items and in identifying the domains of knowledge and practice the examination must reflect. Another criterion of credibility is recognition by the National Organization for Certifying Agencies (NOCA). For example, CCMC is recognized by NOCA.[4]

M. The benefits of certification in case management are many, of which the following are of prime importance:

1. Certifications provide a standard of knowledge for employers of case managers.

2. They also provide a standard and assurance to the consumer and public that the case manager has a sufficient level of knowledge, skills, and competence.

3. In addition, they safeguard the public and provide a recognized benchmark for health care workers and consumers of case management services.

4. Certifications are an indication that the person certified is knowledgeable, informed, and current in his or her area of practice.

N. A case manager should choose a specific certification depending on his or her job function and responsibilities matched to the requirements of the certification and certifying agency.

■ SELECT CERTIFICATIONS IN CASE MANAGEMENT

A. The oldest certification in case management is the CCM that is offered by the CCMC.

---

[4] For information on how to assess the credibility of case management certifying agencies, refer to the CCMC Website: *www.ccmcertification.org*.

1. The CCM is the first certification developed specifically for case managers regardless of professional specialty; that is, it is multidisciplinary.
2. In 1992, the National Case Management Task Force organized a meeting with representatives of various national organizations (stakeholders of case management) with interest in case management. This meeting was organized because of the growing concern that there were no standards or qualifications for people calling themselves case managers.
3. In the early 1990s, case management was a "loose cannon" with no protection for the case manager or the consumer.
4. Consensus was reached in the 1992 meeting to appoint the Commission of Insurance Rehabilitation Specialists (now known as the Commission for Disability Management Specialists) to develop a certification for individual case managers, based on the work of the National Task Force.
5. The work of the National Task Force culminated in the creation of the CCMC and the certification for individual case managers (the CCM).
6. Certification requirements for CCM are as follows (CCMC, 2005):
   a. Good moral character, reputation, and fitness for the practice of case management
   b. Licensure and certification requirements:
      i. License or certification must be based on a minimum educational requirement of a post-secondary degree program in a field that promotes the physical, psychosocial, or vocational well-being of the persons being served.
      ii. The license or certification awarded on completion of the educational program must have been obtained by passing an examination in the area(s) of specialization.
      iii. The license or certification process must grant the holder the ability to legally and independently practice without the supervision of another licensed professional and to perform the following eight essential activities of case management—assessment, planning, implementation, coordination, monitoring, evaluation, outcomes, and general (e.g., case management actions that span all of the essential activities, such as advocacy).
      iv. All licenses and certifications must be current.
   c. Employment experience falls into three categories. The candidate must meet one of them to be eligible for the certification examination:
      i. Twelve months of acceptable full-time case management employment or equivalent under the supervision of a CCM for the 12 months.
      ii. Twenty-four months of acceptable full-time case management employment or equivalent. Supervision by a CCM is not required under this category.
      iii. Twelve months of acceptable full-time case management employment or its equivalent as a supervisor, supervising the activities of individuals who provide direct case management services.
   d. All experience must be verifiable by a manager, supervisor, or employer. Self-employment is acceptable but also must be verified.

e. To qualify as acceptable employment, the applicant must demonstrate as part of his or her employment the eight essential activities of case management (listed earlier) applied to a minimum of five of the following six core components:

    i. Case management concepts

    ii. Case management principles and strategies

    iii. Psychosocial and support systems

    iv. Health care management and delivery

    v. Health care reimbursement

    vi. Vocational concepts and strategies

f. The core components must be applied across a continuum of care, involve interactions with the client's health care system (including physicians, family members, third-party payers, employers, and other care providers), and deal with the client's broad spectrum of needs.

7. The continuum of care is defined in the CCMC certification guide (and is required to be applied by case managers in their practice) as "match[ing] the ongoing needs of individuals being served by the case management process with the appropriate level and type of health, medical, financial, legal, and psychosocial care for services within a setting or across multiple settings" (CCMC, 2005, p. 6).

8. The CCM examination is administered twice a year. This certification is the most widely held certification by case managers—more than 30,000 case managers have been certified by CCMC to date since 1993. Applicants who successfully pass the examination use the designation CCM.

B. Nursing Case Management (Cm) is another certification/credential available in case management and offered by the ANCC (ANCC, 2006).

1. Eligibility requirements to sit for the Cm examination are:

a. Hold an active RN license in the United States or its territories

b. Currently hold an associate, a diploma, baccalaureate, or higher degree in nursing.

c. Have functioned within the scope of a registered nurse and in the capacity of a case manager for a minimum of 2000 hours of practice within the past 2 years.

2. The Cm nurse case manager examination is administered twice a year by the ANCC. The first examination was offered in 1997.

3. Applicants who successfully pass the examination use the designation RN, Cm. The person must be recertified every 5 years.

C. Another certification is the Care Manager Certified (CMC) offered by the National Academy of Certified Care Managers.

1. Eligibility requirements to sit for the CMC examination are:

a. A master's degree in social work, nursing, gerontology, counseling, or psychology

b. Two years of supervised, paid, full-time care/case management experience

    c. Experience must include personal, face-to-face interviewing, assessment, care planning, problem solving, and follow up, or

    d. Applicants with a bachelor's degree in social work, nursing, gerontology, counseling, or care management; and

    e. Four years of paid, full-time work experience with clients in practice settings of social work, nursing, mental health, counseling, or care management. Two of those years must be supervised, paid, full-time care management experience, or

    f. Applicants with a high school diploma or any degree in an area not related to care management; and

    g. Six years of paid, full-time, direct experience with clients in social work, mental health, nursing, counseling or care management; 2 of those years must be supervised.

  2. The first examination for care manager certified was administered in 1996. The person must be recertified every 3 years.

D. The Certified Case Management Administrator (CCMA) is offered by the Center for Case Management and focuses on case managers in leadership positions (Center for Case Management, 2006).

  1. Candidates for the CCMA are case management administrators who supervise employees or who perform the functions listed below. If applying as an experienced case manager, candidates must perform at least eight of the following functions on a daily basis (Center for Case Management, 2006):

    a. Identifying cases

    b. Comprehensively assessing a client's situation

    c. Evaluating and coordinating the plan of care

    d. Matching client resources to client needs

    e. Monitoring delivery of services

    f. Using critical thinking skills, prioritizing appropriately, and managing time wisely

    g. Measuring and evaluating financial, clinical, functional, and satisfaction outcomes

    h. Maintaining accountability for financial, clinical, functional, and satisfaction outcomes

    i. Displaying effective leadership in the performance of current role

    j. Communicating effectively

    k. Evaluating and responding to the needs of clients, clinicians, and the community

  2. Eligibility requirements to sit for the CCMA examination are a master's degree and 1 year of experience in case management administration; or a master's degree and 3 years of experience as a case manager; or a bachelor's degree and 5 years of experience as a case manager.

  3. Recertification is required every 5 years.

  4. The certification examination is administered manually and is composed of a maximum of 200 multiple-choice, objective questions. The content addresses the following topics:

   a. Identification of at-risk population—20%
   b. Assessment of clinical system components—10%
   c. Development of strategies to manage at-risk populations—10%
   d. Assessment of organizational culture—15%
   e. Market assessment and strategic planning—15%
   f. Human resource management—10%
   g. Outcomes measurement, monitoring, and management—20%
5. The examination for case management administrators was first administered in 1998. Individuals who successfully pass the examination use the designation CMAC (Case Management Administrator Certified).

E. There are many other certifications for individuals working in health care. To determine credibility of certification, refer to the section Certification for Case Managers presented earlier in this chapter. See Table 13-3 for a listing of certifications and contact information.

F. There are many credentials case managers use after they obtain certification in case management practice. The following are some examples:
   1. A-CCC—Continuity of Care Certification, Advanced
   2. ACM—Accredited Case Manager
   3. CASWCM—Certified Advanced Social Work Case Manager
   4. CCM—Certified Case Manager
   5. CDMS—Certified Disability Management Specialist
   6. CMAC—Case Management Administrator Certification
   7. CMC—Care Manager Certified
   8. CMCN—Certified Managed Care Nurse
   9. CPDM—Certified Professional in Disability Management
   10. CPUM—Certified Professional in Utilization Management
   11. CPUR—Certified Professional in Utilization Review
   12. CSWCM—Certified Social Work Case Manager
   13. RNCM—Registered Nurse Case Manager

■ URAC ACCREDITATION OF ORGANIZATIONS PERFORMING CASE MANAGEMENT

A. Accreditation is the process of reviewing all aspects of an organization, program, or service for the purpose of evaluating whether it meets published and nationally recognized standards of providing quality services.

B. Accreditation is a voluntary process and applies specific standards determined by the agency.

C. In June 1999, URAC adopted accreditation standards for organizations performing case management.
   1. URAC used an expert panel/advisory committee with representatives from all case management stakeholders to develop the standards.

TABLE 13-3

Case Certifications and Contact Information

Certification	Acronym	Specialization	Sponsoring Organization	Contact Information
Accredited Case Manager Hospital Setting	ACM	Case management	National Institute for Case Management, Inc.	National Institute for Case Management, Inc. 10310 West Markham, Suite 209, Little Rock, AR 72205, 501-227-5400
Advanced Certification Continuity of Care	A-CCC	Multidisciplinary discharge planners, case managers	National Board for Continuity of Care Certification	National Board for Continuity of Care Certification, 638 Prospect Ave., Hartford, CT 06105, 203-586-7525
American Board of Disability Analysts	ABDA	Rehabilitation medicine, case management	American Board of Disability Analysts	ABDA Central Office, Park Place Medical Building, 345 24th Ave. N, Suite 200, Nashville, TN 37203, 615-327-2984
American Board of Quality Assurance and Utilization Review Physicians	ABQAURP	Utilization management for physician and allied health	American Board of Quality Assurance and Utilization Review Physicians, Inc.	American Board of Quality Assurance and Utilization Review Physicians, Inc., 6640 Congress St., New Port Richey, FL 34653, 800-998-6030
Care Manager Certified	CMC	Gerontology, counseling, social work, mental health	National Academy of Certified Care Managers	National Academy of Certified Care Managers, P.O. Box 669, 244 Upton Rd. Cholchester, CT 06415-0669, 800-962-2260
Case Management Administration Certified	CMAC	Case management administration	Center for Case Management, Inc.	Professional Testing Corporation, 1350 Broadway, 17th Floor, New York, NY 10018, 212-356-0660
Certified Case Manager	CCM	Multidisciplinary case managers	Commission for Case Management Certification	Commission for Case Manager Certification, 300 N. Martingale Road, Suite 460, Schaumburg IL, 60173, 847-944-1330
Certified Disability Management Specialist	CDMS	Disability managers Insurance-based insurance rehabilitation specialists Vocational counselors	Certified Disability Management Specialist Commission	Certified Disability Management Specialist Commission, 300 N. Martingale Road, Suite 460, Schaumburg IL, 60173 847-944-1335

Certification	Acronym	Applies to	Organization	Contact
Certified Managed Care Nurse	CMCN	Nurses in managed care	American Board of Managed Care Nursing	American Board of Managed Care Nursing, 4435 Waterfront Drive, Suite 101, Glen Allen, VA 23060, 804-747-9698
Certified Nursing Case Manager	RN, Cm	Nurse case manager	American Nurse Credentialing Center	American Nurse Credentialing Center, 8515 Georgia Ave., Suite 400, Silverspring, MD 20910-3492, 800-284-2378
Certified Occupational Health Nurse–Case Manager	COHN-CM	Occupational health nursing case management	American Board for Occupational Health Nurses, Inc.	American Board for Occupational Health nurses, 201 E. Ogden Ave., Suite 114, Hinsdale, IL 60521, 630-789-5799
Certified Professional Disability Management	CPDM	Disability managers	Insurance Educational Association	Insurance Educational Association, 2670 North Main St., Suite 350, Santa Anna, CA 92705, 800-655-4432
Certified Professional in Healthcare Quality	CPHQ	Quality managers, utilization managers, risk managers	Healthcare Quality Certification Board of the National Association for Healthcare Quality	Healthcare Quality Certification Board of the National Association for Healthcare Quality, PO Box 19604, Lenexa, KS 66285-9604, 800-346-4722
Certified Professional Utilization Review	CPUR	Utilization managers, case managers	McKesson Health Solutions	InterQual, 44 Lafayette Road, PO Box 988, North Hampton, NH 03862
Certified Rehabilitation Counselor	CRC	Rehabilitation counseling, case managers	Commission on Rehabilitation Counselor Certification	Commission on Rehabilitation Counselor Certification, 300 N. Martingale Rd., Suite 460, Schaumburg, IL 60173, 847-944-1325
Certified Rehabilitation Registered Nurse, Certified Rehabilitation Nurse–Advanced	CRRN, CRRN-A	Rehabilitation nurses and Rehabilitation Nurse Care Managers	Rehabilitation Nursing Certification Board	Rehabilitation Nursing Certification Board, 4700 W. Lake Avenue, Glenview, IL 60025, 800-229-7530
Professional, Academy for Healthcare Management Fellow, Academy for Healthcare Management	PAHM, FAHM	Managed care	Academy for Healthcare Management	Academy for Healthcare Management, 2300 Windy Ridge Parkway, Suite 600, Atlanta, GA 30339, 800-667-3133

2. Organizations represented included the CMSA, CCMC, ANA, American Medical Association, American Association of Health Plans, URAC-accredited companies, Association of Managed Healthcare Organizations, health care business representatives, Washington Business Group on Health, American Health Quality Association, American Hospital Association, Blue Cross Blue Shield Association, Centers for Medicare and Medicaid Services (CMS), and representatives from the Department of Defense.
3. The resulting URAC standards are the first to specifically address case management organizations and to set what constitutes a quality case management organization, program, or service.

D. To date, URAC has accredited hundreds of organizations that provide all types of case management services, in both health care and workers' compensation settings. The purpose of this accreditation is to help ensure that the case management services offered by these organizations are of the highest quality (URAC, 2006).

E. URAC designed the standards to fit organizations that provide telephonic or onsite case management services in conjunction with a privately or publicly funded benefits program across settings and specialties. Accreditation or certification is available depending on the type of organization and services being offered.

F. URAC's accreditation process addresses a set of standards that are considered core to all URAC accreditation programs.
1. These standards address several key organizational management functions that are important for any health care organization.
2. The core standards provide the basic structures and process any organization must have to maintain a level of quality expected in a URAC-accredited organization.
3. Each accreditation program also includes additional standards specific to the program. For example, case management programs must meet the core standards as well as the specific case management standards.

G. The URAC core standards address several critical areas of basic structure and processes including organizational structure, personnel management, operations, quality improvement, oversight of delegated responsibilities, and consumer protection (URAC, 2006).
1. According to the organizational structure standard, the organization must define:
   a. Its structure and oversight responsibility and how it maintains policies and procedures that govern all aspects of the operation
   b. The job descriptions
   c. Licensure required for certain personnel
   d. A regulatory compliance program that ensures it is conducting business in accordance with applicable federal and state laws
   e. Confidentiality and conflict of interest policies
   f. Other requirements such as a structured quality management program and processes to protect the safety and welfare of consumers

2. According to the personnel standard, the organization must ensure that:
   a. Written job descriptions for all staff clearly define the following qualifications—education, training, professional experience, expected professional competencies, appropriate licensure/certification requirements, scope and role of responsibilities.
   b. Credentials of licensed or certified personnel are verified
   c. A clear orientation, training, and evaluation program exists and that staff members be given the necessary guidelines to do their job
3. According to the operations and process standard, the organization is expected to:
   a. Establish communication methods across all departments and disciplines to promote collaboration
   b. Coordinate internal activities
   c. Provide quality services
   d. Have systems and processes in place for information management, business relationships, clinical oversight, regulatory compliance, and incentive programs
4. According to the quality improvement standard, the organization must:
   a. Maintain a quality management program that promotes objective and systematic monitoring and evaluation of consumer and client and health care services
   b. Implement its own quality management program that assists the organization in focusing its unique needs and efforts
5. According to the delegation of responsibilities standard, the organization must:
   a. Maintain responsibility and oversight for any function it delegates to another entity
6. According to the consumer satisfaction and protection standard, the organization is expected to:
   a. Communicate with consumers and clients clearly and accurately
   b. Represent information about the organization's services and how to obtain these services
   c. Have a complaint or grievance mechanism in place
   d. Have a process to respond quickly in situations that create an immediate threat to the safety or welfare of consumers

H. The URAC standards that are specific to case management program accreditation cover several critical operational categories. The standards include those described below (URAC, 2006):
   1. Scope of services standard, which addresses the availability of:
      a. Written policies and procedures
      b. A definition of case management
      c. A description of types of consumers served

    d. A description of the delivery model for case management services

    e. A description of qualifications for case management staff

2. Case management staff standard, which addresses the availability of:

    a. Guidelines for reasonable caseload of case managers

    b. Sufficient personnel to provide services to consumers

    c. Licensed physicians available for consultations with case managers

    d. Individuals who directly supervise case managers. These are encouraged to have a bachelor's (or higher) degree in a health-related field; licensure as a health professional, certification as a case manager, or professional certification in a clinical specialty; and five years' experience as a case manager.

    e. A process or program for training and education of case managers that focuses on:

       i. Current principles, procedures, and knowledge of case management based on nationally recognized standards

       ii. Knowledge of the organization's policies and procedures, state requirements, professional roles, health care requirements of specific populations, and URAC standards

       iii. Annual professional education for case managers and the organization to encourage professional development

3. Case management process standard, which addresses the following areas of practice:

    a. Criteria for identifying individuals for case management services

    b. Disclosure to patients information concerning the nature of the case management relationship, the circumstances under which information will be disclosed to third parties, the availability of a complaint process, the availability of written notification of case management activities, any incentive compensation system for case managers based on utilization rates and, upon request, a description of the rationale for selecting case management services

    c. Documentation of the patient's oral consent to services; however, written consent is preferred. (The consent requirement is assumed to be not applicable for workers' compensation case management programs.)

    d. Tools that enable the case manager to collect the information necessary to carry out the case management process

    e. Policies to conduct and document an assessment for each consumer. There must be a case management plan for every consumer that lays out short-term and long-term goals, timeframes for re-evaluation, resources to be used, and collaborative approaches to be used

    f. Conduct of case reviews to promote achievement of case management goals and use of the information for quality management purposes

    g. Policy for resolving disagreements within the organization regarding consumer care options

      h. Criteria for the discharge of consumers or the termination of case management services

   4. Organizational ethics and confidentiality standard, which addresses the organization's responsibilities in the following areas:

      a. Implementation of a policy and procedure to protect the confidentiality of individually identifiable health information and to protect the welfare and safety of consumers and case managers

      b. Implementation of policies and procedures to promote the autonomy of consumer and family decision making

      c. Support for consumer and family decision making by respecting the rights of the consumer to have input into the case management plan, refuse treatment or services, obtain information regarding the criteria for case closure, and so on

      d. Completion of an annual review of policies and procedures supporting the ethical framework for case management

      e. Implementation of policies and procedures that address the organization's obligations to monitor or assist consumers in selecting case management services

   5. Complaints standard that assists the organization in addressing the client needs and concerns.

      a. Policies and procedures through which consumers and providers may submit a complaint must be available.

      b. Policies and procedures for complaints must refer complaints outside the scope of case management responsibilities to the appropriate entity.

I. The URAC accreditation standards assist organizations in the development of policies and procedures that include a definition of case management, the types of consumers served, the delivery model for case management services, and case management staff qualifications and continuing education.

J. The URAC case management accreditation standards provide a solid foundation for effective case management programs. They build on core accreditation standards to enable organizations to successfully:

   1. Train case managers

   2. Identify individuals for case management

   3. Manage and conduct case management activities in an efficient and professional manner

   4. Promote the autonomy of consumer and family decision making

   5. Maintain confidentiality

   6. Delegate responsibility

K. The standards were initially tested in three case management organizations. Today, however, they are nationally recognized and considered reputable.

L. URAC defines a case management organization as an organization or program that provides telephonic or onsite case management services in conjunction with a private or publicly funded benefits program. All such organizations are eligible to apply for accreditation.

M. Case management organizations applying for accreditation participate in a process that entails a rigorous review of four phases; this review takes approximately 8 to 12 months (URAC, 2006).

1. The initial phase, called *building the application*, consists of completing the application forms and supplying supporting documentation, and payment of the application and base fee.

2. In the second phase, called the *desktop review*, the applicant's documentation is analyzed in relation to the URAC standards by one or more URAC reviewers. The documentation includes the organization's formal policies and procedures, organizational charts, position descriptions, contracts, sample template letters, and program descriptions and plans for departments such as quality management and credentialing.

3. In the third phase, the *onsite review*, the accreditation review team (the same team involved in the desktop review) conducts an onsite review to verify compliance with the URAC standards. During this review, the management and leadership team of the case management organization is interviewed about the organization's programs, and staff is observed performing its duties. In addition, audits are conducted and personnel and credentialing files analyzed. Education and quality management programs are reviewed in detail as well.

4. The fourth and last phase, the *committee review*, entails a review of the accreditation process by two URAC committees that include professionals from a variety of areas in health care as well as industry experts selected from or chosen by URAC's member organizations. The committee review process begins with a written summary documenting the findings of the desktop and onsite reviews. This summary is submitted to URAC's accreditation committee for evaluation. An accreditation recommendation is then forwarded to URAC's executive committee, which has the authority to grant accreditation.

N. After reviewing the summary and considering the accreditation committee's recommendation, the executive committee makes a final accreditation determination. Applicants who successfully meet all requirements are awarded a full accreditation, and an accreditation certificate is issued to the organization.

O. Full URAC accreditation lasts 2 years. The accredited case management organization must remain in compliance with the standards throughout the accreditation period.

P. Because there are no other generic case management organization standards, the standards developed by URAC are the standards all organizations—both accredited and nonaccredited organizations—are evaluated against and held to.

■ DIFFERENTIATING INDIVIDUAL FROM ORGANIZATIONAL CERTIFICATION

A. The field of case management has been experiencing a rise in the number of certified case managers and certified (or accredited) programs in case management. This has resulted in confusion about the difference between *individual* and *institution* certification; sometimes they are erroneously used as interchangeable terms (Tahan, 2005).

B. Certification of an individual means that a professional such as a case manager has achieved an advanced level of competence in an area of specialty or practice such as case management.
   1. Certifying an individual care provider/professional is based on the individual meeting certain eligibility criteria prior to sitting for the certification exam provided by a nationally recognized certifying agency, such as the CCMC.
   2. Individuals are certified based on their ability to achieve a passing score on the certification exam.

C. Certification of a program/institution means that an organization has met nationally accepted and recognized standards set forth by a nationally recognized agency, such as URAC.
   1. An institution pursuing certification of a program or service is not obligated to meet any eligibility criteria prior to engaging in the accreditation process.
   2. Certification of a program or service affirms that the institution has a center of excellence in that program or service.
   3. The decision of certification is made based on the institution's ability to demonstrate compliance with the certification (accreditation) standards.

D. Although the credential *certification* is used for both individual case managers and institutions, credentialing an individual case manager takes place in the form of a "certification" and credentialing a program or service occurs in the form of "accreditation."

E. Characteristics of an individual certification are (Tahan, 2005):
   1. It is offered by a nationally recognized agency.
   2. Credentialing is in the form of "certification."
   3. It certifies individual professionals/care providers.
   4. It uses an exam as the basis for certification.
   5. The decision to certify is made based on the individual achieving a passing score on the examination.
   6. It uses nationally recognized standards that focus on the certification exam.
   7. Individuals who pursue certification must meet eligibility criteria first to be able to sit for the exam.
   8. It is science-based.
   9. The offering agency tends to engage in ongoing research activities regarding the certification exam.

10. Certification of an individual does not extend to the institution where he or she works.
11. Certification recognizes the individual care provider as competent in the area of specialty.

F. Characteristics of an organizational certification are:
1. It is offered by a nationally recognized agency.
2. Credentialing is in the form of "accreditation."
3. It certifies a specific program or service in an organization.
4. It uses a national set of standards as the basis for certification.
5. The decision to certify is made based on the institution's ability to demonstrate compliance with the set of standards; a review is completed through a survey process.
6. It uses nationally recognized standards that focus on practice/health care delivery.
7. Institutions may pursue credentialing (certification) at any time—there are no prerequisites.
8. There is no obligation to be science-based; however, the offering agency may use research outcomes in the design of its standards.
9. Certification of the institution/program does not extend to those who work in it.
10. Certification recognizes the program as a center of excellence.

G. Agencies that provide certifications for programs do not normally certify individual professionals; if they happen to do so, different departments within the agency assume responsibility for either of the certifications.

H. There are several agencies that offer accreditation or certification for organizations or case management programs—for example:
1. ACHC—Accreditation Commission for Health Care
2. CARF—Commission on Accreditation of Rehabilitation Facilities
3. JCAHO—Joint Commission on Accreditation of Healthcare Organizations
4. NCQA—National Committee for Quality Assurance
5. URAC—Utilization Review Accreditation Commission

REFERENCES

American Nurses Credentialing Center (ANCC). (2006). Specialty nursing certifications, nursing case management. Website: *http://www.nursingworld.org/ancc/certification/certs/specialty.html*. Retrieved March 13. Silver Spring, MD: American Nurses Association.
Case Management Society of America (CMSA). (2002). *Standards of practice* (rev. ed.). Little Rock, AR: Author.
Cesta, T. G., and Tahan, H. A. (2003). *The case manager's survival guide: Winning strategies for clinical practice*, 2nd ed. St. Louis, MO: Mosby.
Center for Case Management (2006). *Certification for case management administrators*. Website: *http://www.cfcm.com/resources/certification.asp*. Retrieved January 11, 2006.
Commission for Case Manager Certification (CCMC). (2005). CCM Certification Guide. Rolling Meadows, IL: Author.
Kulbok, P. A. & Utz, S. W. (1999). Managing care: Knowledge and educational strategies for professional development (electronic version). *Family and Community Health, 22*(3), 1–11.

Leahy, M., Chan, Fong, Shaw, L. & Lui, J. (1997). Preparation of rehabilitation counselors for case management practice in health care settings. *Journal of Rehabilitation, 63*(3), 53–59.

Moxley, D. (1996). Teaching case management: Essential content for the preservice preparation of effective personnel. *Journal of Teaching in Social Work, 13*(1/2), 111–139.

Stanton, M., & Dunkin, J. (2002). Rural case management: Nursing role variations. *Lippincott's Case Management, 7*(2), 48–58.

Stanton, M., Swanson, C. and Baker, B. (2005). Development of a military competency checklist for case management. *Lippincott's Case Management, 10*(3), 128–135.

Stanton, M., Swanson, M., Sherrod, R. A., & Packa, D. (2005). Case management evolution: From basic to advanced practice role. *Lippincott's Case Management, 10*(6), 274–284.

Tahan, H. A. (2005). Clarifying certification and its value for case managers. *Lippincott's Case Management, (10)*1, 14–21.

Utilization Review Accreditation Commission (URAC). (2006). Case management accreditation and certification program overview. Website: *http://www.urac.org/prog_accred_CM_po.asp?navid=accreditation&pagename=prog_accred_CM.* Retrieved March 13. Washington, DC: American Accreditation Health Care Commission/URAC.

SUGGESTED READING

Benner, P., Tanner, C., & Chesla, C. (1996). *Expertise in nursing practice.* New York: Springer.

Gardner, S. (1999). Academy for Health Care Management offers managed care programs. *Inside Case Management, 6*(2), 12–21.

Mullahy, C., & Jensen, D. (2004). *The case manager's handbook*, 3rd ed. Sudbury, MA: Jones and Bartlett.

Smith, D., et al. (1998). *Case management 101—A training guide.* Los Angeles: AMS Press.

St. Coeur, M. (1967). *Case management practice guidelines.* St Louis: Mosby.

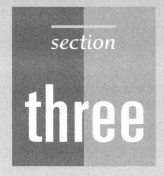

section

three

Case Management Tools

chapter

14

Case Management Plans, Clinical Pathways, and Protocols

Mary Jane McKendry

LEARNING OBJECTIVES

Upon completion of this chapter, the reader will be able to:

1. List the components of a case management care plan.
2. Define important terms and concepts related to developing a successful case management care plan.
3. Identify critical multidisciplinary and cross-functional relationships essential for successful execution of a case management care plan.
4. Describe how to identify appropriate, measurable, and achievable case management plan goals and outcomes.

IMPORTANT TERMS AND CONCEPTS

Acuity
Advocacy
Algorithm
Assessment
Case Management Care Plan
Clinical Pathway
CMAG Guidelines

Dashboard
Development
Evaluation
Evidence-Based Criteria and/or
  Guidelines
Facilitation
Goal (Measurable)

Implementation
Interdisciplinary
Intervention
Monitoring
Outcome
Planning
Problem Identification

Problem Statement
Protocol
Resource
Resource Consumption
Risk Stratification
Utilization Management
Variance

■ INTRODUCTION

A. As the roles of case managers expand and transform in response to changes in the health care marketplace, many case managers find that the traditional goals of case management (CM) seem incongruent with current responsibilities. Often case managers feel conflicted as they try to deliver patient-centered care, while at the same time attempting to reduce costs and control resource utilization.

B. In reality, case managers are trying to meet the goals of many different customers at the same time. For example, keeping care patient-centered is necessary, but so is reducing variation, duplication, and fragmentation of care. Similarly, it is imperative that case managers help patients access appropriate resources to maintain their individual optimal level of wellness; on the other hand, utilization and costs must be addressed and controlled. Helping patients access appropriate resources at the right time results in cost savings and appropriate utilization of resources.

C. It may be possible to achieve balance in both the patient-centered and system-centered goals of CM. In doing this, we start to identify the complexity of the case manager's job and to understand that case managers need a care road map to guide the successful resolution of any identified needs or issues. Consider that perhaps case managers need to have not only clinical skills but also business skills. In this context, system-centered goals may address data gathering and analysis, reducing clinical variation, meeting expectations for timeframes, and addressing available resources, while patient-centered goals may address accessing appropriate care in a timely manner, providing education and tools to ensure patient empowerment, and encouraging patient self-management (Padgett, 1998).

D. Today, the consumers of CM services require well-defined and well-managed plans of care that effectively and efficiently address resource utilization, while at the same time ensure the access to, and quality of, care. By utilizing collaborative approaches for CM care planning, case managers can create a "dashboard" to assist them in meeting the goals and responsibilities of CM; the needs of the patient; and the needs of other CM customers such as employers, health plans, health care facilities, etc. A dashboard is an internal management reporting system for a department or program (in this instance, CM) that provides high-level executive summary reports of the program.

E. Through the use of dashboard reports, users will be able to see if, how, and where the CM company or department is progressing (or not progressing) in its improvement efforts.

F. This chapter on CM plans provides an overview of CM plan design, reviews tools available to assist in evidence-based CM plan development, and discusses strategies for developing comprehensive, multidisciplinary plans of care.

■ KEY DEFINITIONS

A. Algorithm—A binary decision tree that guides step-by-step assessments and interventions. Algorithms are generally most useful for high-risk groups as they are known for their specificity (very specific) and generally do not allow for provider/patient flexibility. Often utilized to manage a specific process, control care practices, or address an individual problem. Algorithms may incorporate research methodology to measure cause and effect (Wojner, 2001).

B. Case management care plan (CM plan)—"A comprehensive plan that includes a statement of problems/needs determined upon assessment; strategies to address the problems/needs; and measurable goals to demonstrate resolution based upon the problem/need, the time frame, the resources available, and the desires/motivation of the client/family" (CMSA, 2002, p. 21).

C. Clinical pathway—A structured, multidisciplinary CM plan designed to support the implementation of specific clinical guidelines and protocols. Clinical pathways are computational maps or algorithms that guide the healthcare team, especially the non-physician care team members, on the usual treatment patterns related to common diagnoses, conditions, and/or procedures.
   1. Clinical pathways are designed to support clinical management, clinical and nonclinical resource management, clinical audit, and financial management.
   2. Clinical pathways promote quality care and decrease costs by standardizing treatment methods within clinical processes, while at the same time endeavoring to improve the continuity and coordination of care across different disciplines.
   3. Clinical pathways also are known by many synonyms including integrated care paths, multidisciplinary pathways of care, care maps, critical pathways, collaborative pathways, or care paths (McKendry, 2004; Open Clinical, 2006).

D. Evidence-based criteria/guidelines—Evidence-based criteria are based on the premise of evidence-based medicine (EBM) and are systematically developed statements to assist practitioners and patients in making decisions about appropriate healthcare for specific clinical circumstances. (Field and Lohr, 1990).
   1. Evidence-based guidelines are generally designed for use by physicians, nurse practitioners, and physician assistants. They help promote

quality of care by monitoring performance and identifying improvement opportunities.

2. Guidelines commonly apply to a general health condition. To be defensible, guideline development must be able to demonstrate:

a. A development process that is open, documented, and reproducible;

b. That the resultant product can be of use to both clinicians and patients;

c. That the concept of appropriateness of services is well reflected in the guideline; and

d. That the guideline relates specifically to clearly defined clinical issues ("Proof and Policy," 2001).

E. Protocol—Guidelines designed to address specific therapeutic interventions for a given clinical problem. Protocols are less specific than algorithms and do allow for minimal provider flexibility via treatment options. They are multifaceted and therefore can be used to drive practice for more than one discipline. Like algorithms, they may incorporate research methodology to measure cause and effect (Wojner, 2001).

■ CM CARE PLANNING AND PLANS OF CARE

A. What is CM care planning if not an essential part of health care? Yet it is often misunderstood or even regarded as a waste of time and effort.

B. Historically, CM was often viewed as a social worker function. In the late 1980s, CM care planning became more of a nursing responsibility. Conceptualizing CM as either social work or nursing is inaccurate; doing so does not effectively involve all members of an interdisciplinary care team. Case managers understand that CM care planning must include all disciplines/members of the health care team involved in the care of a patient. According to the Case Management Society of America (CMSA) CM care planning is a case manager's primary function.

C. Fundamental components for appropriate CM care planning can be found in CMSA's standards of practice and include:

1. The use of evidence-based criteria whenever possible;

2. A fiscally responsible CM plan that enhances quality, access, and cost outcomes;

3. Direct communication with the patient and their family/support structure;

4. Direct and/or indirect communication with members of the health care team, including the patient's physician(s);

5. Education for the patient and their family/support structure so that informed decision making can occur;

6. Contingency planning to anticipate health and service complications;

7. Ongoing assessment and re-evaluation of the patient's health and progress; and

8. A CM plan that is dynamic and adaptable to changes occurring both over time and through various settings (CMSA, 2002).

D. CM care planning should be action oriented and time specific. The end result of CM care planning is a patient-centered CM plan. Consequently, one of the most significant responsibilities for a case manager is the development of a CM plan. The CM plan must be able to:

1. Be individualized yet focus on multidisciplinary care requirements;
2. Work for the patient and their family/support structure, physicians, and other members of the health care team;
3. Be consistent with an individual's needs, preferences, and values; and
4. Demonstrate that the patient understands and has agreed with the CM plan.

E. The effective CM plan is a specific document that delineates:

1. Individual care needs (both diagnostic and therapeutic),
2. Actions required (actions by the CM and/or by the patient),
3. Short- and long-term goals and timeframes for attainment, and
4. Anticipated outcomes.

■ CM PLAN DEVELOPMENT—PATIENT ASSESSMENT

A. Developing a patient-specific process should follow a logical progression.

B. The first step in CM care planning is an accurate and thorough needs assessment. The assessment begins with an accurate determination of the patient's current status and includes an evaluation of the patient's:

1. Physical needs
2. Acuity, comorbidity, polypharmacy
3. Psychological needs
4. Social, environmental, and cultural needs
5. Care coordination requirements
6. Potential resource consumption
7. Support structure
8. Quality indicators
9. Health plan benefit design
10. Evaluation/assessment of potential or present safety issues
11. Community resources

C. Once a current patient status is determined, the case manager must ask three fundamental questions:

1. What are we trying to accomplish? What are the goals for improvement and are they measurable?
2. How do we know that a planned approach (intervention) will result in an improvement/goal attainment?
3. What measurable approach (intervention) can be made that will result in an improvement? Who will do what, for what purpose, and at what frequency?

D. Answering these questions help case managers formulate CM plans that are individualized; contain reasonable goals; and have achievable, measurable, and time-bound outcomes.

E. Let's look at these questions in more detail to understand how they can help formulate a CM plan.

1. What are we trying to accomplish?
   a. This question may drive one or multiple goals. Additionally, the CM plan's priorities may begin to emerge and primary and secondary goals are more easily defined. Examples of goals that may be identified include:
      i. Patient education related to specific aspects of care/self-management, disease condition, medications, etc.
      ii. Patient empowerment
      iii. Patient self-management of activities of daily living (ADLs)
      iv. Respite care
      v. Transportation to/from required medical services such as dialysis or physical therapy
      vi. Glycemic control for patients with diabetes
      vii. Reduction in emergency room utilization
      viii. Appropriate family/social support structure in place
      ix. Access to required nutritional, medical, pharmaceutical, or other needs
      x. Successful return to work
   b. How are the above goals measured? What about the timeframes for accomplishment? Are they short-term or long-term goals? By answering these questions we obtain useful patient-centered information that allows us to write specific statements of expected goals and determine if goals are immediate, short-term, or long-range. It is important to realize that goals contain functional and measurable information such as:
      i. A general description of purpose—stating the aim clearly
      ii. The specific focus—performed by whom, taking place where, requiring what
      iii. Numerical targets—timeframes for completion that are based on measurable data
   c. Goals should be considered targets of achievement that are specific, measurable, attainable, relevant, and time bound.
   d. However, since patients cannot or do not always conform to plans of care, it is essential to remember that goals must be flexible enough to be modifiable.

2. How do we know that a planned approach (intervention) will result in an improvement?
   a. This question guides the formulation of action items, which are more commonly known as interventions (e.g., CM activities), as well as the identification of problems and the formulation of problem lists.

b. Basically, this question is asking the case manager to determine what interventions will actually result in improvements or in meeting the goal(s) defined. In other words, will the interventions planned actually positively affect the patient's overall well-being?

c. Once problems are determined and interventions are decided upon, the following additional questions should be asked of each problem recognized and intervention established:

    i. Will this problem get better?

    ii. Can we make this problem get better by the intervention(s) decided on?

    iii. If a problem is not likely to improve or resolve, will the planned intervention(s) reduce the risk of complications or prevent the problem from getting worse?

    iv. If a problem is not likely to improve and, in fact, deterioration is inevitable, can the planned intervention(s) provide for optimal quality of life, comfort, and dignity for the patient? (Sox, 2006)

    v. Is each defined intervention both measurable and realistic?

d. Interventions may include components of physician/health care provider orders, facility protocols, best-practices standards, or accepted critical pathways.

e. However, all CM plans of care should have interventions that reflect tasks that case managers can actually accomplish and should demonstrate the value of CM involvement. For example, if a physician orders nutritional supplements, the CM interventions would be focused on patient education, strategies for obtaining the nutritional supplements ordered, methods to determine that the patient receives and utilizes the nutritional supplements, and so on.

3. What measurable approach (intervention) can be made that will result in an improvement?

a. This question helps define what the outcomes of the CM plan should be. Just as interventions need to reflect actual tasks that are performed by case managers and/or require CM involvement, outcomes must be discipline specific.

b. The outcomes of a CM plan must objectively measure the patient outcomes that were most influenced by the case manager's involvement, demonstrate the effectiveness of defined interventions, and be variable, depending on many factors such as:

    i. General health status

    ii. Age

    iii. Specific diagnosis

    iv. Functional status

    v. Psychological/cognitive status

    vi. Cultural/ethnic factors

    vii. Severity of illness

    viii. Available resources

c. As these factors demonstrate, outcomes, although needing to be measurable and reportable, need to be patient specific. According to Storfjell and Jessup, "Errors have been made in evaluating the cost-effectiveness of many case management programs, including the following: insufficient or excessive 'doses or inputs' of case management have been used, the time period for evaluating the 'outputs' or results has been insufficient, case management has been only part of the intervention, and/or combined costs of case management services have not been adequately identified"(Cohen and DeBack, 1999, p. 53).

4. This type of thinking, coupled with the diversity of case management practice settings has propelled case managers into utilizing outcomes that are specific to not only their patients' needs but also the environment in which they work. In this way, case managers can best reflect their involvement, directly and indirectly, with patient care. The ultimate purpose of the CM plan is to guide all who are involved in the care of a specific patient to provide the most appropriate treatment in order to ensure optimal outcomes.

■ CM PLAN DEVELOPMENT—ASSESSMENT

A. Developing a patient-specific CM plan requires the use of information gathered during the patient assessment; contract-specific performance metrics; and organization-specific protocols, algorithms, or other evidence-based tools.

B. Standardization of CM plans allows for outcomes reporting.

C. Outcomes reporting in turn demonstrates both the value and return on investment (ROI) of case manager involvement. This process is accomplished differently in various organizations:
1. Some organizations automate their CM plans utilizing software applications designed to gather certain data, determine specific patient risk, and measure specific results.
2. Other organizations develop their own automated patient-specific CM plans based on the patient population served, industry best-practice recommendations, contract-specific requirements, and performance metrics.
3. Still other organizations utilize templates and workflows to develop individualized CM plans that encompass patient populations, best-practice recommendations, contract-specific requirements, and performance metrics.

D. The ideal CM plan addresses patient-specific needs, patient acuity, insurance contract-specific performance requirements, quality indicators/best-practice recommendations, resource consumption, and standardization methodology.

■ CM PLAN DEVELOPMENT—STRATEGIES

A. Pulling this all together requires strategies that help case managers address the seemingly contradictory requirements that CM plans be both patient-specific and standardized.

B. Some of the strategies that can help case managers accomplish this complex task include:

1. Patient-specific needs—When developing a CM plan that is patient-specific the case manager must evaluate many data inputs collected during the assessment. These consist of the following:

   a. Patient acuity/severity of illness,

   b. Availability of family or other support structure,

   c. Functional abilities/limitations,

   d. Services required, and

   e. Benefits available.

2. The case manager has to focus on the type of organization he or she works for and the type and amount of care for which the organization is responsible. This information is vital for recognizing both the timing and the amount of necessary care coordination with other organizations. An example of this is the case manager of an acute care hospital coordinating services with the case manager from a home health organization.

3. Patient acuity—Understanding patient acuity helps to determine the types and frequency of interventions performed by the care manager. Patient acuity is often determined by some type of identification or stratification process and includes:

   a. Current illness or injury,

   b. Comorbid conditions,

   c. Complex medical needs,

   d. Medication management/polypharmacy,

   e. Social support structure, and/or

   f. Psychological/cognitive status.

4. Contract-specific performance metrics—Recognizing contractually defined performance metrics are essential for the development of effective CM plans. Organizations contract to provide specific services to specific populations. Likewise, individual case managers contract to perform specific services for either individual patients or groups of patients.

   a. Generally, contract requirements are defined as performance measures or metrics. Incorporating these performance metrics into CM plan development helps case managers meet both patient and organizational needs as well as demonstrate the value of CM involvement.

   b. Performance metrics include types of services to be provided, timeframe requirements to perform services, guidelines for patient participation in CM, and anticipated outcomes from services provided.

5. Quality indicators/best-practice recommendations—Case managers, by the very nature of their involvement are uniquely positioned to assess the quality of health care services. Focusing on appropriate quality indicators and best-practice recommendations is directly

linked to developing appropriate anticipated outcomes. If quality care is delivered, patients have the optimal chance for the best available outcome.

C. CMSA designates quality of care as a performance indicator for CM involvement. In CMSA's standards of practice, CM is considered "an appropriate, timely, and beneficial service which promotes quality, cost-effective healthcare outcomes for the patient/family" (CMSA, 2002, p. 17).

  1. Promotion of quality-based outcomes via the use of quality indicators such as "improved functional status, improved clinical status, enhanced quality of life, client satisfaction, adherence to the treatment plan, improved patient safety, cost savings, and client autonomy" (CMSA, 2002, p. 17) are important to a CM program.

  2. It is also recommended that case managers engage in strategies to measure improvements in quality of care that directly result from CM interventions.

  3. Quality indicators and best-practice recommendations are directly linked to standardization methodology (discussed further below) and are an important strategy for CM plan development. It is important to remember that CM is regarded as a means to ensure effective quality outcomes and is an area of accountability for case managers.

  4. Addressing these expectations can be accomplished by utilizing quality indicators as outcomes measures.

  5. According to the Commission for Case Manager Certification's glossary of terms, a quality indicator is a "predetermined measure for assessing quality, a metric" (CCMC, 2005, p. 8). Quality indicators can be based on:

     a. Industry recommendations such as evidenced-based guidelines or practice standards,

     b. Organizational performance metrics,

     c. Contractual obligations,

     d. Standardized measures such as the Short Form (SF) 36 or the Minimum Data Set and Care Screening (MDS) instrument for Medicare beneficiaries, or

     e. Other recognized indicators.

  6. Quality indicators, while vital for demonstrating improved outcomes, are applied to the general, not the particular. Therefore, case managers must still create patient-specific parameters within the framework of each quality indicator as well as assure that each intervention describes what the case manager function is and how it will support the quality outcome.

D. Resource Consumption—One vital responsibility often overlooked but essential in CM plan development is resource consumption. CM plans should address anticipated resources needed but also be cognizant of benefits available to provide for these resources. Alternate funding sources as additional means to obtain resources should be included as well.

1. Resource consumption is critical because case managers have responsibility for resource management and stewardship, which includes:
   a. Evaluating safety, effectiveness, cost, and potential outcomes for patients;
   b. Referring, outsourcing, and otherwise delivering care based on ongoing health care needs of the patient;
   c. Linking patients with appropriate resources;
   d. Ensuring access to and coordination of health care services;
   e. Modifying services when possible to meet the patient's health needs; and
   f. Promoting the effective and efficient use of health services and financial resources (CMSA, 2002, pp. 19–20).
2. Case managers should include all necessary resource needs—but *only* the necessary resources. It becomes imperative to identify anticipated end results, monitor progress toward goals, and adapt the CM plan as necessary.

E. Standardization methodology—The pressure to demonstrate accountability for care delivered is at the forefront of the health care industry. However, health care quality reporting presents somewhat of a dilemma.
   1. Report cards, balanced scorecards, regulatory surveys, and so on, focus primarily on systems and processes. Yet, case managers are expected to be accountable for their involvement in the delivery of health care services and the assurance of quality and cost-effective outcomes.
   2. So how do case managers address accountability utilizing standardization methodology? By understanding what standards are applicable for the case managers' areas of practice and by encompassing the aspects of those standards that are the most appropriate for incorporation into CM interventions.
   3. Some standards that case managers may want to review include:
      a. Accreditation standards applicable to CM
      b. Health Plan Employer Data and Information Set (HEDIS)
      c. Minimum Data Set and Care Screening (MDS)
      d. Outcomes and Assessment Information Set (OASIS)
   4. While there are many other standards that are applicable depending on the area of CM practice, the important aspect for case managers to recognize is to encompass essential components of applicable standards in the CM plan development. In this way, case managers will be better able to demonstrate accountability.

F. In developing CM plans, case managers must use all strategies available for creating patient-specific, standardized CM plans that have realistic, achievable goals. These CM plans, once developed, become the means of reporting outcomes and demonstrating case manager accountability. By performing a thorough needs assessment, the framework for an effective CM plan is in place.

■ PROBLEM LIST IDENTIFICATION

A. Once an assessment is completed and the framework for the CM plan is in place, a problem list needs to be reviewed and finalized. This list is based on patient's and family's identified needs and may be:

1. Singularly focused—e.g., specific clinical outcomes such as return to independent ADLs following hip replacement surgery; or
2. Multi-focused—e.g., specific clinical outcomes, transportation issues, and appropriate family/support structure following hip replacement surgery.

B. The problem list can include patient strengths and weaknesses; family/relationship problems; cultural concerns; psychological and cognitive concerns; clinical needs; and other social, financial, and compliance concerns.

C. When the problem list is completed, the case manager must review each problem and once again ask and answer one or more of the following questions:

1. Will this problem get better? If so, then the intervention(s) and goal(s) for that problem should address the anticipated outcome. And, timelines should be incorporated in stages so that evaluation can demonstrate realistic, measurable improvements and outcomes.
   a. An example of this type of problem and interventional focus would be self-care deficit related to hip surgery; and the interventions may include rehabilitation therapy services and returning to independent ADL status.
2. Can we keep this problem from getting any worse or developing complications? If so, then the intervention(s) and goal(s) should focus on the prevention and/or minimization of complications or decline. Again, specific and measurable outcomes should be incorporated that are clearly related to the problem(s).
   a. An example of this type of problem and interventional focus would be a patient with diabetes. While you cannot make diabetes go away, you can help the patient reduce complications of this disease state and potentially avoid or slow the progression. Interventions may include helping the patient maintain blood glucose levels within acceptable ranges as defined by the attending physician.
3. What can we do to provide optimal quality of life, comfort, and dignity for this person? If the patient's problems will, most likely, not improve and deterioration is inevitable, then the goal(s) and intervention(s) must reflect the status of the patient and the measures must be appropriate for the types of interventions at hand.
   a. An example of this type of problem and interventional focus would be the nutritional needs of a patient with a terminal condition. Interventions may be to maintain nutritional status to the best ability of the patient utilizing supplements that are tolerable to the patient (Sox, 2006).

D. As the problem list is better defined, the goals, interventions, and outcomes should also be closely aligned to the problem(s) identified. Interventions and approaches to CM include physician/provider orders, facility/organizational protocols, accepted standards of practice, and defined care paths and algorithms.

■ CM PLAN IMPLEMENTATION

A. Implementation of the CM plan requires the involvement and understanding of all who are or will be responsible for certain CM plan actions or activities.

B. The CM plan implementation involves the patient, family/support structure, facilities, ancillary care providers, physician treatment team, social service agencies, home service providers, transportation agencies, case managers from the payer organization, and others as indicated.

C. Once the CM plan is developed it should be shared with the patient and primary care providers and any others to whom the patient has granted access. Remember: This is the CM plan for the *patient*. Consequently, patients must be aware of and in agreement with the CM plan goals, recognize their role in achieving optimal outcomes, and understand what they need to do to be in compliance with the defined CM plan.

D. When working with providers and other members of the health care team, it is important to share that the patient is in agreement with and has helped in the development of the CM plan. Further, by sharing with providers some of the patient's anticipated goals and identifying the providers' role in helping the patient succeed, the providers are able to take a more interactive role in the successful outcomes defined in the CM plan.

E. Examples of working with providers and other members of the health care team include:
   1. Obtaining laboratory results to evaluate clinical status;
   2. Obtaining results of physician visits and changes in orders/medical treatment plans;
   3. Coordinating transportation to necessary services;
   4. Coordinating nutritional services such as Meals-on-Wheels, and
   5. Facilitating home health, durable medical equipment, and other ancillary services.

F. For the successful implementation of a patient CM plan the case manager must involve all who are required to make the CM plan a success. The purpose of the CM plan is to guide the CM and the patient toward actions and interventions that will facilitate problem resolution (or to mitigate the consequences of problems) and goal attainment.

■ EVIDENCE-BASED MEDICINE

A. Case managers, when practicing utilization management (UM) must use evidence-based clinical practice guidelines; it is the physician's responsibility to utilize evidence-based medicine. This section reviews the types of tools available for use and helps clarify the differences between the tools. Often times, these tools are referenced interchangeably.

B. In reality, evidence-based CM tools have subtle differences and therefore should be used differently when developing plans of care.

C. Another important distinction that often is overlooked is that the tools are just that—"tools"—to assist case managers in accomplishing their goals. However, they are not, in themselves, case management.

D. Evidence-based medicine (EBM)—The integration of best research evidence coupled with clinical expertise and current practice standards. EBM is used as the basis for medical decision making. Medical recommendations based on research evidence can be formed as either guidelines or standards/protocols.

E. Clinical practice guidelines
   1. Are systematically developed statements to assist practitioner and patient decisions about appropriate health care for specific clinical circumstances (Field & Lohr, 1990). As defined, defensible guidelines require four critical concepts ("Proof and Policy," 2001):
      a. The development process is open, documented, and reproducible;
      b. The resulting output is of use to both providers and patients;
      c. The concept of appropriateness of services is reflected; and
      d. The guideline is related to clearly defined clinical issues.
   2. One of the most important attributes of Clinical Practice Guidelines is validity. This means that guidelines should, when followed, lead to the expected clinical, quality, and cost outcomes. Guidelines are considered *recommendations* for best practices.

F. Clinical standards/protocols—Clinical standards are practices that are medically necessary and services that any practitioner under any circumstances would be required to render. Where guidelines are meant to be flexible, standards are meant to be inflexible and should be followed. In addition, when formulating standards they require a higher bar than guidelines ("Proof and Policy," 2001). Standards or protocols are more specific and define a rigid set of criteria outlining the management steps for a single clinical condition.

G. Case Management Adherence Guidelines (CMAG)
   1. Designed to:
      a. Assist case managers in more effectively improving patient adherence to their medication regime work and facilitate health behavioral change
      b. Help case managers in the assessment, planning, facilitation, and advocacy of patient adherence
      c. Provide an interaction and management algorithm to assess and improve the patient's knowledge and his/her motivation to take medications as they are prescribed
   2. Based on concepts presented by the World Health Organization (WHO)
   3. Guidelines focus on two key areas required for adherence:
      a. Motivation
      b. Knowledge

    4. System of assessment
        a. Uses tools that classify individuals into motivation and knowledge categories, and place the individual into a four-quadrant system of adherence intention and interventions
        b. Goal is to move the individual to a higher degree of adherence intention
    5. CMAG includes:
        a. CMAG Workbook
        b. Online tool: CMAGTracker

■ CLINICAL PATHWAYS

A. Known by a variety of synonyms including *care paths, integrated clinical pathways, collaborative care paths, care maps, multidisciplinary action plans,* and *multidisciplinary pathways of care.*

B. These tools are health care provider–specific documents that outline key elements of the day-to-day care activities (both diagnostic and therapeutic) required by a typical patient with a particular diagnosis.

C. Clinical pathways may be developed to show current practice parameters, recommended "best practices," or a combination of both.

D. Other components of clinical pathways may include target lengths of stay and anticipated alternate levels of care.

E. Clinical pathways incorporate multidisciplinary care needs and are intended to be used by multidisciplinary care teams. Team members may include physicians, nurses, social workers, physical therapists, occupational therapists, nutritionists, pharmacists, respiratory therapists, ethicists, clergy, and others.

F. The four main components of clinical pathways are:
    1. A timeline;
    2. Identified categories of care and/or activities and their interventions;
    3. Immediate, intermediate, and long-term outcome criteria; and
    4. Some type of allowance for deviations and variances that can be documented and analyzed.

G. Care activities or elements of patient care addressed in clinical pathways may include:
    1. Assessment of the patient and monitoring
    2. Tests and procedures
    3. Care facilitation/coordination, including important milestones
    4. Consultations and referrals
    5. Medications
    6. Intravenous therapy
    7. Activity
    8. Nutrition
    9. Patient/family education

10. Treatments (e.g., medical, surgical, or nursing interventions)
11. Wound care
12. Physical and occupational therapy
13. Pain management
14. Outcome indicators and projected responses to care/expectations
15. Safety
16. Discharge planning
17. Psychosocial assessment
18. Variance identification and management

H. Clinical pathways do not always address all of the elements of care shared above. Each organization may decide on its own policy and procedure, format, and content.

I. These elements of care are not a standardized list of categories. Health care organizations and providers using clinical pathways may decide on their own list; however, it is important to have an organization-specific standard for everyone to follow to eliminate confusion.

J. Clinical pathways may have a "preprinted order set" attached to them or built into the pathway itself.

K. While clinical pathways are often viewed as practice guidelines, protocols, or algorithms, they differ in their focus as they are clearly inclusive in their requirements for care coordination and the use of multidisciplinary care teams.

■ ALGORITHMS

A. Algorithms are schematic models used to support clinical decision pathways. Structured in a yes/no schema, the decision points depend on certain characteristic or diagnostic and treatment options. Algorithms are simple decision trees, and although useful clinical tools they are not exhaustive nor do they account for all patient-related variables. Therefore, they are intended as guides only for disease states, clinical settings, insurance issues, or economics of care.

B. Clinical algorithms are flow charts that represent a sequence of clinical decisions. Effective algorithms are those that represent the latest scientific evidence and expert consensus, and include protocol charts for guiding step-by-step care of a specific health condition, medical procedure, or problem.

C. Regardless of what tool or combination of tools a case manager uses in the CM plan development process it is essential that the case manager uses the tool(s) as guidelines only. Yet, these tools remain essential for the standardization of CM plan development, which in turn allows for data collection and reporting, provides the basis for demonstrating the value of CM services, and demonstrates the return on investment of CM involvement.

■ BENEFITS OF CM PLANS

A. CM plans, in any form—whether clinical pathway, care map, multidisciplinary actions plan, algorithm, or other format—are known to improve communication among health care providers and with the patient and family; proactively delineate processes of care and expected outcomes; focus on the patient and family; identify perform-ance expectations; ensure quality; define accountability; and improve documentation.

B. CM plans define a consistent standard of care for a specific condition, event, or process. This makes it easier for the case manager to maintain continuity and consistency in care with clear expectations of the roles and responsibilities of the various health care professions involved in the provision of care.

C. CM plans function as tools that facilitate the coordination of care across the continuum of care and settings and for collaboration between the case manager and varied staff from across the continuum.

D. CM plans also are used as a strategy for ensuring adherence to standards of regulatory and accreditation agencies.

E. CM plans can be used as tools for training and education of less-experienced health care professionals, students, and newly hired staff.

F. CM plans may be used in the negotiation of managed care contracts and reimbursement rates.

■ CASE MANAGEMENT AND UTILIZATION MANAGEMENT

A. A comprehensive, patient-specific CM plan must address all the applica-ble aspects of the patient's care. Moreover, case managers have an obli-gation to manage resources appropriately and effectively. In this vein, UM (Chapter 11), transitional planning (Chapter 10), and CM should work hand in hand to comprehensively manage patient and family needs and health care resources. Although the integration of UM and CM is the topic of much discussion, it has been accomplished in several facilities.

B. UM is the process of determining whether all aspects of a patient's care, at every level, are both medically necessary and appropriately deliv-ered. Depending on benefit design, a patient's health care services may be subject to one or more of three utilization review (UR) categories. These are:
   1. Prospective UR—review of a request for services prior to the utiliza-tion of those services
   2. Concurrent UR—review of services during an episode of care, illness, or injury
   3. Retrospective UR—review of services after care has already been com-pleted

C. These three review strategies are important in helping to understand the resources required to meet a patient's care needs for a given episode of care and at a given level of care or setting. Most often, UM uses some type of clinical screening criteria or critical pathways as guidelines for the review process.

D. Generally, UM is a non-physician function within the health care continuum. However, physicians can get involved in UM activities when the health care team believes that services not approved by a third-party insurer are warranted. In such situations, a case manager may seek the assistance of a physician in addressing service approval. The case manager may use CM plans as clinical screening criteria.

E. The understanding of the role of UM is critical for recognizing that although standard processes are in place, even UR needs the flexibility to be patient specific.

F. While some case managers perform UM functions and others do not, incorporating some aspects of UM processes into CM and care plan development is a strategy to consider. How can UM become a strategy of CM plan development? The goals of UM can create synergies for CM practice. UM goals may include:
   1. Objectively screening for the most appropriate treatments and services,
   2. Documenting the need for requested treatments and services,
   3. Assisting in the timely access to care,
   4. Ensuring safe transitions to alternate levels of care utilizing objective screening criteria, and
   5. Allowing early identification of the patient's discharge and/or transfer needs.

G. In looking at these goals, synergies begin to emerge. By integrating UM goals into CM, care planning objectives, case managers can:
   1. Improve communications with care team members,
   2. Increase coordination of care and services allowing for a more seamless transition for the patient,
   3. Ensure more effective use of health plan benefits,
   4. Share resource tools,
   5. Coordinate efforts such as transitioning the patient to an alternate level of care or obtaining home care services and products,
   6. Reduce/decrease duplication of efforts for approval of certain service requests, and
   7. Reduce costs associated with the delivery of health care services.

H. These synergies can be seen as additional strategies for helping case managers meet the challenges of creating and utilizing patient CM plans that are not only patient specific but also standardized. UM can be seen as another tool that case managers may use as a guide to help identify the appropriateness and the timeliness of patient care services.

REFERENCES

Case Management Society of America (CMSA). (2002). *Standards of practice for case management.* Little Rock, AR: Author.

Cohen, E., & DeBack, V. (1999). *The outcomes mandate: Case management in health care today.* St Louis, MO: Mosby.

Commission for Case Manager Certification (CCMC). (2005). *Glossary of terms.* Rolling Meadows, IL: Author. Website: *www.ccmcertification.org.* Retrieved January, 2006.

Field, M. J., & Lohr, K. N. (1990). *Clinical practice guidelines: Directions for a new program.* Washington, DC: National Academy Press.

McKendry, M. J. (2004). *Certified professional in utilization management.* Newton, MA: McKesson Health Solutions.

Open Clinical. (2006). Evidence-based medicine; clinical practice guidelines; clinical pathways. Website: *www.openclinical.org.* Retrieved January, 2006.

Padgett, S. M. (1998). Dilemmas of caring in a corporate context: A critique of nursing case management. *Advances in Nursing Science, 20*(4), 1–12.

Proof and Policy from Medical Research Evidence. (2001). *Journal of Health Politics, Policy, and Law, 26*(April), 2. Website: *www.ahrq.gov.* Retrieved January, 2006.

Sox, H. (2006). What is a CM plan? *Nursing CM Plans.* Website: *www.careplans.com.* Retrieved January, 2006.

Specialist Library, Health Management. Clinical guidelines: A brief introduction. *Care Pathways.* Website: *http://libraries.nelh.nhs.uk/health.* Retrieved January, 2006.

Wojner, A. (2001). *Outcomes management: Applications to clinical practice.* St. Louis, MO: Mosby.

SUGGESTED READING

Agency for Healthcare Research and Quality. National guidelines clearinghouse. Website: *www.guideline.gov.* Retrieved January, 2006.

American College of Physicians. Algorithms. Website: *www.acponline.org.* Retrieved January, 2006.

Case Management under Connecticut Partnership Plans. *Case Management.* Website: *www.CTpartnership.org.* Retrieved January, 2006.

Commission for Case Manager Certification. (2005). *Code of professional conduct for case managers.* Rolling Meadows, IL: Author.

Leighton, J. (2002). *Case management today: Strategies for thriving, rather than surviving.* Marlborough, MA: McKesson Health Solutions.

Margolis, C. Z. (1983). Use of clinical algorithms. *Journal of the American Medical Association, 249,* 5. Website: *http://juma.ama-assn.org.* Retrieved January, 2006.

McKendry, M. J., & Hubbard, J. (2004). *Certified professional in utilization review.* Newton, MA: McKesson Health Solutions.

National Association of Social Workers (NASW). (2004). *Specialty certification in case management.* Baltimore, MD. Website: *www.nasw.org.* Retrieved January, 2006.

Ohio Bureau of Workers' Compensation. Medical management. Website: *www.ohiowc.com.* Retrieved January, 2006.

Satinsky, M. (1995). *An executive guide to case management strategies.* Chicago, IL: American Hospital Publishing.

Snowden, F. (Ed.) (2002). *Medical case management: Forms, checklists, and guidelines.* Gaithersburg, MD: Aspen.

15 Information Systems in Case Management

Dee McGonigle
Kathleen Mastrian

LEARNING OBJECTIVES

Upon completion of this chapter, the reader will be able to:

1. Describe information systems (IS).
2. Assess the goals of case management information systems (CMIS).
3. Explore the benefits of an automated CMIS and how case management informatics support standards of care.
4. Delineate the features and functions required in CMIS that are necessary to support case management practice.
5. Describe the data requirements of CMIS.
6. Assess the limitations of CMIS.
7. Describe how CMIS process case management data used to measure the effectiveness of case management outcomes.
8. Explore the process of selecting and implementing a CMIS.
9. Examine the impact of the Electronic Health Record (EHR) on CMIS.
10. Assess selected information technology solutions available for medication reconciliation.
11. Investigate other technology tools available to the case manager.

IMPORTANT TERMS AND CONCEPTS

Algorithm	Input
Artificial Intelligence (AI)	Interface
Bandwidth	Interoperability
Batch Processing	Knowledge
Case Management (CM)	Knowledge Base
Case Management Information	Networks
Systems (CMIS)	Nomenclature
Critical or Clinical Pathways	Outcomes Analysis
Data	Output
Data Mart	Population Level
Data Mining or Knowledge-Discovery	Protocols
in Databases (KDD)	Query
Data Model	Remote Access
Data Warehouse	Return on Investment (ROI)
Database	Rule-Based Systems
Decision Support System (DSS)	Scalability
Digital Divide	Software
Disease Management (DM)	Tacit Knowledge
Domain	Technology
Explicit Knowledge	Telecommunications Network
Extended Care Pathway (ECP)	Telemedicine
Feedback	Terminology
Hardware	Throughput
Health Care Informatics	Usability
Heuristics	Value Chain
Information	Variance
Information Systems (IS)	Wisdom
Information Technology (IT)	Workflow
Individual Level	

■ INTRODUCTION

A. Case managers and the care management team have numerous tools at their disposal to assist in the efficient performance of their work. These tools include guidelines, practice standards, pathways, critical pathways, and "tickler" or reminder systems. Case managers traditionally have relied on guidelines to simplify and standardize their interactions with the patient. Since many organizations have migrated their traditional paper-based systems to computer-based systems, case managers must be prepared to fully appreciate and utilize the functionality of these increasingly sophisticated systems.

This chapter is a revised version of what was previously published in the first edition of *CMSA Core Curriculum for Case Management*. The contributors wish to acknowledge Nancy Nasuti Whipple, as some of the timeless material was retained from the previous version.

B. This chapter focuses on automated case management information systems (CMISs) that are designed to streamline the case manager's workflow and eliminate much of the "busy work" that comes with managing patients, such as duplicate documentation, photocopying files to share with associates, placing "yellow stickies" everywhere to remember interventions, and filling out numerous forms to authorize services. The power of a CMIS comes from its ability to efficiently facilitate data collection, data storage, data sharing, data retrieval, information generation, and decision-making functions. These systems are purposefully designed to bring people, data, information, and procedures together for the purpose of managing information to support case management at the individual, team, and organizational levels.

C. CMISs are rapidly becoming key elements of case management, disease management (DM), and medication reconciliation. These systems encompass computer networks, the Internet, and telecommunication networks including telephonics. The Internet provides potent resources including Internet-based communication to the patient and providers, as well as tools to explore this vast new frontier of information. Currently, most of these tools are simply used for data collection or information gathering. With the exception of computer-based demand management, the majority of these tools do not support decision making based on the information gathered. Case managers independently determine which actions to take. New CMISs are incorporating more decision-making tools and artificial intelligence (AI).

D. The use of CMISs to enhance the value chain is extremely important since an organization's primary goal when using any tool is to produce results that are valued by its customers. Customers include not only the patients but also the users of the tools, the providers of services, and the organization's management. The concept of a "value chain," as defined by Koulopoulos and Champy (2005) is "the coordinated series of activities leading to the creation and delivery of any product or service that is deeply embedded in the collective wisdom of today's business leaders" (p. 24). Recklies (2001) describes the importance of value chain analysis in linking an organization's activities with its competitive advantage. This evaluation of each activity and determining the value added creates the value chain. The Society of Management Accountants of Canada (1999) defined value chain as, "how customer value accumulates along a chain of activities that lead to an end product or service" (p. 2). The rapid change over the last 10 to 15 years in the business market due to the evolution of ecommerce and a global marketplace have impacted the way value chains are perceived and developed. Current value chains reflect more complexity than did their recent predecessors. In the health care industry, the entire service path from organization to the end user, or patient, constitutes a value chain. Health care value can be calculated by factoring the overall financial, time, resource, and problem costs into improved clinical, economic, service, and humanistic outcomes.

E. In today's era of cost containment, case management organizations of all sizes and structures cannot afford *not* to automate, and today's case managers must be computer literate (Daus, 1997). The terms *medical* and *nursing informatics* should be expanded to include all levels of health care and be termed *health care informatics*. Health care informatics is becoming pervasive in all areas of the health care delivery system. Case managers must become knowledgeable in all aspects of health care informatics to maximize the benefits of these systems. They must be open to whatever technology is available to them, be consistent and persistent in using them to their maximum potential, and generate ideas to improve and enhance these systems.

F. The return-on-investment (ROI) issue continues to loom and will not go away in the difficult economic times health care is experiencing. Case managers are encountering heavier caseloads, both in the quantity and the complexity of their cases, and they are increasingly required to justify their own value. Tools are needed to be able to provide proof of effectiveness. CMISs are increasing their capability to gather information to provide indicators of the value of case management in beneficial outcomes for their patients and in the health care industry.

G. Case managers who use computer-based CMISs estimate that they can complete a comprehensive plan in one third to one half of the time previously required (Smith, 1998). As case managers become more adept at the use and integration of CMISs in their work they continue to demand more functionality from the systems they use. This pushing of the envelope will cause CMISs to continue to evolve to enhance the valuable work of the case manager.

H. Usability is a key factor in the success of any CMIS. The users who work with the systems arc the most important resource in helping developers understand current needs as well as new and innovative approaches to enhance the work of the case manager and to meet the ultimate goal— successful patient outcomes. Career opportunities are available for case managers and other health care providers to work as consultants to developers of information systems (IS) and organizations who wish to use this technology.

■ KEY DEFINITIONS

A. Algorithms—Flow diagrams that consist of branching logic pathways that permit the application of defined criteria to the task of identifying a terminus. The terminus can be an identification, a classification, or an activity (Horan, 1994). Algorithms, both formally and informally defined, have been used in health care for many years—for example, the algorithm for approaching an unconscious heart attack victim. Algorithms have been criticized as being too rigid. Opponents say that patients are too variable to fit into any one box. Another criticism is that algorithms impose too many restrictions, preventing the health care professional from using his or her own expertise. However, any reasonable system that incorporates algorithms provides the ability to override decisions made by the algorithm or to customize any embedded algorithm.

B. Database—A collection of data or records that is stored in a systematic fashion that allows you to search through the data for specific aims. You can run a query (ask or request information) from the database. For example, you could ask: How many people have asthma? How many people have been readmitted following an appendectomy?

C. Data mart—A subset of a data warehouse that supports a specific business process and is limited in its scope or capacity. For example, it could be tailored for the decision support applications needed by specific end user(s).

D. Data mining—According to Wikipedia, data mining is also known as knowledge-discovery in databases (KDD). This is the practice of automatically searching for meaningful patterns and relationships among data. For example, data mining could help to identify patients at risk based on their lifestyle/behaviors and medical history.

E. Data model—A chart, map, or diagram that illustrates the data entities of a database and their relationships.

F. Data warehouse—A collection of enterprisewide business information garnered from many sources in the organization. This information covers all aspects of the organization's products or services, processes, and customers. It is the integration of many resources (databases and other informational sources) into one, single repository or warehouse. This singular access point is capable of being queried, processed, or analyzed.

G. Decision support system—A decision support system (DSS) enriches a case manager's professional judgment by quickly verifying or invalidating business decisions. The user has at his or her fingertips all of the pertinent elements needed for evaluation.
1. The heart of a DSS system is a medical information warehouse containing all of the information about the patient, as well as data and outcomes of patients identified as having similar medical conditions (Dietzen, 1997).
2. Data come from a variety of sources (e.g., laboratories, pharmacy, authorizations), although the majority of information comes from claims. Data must be organized in a way that facilitates easy retrieval for meeting the identified business needs.

H. Digital divide—There is a gap between those who know how to use computers and the IS available to them to obtain vital, timely information they need, versus those who do not have access or do not know how to use the systems well enough to reap these same benefits. According to Jessup and Valacich (2006), "In the new economy there is a digital divide, where those with access to information technology have great advantages over those without access to information technology" (p. 8).

I. Domain—This term has different meanings; it could mean a field of study, the acceptable values for data attributes, or the knowledge area addressed by an expert system. As the acceptable value, according to Stair and Reynolds (2006), "The domain for an attribute such as gender would be limited to male or female" (p. 202).

J. Entity—A thing about which we collect and maintain data such as a person, place, item, or event. For example, a CMIS could include entities named *patient, medications, primary care physician,* etc.

K. Explicit knowledge—Information that can be documented, archived, and standardized such as manuals, documents, procedures, and stories.

L. Extended care pathway (ECP)—A set of policies and procedures that providers use to address a specific disabling chronic condition over time and across various service settings. It is a standardized approach to the multidisciplinary care of an individual with a particular diagnosis. An ECP is designed to increase the continuity of care between settings, and thereby improve both the quality and cost effectiveness of care. ECPs indicate what key events are necessary for patients to meet expected outcomes. They are tools to be used for managing, monitoring, and evaluating care (National Health Care Consortium [NHCC], 1995).

   1. ISs were important forerunners to the formulation of ECPs, because they standardized information and guided case managers toward similar practices.

   2. The challenge to link acute care with the community and long-term care systems is now being addressed. Case management, using such tools as ISs with integrated ECPs, is helping to meet the challenge of supplying this missing link.

M. Health care informatics—The synthesis of discipline-specific science, information management science, cognitive science, and computer science to enhance the "input, retrieval, manipulation, and/or distribution" of health care data with the ultimate goal of creating and disseminating knowledge to improve patient care and advance the discipline (McGonigle and Eggers, 1991, p. 194).

N. Heuristics—Rules, standards, or guidelines, such as "rules of thumb."

O. Protocol—A tool for deciding which care to provide under which circumstances. To assist in decision making, it may contain a decision tree or flow chart. It frequently covers a smaller segment of care rather than the whole illness. It can describe the particular order of events, but in most cases it does not suggest a timeline.

P. Rule-based systems—Systems that generate patient-specific recommendations based on all of the information gathered up to that point.

Q. Tacit knowledge—Knowledge that resides within an individual's mind based on his or her education and experience. It cannot be standardized; rather, it represents implicit processes in the worker's mind that can only be transferred through training.

R. Telemedicine—Accessing health care services using any medium besides hands-on, direct patient contact. Although it can include simple telephonic contact like telephonic triage, the more accepted definition includes the use of computers, video equipment, and remote medical monitoring (Wrinn, 1998b), for example, electrocardiogram (EKG) hook-ups, blood pressure monitoring, quality-of-life assessments, and self-risk assessments. Case managers should be aware of the uses, benefits, and limitations of telemedicine so that they can use the technology in the appropriate way. In addition, case managers can perform long-term monitoring of patients using the same telemedicine tools. This is addressed in detail in Chapter 16.

■ INTRODUCTION TO INFORMATION SYSTEMS (IS)

A. An IS is a combination of hardware, software, telecommunications networks, and the Internet. These interconnected elements "collect (input), manipulate (process), store, and disseminate (output) data and information and provide a feedback mechanism to meet an objective" (Stair and Reynolds, 2006, p. 15). The IS is a purposefully designed system that brings people, data, information, and procedures together for the purpose of managing information to support operations, management, and decision functions important to an individual, team, or organization.

B. Graves and Corcoran (1989) pioneered the focus on nursing data, information, and knowledge. This innovative thinking changed the way documentation and technology were viewed and enhanced the exchange of nursing-related information and knowledge. It is from their classic writings that the data, information, and knowledge triad came to the forefront. Understanding this triad is important because an IS relies on correct input or clean data in order to provide appropriate information. Therefore, at the core of the system are the *data,* or raw facts, that it processes. Data that has been given meaning is considered *information.* Information is processed data that has value beyond the facts or data themselves. Information is a critical resource for organizations, necessary for their day-to-day operation and management. The IS is designed to perform specific functions and must be able to meet the data and information processing needs of individuals, teams, and the organization.

C. According to McGonigle and Goshow (2003), the value of the information generated is directly related to how it helps decision makers achieve their goals currently and prospectively. It is the interplay between the IS's generated information and the knowledge and wisdom of the users or decision makers that makes the process potent. "Knowledge and wisdom are based in the collective organization, teams, and individuals. *Knowledge* is related information or information that has been processed through one's knowledge base of experience, education, and intelligence" (McGonigle and Goshow, Slide 3). Woods (1999) states that "Knowledge adds color to information" (Slide 3). *Wisdom* "is the ability to insightfully use knowledge or experience or understanding to make correct decisions or judgments. Wisdom is an intangible attribute gained through actively experiencing life" (McGonigle and Goshow, Slide 7).

D. According to Stair and Reynolds (2006), "Information systems must be applied thoughtfully and carefully so that society, business, and industry can reap their enormous benefits" (p. 2). The ethical issues inherit with such data collection and the threats to security and privacy must be addressed. These threats affect businesses; however with the sensitive information dealt with in health care, it is paramount that the systems in place are secure. Everyone in health care has a responsibility to make sure that they do not breach the security of these systems, such as giving out their passwords, attempting to access areas that are not available to them, and entering incorrect data.

E. The IS performs an essential and continually intensifying role in society, business, and industry. IS are everywhere in our lives—at the bank, grocery store, etc. Our interaction with these systems becomes routine and seamless after repetitive use. We even have ideas about ways in which these systems can be improved or enhanced to better meet our needs. Health care is just scratching the surface and beginning to reap the benefits of the superior information processing and decision support tools available in our ever-evolving information age.

F. The IS should provide the information users need, when and where it is needed.

■ GOALS OF A CASE MANAGEMENT INFORMATION SYSTEM (CMIS)

A. The goals of a CMIS are derived from the general goals of case management. Case management strives to create a collaborative partnership between providers of services and the service recipients to ensure that services are "appropriate, effective, cost efficient, and focused on patient needs" (Rossi, 2003, p. 17). Thus, the system used to manage case information must allow for collaboration, identification of appropriate services, effectiveness, efficiency, and focus.

B. Case managers need appropriate and timely data about the service recipient. Traditionally, case managers have relied on the patient as the source of timely and accurate data. Owen (2003) estimates that 40% of a provider's time is inappropriately spent looking for critical pieces of case information or in recollecting critical data. A well-designed CMIS can provide access to critical data in a timely and efficient manner.

C. A CMIS needs to be designed for intuitive usability (Hamilton et al., 2004), such that a PC-proficient operator would need little training to master.

D. Newer CMIS systems are designed to meet both individual-level care delivery and population-level management. The traditional individual-level system includes such features as clinical workstations, physician ordering systems, clinical decision support, and drug dispensing. The population-level system is designed to support the collection and analysis of aggregate data through clinical registries, data warehouse development, provision of benchmarking data, and pharmaceutical surveillance (Weiner et al., 2004).

E. A well-designed CMIS will:
1. Eliminate double data entry by the same user; that is, data can be viewed in several places within the system and in several formats
2. Eliminate double data entry by multiple users; permit data-sharing capabilities for all users with appropriate access security in place
3. Provide the ability to run in tandem with other systems and communicate with other systems either in real time (data are accessible as soon as they are entered anywhere in the system or in a legacy system with which the CMIS is integrated) or in batch mode (data are updated on a preset timed periodic schedule); make decision-making data available in real time

4. Provide users with the ability to quickly access the information that is most important to them and to filter out messages, reminders, and other prompts that are not directed to them

5. Act as central repository for all the information about a patient. Patient-centered data include:

   a. Data related to the entire continuum of the illness or disability, such as medical history, psychosocial history, financial status, goals and problems, plan of treatment, and intervention target dates

   b. Data that support the key elements of case management, including assessment, problem and goal definition, planning, monitoring, and evaluation

   c. Data that are easily transmissible among different service providers

6. Act as a central repository for population-level data to:

   a. Provide for long-term population trending and enhance outcome analysis

   b. Provide cost details as well as the clinical causes of patient variances (Favor and Ricks, 1996)

   c. Simplify accreditation updates by tracking the minute details required by regulatory agencies

   d. Generate specific-user–designed reports and charts to facilitate evaluation of case management goals, aggregate relevant data and information, and set milestone reminders for regulatory agency interactions

   e. Provide patient census data

7. Standardize terminology, documentation, data management practices, outcome measurement, and reporting. In the past, each case manager could measure outcomes differently making this process subjective in nature. A CMIS allows objective, standardized reporting over the entire managed population by all case managers.

8. Provide the ability to document and retrieve case manager interventions and cost of care information, and directly relate these activities to patient outcomes and cost savings realized as a direct result of the case manager coordinating the appropriate level of care, at the appropriate site, in the appropriate time frame. In other words, it links the financial aspects of care with clinical data, giving organizations the advantage of knowing what the cost of care is and where specifically dollars are spent.

9. Provide a DSS that turns data into actionable information, leading to additional cost savings. Data must be timely and easily retrievable to be effective as a tool for intervention.

■ BENEFITS AND LIMITATIONS OF AN AUTOMATED CMIS

A. The benefits of using a CMIS can be divided into three categories: workflow, patient care, and organizational.

   1. *Workflow* benefits include support of the case management process (allowing the case manager to focus on the patient and patient outcomes

and not be overwhelmed by clerical tasks); reduction of documentation duplication; elimination of "double-data" entry; generation of reminders or "ticklers" when a case manager intervention is required; improving data entry and storage; improving data access for sharing and reporting; and simplifying and streamlining mundane tasks.

2. *Patient care* benefits include keeping patients from "falling through the cracks"; monitoring and recording the progress of the patient throughout the health continuum; promoting a consistent, best-practice approach to managing patients with similar medical conditions; and incorporating national standards and reducing the variability of case management practices. For example, when a patient with congestive heart failure is discharged from the hospital, scheduling a follow-up visit within 2 weeks seems like a routine task. However, keeping that appointment has implications both clinically and financially. Some studies have shown that if patients wait even 1 month after discharge to follow up with their provider, readmission rates are significantly higher (Barr, 1998). The CMIS can facilitate patient–case manager interaction by maintaining patient contact via communication tools and a database for patient-centered materials. This would enhance communication and information exchange for both the patient and case manager.

3. *Organizational* benefits focus on enhancing the value chain by improving efficiency in the case management process; improving case manager job satisfaction; increasing staff accountability and empowerment; improving patient satisfaction; improving relationships with providers; increasing consistency in providing care; and providing the ability to document and report outcomes. Evaluation of the organization's capacity results from the documentation being integrated, streamlined, simplified, standardized, and reportable.

B. Limitations of the CMIS reflect not only internal limitations such as software, interfacing, and enhancements that may be lacking but also external factors such as decreased data transmission rates or bandwidth that can compromise data sharing and communication.

1. When dealing with people, health care professions are intuitive at times as to the patient's status, and the system cannot replicate or take the place of what is sometimes called the "gut factor." Any decisions made by the system must still be reviewed by a health care professional (McGarvey, 1998).

2. Health care lags behind other industries in information management. Standardization of data across the health continuum at different locations is not yet a reality, although much progress has been made within the last few years with several different initiatives. In an integrated delivery system (IDS), data sharing is less of a challenge because there are no issues of ownership and security. There are teams of people working to standardize our terminology (technical or special terms used) so that we are all referring to the same thing. Until this standardization is used throughout our facilities, it will not be possible to have seamless information along the patient care continuum.

a. Health Level Seven, Inc. (HL7)—HL7 is a nonprofit standards-developing organization accredited by the American National Standards Institute (ANSI). HL7 has developed a standard vocabulary for clinical and health care administrative data.

b. The American Nurses Association (ANA) established the Nursing Information and Data Set Evaluation Center (NIDSEC) in December of 1995. The NIDSEC "Develops and disseminates standards pertaining to information systems that support the documentation of nursing practice, and evaluates voluntarily submitted information systems against these standards" (ANA, 1995, para. 3). This site lists the following currently recognized terminologies (http://www.nursingworld.org/npii/terminologies.htm):

   i. North American Nursing Diagnosis Association, Inc. (NANDA)

   ii. Nursing Interventions Classification System (NIC)

   iii. Nursing Outcomes Classification System (NOC)

   iv. Nursing Management Minimum Data Set (NMMDS)

   v. Clinical Care Classification (CCC) [formerly Home Health Care Classification (HHCC)]

   vi. Omaha System

   vii. Patient Care Data Set (PCDS)

   viii. Perioperative Nursing Data Set (PNDS)

   ix. Systemized Nomenclature of Medicine—Clinical Terms (SNOMED—CT)

   x. Nursing Minimum Data Set (NMDS)

   xi. International Classification of Nursing Practice (ICNP)

   xii. ABC Codes

   xiii. Logical Observation Identifiers, Names, and Codes (LOINC)

c. The Systemized Nomenclature of Medicine (SNOMED)—SNOMED is a complete dictionary of medical terms containing the relationships between the SNOMED terms and other coding systems, such as billing codes and diagnostic codes. Requiring care providers to use the same medical terminology dictionary to capture data allows analyses to be done comparing "apples to apples."

   i. NANDA, NIC, NOC are being merged with SNOMED.

   ii. Read Code is sponsored by the Department of Health and National Health Service in Great Britain. There is an initiative under way to merge SNOMED with Read Code to become the English language standard.

d. Logical Observation Identifiers, Names, and Codes (LOINC)— LOINC is a compendium of terminology developed for standardized nomenclature used in laboratory observations.

e. The Kennedy-Kassebaum Bill, Health Insurance Portability and Accountability Act (HIPAA), mandates development of standards to facilitate exchange of patient information.

3. There is no centralized database for patient data as the patient moves from one management organization to another, one facility to another,

or one provider to another. This lack of standardization makes interfacing, integration, and maintenance difficult or impossible.

■ CMIS AND CASE MANAGEMENT INFORMATICS SUPPORT CASE MANAGEMENT PRACTICE

A. CMIS and health care informatics for case managers support practice from identification, selection, and assignment of patients through patient assessment, identification of problems, planning, monitoring, and evaluation.

1. Identification, selection, and assignment of patients—Case managers are assigned patients by selected identification and selection criteria. Case identification and selection defines the reasons a patient is being cared for by a case manager. Many criteria can be used to identify suitable candidates for case management, including the primary disease or illness, medical complications, exacerbations and comorbidities, the cost of care, psychosocial status, the prevalence of the disease, and the amount of treatment variation. The CMIS can automatically identify patients for case management based on user-defined triggers, or the case manager can review the patient against the criteria to determine the suitability for case management. More organizations are attempting to automate this process so patients are all evaluated in the same way, by the same system criteria, and so no patient falls through the cracks.

2. Patient assessment— Provides the case manager with a method of conducting a thorough and objective analysis of the patient's current status (Case Management Society of America [CMSA], 2002). The case manager can perform baseline, ongoing psychosocial and quality-of-life assessments; administer patient satisfaction surveys; and perform clinical status reviews. In addition, the system can track changes in responses over time. An integral part of the assessment is to move patients with a particular disease or condition into homogeneous subgroups, called *stratification groups*. The system guides the user through the stratification process, applying criteria as appropriate and available, to reduce subjectivity and variability. Patients will naturally move from one stratification group to another as the illness progresses. For example, the population identified as having asthma can be broken down further into the following stratification groups: severe persistent, moderate persistent, mild persistent, and mild intermittent. The system automatically tracks the stratification history and supports a restratification process. The CMIS can alert the case manager to stratification changes for their patients. The CMIS can also alert the case manager to patient assessment results that need immediate attention if, for example, the satisfaction surveys are completed online, negative comments or concerns could trigger an alert for the appropriate case manager. Positive comments can also trigger praise statements sent to the case manager and his or her supervisor. The comments, both negative and positive, are added to a special database for the organization. At the organizational level, these database items can become part of the continuous quality improvement program.

3. Identification of problems—Problems can be defined as issues that may affect the health and functioning of the patient or barriers to effectiveness of their care. Default problems can be automatically assigned to a patient by the system based on the patient's illness and the subgroup to which he or she belongs. The individual patient problems can be filtered through an AI system built into the CMIS to further define and refine necessary case management strategies for that specific patient. AI could be a computer or IS. One example of AI is an *expert system*. A CMIS could use a potent expert system that processes huge amounts of data or recognized information and draws conclusions based on the input. For example, you could input a patient's symptoms and the expert system could provide a diagnosis based on the inputted information or symptoms. Patient problems can also be aggregated into a database to evaluate interventions and outcomes and to establish ROI while assessing existing issues with case managers' workloads based on competing patients' needs.

4. Planning—Involves the identification of immediate, short-term, and long-term goals, as well as coordination of treatment based on identified problems and needs of the patient. Goals can appear in many forms, such as patient centered (e.g., return to previous level of function), case management (e.g., patient's endurance will improve with physical therapy), or clinical (e.g., stabilization of diabetic status with proper use of insulin). The system can keep track of the status of goals. In addition, by using AI, default goals can be defined by the system based on the patient's diagnosis and the subgroup to which they have been assigned. This assignment and the established plan are also routinely monitored to verify that the patient's needs are being addressed.

5. Monitoring—Throughout the course of the patient's continuum of care, the case manager must monitor and assess the patient's status as well as collect information regarding the delivery of services. Many times, patients "fall through the cracks" owing to lack of follow up by their provider. The case manager plays a vital role in proactively monitoring the patient as he or she progresses through critical junctures in the course of the disease. The AI built into the CMIS can define and schedule time-critical interventions and, with the interaction of the case manager, verify that the interventions are being implemented.

6. Evaluation—The case management process requires continuous evaluation. The patient's status and response to treatment is evaluated; the provider's plan of care is evaluated and refined for effectiveness and consistency with established standards; the status of goals is evaluated to determine the progress made; and the case manager must evaluate himself or herself against adopted guidelines and protocols. Evaluation is more meaningful and effective when status and outcomes can be measured consistently and objectively. After each evaluation, the case manager, along with the AI in the CMIS, modifies the intervention strategy or plan as necessary to verify that the patient's needs are being met. This is a dynamic process through which the case manager, patient, and CMIS must all be working together. Adherence or other patient issues must be addressed immediately. The case manager must constantly review and evaluate the process facilitated by the CMIS and

validate that the CMIS is indeed enhancing the process. The case manager is instrumental in suggesting necessary changes in the CMIS to enhance the system as needed and improve patient care.

B. CMIS and health care informatics for case managers support the tracking and analysis of outcomes. *Outcomes* can be defined in a variety of ways, depending on what elements of the patient's health status the case manager has an interest in or can affect.

1. The same bits of data can provide different information to different users based on the way the data are reported (Steinhauser, 1999). For example, a CMIS reports how many patients met their goal of "understanding their disease process" by the target date. Tracking and analysis occur at various levels within the organization:

   a. The case manager looks at the data to determine whether his or her intervention strategy with the patient was appropriate.

   b. The medical director looks at the results of assessments. For example, based on the fact that the patient was unable to recite the basic aspects and goals of his or her treatment, it is determined that the providers were not adequately explaining the disease to the patient or involving him or her in the treatment plan.

   c. The case management director identifies that the target date of the goal was too aggressive, based on the target population.

   d. The health plan uses the data to support the development of a disease management program for the specific disease to promote patient education and improve outcomes.

2. There are many different ways a CMIS system can be used to measure outcomes, beginning from a medical standpoint all the way through to an organizational approach. The most important measure, however, comes from patients, their perception of their outcomes and current health status, their satisfaction with their care, and their ability to help themselves.

   a. Medical—Readmission rates, emergency department visits signifying treatment failure, exacerbations, complications, too-frequent or too-infrequent office visits, lengths of stay (LOSs), mortality.

   b. Case management—Defined processes followed, goals met and variances reported, time-dependent interventions completed, adherence improved (patient and provider), patient knowledge increased.

   c. Patient—Improved quality of life, satisfaction with provider and the care he or she is receiving, and empowerment.

   d. Organizational—Value chain evaluated: cost savings, population profiling, improved working relationships, improved community image.

■ FUNCTIONAL AND NONFUNCTIONAL REQUIREMENTS AND FEATURES OF CMIS

A. *Requirements* refer to a careful analysis of the needs that the system must meet. In other words, what are you expecting to get from your CMIS?

This requires a very careful scrutiny of all of the requirements and validates why the system is needed. This should be based on current needs and to the extent possible, future needs. The next important question becomes, what CMIS *features* will fulfill this framework? This leads the organization to the "how" phase—how will this system be developed? Appropriate vendors (outsourcing) or in-house (insourcing) capabilities must be explored prior to making the decision to buy or build. Specifications for the new system must be formulated. The specification for the new system based on the identified requirements bridges the goals of the developers and the organization's users. A rapport should be established between all users and the developers. Users range from data entry personnel, case managers, other health care professionals to administrators and IT support staff. Sometimes, in systems developed within the organization using its own IS specialists, the developers also become users when they must retrieve information from the system to meet organizational reporting needs. *Functional* requirements describe the processing or functions to be supported by this new system. *Nonfunctional* requirements describe how well this system supports its functional requirements.

1. Functional requirements are based on the users' requirements for the new system. Functional requirements describe how the system will behave or function.
   a. Integration of both clinical and nonclinical components is essential because information is a critical resource in the case management process.
      i. Assessments—The responses to any individual question can be tracked over time. Responses can trigger entries on the to-do list (tickler feature) or generate a goal or problem. For example, if the case manager asks the patient whether he or she is able to tolerate mild activity and the patient responds negatively, the CMIS can generate a problem on the patient's problem list that states "patient has poor stamina" and a goal may appear that states "patient's stamina will improve." The system can also generate a reminder when the time is appropriate to perform an assessment. In addition, notes can be automatically generated that contain the responses to key questions.
      ii. Goals—CMISs can automatically remind the case manager when the target date for a goal is approaching and track the progress toward the goal.
      iii. Problems—CMISs can link problems and goals with plans to resolve each problem.
      iv. Milestones—Again, the CMIS can track the status of patient milestones. Is the patient reaching the milestones by the target dates? If not, what are the primary reasons? Is the case manager performing the appropriate interventions at the designated time once the patient meets a milestone?
   b. Rule-based alerts, messages, and reminders based on information gathered or clinical recommendations—Structured data entry with discrete data elements must be in place to meet this requirement. Reminder rules used in the system assess patient states,

determine what issues need attention, and then generate the system reminders.

    i. Rules can be related to overlooked treatments, preventive care (reducing complications and exacerbations), proper follow up, or monitoring current treatment and interventions (McDonald, Tierney, and Overhage, 1994).

    ii. Reminder rules consist of two parts. The first part, specified by one or more criteria, defines a particular patient state; for example, "The patient is not using inhaler properly." The second part specifies the required response to that state; for example, "Send written instructions on the proper use of inhaler."

    iii. The suggested response can be based on empirical data but more likely is based on anecdotal evidence with its intrinsic uncertainty—that is, what worked "best" in the past. Responses must be re-evaluated based on outcome studies. For example, 1 month after receiving educational material about using inhalers properly, 70% of identified patients still use them incorrectly. A new response may be indicated, such as "Patient receives home visit by asthma specialist to give live demonstration about how to use inhaler, evaluate patient feedback, and reinforce importance of compliance."

    iv. The success of reminder rules depends on an organization's ability to identify, analyze, and select a set of simple principles for building them; for example, "Simplicity is a required attribute." If a developer recommends a more complex rule, there must be proof to support the complexity.

c. Patient education material can be accessed online as well as sent directly to the patient or provider.

d. Tracking of services, admissions, procedures, and equipment approved for the patient

e. Access to real-time updates with other systems within the organization

f. Ability to send messages, referrals, and review requests to other users of the system

g. Ability to scan documents into the system. These may include documents from providers' offices or illustrations.

h. Communication tools to support meaningful dialogues. The CMIS must facilitate collaboration and sharing in real time either through data sharing, text, audio, and/or video interchange. This is another area that is beginning to enhance patient care by providing timely communications among varied levels of personnel responsible for the patient. This is especially paramount with the infusion of telehealth (addressed in Chapter 16).

i. Data sharing and system integration to facilitate networking is imperative. CMIS must afford the ability to interface at all levels of the organization and provider base.

2. Nonfunctional requirements are the guarantee that you will have a functional and controllable system that provides the required functionality

in a dependable or reliable, secure, and stable or uninterrupted manner under most conditions. The ability to meet these criteria distinguishes how well they support the functional requirements. Therefore, the nonfunctional requirements describe how the system will operate. Some of these requirements are listed below.

a. *Performance* refers to the ability to execute and support the functional requirements with minimal errors. Instantaneous key stroke, screen update, and query response times—encounters with patients and with the system can be as short as a minute, so the amount of time documenting the encounter or accessing information relevant to the encounter is extremely limited. The system should perform at "think speed" (Casanova, 1997).

b. *Portability* is the potential to convert data and share user interfaces across various software and hardware environments. The CMIS must have portability and remote access with synchronization to the host system. The data must be able to go with the user. Case managers are no longer spending all of their time behind a desk; onsite visits are an essential part of the assessment process. For case managers, this means visits and meetings in places such as hospitals, patient homes, provider facilities, and home offices. Access to key data should be available at all times. Synchronization of data between remote and on-site systems can occur as needed and should be easy, reliable, and quick.

c. System *availability* refers to the system being available when you need it.

d. *Flexibility*—The CMIS should allow for the customization of system parameters. The system must be flexible enough to support a wide range of environments and unique business processes while reducing variance and subjective reporting. For example, two employer groups subscribe to the same HMO. One group has opted for an aggressive DM program for diabetes, whereas the other has not identified diabetes as a major issue for its employee population.

e. *Security* deals with access to the system and the safekeeping of its contents. There are password protections and authentications necessary for access, and the contents are secure and safe from hackers attempting to access the system dishonestly. Confidentiality of patient data from unauthorized individuals and organizations as well as encryption capabilities and secure electronic data transfer must be guaranteed by the system.

f. *Usability* means that the system has a low error rate, is intuitive or easy to learn, completes tasks quickly, and satisfies its users' needs. Intuitive user navigation is essential. The information must be arranged and accessed in a way that makes sense to the user. "Jumping" from one area to another must be quick, without requiring specific paths or a steep learning curve. Human–technology interfacing or human–computer interaction is an area of study that focuses on how the technology is used and how users interact with the technology to accomplish their tasks. The research and practical applications that arise from this field have impacted how we perceive and implement technological innovations based on the target audience or users.

g. *Reliability* means that the system must be consistent in its operation; the commands must function as specified and the displayed or accessed data must reflect the data in the database.

h. *Backup* and *recovery*—Backup is the copying of files or databases so that the data processed at that time will be preserved in case of an equipment malfunction or other disaster. Recovery means that the backed up data are returned to this original condition on the media used to back it up.

i. *Scalability* means that the system has room to expand. For example, you may begin with hundreds of icons (a small picture or image on your screen that represents a certain program, file, directory, or option) and need several thousand in the future. The system must be able to scale up to meet your expanding needs.

j. *Maintainability* refers to the ease with which the system can be kept in good condition.

B. Features of CMIS

1. AI is becoming critical to creating and managing health care ISs. According to Thomson (2006), there has been unprecedented growth in the scientific understanding of diseases and their treatment regimes without a corresponding ability to apply that knowledge in practice. Systems that can automate, educate, and evaluate practice measures are crucial to safe, effective, efficient, and enhanced patient care capabilities for practitioners who are powerless at times to keep up with this overwhelming knowledge explosion.

An effective case management practice system includes:

a. Standards of practice that are customizable to accommodate variability in practice based on setting

b. A Decision Support System (DSS)

c. An educational system for case managers and other personnel

d. Laboratory systems

e. Pharmacology systems

f. Quality assurance and administration

g. Imaging systems

2. Storage of clinical knowledge, divided into three major categories:

a. Reference—This aspect of clinical knowledge pertains to the underlying medical knowledge, facts, or treatment standards that are used as rationale within the software. It can remain strictly in the background as the clinical justification for the software-driven clinical outputs and may not be visible to the user; or references and facts are visible within the application and serve as resource and support in the form of look-up tables, lists, indices, or glossaries.

b. Informational knowledge—The informational knowledge base conveys data and information about patients and providers. Also included in this category are the various types of patient and user education material, including audio, text, or scripts formatted and accessible through the software as well as clinical data.

c. Software-driven clinical outputs—The last type of clinical knowledge base relates to the actions or recommended actions that stem from software logic. Often, this takes the form of alerts, reminders, or recommendation prompts. To a large extent, this knowledge base is subjective and is based on an extrapolation of clinical facts or a consensus agreement among clinical experts. Risk assessment criteria are also in this category. Based on system-initiated prompts for input, the system makes a decision regarding the intervention strategy or the approach the case manager should take. DSSs are critical to facilitate the appropriate care being provided based on up-to-date clinical information. For example, an algorithm is applied to the treatment, diagnostic, and pharmacy history of a group of patients. The output consists of the following:

   i. A list of patients who are at high risk for developing complications and exacerbations or for requiring a hospital admission in the near future. These patients should be actively managed.

   ii. A list of patients who are relatively stable or at moderate risk. These patients may be enrolled in a DM program or have a case management contact scheduled for every month for follow up and assessment.

   iii. A list of patients who are stable and at low risk for complications. These patients may still benefit from intervention by a case manager in the form of educational material being mailed directly to their homes.

3. Promote awareness of guidelines, pathways, and protocols (Casanova, 1997)

   a. Prompting case managers with reminders (e.g., "follow up with patient regarding adherence to medication regimen")

   b. Providing treatment recommendations tailored to the individual patient (e.g., patient enrollment in a weight-reduction program)

   c. Generating appropriate alerts for immediate issues (e.g., contact physician regarding possible treatment failure)

   d. Allowing access to guideline specifics (e.g., schedule for laboratory tests, office visits, and eye exams)

4. Provide exception tracking when the patient varies from the guideline

5. Facilitate accurate and simplified data entry and collection

6. Support data retrieval for reporting and outcomes measurement

■ CMIS DATA AND DATA CONTENT REQUIREMENTS

A. Data requirements

1. Obviously, the generation of information is the goal of an information system. Data must be transformed into useful information and then converted to knowledge. Data are specific, relevant, comparable, timely, meaningful, and actionable facts that are processed into information.

Information must be provided to the decision makers closest to the "action."

2. Any system must support simplified, accurate data entry. If data entry becomes more cumbersome or error prone, the system will not be used as intended. This could lead to inconsistent data collection, which can then lead to misleading and inaccurate reports. Without consistency, all data are suspect and data integrity is lost.

3. Data must have these core elements:
   a. Integrity
   b. Consistency, i.e., meaning the same thing to all users
   c. Validity
   d. Completeness

4. Data must support health and DM initiatives.
   a. By case manager—Change activity of case manager; change behavior of patient or provider, based on responses to interventions and treatment; change guidelines, protocols, or clinical pathways
   b. By organization—Patient population profiles, cost of treating and managing diseases, outcomes analysis, variance identification, and tracking

5. Data breadth (what) and depth (about whom) as well as completeness (by whom) must be supported consistently for all data collected. Reduce the number of "holes" in the data, making reports more accurate and meaningful.

6. Graphic display of data allows more data to be displayed, making it easier to view and allowing the user to detect trends or track key indicators.

7. Data should be stored in a structured, standardized format that can be aggregated and captured as discrete data for reporting. Queries should be possible that can extract data from multiple files with speed and integrity. The end user cannot wait for days, weeks, or months for information.

8. The same type of information must be available for all patients in a group. Information should be shared among all of the members of the health care team. Collaboration with the provider or patient, or both, will improve outcomes. Once action is taken, assess the impact of that action and compare this impact against alternative actions to determine the best practice.

9. Provide feedback on demand with a user-specified denominator; that is, the subpopulation that will be reviewed.

B. Data content requirements
   1. Patient demographics, including address, contact information, employment or student status, and date of birth
   2. Patient clinical information, including medical directives, primary diagnoses, and allergies
   3. Insurance, including providers, plan, eligibility, coverage, benefits, and authorization

4. May include access to most or all of the following:
   a. Clinical practice database, including interventions and outcomes evaluations
      i. International Classification of Disease (ICD-9) Codes
      ii. Current Procedural Terminology (CPT-4) Codes
      iii. *Diagnostic and Statistical Manual of Mental Disorders,* 4th Edition (DSM-IV) Codes
   b. Table of drugs
   c. Patient claims
   d. Patient pharmacy data (pharmacy benefits manager [PBM])
   e. Provider database
   f. Facility database
   g. Community resources database
   h. Medical dictionary and medical spell-check system
   i. DM database for the latest scientific information about specific diseases
   j. Anatomy and physiology database
   k. Medication reconciliation support with pharmacology database

■ USING CMIS TO MEASURE EFFECTIVENESS OF CASE MANAGEMENT OUTCOMES

A. According to Sullivan (2002), "Integrating the electronic medical record (EMR) systems and other enterprisewide components into a clinical information system (CIS) is usually complicated and expensive. But traditional cost/benefit justifications are not adequate and not even completely applicable" (para. 1).

B. Technology makes it possible to measure the effectiveness of case management outcomes. Consumer demand for high-quality affordable care, organizational return-on-investment (ROI) assessments, and the competition over finite health care resources makes it necessary for the case manager to become an active contributor to revenue goals through knowledgeable, responsible, efficient, and effective practice.

C. There has been an evolution to outcomes-based practice advancing past the clinical pathway to focus on patient outcomes. In order to succeed, the organization must have buy-in at all levels and integrate all of the necessary tools to facilitate adoption of outcomes-based practice. They should not throw away everything that has been in place, but instead, incorporate these tools—such as clinical pathways and treatment protocols—to enhance this process. Automation can facilitate this process by integrating all of the necessary pieces, such as:

1. Clinical pathways
2. Protocols
3. Patient data, including satisfaction surveys, health status, and outcomes
4. Case manager data

5. Physician data
6. Provider data
7. Financial data, including billing and reimbursement information
8. Evaluative strategies and criteria

D. Once all of these items listed above are in place, the dollar amounts can be linked to the patient data and case management practice so the financial formulas can be applied automatically in the system.

E. The use of cost–benefit analysis has continued to skyrocket. This is an approach that can easily show the benefits of case managers' intervention in patient care. Cost should not drive practice; however, in a world that is cost-containment oriented, case managers must be aware that their services must provide a benefit and they must be able to demonstrate this benefit. Many organizations focus on the high-cost, complex cases to show the most benefit; but the day-to-day benefit on all case managed patients should be evaluated in a cost–benefit analysis. "As difficult as they are to cost-justify or quantify, improved patient outcome and satisfaction, health service efficiency, patient access and information access are important benefits that should be factored into the achievements of an integrated solution" (Sullivan, 2002, para. 1). The organization must establish a dollar amount for the tangible and intangible benefits of case management as well as the costs. This process can be automated using IS technology.

F. Current cost–benefit analyses and other ROI calculations are vital to promoting case management and improving patient care. These strategies can easily be automated using the power of CMIS technology based on specific criteria.

■ PROCESS OF SELECTING AND IMPLEMENTING A CMIS

A. Blackmore (2003) suggests tying the CMIS selection process to organizational strategic planning and business process improvement (BPI). By basing the selection of a CMIS on a strategic plan, the selection committee is forced to consider future needs as well as current needs. In the BPI model, two workflow diagrams are constructed to define the "as is" process and the "to be" process. The workflow diagramming helps to identify efficiencies and cost effectiveness and also provides an opportunity to evaluate current workflow processes.

B. A large part of system selection and implementation is to determine whether the technology will be a *transformational* technology requiring a fundamental change in the way work is done in the institution, or an *efficiency* technology, designed to support and streamline current work practices (Pare, 2002). Clearly each type will require specific implementation strategies. The two workflow diagrams described above will help to determine the type of system needed.

C. Will the CMIS be proprietary or designed to facilitate interagency use? Interagency use will require specific planning to develop a shared language (core terminology and data elements), standardized system functions, and confidentiality standards to protect shared client data (Constantine, 1997). *Proprietary, open source,* and *free software* can be confusing terms. Proprietary software protects its coding by patent or trademark and does not permit it to be modified. It is not free and does not permit distribution. Microsoft Windows would be an example of a proprietary product. Open source software consists of coding that users can view and modify freely. Linux, an operating system, is an example of open source software. According to Defective by Design.org (2006), free software on the other hand provides the user with the *freedom* to use, study, modify, improve, and redistribute the software; they contend that, "'Free software" is a matter of liberty, not price. To understand the concept, you should think of 'free' as in 'free speech,' not as in 'free beer'" (para. 2).

D. Will the system be client centered or agency centered? Fitch (2004) proposes the use of general systems theory to develop a web-based model for client control of case information. In the proposed model, the client/family controls access to a central database of client information and can direct agencies to their personal web page and provide access codes to retrieve information.

E. Weiner et al. (2004) studied selection and implementation of a CMIS in five IDSs. They offer several conclusions for consideration:
   1. Client-level system functions were more likely to be used than were population-level system functions.
   2. Leadership for implementation must come from senior management to provide a strategic, system-level, business-based perspective on IT decision making.
   3. A phased approach provides the opportunity to improve the process for each successive implementation, but may delay the realization of benefits and the weaning of users from the legacy system.
   4. Two organization challenges that emerged were the seamless integration of IS in the face of vendor resistance to interoperability and the difficulty of accurately capturing and calculating return on investment.

F. Pare (2002) also studied the process of implementing clinical IS and developed several key propositions for consideration:
   1. The successful implementation of CMIS represents a purposeful process where change agents socially construct envisioned goals, anticipate challenges ahead, and capitalize on opportunities (para. 38).
   2. The selection and effectiveness of an implementation strategy depends on the background, skills, beliefs, and motivation of key actors involved in the process (para. 39).
      a. Key actors' beliefs regarding courses of action that should be adopted are constrained or strongly influenced by the context of a given project (para. 41).
      b. The process of implementing CIS is likely to be characterized by a certain indeterminacy. Every implementation project has a life of its own and cannot be perfectly controlled or predicted (para. 45).

G. Malato and Kim (2004) studied resistance to change during the implementation of a computerized medication system. They describe the following implementation challenges:

1. Training issues associated with end-user technology anxiety and negative experiences during implementation

2. Perceptions of flaws in the technology resulting in circumvention tactics.

3. Perceptions of a lack of participation in design of a system leading to resistance to change.

4. Strategic and structural flexibility as necessary for identifying and managing the "black holes"—those unanticipated process flaws in the technology that emerge during implementation.

H. At present, there is an explosion of medical informatics systems and, specifically, software to support case management. The Employer Health Register Directory of Products and Services lists more than 55 different companies providing case management software. A key consideration when selecting a vendor for a "one off" (off-the-shelf) system is the financial stability of the company and their product support history. Vendors should also be willing to provide a list of other users to allow for networking with others who have implemented the product. Networking with other case managers as well as exploring vendor presentations at national conferences can also be beneficial (Blackmore, 2003).

I. Appoint key individuals to participate in selecting the CMIS system. The selection team must at minimum include senior-level management representation, IT staff, and end-user representation. Select members to ensure that all stakeholders are adequately represented; make certain that those selected are committed and enthusiastic about the project.

J. A pivotal decision for an organization is "buy or build?" It is important to realize that no one software program will meet 100% of the needs of an organization.

1. Explore vendors formally via request-for-information (RFI) and request-for-proposal (RFP) processes.

a. Use workflow analyses developed by the multidisciplinary team and craft an RFI.

b. Compare the RFI responses to narrow down the vendor list and invite several for an onsite demonstration.

c. Develop a formal RFP and consider having the vendor demonstrate a second time using a typical case from the organization.

d. See sample vendor rating tool at www.aafp.org/fpm/20050200/55howt.html#box_e and sample RFP outline at www.aafp.org/fpm/20050200/55howt.html#box_b.

K. Planning for implementation

1. Identify a specific planning team. Define the role of each team member and the meeting schedule. Each team member must be committed to attending all relevant meetings and to performing action items that are identified in these meetings. More time spent at the beginning of

the process will yield time savings after implementation because fewer changes will need to be made.

2. Create a timeline project plan that identifies resources that must be used at each phase.

3. Standardize processes, terms, and data elements such as goal definitions, target dates, measuring tools, and intervention strategies. Map existing case management processes to system functions.

4. Rewrite any policies, procedures, or job descriptions that are changing as a result of the system.

5. Assign an administrator who understands the functional and technical sides of the system. The administrator will be responsible for setting up configurable parameters and communicating problems and requests to the vendor.

6. Hardware is typically the smallest expense in implementing a system. Equipment purchased should support the current data storage needs and processing power and the projected needs for the next 5 years.

7. Train super-users (Experts in organizations who answer queries and support trainees) early.

   a. Set up a test environment that mimics the real world. Verify that the system performs as expected.

   b. For the first group to use the system live, choose a pilot group made up of people who are excited about the project, comfortable with technology, and possess good communication skills. Gradually add small groups and anticipate an initial drop in productivity.

8. Identify an "executive sponsor" to provide motivation and incentive to participate and cooperate.

9. Monitor system performance and users' perceptions and acceptance.

   a. Review processes for optimization and enhancement opportunities as well as creative new ways to use the system.

   b. Keep an open path of communication for feedback from users and among users to share ideas.

   c. Be alert for saboteurs and circumventors.

■ ELECTRONIC HEALTH RECORD

A. In 2004, President Bush set a goal to establish an electronic health record (EHR) for each U.S. citizen by 2014 and created the office of National Coordinator of Health Information Technology.

B. Lack of a health industry standard to describe an electronic representation of patient health information has led to confusion among providers and patients alike. Fishman (2005) describes nine different names and acronyms related to electronic health data. They include document management system, automated medical record, electronic patient record (EPR), computerized patient record (CPR), computerized medical record, continuity of care record (CCR), personal health record (PHR), electronic medical record (EMR), and electronic health record (EHR).

C. Leslie (2005) suggests that the needs for electronic management of health data are increasingly complex and require easy storage, capture, retrieval, search capability, and sharing among multiple providers. She maintains that current EHRs are primarily clinician-centric in that they are designed to enhance the clinician's practice and are patient-centric only in that they contain a single patient's information. She advocates the development of a PHR (patient health record) on a USB memory stick managed primarily by the patient in collaboration with the providers. This bottom-up, consumer-driven model requires the patient to be a managing partner in health care and allows the patient to determine access to private health information.

D. The American Health Information Management Association has developed a website in the United States to assist in the development of a personal health record (www.myphr.com/). The site includes tips for collecting information and downloadable forms for organizing information.

E. It is clear that interoperability among health care organizations is required for electronic management of patient records. Many physicians have resisted the conversion to EHRs in their practices because of the lack of standardization, high costs, lack of information about selecting and implementing an electronic system, concerns about HIPAA, and the fear that the system life cycle would be too short to realize an ROI. Adler (2005) provides detailed information about selecting an EHR, including vendor rating forms, an RFP outline (see Process of Selecting and Implementing a CMIS, Section J1, above), and an EHR functionality checklist.

■ IT SOLUTIONS FOR MEDICATION RECONCILIATION

A. Medication reconciliation is one of 14 National Patient Safety Goals implemented in 2006 by the Joint Commission on Accreditation of Healthcare Organizations (JCAHO).

B. Medication reconciliation is a process where all medications taken by a patient are reconciled; that is, examined and monitored for compatibility, necessity, and safety across the continuum of care. The goal is to reduce the number of adverse drug events.

C. There is still a disconnect between inpatient and outpatient care. It is paramount that continuity and interoperability be achieved for the patient's sake. Thompson (2005), states that "Interoperability in health care, according to the National Alliance for Health Information Technology, is the ability of different information technology systems and software applications to communicate, to exchange data accurately, effectively, and consistently, and to use the information that has been exchanged" (para. 3). The diverse medication coding systems and system-specific description of drug regimens must be unraveled and interfaced to promote patient safety and facilitate medication reconciliation. Case managers must become proactive in the development of ISs that address their patient's needs and promote safety.

D. Hospital admission is viewed as one logical place for this data collection and reconciliation. In addition, reconciliation is important during any transition that a patient makes, either within the hospital setting to another unit or upon discharge to another facility or to the community. According to Knowlton (2006), the New Jersey Health Care Quality Institute (NJHCQI) has modeled a Patient Safety Reporting System (PSRS) through which any member of a patient's health care team can fill out an online web form with specific information about an incident he or she is aware of that did or could have breached patient safety. Patients are also encouraged to participate. This is an anonymous and confidential reporting system. The PSRS supplements the mandatory reporting system and helps to identify "near misses as well as system defects and human errors which would otherwise go unnoticed" (p. 17). Reviewing these reports heightens our awareness and should help us be more proactive in the safety aspect of care. It is important that medication errors as well as problems with the IS responsible for facilitating medication reconciliation be identified, reported, and disseminated for changes to be made to protect our patients.

E. Technology can aid in the process in a number of ways. First, technology can prompt the case manager to ensure that a complete list of all medications including over the counter and herbal supplements and vitamins is collected within 24 hours of admission. Those who have reported implementation of such a system advocate using a single form to assess medications, to track the physician's review and action (e.g., continue, switch to a new medication, or discontinue), and to act as an order form for the pharmacy. The pharmacy can compare the medication assessment form to a drug database to screen for incompatibility of medications.

F. Issues associated with implementation of medication reconciliation include buy-in from all actors and specific designation of persons responsible to collect data and track the process. In addition, patients may not accurately recall medications, or they do not take them as prescribed. They may use multiple doctors and multiple pharmacies, or "share" medications with friends. Obviously, the accuracy of the reconciliation may be affected by faulty or incomplete data collection.

G. A new approach has recently been reported where a company has offered to electronically provide outpatient medication records to inpatient clinicians. This approach is patient centered in that the medication record belongs to the patient and will follow him or her across the continuum of care (Sipkoff, 2005).

■ **OTHER TECHNOLOGY TOOLS AVAILABLE TO THE CASE MANAGER**

A. As CMISs continue to evolve, more and more technology tools are becoming integrated, such as the Internet. Software is being honed to meet our needs in an integrated and fluid way involving intuitive capabilities and potent infrastructures. There are many packages on the market that allow users to search the Internet within their environment, and capture, reference, annotate, highlight, and even share this information with other users. These capabilities continue to advance our quest for timely and accurate data, information, and knowledge. The Internet has been a boon for people searching out information, and its value to case managers is no exception. A significant component of the Internet, the World Wide Web (WWW), has revamped our data-gathering methods and ignited the information explosion. Case managers use the Internet and WWW to:

1. Stay abreast of the current regulatory requirements, accreditation criteria, and standards of care as set by government and nongovernment disease-focused agencies (e.g., National Committee for Quality Assurance, American Accreditation Health Care Commission, Health Plan Employer Data and Information Set, Joint Commission on Accreditation of Healthcare Organizations)

2. Research the latest guidelines. This information can be included in any program-specific guidelines you have created within your own organization.

3. Access online journals and practice-based materials that include studies that support best-practice methods of treatment. Again, this information can be included in guidelines you have created or are using.

4. Obtain copies of public domain assessment tools; for example, a quality-of-life assessment tool

5. Search the Internet using metasearch tools such as dogpile.com to locate needed information. Share favorite sites and information with colleagues.

6. Review patient education material and recommend reviewed sites and materials to your patients and colleagues

7. Access health care statistics to help you plan your organization's case management needs for the future

8. Allow early-stage access to patient information—Case managers can communicate directly with the patient, physician, or hospital to gather information and to manage the services required. The biggest obstacles to this functionality are patient access, technology skills, security, and patient confidentiality and other legal issues.

9. Identify resources for treatment (i.e., specialists, clinics, equipment, and providers)

10. Attend conferences or seminars on the WWW (called *Webinars*) without leaving the organization. The organization's intranet (network designed just for that organization's use) should also have online events and training you can attend.

B. Claims review systems may not be directly used by the case manager but they can still have a significant impact on how case managers do their jobs.

1. Identify which providers are outliers.

2. Identify which diagnoses are the biggest consumers of health care dollars and could benefit from case management.

3. Identify which procedures are ordered inappropriately. The results of this investigation may lead to a policy that anytime this procedure is ordered, it must be pre-approved.

4. Identify which procedures are not performed when a particular condition or diagnoses warrants it; may lead to a case manager working with a provider to ensure consistency of care.

5. If claims can be reviewed in a timely fashion, they can be used to help identify patients who may benefit from case management interventions.

C. Electronic medical records (EMRs) contain data that can be shared among all providers, delivery locations, and case managers in a standardized, fully automated format (Shaffer, 1999). As EMRs have become more widespread, patients are able to be identified by more clinical criteria. For example:

1. Vital signs out of normal range for a user-defined period of time

2. Laboratory values out of normal range for a user-defined period of time

3. Any combination of vitals signs, laboratory values, diagnoses, procedures, and medications

D. Red flags—Indicators for case management (Kongstvedt, 1996). In the basic system, claims or authorizations are analyzed. User-defined criteria are used to identify patients who would benefit from case management. For example:

1. Patients with admissions lasting longer than "x" number of days

2. Patients with specific diagnoses

3. Patients with a specified procedure ordered or performed

4. Patients whose cost for the current episode exceeds "x" number of dollars

5. Patients receiving "x" number of services during a user-defined period of time

E. More sophisticated systems may look at combinations of events. For example:

1. Patients with a specific diagnosis and on a specific medication

2. Patients with a specific diagnosis and a specific procedure ordered

3. Patients who do not refill a maintenance prescription at the appropriate time

4. Patients who refill a prescription more often than indicated

F. Hardier communication tools that permit audio and video conferencing as well as application sharing to facilitate team work and enhance continuity of care. This collaborative edge really fosters a patient-centered approach and should keep everyone in the loop. The power of these tools is described in Chapter 16 on telehealth.

REFERENCES

Adler, K. (2005). How to select an electronic health record system. *Family Practice Management*, 12(2), 55–62. Retrieved from ABI/INFORM Global database (Document ID: 795118311).

American Nurses Association (ANA). (1995). Nursing Information and Data Set Evaluation Center (NIDSEC). Website: *www.nursingworld.org/nidsec/*. Retrieved January 30, 2006.

Barr, C. E. (1998). The role of information technology in disease management supporting identification of best practices. *Disease Management*, 1(3), 121–132.

Blackmore, P. (2003). Case management and technology. In P. Rossi (Ed.), *Case Management in health care* (pp. 33–54). Philadelphia, PA: Saunders.

Casanova, J. (1997). *Tools for the task: The role of clinical guidelines.* Tampa, FL: Hillsboro Printing.

Case Management Society of America (CMSA). (2002). *Standards of practice for case management.* Little Rock, AR: Author.

Constantine, N. (1997, July 29). *Development of uniform standards for interagency data sharing, case management information systems, and data confidentiality: Che California interagency data collaboration.* Paper Presented at Centers for Disease Control and Prevention, National Center for Health Statistics Joint Meeting of the Public Health Conference on Records and Statistics and the Data Users Conference, Washington, DC.

Daus, C. (1997). Software solutions: Case management gets automated for success. *Case Review, 3*(2), 54–56.

Defective by Design.org. (2006). The free software definition. Website: *www.gnu.org/philosophy/free-sw.html.* Retrieved July 18, 2006.

Dietzen, J. (1997). Decision support systems: Technology enhancing case management. *The Journal of Case Management, 3*(6), 12–17.

Favor, G., & Ricks, R. (1996). Preparing to automate the case management process. *Nursing Case Management, 1*(3), 100–106.

Fishman, E. (2005). Terminology in the health care records industry. Web site: *www.emrconsultant.com/emr_terminology.php.* Retrieved Jan. 30, 2006.

Fitch, D. (2004). *Client-controlled case information: A general system theory perspective. Social Work, 49*(3), 497–505. Retrieved from Research Library Core database (Document ID: 670972151).

Graves, J., & Corcoran, S. (1989). The study of nursing informatics. *Image: Journal of Nursing Scholarship, 21*(4), 227–231.

Hamilton, C., Jacob, J., Koch, S., & Quammen, R. (2004). Automate best practices with electronic healthcarehealth care records. *Nursing Management, 35*(2), 40E–40F. Retrieved from ABI/INFORM Global database (Document ID: 551919561).

Horan, D. (1994). Use of algorithms in clinical guideline development. *Clinical practice guideline development methodology perspectives.* Washington, DC: U.S. Department of Health and Human Services.

Jessup, L., & Valacich, J. (2006). *Information systems today: Why IS matters* (2nd ed.). Upper Saddle River, NJ: Pearson/Prentice-Hall.

Knowlton, D. (2006). Why nurses matter in the fight to reduce preventable medical errors. *The Institute for Nursing Newsletter, 2*(1), 17.

Kongstvedt, P. (1996). *The managed health care handbook.* Gaithersburg, MD: Aspen.

Koulopoulos, T., & Champy, J. (2005). Building digital value chains. *Optimize, 4*(9), 24–34.

Leslie, H. (2005). Commentary: The patient's memory stick may complement electronic health records. *Australian Health Review, 29*(4), 401–405. Retrieved from ABI/INFORM Global database (Document ID: 930870391).

Malato, L., & Kim, S. (2004). End-user perceptions of a computerized medication system: Is there resistance to change? *Journal of Health and Human Services Administration, 27*(1/2), 34–55. Retrieved from ABI/INFORM Global database (Document ID: 839715371).

McDonald, C., Tierney, W., & Overhage, J. (1994). Computer based reminder rules, data bases, and guideline development. *Clinical practice guideline development methodology perspectives.* Washington, DC: U.S. Department of Health and Human Services.

McGarvey, L. (1998). Technology's role in case management. *The Case Manager, 9*(2), 69–72.

McGonigle, D., & Eggers, R. (1991). Establishing a nursing informatics program. *Computers in Nursing 9*(5), 174–179.

McGonigle, D., & Goshow, C. (2003). The data to wisdom pathway. Website: *www.eaa-knowledge.com/eaa/The Data to Wisdom Pathway.ppt.* Retrieved January 31, 2006.

National Health Care Consortium. (1995). *Conceptualizing, implementing and evaluating extended care pathways.* Bloomington, MN: Author.

Owen, M. (2003). Changes in case management. In P. Rossi (Ed.), *Case management in health care* (pp. 19–32). Philadelphia, PA: Saunders.

Pare, G. (2002). Implementing clinical information systems: A multiple-case study within a US hospital. *Health Services Management Research, 15*(2), 71. Retrieved from ABI/INFORM Global database (Document ID: 118577259).

Recklies, D. (2001). The value chain. Website: *www.themanager.org/Models/ValueChain.htm.* Retrieved October 24, 2005.

Rossi, P. (2003). *Case management in health care,* 2nd ed. Philadelphia: Saunders.

Shaffer, C. (1999). Case management law. *Continuing Care, 18*(4), 14–16.

Sipkoff, M. (2005, Dec 12). RxHub and Siemens join to offer drug reconciliation. *Drug Topics.* Website: *www.drugtopics.com/drugtopics.* Retrieved Jan 23, 2006.

Smith, R. (1998). Simplifying tasks: Computer software programs increase efficiency for case managers. *Case Review, 4*(3), 42.

Society of Management Accountants of Canada (1999). Value chain analysis for assessing competitive advantage. Website: *www.cma-canada.org/download/smap/csc/Value_Chain_Assessing_Comp_ Advantage.pdf.* Retrieved October 24, 2005.

Stair, R., & Reynolds, G. (2006). *Principles of information systems,* 7th ed. Boston: Thomson Course Technology.

Steinhauser, K. (1999). Tracking numbers. *Continuing Care, 18*(2), 16–21.

Sullivan, A. (2002). Connected EMRs yield measureable ROI. *HealthcareHealth care Informatics Online,* Website: *www.healthcarehealth care-informatics.com/issues/2002/05_02/casereport.htm.* Retrieved January 29, 2006.

Thompson, C. (2005). Interoperability may aid medication reconciliation. Website: *www. ashp.org/news/ShowArticle.cfm?id=13538.* Retrieved January 22, 2006.

Thomson, R. (Ed.). (2006). Open Clinical. Website: *www.openclinical.org/home.html.* Retrieved January 28, 2006.

Weiner, B., Savitz, L., Bernard, S., & Pucci, L. (2004). How do integrated delivery systems adopt and implement clinical information systems? *Health Care Management Review, 29*(1), 51N66. Retrieved ABI/INFORM Global database (Document ID: 543097111).

Wikipedia, The Free Encyclopedia. (2006). Data mining. Website: *www.wikipedia.org/wiki/Data_ mining.* Retrieved January 30, 2006.

Woods, W. (1999). Information, knowledge and wisdom. Website: *www.cali.org/conference/1999/ postconf/WOODS/index.htm.* Retrieved January 22, 2006.

Wrinn, M. (1998a). A new frontier for case management: Outcomes measurement. *Continuing Care, 17*(6), 16.

Wrinn, M. (1998b). The emerging role of telehealth in health care. *Continuing Care, 17*(8), 18–19.

SUGGESTED READING

Baker, L. (2005). Benefits of interoperability: A closer look at the estimates. *Health affairs: Web exclusives, 24,* 22–25. Retrieved from ABI/INFORM Global database (Document ID: 911043501).

Basch, P. (2005). Electronic health records and the national health information network: Affordable, adoptable, and ready for prime time? *Annals of Internal Medicine, 143*(3), 227–228. Retrieved from Health Module database (Document ID: 877306001).

Brailer, D. (2005). Interoperability: The key to the future health care system. *Health affairs: Web exclusives, 24,* 19–21. Retrieved from ABI/INFORM Global database (Document ID: 911043491).

Bristol, N. (2005). The muddle of U.S. electronic medical records. *The Lancet, 365*(9471), 1610–1611. Retrieved from Research Library Core database (Document ID: 839281831).

Campazzi, E., & Lee, D. (1997). *How to assess clinical guidelines, tools for the task: The role of clinical guidelines.* Tampa, FL: Hillsboro Printing.

Drazen, E., & Metzger, J. (1999). *Strategies for integrated health care.* San Francisco: Jossey-Bass.

Gebhart, F. (2005, Jan 24). Setting up a medication reconciliation system. *Drug Topics.* Retrieved Jan 23, 2006, from Proquest Database.

Goldschmidt, P. (2005). HIT and MIS: Implications of health information technology and medical information systems. *Association for Computing Machinery. Communications of the ACM, 48*(10), 68–74. Retrieved from ABI/INFORM Global database (Document ID: 903466311).

Hammond, W. (2005). The making and adoption of health data standards. *Health Affairs, 24*(5), 1205–1213. Retrieved from ABI/INFORM Global database (Document ID: 899710811).

Himmelstein, D., & Woolhandler, S. (2005). Hope and hype: Predicting the impact of electronic medical records. *Health Affairs, 24*(5), 1121–1123. Retrieved from ABI/INFORM Global database (Document ID: 899710751).

James, B. (2005). E-health: Steps on the road to interoperability. Health *Health affairs: Web exclusives, 24,* 26–30. Retrieved from ABI/INFORM Global database (Document ID: 911043511).

Kelly, J., & Bernard, D. (1996). *Disease management: A systems approach to improving patient outcomes.* Chicago: American Hospital Publishing.

Ketchum, K., Grass, C., & Padwojski A. (2005). Medication reconciliation. *American Journal of Nursing, 105*(11), 78–85.

Lykowski, G., & Mahoney, D. (2004). Computerized provider order entry improves workflow and outcomes. *Nursing Management, 35*(2), 40G–40H. Retrieved from ABI/INFORM Global database (Document ID: 551919631).

McAdams, S. (2005). Beyond electronic health records: Quality outcomes management. *Physician Executive, 31*(4), 12–15. Retrieved from ABI/INFORM Global database (Document ID: 904923681).

Nash, D., & Todd, W. (1997). *Disease management, a systems approach to improving patient outcomes* (pp. 52–53). Chicago: American Hospital Association.

Ollier, D., & Weber (2005). The state of the electronic health record in 2005. *Physician Executive, 31*(4), 6–10. Retrieved from ABI/INFORM Global database (Document ID: 904923761).

Pronovost, P., Weast, B., & Schwarz M. (2003). Medication reconciliation: A practical tool to reduce the risk of medication errors. *Journal of Critical Care, 18*(4), 201–205.

Raghupathi, W., & Tan, J. (2002). Strategic IT applications in health care. *Association for Computing Machinery. Communications of the ACM, 45*(12), 56–61. Retrieved from ABI/INFORM Global database (Document ID: 266894581).

Shortliffe, E. (2005). Strategic action in health information technology: Why the obvious has taken so long. *Health Affairs, 24*(5), 1222–1233. Retrieved from ABI/INFORM Global database (Document ID: 899710601).

Tang, P., & Lansky, D. (2005). The missing link: Bridging the patient–provider health information gap. *Health Affairs, 24*(5), 1290–1295. Retrieved from ABI/INFORM Global database (Document ID: 899710641).

Taylor, R., Bower, A., Girosi, F., & Bigelow, J. (2005). Promoting health information technology: Is there a case for more-aggressive government action? *Health Affairs, 24*(5), 1234–1245. Retrieved from ABI/INFORM Global database (Document ID: 899710831).

Walker, J. (2005). Electronic medical records and health care transformation. *Health Affairs, 24*(5), 1118–1120. Retrieved from ABI/INFORM Global database (Document ID: 899710531).

Walker, J., Pan, E., Johnston, D., & Adler-Milstein, J. (2005). The value of health care information exchange and interoperability. *Health affairs: Web exclusives, 24*, 10–18. Retrieved from ABI/INFORM Global database (Document ID: 911043481).

Whittington, J., & Cohen, H. (2004, Jan–Mar). Of health care's journey in patient safety. *Quality Management in Health Care, 13*. Retrieved Jan 24, 2006, from ProQuest Database.

WEB-BASED RESOURCES

American Health Information Management Association—*www.ahima.org*
American Medical Informatics Association—*www.amia.org*
American National Standards Institute—*www.ansi.org/*
Certification Commission for Health Information Technology—*www.cchit.org/*
College of Healthcare Information Management Executives—*www.cio-chime.org/index.asp*
Department of Health and Human Services—*www.dhhs.gov/*
eHealth Initiative—*www.ehealthinitiative.org*
EMR Consultant Site—*www.emrconsultant.com/index.php*
Healthcare Information and Management Systems Society—*www.himss.org*
Health Insurance Portability and Accountability Act (of 1996)—*www.cms.hhs.gov/hipaa/*
Medical Records Institute—*www.medrecinst.com/*
National Alliance for Health Information Technology—*www.nahit.org*
National Health Information Infrastructure—*aspe.hhs.gov/sp/nhii/index.html*
Systematized Nomenclature of Human Medicine and Systematized Nomenclature of Medicine—Clinical Terms—*www.snomed.org*

16 Telehealth and Telemedicine in Case Management

Dee McGonigle

Kathleen Mastrian

Robert Pyke

LEARNING OBJECTIVES

Upon completion of this chapter, the reader will be able to:

1. Describe telehealth, telenursing, and telemedicine.
2. Explore the benefits of and barriers to telehealth practice.
3. Assess the impact of the World Wide Web and the Internet on case management practice.
4. Explore the online telehealth resources for the case manager and the consumer of case management services.
5. Demonstrate how to evaluate Web sites and their resources.
6. Assess telephonic case management and home-based telehealth monitoring technology.
7. Explore the future of telehealth in case management practice.

IMPORTANT TERMS AND CONCEPTS

Acoustic Data Transmission
Analog
Asynchronous
Audio
Bandwidth

Broadband
Case Management (CM)
Component Video
Composite Video
Data

Data Warehouse	Plain Old Telephone System
Database	(POTS)
Digital	Point to Point
Digital Camera	Protocols
Digital Divide	Real Time
Disease Management (DM)	Resolution
Download	Software
Encryption	Synchronous
Feedback	Technology
Hardware	Technology Infrastructure
Home Tele-Health (HTH)	Telecare
Information Systems (IS)	Telehealth (TH)
Information Technology (IT)	Tele-Imaging
Input	Telemedicine (TM)
Integrated Services Digital Network	Telenursing (TN)
(ISDN)	Telepatient
Interactive Tele-Video (IATV or ITV)	Telepharmacy
Monitoring Center/Station	Telephone Triage
Networks	Telephonic Case Management
Online	Upload
Pendant	Wireless

■ INTRODUCTION

   A. Definition of telehealth/telemedicine

      1. "Defined simply, telehealth and telemedicine involve the use of electronic communication technology as a method of delivering both health education and medical care" (CTTC, 2003, para. 1).

      2. Other definitions include a broader range, such as using "telecommunications and information technologies to share information, and to provide clinical care, education, public health, and administrative services at a distance" (OAT, 2006, para. 1).

      3. "Dissolving barriers such as distance, time, geography, weather, and economics, tele-health and tele-medicine (TH/TM) applications are designed to bring services to the clients rather than the traditional formula of clients to services" (CTTC, para. 1). This is an important aspect of telehealth (TH) since "the common goal of any tele-application is to increase access and ease of care, especially for under-served and isolated populations" (CTTC, para. 1).

   B. History of TH

      1. Craig and Patterson (2005) suggest that most of the advances in telemedicine (TM) have taken place in the last 20 to 30 years. However, they

This chapter is a revised version of what was previously published in the first edition of the *CMSA Core Curriculum for Case Management*. The contributors wish to acknowledge Nancy Nasuti Whipple, as some of the timeless material was retained from the previous version.

also point out that bonfires were used in the Middle Ages to transmit information about bubonic plague from one village to neighboring villages.

2. Postal services and telegraphy, developed in the mid-19th century, and then the telephone, all aided in the transmission of medical information across a distance.

3. The earliest known transmission of stethoscope sounds by telephone is thought to be 1910.

4. Radio communications (first by Morse code, followed by voice) near the end of the 19th century were used for medical support for seamen. They describe the development of the Seaman's Church Institute of New York (1920) and the International Radio Medical Center (1938) as two early organizations providing medical consultations to passengers and crews of ships. These services were later expanded to air travel.

5. Venable (2005) describes the connection of seven state hospitals in four states via a closed-circuit telephone system in the 1950s. This program was supported by the National Institute of Mental Health. Craig and Patterson (2005) suggest that TM developed further because of organizations with special interests (e.g., NASA).

6. In the 1950s, the television was first used to help medical personnel monitor patients remotely in clinical situations. In 1964, the first interactive, closed-circuit television system was established.

7. TM developed further as remote rural locations were connected by interactive video with health care providers.

8. More recent developments include the move from analog to digital transmissions, falling costs of computing, and the explosion of mobile phones and satellite communications.

■ KEY DEFINITIONS

A. Acoustic data transmission—Transmitting or sending voice or other sounds via telephone lines, video cable, or any other media.

B. Bandwidth—Capacity for data transfer or the capacity of a medium to transmit data. For example, video transmissions use more bandwidth than do data transmissions.

C. Broadband—Two or more signals share the same medium; high-capacity communications medium enabling the transmission of data, audio, and video; high data transmission rate.

D. Component video—A type of analog video information or a way of communicating using higher resolution and high-quality color image or video transmission.

E. Composite video—A way of communicating that conserves bandwidth but results in a lower resolution and poorer quality color image or video transmission.

F. Encryption—Encoding information to make it obscure or unreadable without special knowledge or code; used to ensure security prior to transmission.

G. Health telematics (Craig and Patterson, 2005)—Refers to the use of both information and communication technologies. The use of the term in the literature is modeled after medical or nursing informatics.

H. Home telehealth or telehomecare (Dansky, Ajello, and Duncan, 2005)—Refers to the remote delivery of services in the patient's home.

I. Pendant—A hanging object worn around the neck that contains a mini-transmitter.

J. Telecare (Craig et al., 2005)—The provision of both nursing and community support.

K. Tele-ophthalmology (Kumar and Yogesan, 2005)—Refers to remote, electronic provision of eye-care services.

L. Telepharmacy (Reed, 2005)—Refers to remote control of dispensing and inventory of drugs at a distance. The program was piloted in Alaska and links a rural clinic with a pharmacist in Anchorage.

■ INTRODUCTION TO TELEHEALTH, TELENURSING, AND TELEMEDICINE

A. According to the American Telemedicine Association (ATA, 2005), TM does not constitute a separate or distinct medical specialty: "Products and services related to telemedicine are often part of a larger investment by health care institutions in either information technology or the delivery of clinical care" (ATA, para. 1).

B. TM encompasses different types of programs and services provided for the patient. Each component involves different providers and consumers.

C. Telenursing (TN) has been defined "as the practice of nursing over distance using telecommunications technology" (NCSBN, 1997, para. 2). According to the International Council of Nurses (ICN), "Advances in telecommunications technologies are revolutionizing education and health services globally, including the provision of nursing services" (2006, para. 1). "The nurse engages in the practice of nursing by interacting with a client at a remote site to electronically receive the client's health status data, initiate and transmit therapeutic interventions and regimens, and monitor and record the client's response and nursing care outcomes" (NCSBN, para. 2). "Decreasing time and distance, these advances increase access to health and health care, especially to underserved populations and those living in rural and remote areas" (ICN, para. 1). "The value of telenursing to the client is increased access to skilled, empathetic and effective nursing delivered by means of telecommunications technology" (NCSBN, para. 2).

D. TN has been around for some time now. Nurses have provided health information and nursing advice over the telephone for several decades. This telephonic beginning is evolving with the technological advances. Teledelivery of nursing care encompasses primary prevention strategies through tertiary prevention support. Nurses are diagnosing, treating, and educating their patients using teledistance technologies that afford the patients professional care without a local provider. This is improving the quality of health in populations from underserved areas as well as in developing countries needing TH support.

E. According to Field, Meyer, and Rivera (2006), "Telemedicine offers a potential for individualized, frequent contacts between nurse and patient in a novel setting that increases access to care, and may improve patient care in a manner that is cost-effective for the health care system" (para. 5). Case managers live in a world of paper, computers, and telephones. Being able to extend their practice and enhance patient contact is paramount. Field et al. feel that "The audio and video connections of telemedicine enable a degree of personal interaction not possible through telephone or written communication" (para. 5).

F. For the case manager, TM could include simple telephonic contact such as telephone triage; monitoring, as in EKG hookups and blood pressure; as well as quality-of-life assessments and self-risk assessments. The idea of incorporating long-term monitoring into the case manager's repertoire enhances patient care and support through the continuum as well as providing valuable information to document patient outcomes, decreased sequelae, and return on investment (ROI).

G. Case managers use the telephone, emails, letters, and faxes when contacting their patients, the patient's employer (workers' compensation), insurance companies, physicians, and other healthcare providers.

H. TM addresses such services as patient consultation and monitoring, specialist referral and consultation, educational materials, and online discussion and support groups.

I. A TH system is composed of numerous delivery mechanisms or elements.
   1. According to ATA (2005), there are several delivery mechanisms:
      a. "Hub-and-spoke" networks where the *hub* is the main hospital and the *spokes* are the remote clinics
      b. Point-to-point connections that use private networks and outsource or contract out the clinical services to independent service providers
      c. Home-to-monitoring center linkages for homebound patients, those at risk for sequelae, and those who need frequent monitoring
      d. Internet or Web-based e-health patient service sites that provide direct consumer outreach services over the Internet including education, direct patient care, and consultations

2. British Columbia (2001), describes a TH system as being divided into three distinct elements that integrate the services between remote and main sites:
   a. TH users and providers (people)
   b. TH application technology
   c. Telecommunications and network links

■ TH LEGISLATION

A. The Medicare Telehealth Enhancement Act of 2005 (HR 2807) was designed to address the current limitations preventing TH from realizing its full capabilities and provide $30 million for TH initiatives (CTeL, 2005).

B. Legislative impacts affect case management (CM) practice and case managers must be aware of proposed bills and acts. There have been two important acts that never became law. The Telehealth Improvement Act of 2004 was proposed as a way to strengthen TH programs. The significant aspects of this proposed legislation included removing the requirement of a rural location for the telecare originating sites and expanding those organizations that would be able to offer services. The Medicare Telehealth Validation Act of 2003 was designed to improve TH services under Medicare. This proposed legislation directed the Secretary to support and assist with multi-state practitioner licensure and expansion of access in rural, frontier, and medically underserved areas using telecare services. Case managers must be aware of the impact of legislative authority on their practice and the range of quality services available to their clients as skilled nursing facilities, clinics, assisted living, and other county and community agencies begin to provide telecare.

C. Health care Safety Net Amendments of 2002—This bill amended the Public Health Service Act to reauthorize and strengthen the health centers program and the National Health Service Corps, and to establish the Healthy Communities Access Program, which will help coordinate services for the uninsured and underinsured, and for other purposes. It became a law October 26, 2002.

D. Legislation issues remain blurry
   1. Practicing
      a. across state lines
      b. in foreign countries
   2. Reimbursement schema
   3. Protection from fraud and abuse

■ BENEFITS OF TH

A. Hjelm (2005) summarized opinions and perceptions about the benefits of TM, cautioning that there is still limited data supporting clinical and cost effectiveness. He identified the potential benefits as improved access to information for health professionals, patients, and the general population; provision of care not previously deliverable; improved access to services and increasing care delivery because of speed, convenience, time savings, and better connections between primary, secondary, and tertiary care; improved professional education; quality control of screening programs; and reduced health care costs. Costs will also be discussed in the barriers section of this chapter. The following sections provide in-depth discussion of the two main benefits of TH—improved clinical outcomes and access to health care.

B. Improved clinical outcomes

1. Informedix (2006) has a Med-eMonitor System that could be the medication compliance and adherence solution for disease management (DM) programs as well as drug trials. This system integrates a "portable patient-interactive monitoring device, hardware, software, and networked communications system to enable CATV programs, pharmaceutical and biotechnology companies, and medical researchers to efficiently monitor and manage patients' medication compliance, protocol adherence, clinical response, and drug safety" (Informedix, para. 7). According to Informedix, this system "improved mean medication adherence rates to over 92% compared to a baseline medication adherence rate of 40%" (para. 2). They also found that it decreased "Hemoglobin A1c (HbA1c) levels by an average of 18.5% in a 3-month period (p<.002), in a medication management program involving Type II Diabetes patients in Montana" (para. 2). This will have a tremendous effect on health care initiatives and costs since "a reduction in HbA1c is associated with improved lifespan and morbidity and a significant reduction in health care costs in the treatment of diabetes patients" (para. 2).

2. Shea et al. (2006) compared diabetes control outcomes in a group who received CM and monitoring via a home telemedicine unit (HTU) with a control group who received usual care by their primary physician. The HTU provided videoconferencing, remote data upload and monitoring of blood glucose and blood pressure; a Web portal for data storage and access by both patients and clinicians, and messaging with nurse case managers; and access to an educational Website. They report positive and statistically significant differences in clinical outcomes (hemoglobin A1c, blood pressure, and LDL cholesterol) between the TM and usual care groups at one year follow up.

3. Conversely, Farmer et al. (2005) were unable to demonstrate statistically significant differences in hemoglobin A1c between their TH and usual care groups of young adults with Type 1 diabetes. However, they report that the TM system was equally effective in monitoring patients and that patients valued and accepted the system.

4. TM can be used to facilitate home monitoring of chronic diseases such as diabetes, hypertension, renal disease, and dialysis; to aid in the provision of home nursing services; and to facilitate home births (Hjelm, 2005).

5. A remote continuous real-time wireless monitoring system for cardiology was tested on ten healthy volunteers. Researchers were able to demonstrate high reliability and efficacy of the system using Bluetooth technology, telemetry, and a mobile phone. Volunteers were also asked to keep a diary of activities during the testing period. Some interference with data collection was noted during peak network times and when the subject was in a moving vehicle (Jasemian and Arendt-Nielsen, 2005).

6. Venable (2005) suggests that TM may help prevent two of the most common medical errors—inaccurate diagnosis and failure to prevent injury through access to specialty consultation.

7. The efficacy of using store-and-forward (SAF) technology in addition to live videoconferencing with patients who needed dermatology diagnostic services was investigated by Baba, Seçkin, and Kapdagli (2005). They concluded that the combination of SAF and videoconferencing provided the most accurate diagnosis. In addition, 85% of the subjects were satisfied with the TM dermatology service and would participate in teledermatology in the future. Of them, 82% would want future consultations to also include the videoconferencing with the dermatologist.

C. Access to health care
1. One of the most well-known uses of TM is for off-hour diagnostic radiology services. Linking radiologists who reside in various time zones allows for prompt diagnosis and treatment of patients (Schindler, 2005).

2. Tele-ophthalmology services to Africa via a dedicated Internet site in a London-based eye hospital are described by Kumar et al. (2005). The network primarily provides clinical consultations for diagnosis and treatment, but has also been used for surgical telemonitoring (real time) and education of physicians in remote countries.

3. Rao (2005) describes a successful use of TM in India where there are inadequate numbers of hospital beds for the large population, few physicians practicing in rural areas where two-thirds of the population resides, and high maternal/child mortality rates. The initial project, developed in conjunction with the space program, focused on transmission of medical images, ECGs, and patient history to a specialist who suggests treatment to the patient. It has expanded to include assistance to remote physicians for complicated medical procedures, mobile TM in ambulances for better prehospital care, ophthalmology, and disease prevention and health promotion.

4. Daly et al. (2005) report on the efficacy of using TH to satisfy the physician visit rules for nursing home residents. They compared the data collected by a remote operator using a mobile electronic system (computer, monitor, live video and audio, stethoscope, otoscope, EKG, dermascope, and dentalscope) with data obtained in immediate live visits by the physician. Results indicated a high correlation between live and remote assessments of nursing home residents.

Reimbursement for remote visits remains an issue and will be discussed under barriers.

5. TM can also be effective in monitoring the health of prison populations, in reporting and tracking infectious diseases, and in supporting advanced practice nurses as they deliver care in rural areas. Nurse practitioners have performed advanced colorectal screenings while consulting with a physician specialist and provided chronic disease care management in cases of congestive heart failure, diabetes, and asthma. (Reed, 2005).

6. Case managers in home-based TH
   a. Home-based TH features telemonitoring. This is such an important aspect of telecare because it helps to keep patients on track while providing up-to-date measures of their health status.
   b. Telehomecare is becoming more prevalent. Case managers will increasingly continue to coordinate and collaborate in the delivery of telehomecare.
   c. Examples where home-based TH can be used.
      i. Assessments
      ii. Consultations
      iii. Interventions
         a. Telemonitoring
         b. Reinforcement or positive feedback sessions
         c. Family video-conferencing/counseling
      iv. Evaluations

7. Telephonic case management (TCM)
   a. Traditionally, case managers have practiced using the plain old telephone system (POTS). In the past, TCM practice used only audio conversations with the patient, significant others, and other health care professionals.
   b. TCM has been known for its
      i. Frequent telephone contacts
      ii. Short health assessments
      iii. Follow-up evaluations
      iv. Incorporation of fax technology
   c. Current TCM is augmented with the evolving capabilities of telephone technology.
      i. Transfer voice and data
      ii. Internet and data transfer
      iii. Sending and receiving monitoring inputs
   d. TH incorporates TCM into a comprehensive care strategy.

■ BARRIERS TO TH

A. Hjelm (2005) listed the barriers to TH/TM as a potential breakdown in the relationship between health professional and patient (especially depersonalization) and among health professionals; issues related to the accuracy and quality of health information; and organizational (resistance to change) and bureaucratic issues. Specific documentation of additional barriers is included below.

B. Security of data
1. Shea et al. (2005) safeguarded patient data for their HTUs by use of a firewalled subnet for dedicated servers, encryption of all Internet data transfers, secure socket layer encryption for Web access, and authentication protocols for clinician access.
2. Venable (2005) advocates for the development of national standards for the security and transmission of private patient information during a TH service.

C. The digital divide
1. Equality of access to computers and the Internet and the acquisition of skills necessary to become proficient may be barriers to the implementation of TH.
2. Shea et al. (2005) did not require the subjects receiving home TH to be computer literate. Grant restrictions required that participants reside in medically underserved areas. They report that despite low education levels and little or no computer savvy, most subjects were able to learn the skills necessary to remain in the study. Resistance to the technology was reported among some of the primary care physicians who insisted on the use of telephone and fax communications with nurse case managers rather than web-based messaging.

D. Cost
1. Shea et al. (2005) report the cost of the home TM unit used in their study as $3,425. Additional costs include training, maintenance, and support for both the provider and the recipient. At present, most insurers are resistant to reimbursement for TM services because the clinical effectiveness has not been empirically demonstrated to their satisfaction.
2. Dansky et al. (2005) reviewed TH marketing strategies used by home health agencies. They identified three common organizational goals—clinical excellence, technological preeminence, and cost containment. They urge organizations to clearly assess their potential market, align organizational goals to accommodate TH, and seek grant funding for technology and start up. One advantage of implementing TH is that clinicians can potentially provide services to a greater number of clients thus increasing revenues. The authors, however, caution against using cost containment as part of the organizational marketing strategy as it may backfire if clients believe they are receiving substandard services.

E. Reimbursement for services
1. We are making advances in the reimbursement arena. According to the ATA (2005), "Even in the reimbursement fee structure, there is usually no distinction made between services provided on site and those provided through telemedicine, and often no separate coding required for billing of remote services" (para. 1).

2. A Medicare and Medicaid services bulletin issued December 23, 2005, lists the approved Medicare Telehealth Services as consultations, office or other outpatient visits, individual psychotherapy, pharmacological management, psychiatric diagnostic interview examination, end-stage renal disease services, and individual medical nutrition therapy. Approved practitioners are physicians and physician's assistants; advanced practice nurses including nurse practitioners, nurse midwives, and clinical nurse specialists; clinical psychologists; clinical social workers; and nutrition specialists or dieticians. In all cases, except for the demonstration projects in Alaska and Hawaii (allowing asynchronous SAF technology), the TH service delivery must include synchronous audio and video interaction between the patient and the qualified service provider. Additional restrictions include that patients reside in specifically designated areas (such as rural or medically underserved) and that the services originate in a physician's office, hospital, clinic, or federally qualified health center.

3. Venable (2005) summarized several other reimbursement issues related to Medicare. There is a concern for the potential of abuse of TM by grouping patients together in the videoconference, but billing services separately. Another potential problem is that rural practitioners may be driven out of practice or rural hospitals and clinics will be usurped by TH services.

4. Health insurance adaptation is necessary. Payment coverage by third-party insurers varies, but the benefits and potential cost savings of TH services are being slowly recognized and reimbursed. Venable (2005) advocates the passage of specific legislation requiring insurers to reimburse for TH services.

F. Licensure to practice TM

1. About 30 states require licensure specifically for the practice of TM. The difficulties lay in the fact that TM may be practiced across state lines. The Health Care Safety Net Amendment of 2002 provides authorization for grants to state licensing boards "to facilitate cooperation between different States in developing and implementing policies that will reduce statutory and regulatory barriers to telemedicine" (Section 102).

2. Currently, many states require that a practitioner be licensed in that state in order to provide services. The requirement of full licensure in multiple jurisdictions creates an unnecessary burden (cost, time, requirements for relicensure) for practitioners and may discourage them from practicing TH. Venable (2005) advocates for a national licensure system with national organization oversight. The ideal system from Venable's perspective is a requirement of dual licensure. That is, a TM practitioner must hold a full professional license in a state, and a separate national TM license. This alternative allows individual states to continue to monitor and maintain practice standards and removes the barrier to TH consultations across state lines. Alternatives to national licensure could include a registration system allowing for part-time practice in another state, lim-

ited licensure designed to allow specific interventions within a state, and a mutual recognition system among states.

G. Standard of care issues

1. Venable (2005) points out that standard of care legislation that holds to a standard professional practitioners in similar conditions and comparable surroundings may not hold true in TH/TM cases where the consultation has taken place across a state line.

2. Liability is an issue. Is the practitioner held to the standard of care where the patient resides, or is the patient considered to be electronically present in the state where the practitioner is located? Venable (2005) argues for the development of a national standard of care for TH practitioners. This becomes especially important in malpractice issues and needs to be fairly developed to protect both patients and practitioners.

H. Limitations of TH

1. Securing transmissions—the ability to have secure and private transmissions as well as being able to link and sustain the linkage. Is there liability of the provider of the technology services and network operators?

2. Access to TH equipment and centers

3. Ease of use as well as potential uses may not be known to all personnel. Personnel using telecare equipment must be educated on its uses and capabilities to use the technology to its full potential as well as be knowledgeable about its limitations.

■ WORLD WIDE WEB (WWW) AND INTERNET IMPACT ON CM

A. Both the WWW and the Internet have had a tremendous impact on CM practice. Through the Internet, case managers can interact with their patients via text (email and instant messaging) and audio and/or video conferencing. These tools have provided a connection between case managers and patients that is unprecedented.

B. The WWW has provided a wealth of information that patients and case managers access. Case managers must be diligent in their surveillance of Web sites that are suitable for patients as well as reviewing those that patients share with them. Case managers should build a resource bank of helpful patient sites for the various patient populations that they manage.

C. Case managers should also build a resource bank of informational Web sites to share with other health care professionals. Information sharing among practitioners involved in a single case can help to ensure consistency and continuity of care.

D. The future of TH in CM practice

1. As TH and telecare practices continue to evolve with CM practice, case managers will need to understand and use TH strategies with their patients. From in-home monitoring through full audio and visual health visits, the case manager of the future will provide unique telecare experiences for individual patients.

2. The future integration of TH, TM, and TN will continue to improve the quality of health in populations from underserved areas as well as developing countries needing TH support.
3. TH is here to stay and its use will only increase as practitioners become more and more confident and capable in telecare delivery.

■ EVALUATING WEB SITES

A. According to McGonigle (2002), there are many ways to evaluate Web sites. Here is her five-step plan.
  1. Step 1—Authority
     a. Who is/are the author(s)?
     b. Describe each author's authority or expertise.
     c. Are professional qualifications afforded?
     d. How can you contact the author(s)?
     e. Who is the site's sponsor?
     f. Is the site copyright protected?
  2. Step 2—Timeliness and continuity
     a. When were the site materials created?
     b. When did the site become active on the WWW?
     c. When was it last updated/revised?
     d. Are the links up to date?
     e. Are the links functional?
     f. When was data gathered?
     g. What version/edition is it?
  3. Step 3—Purpose
     a. Who is the targeted audience?
     b. What is the purpose?
     c. Are the goals/aims/objectives clearly stated?
  4. Step 4—Content: accuracy and objectivity
     a. Does the information provided meet the purpose?
     b. Who is accountable for accuracy?
     c. Are the cited sources verifiable?
     d. What is the content value of this site in terms of your topical needs?
     e. How complete and accurate is the content information and links?
     f. Is the site biased?
     g. Does it contain advertisements?
  5. Step 5—Structure and access
     a. Does the site load quickly?
     b. Do multimedia, graphics, and art used on the page serve a purpose or are they just decorative or fun?
     c. Is there an element of creativity?

     d. Is there appropriate interactivity?

     e. Is the navigation intuitive?

     f. Are there icons?

     g. Is this a secured site?

B. Based on the answers to each evaluative step above, you should have a clear picture as to the significance and value of the site as it relates to your topical needs. This is a tool that can be easily implemented. See Table 16-1 for a list of useful evaluative Web sites.

C. Brown (2005) provides a comprehensive listing of electronic and print resources for TH information, and organizations and listserves for TH professionals. It is important to note that there are two peer-reviewed journals that have been in existence for more than ten years— *Journal of Telemedicine and Telecare* and *Telemedicine Journal and e-Health.*

D. For a list of online telehealth resources, see Table 16-2.

TABLE 16–1
Evaluative Web Sites

"How to Critically Analyze Information Sources," revised October 6, 2004. Originally by Joan Ormondroyd, then updated by Michael Engle and Tony Cosgrave, Reference Services Division, Olin and Uris Libraries at Cornell University.	*http://www.library.cornell.edu/okuref/ research/ skill26.htm*
"Evaluating Internet Research Sources." Robert Harris uses the CARS Checklist for information quality.	*http://www.virtualsalt.com/evalu8it.htm*
"Ten C's for Evaluating Internet Sources," revised June 19, 2003. Contact Betsy Richmond at the University of Wisconsin–Eau Claire.	*http://www.uwec.edu/library/Guides/tencs. html*
"Evaluating Internet Resources," Trudi Jacobson, Coordinator of User Education Programs and Laura Cohen, Network Services Librarian University At Albany Libraries.	*http://library.albany.edu/internet/evaluate. html*
"The A B C Ds of Evaluating Internet Resources," modified October 31, 2005. Contact Janet Hogan at Binghamton University Libraries.	*http://library.lib.binghamton.edu/search/ evaluation.html*
Health on the Net Foundation	*http://www.hon.ch/*

Caveat: URLs come and go on the ever-evolving WWW. All of the URLs within this section were available on January 16, 2006 and reflected the content cited at that time. There are no guarantees, though, that these sites will remain on the WWW in this form.

TABLE 16–2
Online Telehealth Resources

For Case Managers

CTeL (Center for Telehealth and e-Health Law)	http://www.ctel.org/
CTTC (California Telehealth and Telemedicine Center)	http://www.pageweavers.com/cttc/
ICN (International Council of Nurses)	http://www.icn.ch/matters_telenursing.htm
OAT (Office for the Advancement of Telehealth)	http://telehealth.hrsa.gov/welcome.htm
Telehealth information resources	http://www.uchsc.edu/ahec/mapp/telehealth/index.htm
Telehealth school based	http://eahec.ecu.edu/telehealth/links.html
ZUR Institute: Telehealth and e-Therapy Online Resources	http://drzur.com/telehealthresources.html
Behavioral healthcare and telehealth	http://www.umdnj.edu/psyevnts/pointers.html
ATA (American Telemedicine Association)	http://www.americantelemed.org/index.asp
TIE (Telemedicine Information Exchange)	http://tie.telemed.org/links/international.asp
hcPro The Healthcare Compliance Company	http://www.hcpro.com/case-management/
Disease management via telehealth	http://www.itelehealthinc.com/diseasemanage.asp

For Consumers of Telehealth Case Management Services

Centers for Medicare and Medicaid Services (CMS) overview of telemedicine	http://www.cms.hhs.gov/telemedicine/
Case Management Society of Australia: What is case management?	http://www.cmsa.org.au/definition.html
Case management for caregivers	http://www.aoa.gov/prof/aoaprog/caregiver/careprof/progguidance/background/program_issues/fin-noelker.pdf
Case manager defined by patient population, such as adolescent mental health, health care, legal mesothelioma, mental health, and nursing home abuse	http://www.topicalterminology.com/dictionary/Case+Manager
ATA (American Telemedicine Association): About telemedicine	http://www.atmeda.org/news/library.htm
The Telemedicine Information Exchange (TIE)	http://tie.telemed.org/
Asthma In-home Monitoring (AIM)	http://tie.telemed.org/programs/showprogram_t2.asp?item=2839
Informatics for Diabetes Education and Telemedicine	www.ideatel.org/casemanagement.html
Division of e-Health and Telemedicine	http://telemedicine.georgetown.edu/eHealth/DesktopDefault.aspx

For Home Telemedicine and Telehomecare

ECU Telemedicine Center, Brody School of Medicine	http://www.ecu.edu/telemedicine/home_care.htm
TIE (Telemedicine Information Exchange) Home Telehealth	http://tie.telemed.org/homehealth/

TABLE 16–2
Online Telehealth Resources (*continued*)

For Home Telemedicine and Telehomecare

Virtual Medical Worlds Home Telemedicine Project	*http://www.hoise.com/vmw/00/articles/vmw/ lv-vm-05-00-12.html*
Telecare: Telemedicine for Home-bound Clients	*http://www.hometelecare.info/publica_1.htm*
Rural Telemedicine Data/Image Transfer Methods	*http://home.uchicago.edu/~gevann/Rural-TelemedData.pdf*
University of Iowa Nursing Home Telemedicine	*http://www.uihealthcare.com/depts/med/ familymedicine/research/geriatrics/ telemedicine.html*

All of these resources were retrieved on February 28, 2006, and reflected the intended content at that time.

REFERENCES

American Telemedicine Association (ATA). (2005). Defining telemedicine. Website: *www.american-telemed.org/news/definition.html*. Retrieved February 14, 2006.

Baba, M., Seçkin, D., & Kapdagli, S. (2005). A comparison of teledermatology using store-and-forward methodology alone, and in combination with Web camera videoconferencing. *Journal of Telemedicine and Telecare, 11*(7), 354–360. Retrieved from ProQuest Psychology Journals database (Document ID: 926130421).

British Columbia, The Information Management Group, Corporate Shared Services, Ministry of Health Planning and Ministry of Health Services. (2001). Telehealth projects: A practical guide. Website: *www.healthservices.gov.bc.ca/cpa/publications/practicalguide.pdf*. Retrieved February 14, 2006.

Brown, N. (2005). Information on telemedicine. *Journal of Telemedicine and Telecare, 11*(3), 117–126. Retrieved from ProQuest Psychology Journals database (Document ID: 840267431).

California Telehealth and Telemedicine Center (CTTC). (2003). Terms. Website: *www.pageweavers.com/cttc/t_terms.html*. Retrieved February 8, 2006.

Center for Telehealth and E-Health Law (CTeL). (2005). Telehealth and emerging technologies. Website: *www.ctel.org/Telehealth.html*. Retrieved February 8, 2006.

Craig, J., & Patterson, V. (2005). Introduction to the practice of telemedicine. *Journal of Telemedicine and Telecare, 11*(1), 3–9. Retrieved from ProQuest Psychology Journals database (Document ID: 805776671).

Daly, J. M., Jogerst G., Jung-Yong, P., Yun-Deok, K., & Taehee, B. (2005). A nursing home telehealth system: Keeping residents connected. *Journal of Gerontological Nursing, 31*(8), 46–51. Retrieved from database (Document ID: 878036341).

Dansky, K., Ajello, J., & Duncan, D. (2005). Marketing telehealth to align with strategy. *Journal of Healthcare Management, 50*(1), 19–31. Retrieved from ABI/INFORM Global database (Document ID: 788326961).

Farmer, A. J., Gibson, O., Dudley, C., Bryden, K., et al. (2005). A randomized controlled trial of the effect of real-time telemedicine support on glycemic control in young adults with type 1 diabetes (ISRCTN 46889446). *Diabetes Care, 28*(11), 2697–2702. Retrieved from Health Module database (Document ID: 924546891).

Field, L., Meyer, S., & Rivera, J. (2006). The telemedicine nurse case manager perspective. Website: *www.ideatel.org/syllabus/manager.html*. Retrieved February 6, 2006.

Health Care Safety Net Amendments of 2002. (n.d.). Website: *www.govtrack.us/congress/bill.xpd?tab=summary&bill=s107-1533*. Retrieved February 19, 2006.

Hjelm, N. (2005). Benefits and drawbacks of telemedicine. *Journal of Telemedicine and Telecare, 11*(2), 60–70. Retrieved from ProQuest Psychology Journals database (Document ID: 820279421).

Informedix, Inc. (2006). InforMedix' Med-eMonitor improves patient medication adherence to over 92%, reduces hemoglobin A1c levels by 18.5%, in type II diabetes medication management program. Rockville, MD., Feb 13, 2006, (BUSINESS WIRE). Website: *http://investor.informedix.com/newsrelease.asp?news=2130953533&ticker=IFMX&lang=EN&ny=on*. Retrieved February 13, 2006.

International Council of Nurses (ICN). (2006). Telenursing. Website: *www.icn.ch/matters_telenursing.htm*. Retrieved February 6, 2006.

Jasemian, Y., & Arendt-Nielsen, L. (2005). Evaluation of a realtime, remote monitoring telemedicine system using the Bluetooth protocol and a mobile phone network. *Journal of Telemedicine and Telecare, 11*(5), 256–260. Retrieved from ProQuest Psychology Journals database (Document ID: 892867031).

Kumar, S., & Yogesan, K. (2005). Internet-based eye care: VISION 2020. *The Lancet, 366*(9493), 1244–1245. Retrieved from Research Library Core database (Document ID: 912320331).

McGonigle, D. (June 2002). How to evaluate web sites. *Online Journal of Nursing Informatics (OJNI), 6*(2). Website: *http://eaa-knowledge.com/ojni/ni/602/web_site_evaluation.htm*. Retrieved January 16, 2006.

National Council of State Boards of Nursing (NCSBN). (1997). Telenursing: A challenge to regulation. Website: *www.ncsbn.org/resources/complimentary_ncsbn_telenursing.asp*. Retrieved February 8, 2006.

Office for the Advancement of Telehealth (OAT). (2006a). Grantees directory. Website: *http://telehealth.hrsa.gov/grants/04/grantee.htm*. Retrieved February 8, 2006.

Office for the Advancement of Telehealth (OAT). (2003b). Telemedicine licensure report. Website: *http://telehealth.hrsa.gov/lincensure.htm*. Retrieved February 8, 2006.

Rao, R. (2005). Telemedicine takes health care to India's rural areas. *Appropriate Technology, 32*(4), 25–27. Retrieved from ABI/INFORM Global database (Document ID: 977801451).

Reed, K. (2005). Telemedicine: Benefits to advanced practice nursing and the communities they serve. *Journal of the American Academy of Nurse Practitioners, 17*(5), 176–180. Retrieved from database (Document ID: 874910681).

Schindler, E. (2005). Mouse calls. *NetWorker, 9*(4), 11–13. Retrieved from ABI/INFORM Global database (Document ID: 957721091).

Shea, S., Weinstock, R., Starren, J., Teresi, J., Palmas, W., Field, L., Morin, P., Goland, R., Izquierdo, R., Wolff, L., Ashraf, M., Hilliman, C., Silver, F., Meyer, S., Holmes, D., Petkova, E., Capps, L., & Lantigua, R. (2006). A randomized trial comparing telemedicine case management with usual care in older, ethnically diverse, medically underserved patients with diabetes mellitus. *Journal of American Medical Informatics Association, 13*, 40–51. Website: *www.jamia.org/cgi/content/short/13/1/40*. Retrieved February 6, 2006.

Venable, S. (2005). A call to action: Georgia must adopt new standard of care, licensure, reimbursement, and privacy laws for telemedicine. *Emory Law Journal, 54*(2), 1183–1217. Retrieved from Law Module database (Document ID: 875322011).

TELEHEALTH READING LIST

Textbooks

Bauer, J. (1999). *Telemedicine and the reinvention of health care.* McGraw-Hill.

Coiera, E. (1998). *Guide to medical informatics, the Internet, and telemedicine.* Chapman and Hall Medical.

Darkins, A. W., & Carey, M. A. (2000). *Telemedicine and telehealth: Principles, policies, performance and pitfalls.* New York: Springer.

Englebardt, S. P., & Nelson, R. (2002). *Health care informatics: An interdisciplinary approach.* Mosby.

Fleisher, L. D., & Dechene, J. C. (2005). *Telemedicine and e-health law.* New York: Law Journal Press.

Negroponte, N. (1995). *Being digital.* New York: Knopf.

Simmons, S. C., West, V. L., & Chimiak, W. J. (2003). Telecommunications and videoconferencing for psychiatry. In *Telepsychiatry and e-mental health.* London: Royal Society of Medicine Press.

Journal Articles and Reports

Abbott, K. C., Boocks, C. E., Sun, Z., Boal, T. R., & Poropatich, R. K. (2003). Walter Reed Army Medical Center's Internet-based electronic health portal. *Military Medicine, 168*(12), 986–991.

American Nurses Association. (1999). *Core principles on telehealth.* Washington, DC: American Nurses Publishing. Website: *http://www.nurse.org/acnp/telehealth/th.ana.core.shtml.*

Ashley, R. C. (2002). Telemedicine: legal, ethical, and liability considerations. *Journal of the American Dietetic Association, 102*(2), 267–269.

Barker, G. P., Krupinski, E. A., Schellenberg, B., & Weinstein, R. S. (2004). Expense comparison of a telemedicine practice versus a traditional clinical practice. *Telemed Journal and E Health, 10*(3), 376–380.

Benger, J. R., Noble, S. M., Coast, J., & Kendall, J. M. (2004). The safety and effectiveness of minor injuries telemedicine. *Emergency Medicine Journal, 21*(4), 438–445.

Bolch, E. (2004). America's health care system in crisis: the case for telemedicine. *Caring, 23*(7), 6–9, 11.

Brebner, E. M., Brebner, J. A., Ruddick-Bracken, H., Wootton, R., & Ferguson, J. (2003). The importance of setting and evaluating standards of telemedicine training. *Journal of Telemedicine and Telecare, 9*(Suppl 1), S7–9.

Campbell, J. D., Harris, K. D., & Hodge, R. (2001). Introducing telemedicine technology to rural physicians and settings. *Journal of Family Practice, 50*(5), 419–424.

Capalbo, S. M., & Heggem, C. N. (1999). Innovations in the delivery of health care services to rural communities: Telemedicine and limited-service hospitals. *Rural Development Perspectives, 14*(3), 8–13.

de la Torre, A., Hernandez-Rodriguez, C., & Garcia, L. (2004). Cost analysis in telemedicine: Empirical evidence from sites in Arizona. *Journal of Rural Health, 20*(3), 253–257.

Demiris, G., Oliver, D. R., Fleming, D. A., & Edison, K. (2004). Hospice staff attitudes towards telehospice. *American Journal of Hospice and Palliative Care, 21*(5), 343–347.

Eron, L., King, P., Marineau, M., & Yonehara, C. (2004). Treating acute infections by telemedicine in the home. *Clinical Infectious Disease, 39*(8), 1175–1181.

Federal Communications Commission. (2004). *Lands of opportunity: Bringing telecommunications services to rural communities.* Washington, DC. Website: *http://www.fcc.gov/cgb/rural/Ruralbook120204.pdf.*

Fox, S., & Fallows, D. (2003). *Internet Health Resources: Health searches and email have become more commonplace, but there is room for improvement in searches and overall Internet access.* Pew Internet & American Life Project; Washington, DC. Accessed July 16, 2003. Website: *www.pewinternet.org/reports/pdfs/PIP_Health_Report_July_2003.pdf.*

Fox, S., & Rainie, L. *The online health care revolution: How the web helps Americans take better care of themselves.* Pew Internet & American Life Project; Washington, DC. Accessed November 26, 2000. Website: *www.pewinternet.org/reports/pdfs/PIP_Health_Report.pdf.*

Givens, G. D., Blanarovich, A., Murphy, T., Simmons, S., Balch, D., & Elangovan, S. (2004). Internet-based tele-audiometry system for the assessment of hearing: A pilot study. *Telemedicine Journal and E-Health, 9*(4), 375–378.

Goldberg, L. R., Piette, J. D., Walsh, M. N., Frank, T. A., Jaski, B. E., Smith, A. L., Rodriguez, R., Mancini, D. M., Hopton, L. A., Orav, E. J., & Loh, E. (2003). Randomized trial of a daily electronic home monitoring system in patients with advanced heart failure: the Weight Monitoring in Heart Failure (WHARF) trial. *American Heart Journal, 146*(4), 705–712.

Grigsby, J., Rigby, M., Hiemstra, A., House, M., Olsson, S., & Whitten, P. (2002). The diffusion of telemedicine. *Telemedicine Journal and e-Health, 8*(1), 79–94.

Gustke, S. S., Balch, D. C., West, V. L., & Rogers, L. O. (2000). Patient satisfaction with telemedicine. *Telemedicine Journal, 6*(1), 5–13.

Hailey, D., Ohinmaa, A., & Roine, R. (2004). Study quality and evidence of benefit in recent assessments of telemedicine. *Journal of Telemedicine and Telecare, 10*(6), 318–324.

Hersh, W., Helfand, M., Wallace, J., Kraemer, D., Patterson, P., Shapiro, S., & Greenlick, M. (2002). A systematic review of the efficacy of telemedicine for making diagnostic and management decisions. *Journal of Telemedicine and Telecare, 8*(4), 197–209.

Hicks, L. L., Boles, K. E., Hudson, S. T., Koenig, S. E., Madsen, R. W., Kling, B. W., Tracy, J. A., Mitchell, J. A., & Webb, W. D. (2000). An evaluation of telemedicine satisfaction among health care professionals. *Journal of Telemedicine and Telecare, 6*(4), 209–215.

Hood, M. M. (2004). Crisis in the countryside: Networking and telemedicine are crucial for health care facilities in rural America. *Health Progress.* Website: *http://www.chausa.org/PUBS/PUBSART.ASP?ISSUE=HP0403&ARTICLE=G.*

Institute of Medicine. Quality through collaboration: The future of rural health care. Washington, DC: National Academies Press. Website: *http://www.nap.edu/books/0309094399/html/.*

Jaatinen, P. T., Forsström, J., & Loula, P. Teleconsultations: (2002). Who uses them and how? *Journal of Telemedicine and Telecare, 8*, 319–324.

Jacklin, P. B., Roberts, J. A., Wallace, P., Haines, A., Harrison, R., Barber, J. A., Thompson, S. G., Lewis, L., Currell, R., Parker, S. & Wainwright, P. (2003). Virtual outreach: Economic evaluation of joint teleconsultations for patients referred by their general practitioner for a specialist opinion. *BMJ, 327*(7406), 84.

Jennett, P., Jackson, A., Healy, T., Ho, K., Kazanjian, A., Woollard, R., Haydt, S., & Bates, J. (2003). A study of a rural community's readiness for telehealth. *Journal of Telemedicine and Telecare, 9*(5), 259–263.

Jennett, P. A., Scott, R. E., & Hunter, J. (2004). Models of telehealth : An invitational workshop. CANARIE Inc. Website: *http://www.canarie.ca/conferences/telehealth/report.pdf.*

Johnson, L. J. (2003). Malpractice consult: Legal risks of telemedicine. *Medical Economics,* 101.

Kane, B., & Sands, D. Z. (1998). Guidelines for the clinical use of electronic mail with patients. *Journal of the American Medical Informatics Association, 5*(1), 104–111.

Krupinski, E., Nypaver, M., Poropatich, R., Ellis, D., Safwat, R., & Sapci, H. (2002). Clinical applications in telemedicine/telehealth [review]. *Telemedicine Journal and e-Health, 8*(1), 13–34.

List of medicare telehealth services. (2005). Website: *www.cms.hhs.gov/Transmittals/downloads/R43BP.pdf.* Retrieved February 19, 2006.

Malasanos, T. H., Burlingame, J. A., & Muir, A. (2004). Advances in telemedicine in the 21st century. *Advances in Pediatrics, 51,* 131–169.

Mangrulkar, R., Athey, B., Brebner, E., Moidu, K., Pulido, P., & Woolliscroft, J. (2002). Telemedicine and medical/health education. *Telemedicine Journal and E-Health, 8*(1), 49–60.

Menachemi, N., Burke, D. E., & Ayers, D. J. (2004). Factors affecting the adoption of telemedicine: A multiple adopter perspective. *Journal of Medical Systems, 28*(6), 617–632.

Nesbitt, T. S., Marcin, J. P., Daschbach, M. M., & Cole, S. L. (2005). Perceptions of local health care quality in seven rural communities with telemedicine. *Journal of Rural Health, 21*(1), 79–85.

Nitzkin, J. L., Zhu, N., & Marier, R. L. (1997). Reliability of telemedicine examination. *Telemedicine Journal, 3,* 141–158.

Noel, H. C., Vogel, D. C., Erdos, J. J., Cornwall, D., & Levin, F. (2004). Home telehealth reduces healthcare costs. *Telemedicine Journal and E Health, 10*(2), 170–183.

Sisk, J. E., & Sanders, J. H. (1998). A proposed framework for economic evaluation of telemedicine. *Telemedicine Journal, 4,* 31–37.

Stamm, B. H., & Perednia, D. A. (2000). Evaluating psychosocial aspects of telemedicine and telehealth systems. *Professional Psychology: Research & Practice, 31,* 184–189.

Stamm, B. H. (2003). Bridging the rural-urban divide with telehealth and telemedicine. In *Rural behavioral health care: An interdisciplinary guide* (pp. 145–155). Washington, DC: American Psychological Association.

Strode, S. W., Gustke, S., & Allen, A. (1999). Technical and clinical progress in telemedicine. *Journal of the American Medical Association, 281*(12), 1066–1068.

Whitten, P., & Adams, I. Success and failure: (2003). A case study of two rural telemedicine projects. *Journal of Telemedicine and Telecare, 9*(3), 125–129.

Wikipedia: The Free Encyclopedia. (2006). Telehealth. Website: *http://en.wikipedia.org/ wiki/Telehealth.* Retrieved February 28, 2006.

SPECIALTIES READING LIST

Cardiology

Bonvini, R. F., Caoduro, L., Menafoglio, A., Calanca, L., von Segesser, L., & Gallino, A. (2002). Telemedicine for cardiac surgery candidates. *European Journal of Cardiothoracic Surgery, 2*(3), 377–380.

Casey, F., Brown, D., Craig, B. G., Corrigan, N., McCord, B., Rogers, J., Mulholland, H. C., & Quinn, M. (1998). Value of a low-cost telemedicine link in the remote echocardiographic diagnosis of congenital heart defects. *Journal of Telemedicine and Telecare, 4*(Suppl 1), 46–48.

Chronaki, C., Kostomanolakis, S., Lelis, P., Lees, P. J., Chiarugi, F., Tsiknakis, M., & Orphanoudakis, S. C. (2000). Integrated teleconsultation services in cardiology. *IEEE Computers in Cardiology, 27,* 175–178.

Cloutier, A., & Finley, J. (2004). Telepediatric cardiology practice in Canada. *Telemedicine Journal and e-Health, 10*(1), 33–37.

Cotton, J. L., Gallaher, K. J., & Henry, G. W. (2002). Accuracy of interpretation of full-length pediatric echocardiograms transmitted over an integrated services digital network telemedicine link. *Southern Medical Journal, 95*(9), 1012–1016.

McConnell, M. E., Steed, R. D., Tichenor, J. M., & Hannon, D. W. (1999). Interactive telecardiology for the evaluation of heart murmurs in children. *Telemedicine Journal, 5*(2), 157–161.

McCue, M. J., Hampton, C. L., Malloy, W., Fisk, K. J., Dixon, L., & Neece, A. (2000). Financial analysis of telecardiology used in a correctional setting. *Telemedicine Journal and e-Health, 6*(4), 385–391.

Sable, C. A., Cummings, S. D., Pearson, G. D., Schratz, L. M., Cross, R. C., Quivers, E. S., Rudra, H., & Martin, G. R. (2002). Impact of telemedicine on the practice of pediatric cardiology in community hospitals. *Pediatrics, 109*(1), e3.

Shanit, D., Cheng, A., & Greenbaum, R. A. (1996). Telecardiology: Supporting the decision-making process in general practice. *Journal of Telemedicine and Telecare, 2*(1), 7–13.

Tsagaris, M. J., Papavassiliou, M. V., Chatzipantazi, P. D., Danis, D., Dendrinou, M. S., Tsantoulas, D. J., & Loannidis, P. G. (1997). The contribution of telemedicine to cardiology. *Journal of Telemedicine and Telecare, 3*(Suppl 1), 63–64.

Zhang, R., Yamauchi, K., Nonogawa, M., Ikeda, M., Zhang, W., & Huang, D. (2004). A telemedicine system for collaborative work on radiographic coronary video-images. *Journal of Telemedicine and Telecare, 10*(3), 152–155.

Dermatology

American Academy of Dermatology. (2001). American academy of dermatology association position statement on telemedicine. Accessed November 23, 2001. Website: *http://www.aadassociation.org/telemedicine.html.*

Burdick, A. E., & Hu, S. (2003). U.S. teledermatology survey: American Telemedicine Association. Website: *http://www.atmeda.org/ICOT/sigtelederm.SIGSurveyDatabase2003-v.2.pdf.*

Norton, S. A., Burdick, A. E., Phillips, C. M., & Berman, B. (1997). Teledermatology and underserved populations. *Archives of Dermatology, 133*(2), 197–200.

Pak, H. S., Harden, D., Cruess, D., Welch, M. L., Poropatich, R./National Capital Area Teledermatology Consortium. (2003). Teledermatology: An intraobserver diagnostic correlation study, Part I. *Cutis, 71*(5), 399–403.

Pak, H. S., Harden, D., Cruess, D., Welch, M. L., Poropatich, R./National Capital Area Teledermatology Consortium. (2003). Teledermatology: An intraobserver diagnostic correlation study, Part II. *Cutis, 71*(6), 476–480.

Pak, H. S., Welch, M., & Poropatich, R. (1999). Web-based teledermatology consult system: Preliminary results from the first 100 cases. *Studies in Health Technology and Informatics, 64*, 179–184.

Phillips, C. M., Burke, W. A., & Allen, M. H. (1998). Reliability of telemedicine in evaluating skin tumors. *Telemedicine Journal, 4*(1), 5–9.

Phillips, C. M., Burke, W. A., Bergamo, B., & Mofrad, S. (2000). Review of teleconsultations for dermatologic diseases. *Journal of Cutaneous Medicine and Surgery, 4*(2), 71–75.

Roth, A. C., Reid, J. C., Puckett, C. L., et al. (1999). Digital images in the diagnosis of wound healing problems. *Plastic Reconstructive Surgery, 103*, 483–486.

Wootton, R., & Oakley, A. (2002). *Teledermatology.* London: Royal Society of Medicine Press.

Emergency Medicine, Trauma, and Disaster Response

Benger, J. R., Noble, S. M., Coast, J., & Kendall, J. M. (2004). The safety and effectiveness of minor injuries telemedicine. *Emergency Medicine Journal, 21*(4), 438–445.

Benner, T., Schachinger, U., & Nerlich, M. (2004). Telemedicine in trauma and disasters: From war to earthquake: Are we ready? *Studies in Health Technology and Informatics, 104*, 106–115.

Boulanger, B., Kearney, P., Ochoa, J., Tsuei, B., & Sands, F. (2001). Telemedicine: A solution to the follow-up of rural trauma patients? *Journal of the American College of Surgeons, 192*(4), 447–452.

Brebner, E. M., Brebner, J. A., Ruddick-Bracken, H., Wootton, R., Ferguson, J., Palombo, A., Pedley, D., Rowlands, A., & Fraser, S. (2004). Evaluation of an accident and emergency teleconsultation service for north-east Scotland. *Journal of Telemedicine and Telecare, 10*(1), 16–20.

Gomez, E., Poropatich, R., Karinch, M. A., & Zajtchuk, J. (1996). Tertiary telemedicine support during global military humanitarian missions. *Telemedicine Journal, 2*(3), 201–210.

Haskins, P. A., Ellis, D. G., & Mayrose, J. (2002). Predicted utilization of emergency medical services telemedicine in decreasing ambulance transports. *Prehospital Emergency Care, 6*(4), 445–448.

Hicks, L. L., Boles, K. E., Hudson, S. T., Madsen, R. W., Kling, B. W., Tracy, J. A., Mitchell, J. A., & Webb, W. D. (2001). Using telemedicine to avoid transfer of rural emergency department patients. *Journal of Rural Health, 17*(3), 220–228.

Jones, S. M., Milroy, C., & Pickford, M. A. (2004). Telemedicine in acute plastic surgical trauma and burns. *Annals of the Royal College of Surgeons of England, 86*(4), 239–242.

Ricci, M. A., Caputo, M., Amour, J., Rogers, F. B., Sartorelli, K., Callas, P. W., & Malone, P. T. (2003). Telemedicine reduces discrepancies in rural trauma care. *Telemedicine Journal and e-Health, 9*(1), 3–11.

Servadei, F., Antonelli, V., Mastrilli, A., Cultrera, F., Giuffrida, M., & Staffa, G. (2002). Integration of image transmission into a protocol for head injury management: A preliminary report. *British Journal of Neurosurgery, 16*(1), 36–42.

Simmons, S. C., Murphy, T. A., Blanarovich, A., Workman, F. T., Rosenthal, D. A., & Carbone, M. (2003). Telehealth technologies and applications for terrorism response: A report of the 2002 coastal North Carolina domestic preparedness training exercise. *Journal of the American Medical Informatics Association, 10*(2), 166–176.

Tachakra, S., Jaye, P., Bak, J., Hayes, J., & Sivakumar, A. (2000). Supervising trauma life support by telemedicine. *Journal of Telemedicine and Telecare, 6*(Suppl 1), 7–11.

Pathology

Cross, S. S., Dennis, T., & Start, R. D. (2002). Telepathology: Current status and future prospects in diagnostic histopathology [Review]. *Histopathology, 41*(2), 91–109.

Della Mea, V., Cataldi, P., Pertoldi, B., & Beltrami, C. A. (2000). Combining dynamic and static robotic telepathology: A report on 184 consecutive cases of frozen sections, histology and cytology. *Analytical Cellular Pathology, 20*(1), 33–39.

Dierks, C. (2000). Legal aspects of telepathology. *Analytical Cellular Pathology, 21*(3–4), 97–99.

Lanschuetzer, C. M., Pohla-Gubo, G., Schafleitner, B., Hametner, R., Hashimoto, T., Salmhofer, W., Bauer, J. W., & Hinter, H. (2004). Telepathology using immunofluorescence/immunoperoxidase microscopy. *Journal of Telemedicine and Telecare, 10*(1), 39–43.

Lee, E. S., Kim, I. S., Choi, J. S., Yeom, B. W., Kim, H. K., Ahn, G. H., & Leong, A. S. Y. (2002). Practical telepathology using a digital camera and the Internet. *Telemedicine Journal and e-Health, 8*(2), 159–165.

Marchevsky, A. L., Lau, S. K., Khanafshar, E., Lockhart, C., Phan, A., & Fishbein, M. C. (2002). Internet teleconferencing method for telepathology consultations from lung and heart transplant patients. *Human Pathology, 33*(4), 410–414.

Morgan, M. B., Tannenbaum, M., & Smoller, B. R. (2003). Telepathology in the diagnosis of routine dermatopathologic entities. *Archives of Dermatology, 139*(5), 637–640.

Oberbarnscheidt, P., Hufnagl, P., Guski, H., Hauptmann, S., & Dietel, M. (2000). Analysis of errors in telepathology. *Electronic Journal of Pathology and Histology, 6*(3), 109–121.

Schwarzmann, P., Binder, B., & Klose, R. (2000). Technical aspects of telepathology with emphasis on future development. *Analytical Cellular Pathology, 21*(3–4), 107–126.

Settakorn, J., Kuakpaetoon, T., Leong, F. J. W.-M., Thamprasert, K., & Ichijima, K. (2002). Store-and-forward diagnostic telepathology of small biopsies by e-mail attachment: A feasibility pilot study with a view for future application in Thailand diagnostic pathology services. *Telemedicine Journal and e-Health, 8*(3), 333–341.

Weinstein, R. S., Descour, M. R., Liang, C., Bhattacharyya, A. K., Graham, A. R., Davis, J. R., Scott, K. M., Richter, L., Krupinski, E. A., Szymus, J., Kayser, K., & Dunn, B. E. (2001). Telepathology overview: From concept to implementation. *Human Pathology, 32*(12), 1283–1299.

Winokur, T. S., McClellan, S., Siegal, G. P., Redden, D., Gore, P., Lazenby, A., Reddy, V., Listinsky, C. M., Conner, D. A., Goldman, J., Grimes, G., Vaughn, G., and McDonald, J. M. (2000). Prospective trial of telepathology for intraoperative consultation: Frozen sections. *Human Pathology, 31*(7), 781–785.

Pediatrics

Britton, C. V., Anderson, M. R., Berkowitz, C. D., Friedman, A. L., Goodman, D. C., Outwater, K. M., Pan, R. J. D., Sowell, D. R., McGuinness, G. A., Dunston, F. J., Stoddard, J. J., Tunnessen, W. W., Woodhead, J. C., & Jewett, E. A. (2003). Scope of practice issues in the delivery of pediatric health care. *Pediatrics, 111*(2), 426–435.

Bynum, A. B., Cranford, C. O., Irwin, C., & Denny, G. S. (2002). Participant satisfaction with a school telehealth education program using interactive compressed video delivery methods in rural Arkansas. *Journal of School Health, 72*(6), 235–242.

Caban-Martinez, A. J., & Caban-Alemany, A. J. (2002). Medical informatics in a pediatric ambulatory practice. *International Pediatrics, 17*(4), 198–202.

Cloutier, A., & Finley, J. (2004). Telepediatric cardiology practice in Canada. *Telemedicine Journal and e-Health, 10*(1), 33–37.

Grigsby, R. K., McSwiggan-Hardin, M., Pursely-Crotteau, S., Adams, L. N., Bell, W., Stachura, M. E., & Kanto, W. P. (2000). Use of telemedicine for children with special health care needs. *Pediatrics, 105*(4), 843–847.

Izenberg, N., & Lieberman, D. A. (1998). The Web, communication trends, and children's health: Part 2: The Web and the practice of pediatrics. *Clinical Pediatrics, 37*(4), 215–221.

McConnell, M. E., Steed, R. D., Tichenor, J. M., & Hannon, D. W. (1999). Interactive telecardiology for the evaluation of heart murmurs in children. *Telemedicine Journal, 5*(2), 157–161.

Sable, C. A., Cummings, S. D., Pearson, G. D., Schratz, L. M., Cross, R. C., Quivers, E. S., Rudra, H., & Martin, G. R. (2002). Impact of telemedicine on the practice of pediatric cardiology in community hospitals. *Pediatrics, 109*(1), e3.

Spooner, S. A., & Gotlieb, E. M./Steering Committee on Clinical Information Technology. (2004). Telemedicine: Pediatric applications. *Pediatrics, 113*(6), e639–e643.

Urbach, J., Elishkevitz, K., Rotstein, R., Rozenblat, M. V., Mardi, T., Shapira, I., Brandski, D., & Berliner, S. (2003). Telemedicine-based application for the detection of inflammation in pediatrics. *Telemedicine Journal and e-Health, 9*(3), 241–246.

Whitten, P., Kingsley, C., Cook, D., Swirczynski, D., & Doolittle, G. (2001). School-based telehealth: An empirical analysis of teacher, nurse, and administrator perceptions. *Journal of School Health, 71*(5), 173–179.

Wootton, R., & Batch, J. (2004). *Telepediatrics: Telemedicine and child health.* London: Royal Society of Medicine Press.

Young, T. L., & Ireson, C. (2003). Effectiveness of school-based telehealth care in urban and rural elementary schools. *Pediatrics, 112*(5), 1088–1094.

Physical Medicine and Rehabilitation

Brennan, D., Georgeadis, A., & Baron, C. (2002). Telerehabilitation tools for the provision of remote speech-language treatment. *Topics in Stroke Rehabilitation, 8*(4), 71–78.

Clement, P. F., Brooks, F. R., Dean, B. V., and Galaz, A.(2001). A neuropsychology telemedicine clinic. *Military Medicine, 166*(5), 382–384.

Craig, J. J., McConville, J. P., Patterson, V. H., & Wootton, R. (1999). Neurological examination is possible using telemedicine. *Journal of Telemedicine and Telecare, 5*(3), 177–181.

Diamond, B., Shreve, G. M., Bonilla, J. M., Johnston, M. V., Morodan, J., & Branneck, R. (2003). Telerehabilitation, cognition and user-accessibility. *Neurorehabilitation, 18*(2), 171–177.

Dreyer, N. C., Shaw, D. K., & Wittman, P. P. (2001). Efficacy of telemedicine in occupational therapy: A pilot study. *Journal of Allied Health, 30*(1), 39–42.

Egner, A., Phillips, V. L., Vora, R., & Wiggers, E. (2003). Depression, fatigue, and health-related quality of life among people with advanced multiple sclerosis: results from an exploratory telerehabilitation study. *NeuroRehabilitation, 18*(2), 125–133.

Forducey, P. G., Ruwe, W. D., Dawson, S. J., Scheiderman-Miller, C., McDonald, N. B., & Hantla, M. R. (2003). Using telerehabilitation to promote TBI recovery and transfer of knowledge. *NeuroRehabilitation, 18*, 103–111.

Gammon, D., Sorlie, T., Bergvik, S., & Hoifodt, T. S. (1998). Psychotherapy supervision conducted by videoconferencing: A qualitative study of users' experiences. *Journal of Telemedicine and Telecare, 4*(Suppl 1), 33–35.

Jacobsen, S. E., Sprenger, T., Andersson, S., & Krogstad, J.-M. (2003). Neuropsychological assessment and telemedicine: A preliminary study examining the reliability of neuropsychology services performed via telecommunication. *Journal of the International Neuropsychological Society, 9*(3), 472–478.

Lai, J. C. K., Woo, J., Hui, E., & Chan, W. M. Telerehabilitation: (2004). A new model for community-based stroke rehabilitation. *Journal of Telemedicine and Telecare, 10*(4), 199–205.

Lemaire, E. D., Boudrias, Y., & Greene, G. (2001). Low-bandwidth, Internet-based videoconferencing for physical rehabilitation consultations. *Journal of Telemedicine and Telecare, 7*(2), 82–89.

Palsbo, S. E. (2004). Medicaid payment for telerehabilitation. *Archives of Physical Medicine and Rehabilitation, 85*, 1188–1191.

Russell, T. G., Buttrum, P., Wootton, R., & Jull, G. A. (2003). Low-bandwidth telerehabilitation for patients who have undergone total knee replacement: preliminary results. *Journal of Telemedicine and Telecare, 9*(Suppl 2), S44–47.

Savard, L., Borstad, A., Tkachuck, J., Lauderdale, D., & Conroy, B. (2003). Telerehabilitation consultations for clients with neurologic diagnoses: Cases from rural Minnesota and American Samoa. *NeuroRehabilitation, 18*(2), 93–102.

Scheideman-Miller, C., Clark, P. G., Smeltzer, S. S., Carpenter, J., Hodge, B., & Prouty, D. (2002). Two-year results of a pilot study delivering speech therapy to students in a rural Oklahoma school via telemedicine. *Proceedings of the 35th Annual Hawaii International Conference on System Sciences.* IEEE Computer Society Press, Los Alamitos, CA. 9 pp.

Telehealth starting to make inroads in occ-health; future is virtually limitless: new regulations, lower costs may help growth. (2004). *Occupational Health Management, 14*(3), 25–29.

Verburg, G., Borthwick, B., Bennett, B., & Rumneya, P. (2003). Online support to facilitate the reintegration of students with brain injury: Trials and errors. *Neurorehabilitation, 18*(2), 113–123.

Winters, J. M. (2002). Telerehabilitation research: Emerging opportunities. *Annual Review of Biomedical Engineering, 4*, 287–320.

Psychiatry/Mental Health

American Psychiatric Association. (1998). APA resource document on telepsychiatry via videoconferencing. Website: *http://www.psych.org/pract_of_psych/tp_committee.cfm.*

Day, S. X., & Schneider, P. L. (2002). Psychotherapy using distance technology: A comparison of face-to-face, video, and audio treatment. *Journal of Counseling Psychology, 49*(4), 499–503.

Gemmill, J. (2005). Network basics for telemedicine. *Journal of Telemedicine and Telecare, 11*(2), 71–76. Retrieved from ProQuest Psychology Journals database (Document ID: 820278971).

Glueckauf, R. L., Pickett, T. C., Ketterson, T. U., Nickelson, D. W., & Loomis, J. S. (2003). Telehealth and chronic illness: Emerging issues and developments in research and practice. In S. Llewelyn & P. Kennedy (Eds.), *Handbook of clinical health psychology.* London: Wiley.

Glueckauf, R. (2002). Telehealth and chronic disabilities: New frontier for research and development. *Rehabilitation-Psychology, 47*(1), 3–7.

Hohmann, A. A., & Shear, M. K. (2002). Community-based intervention research: Coping with the "noise" of real life in study design. *American Journal of Psychiatry, 2*, 201–207.

Kennedy, C., & Yellowlees, P. (2000). The effectiveness of telepsychiatry measured using the Health of the Nation Outcome Scale and the Mental Health Inventory. *Journal of Telemedicine and Telecare, 9*(1), 12–16.

Liss, H. J., Glueckauf, R. L., & Ecklund-Johnson, E. P. (2002). Research on telehealth and chronic medical conditions: Critical review, key issues, and future directions. *Rehabilitation-Psychology, 47*(1), 8–30.

Monnier, J., Knapp, R. G., & Frueh, B. C. (2003). Recent advances in telepsychiatry: An updated review. *Psychiatric Services, 54*(12), 1604–1609.

New Freedom Commission on Mental Health. Achieving the promise: Transforming mental health care in America. Final Report. DHHS Pub. No. SMA-03-3832. Rockville, MD: 2003.

NIMH. (2003). Internet-based research interventions in mental health: How are they working? Website: *http://www.nimh.nih.gov/research/interventionsJuly03.cfm.*

Schopp, L., Johnstone, B., & Merrell, D. (2000). Telehealth and neuropsychological assessment: New opportunities for psychologists. *Professional Psychology: Research and Practice, 31*, 179–183.

Stamm, B. H. (1998). Clinical applications of telehealth in mental health care. *Professional-Psychology: Research and Practice, 29*(6), 536–542.

Wootton, R. (2003). *Telepsychiatry and e-Mental Health.* London: Royal Society of Medicine Press.

Specialty Practices in Case Management

Life Care Planning and Case Management

Patricia McCollom

LEARNING OBJECTIVES

Upon completion of this chapter, the reader will be able to:

1. Define life care planning.
2. Define a life care plan.
3. Describe the role of the life care planner.
4. List the activities included in the life care planning process.
5. List three applications for use of a life care plan.
6. Discuss three phases of development of a life care plan.
7. Describe five categories of assessment in the life care planning process.
8. Compare four components of a life care plan with those of a case management plan.

IMPORTANT TERMS AND CONCEPTS

Accessible
Actionable Tort
Assessment
Clinical Practice Guidelines
Deposition

Efficacy of Care
Expert Witness
Exposure
Life Care Plan
Life Care Planner

| Life Care Planning | Medicare Secondary Payer (MSP) |
| Medicare Set Asides (MSA) | Outcome |

■ INTRODUCTION

A. Life care planning is a program recently established for the management of the care, resources, and services required by the catastrophically injured or the person suffering from a chronic condition.

B. Life care planning focuses on promoting the patient's independence and empowerment, as well as the enhancement of the quality of care to ensure a meaningful life for the chronically or catastrophically ill.

C. According to the International Academy of Life Care Planners (IALCP), life care planning is defined as an advanced and collaborative transdisciplinary practice that includes the patient, family, varied care providers, and other parties who are concerned in coordinating, accessing, evaluating, and monitoring the necessary services required for the care of a catastrophically injured or chronically ill client (IALCP, 2006a).

D. Life care planning is a transdisciplinary specialty practice. Each professional, including rehabilitation specialists, nurses, case managers, physicians, social workers, and other allied health personnel, involved in life care planning brings his or her expertise and specialization to the life care planning process and to the life care plan for the ultimate benefit of the patient.

E. The standards of practice for life care planning are developed based on the standards of practice of the individual disciplines that constitute the life care planning team such as nursing, medicine, case management, and rehabilitation.

F. IALCP is the professional organization responsible for the development, maintenance, and promotion of life care planning standards.

■ KEY DEFINITIONS

A. Accessible—A term used to denote buildings/environments that are barrier free, thus allowing all members of society safe entry and exit.

B. Actionable tort— A legal duty imposed by statute or otherwise, owing by a defendant to the person injured.

C. Assessment—The process of collecting in-depth information about a person's situation, family, and functioning to identify an individual's needs in order to develop a comprehensive life care plan. Information should be gathered from all relevant sources (patient, family, caregivers, employers, medical records, etc.).

D. Clinical practice guidelines—Systematically developed statements on medical or nursing practices that assist a practitioner in making decisions about appropriate diagnostic and therapeutic health care services. Practice guidelines are usually developed by authoritative professional societies and organizations.

E. Deposition—The testimony of an individual taken under oath, but not in open court, on the subject at hand, reduced to writing and authenticated, which may be used in court.

F. Efficacy of care—The potential, capacity, or capability to produce the desired outcome through evidence-based findings.

G. Expert witness—An expert qualified to provide court testimony by virtue of knowledge, skill, experience, training, or education.

H. Exposure—The amount of money for goods, care, and services an insurance company owes, when there is liability for the injured/ill person.

I. Life care plan—A dynamic document based on published standards of practice, comprehensive assessment, research, and data analysis, which provides an organized, concise plan for current and future needs, with associated costs, for individuals who have experienced catastrophic injury or have chronic health care needs.

J. Life care planner—A health care professional specifically educated regarding the methodology for life care planning. Professionals engaged in this specialty practice may be nurses, vocational rehabilitation counselors, rehabilitation psychologists, physicians, occupational therapists, social workers, physical therapists, and speech/language pathologists.

K. Outcome—The result and consequence of a health care process. In life care planning, an outcome is used to describe the result of the expected care or services.

■ AIMS OF LIFE CARE PLANNING

A. The aims of life care planning are similar to those of case management and may include the following:
   1. Assist patients in achieving optimal health outcomes
   2. Provide health education to patients and other interested parties
   3. Ensure the appropriate allocation of resources and timely access to necessary and specialty services. This may include the development of alternate care plans.
   4. Communicate accurate and timely cost information for ease of utilization by patients and the life care planning team
   5. Develop measurement tools for the evaluation of outcomes
   6. Ensure that all parties involved, including the patient/family and health care professionals, are well aware of the life care plan, including the goals and expected outcomes
   7. Provide care and services that are cost effective and produce the best possible outcomes
   8. Promote teamwork and collaboration among the varied health care providers involved in the care of the patient; external parties such as employers, lawyers, and community agencies; and insurers or payers.

■ THE PROCESS OF LIFE CARE PLANNING

A. The life care planning process is similar to that of case management. It includes the following activities (IALCP, 2006b):

1. Assessment—Collection and analysis of data about the patient's health condition, injury, finances, and social network.

2. Life care plan development and research—Determination of the content of the life care plan and researching the associated potential cost.

3. Data analysis—Deciding on the patient's care needs and ensuring that the recommended care activities are consistent with national standards.

4. Planning—Organizing the data and content of the life care plan. It also involves the creation of reports including cost projections.

5. Collaboration—Developing effective relationships with other professionals and sharing relevant information with the team to formulate care recommendation.

6. Facilitation—Expediting care and resolving disagreements.

7. Evaluation—Reviewing and revising the life care plan, monitoring use of resources, and ensuring completeness and consistency with standards.

8. Testimony—Participation in legal matters, such as expert sworn testimony, or acting as a consultant to legal proceedings related to determining care needs and costs.

■ ROLE OF THE CASE MANAGER AS A LIFE CARE PLANNER

A. The case managers in a life care planning program are called *life care planners*. They use tools such as the life care plan to provide individualized and comprehensive life care services. In their roles, they project current and future long-term care needs that are congruent with the level of disability evident in the condition of the catastrophically injured or chronically ill individual.

B. Life care planners must possess appropriate educational and licensure requirements and knowledge as defined by their profession and its associated standards and scope of practice.

C. Life care planners must have a foundation of knowledge and appropriate experience in a specialty such as rehabilitation or nursing. According to IALCP (2006b), they:

1. Possess specialized knowledge and skills in researching and critically analyzing health care data and resources

2. Manage and interpret large volumes of information related to the care of an individual patient

3. Work autonomously

4. Attend to details and communicate effectively (both written and verbal communication)

5. Develop positive relationships and partnerships with patients and other health care professionals

6. Create and use networks for gathering necessary information

7. Participate in professional, community, and national organizations
8. Demonstrate professional demeanor

■ THE LIFE CARE PLAN

A. The term *life care plan* was introduced into the health care literature in 1981 by Paul Deutsch and Fred Raffa in a legal publication entitled *Damages in Tort Action*. The publication described how damages could be identified in civil litigation.

B. In 1987, the life care plan was introduced into the field of rehabilitation in *Guide to Rehabilitation* (Deutsch and Sawyer, 1987). The life care plan was identified as part of a rehabilitation evaluation to project the impact of catastrophic injury on an individual's future and was differentiated from a *discharge* plan by its specification of costs for long-term services to meet the needs of the catastrophically injured patient.

C. Communicated in 2000 and revised in 2006, the IALCP published the following definition of the life care plan: *"A life care plan is a dynamic document based upon published standards of practice, comprehensive assessment, research and data analysis, which provides an organized, concise plan for current and future needs with associated costs, for individuals who have experienced catastrophic injury or have chronic health care needs"* (2006b).

D. The life care plan has been utilized in a variety of health care settings, including the legal and ethical domains, to provide information regarding the cost of services needed for the catastrophic and long-term care of an individual. Life care plans focus mainly on rehabilitation planning, services implementation, management of health care costs and funds, transitional/discharge planning, and patient and family education (IALCP, 2006b).

E. An example of a life care plan is shown in Table 17-1.

F. A life care plan is also used as a tool in the administration and litigation of catastrophic injury claims of persons who have long-term health care needs related to a chronic illness. In this case it:
   1. Provides a comprehensive assessment of the current and future medical and rehabilitative needs of a person over his or her lifetime; and
   2. Is used to determine the long-term financial exposure to a carrier or to help evaluate a claim for settlement value.

G. Characteristics that differentiate life care plans from other plans of care are:
   1. Life care plans are projections for *needs* into the future, rather than planned *actions* related to an acute health/illness episode, and describe the specific current need for intervention.
   2. Life care plans include recommendations supported by the literature, research, and clinical practice guidelines, that meet legal requirement and court imposed parameters.
   3. Life care plans are preventive in their approach, relating recommendations to prevention of high cost complications, high cost equipment, replacement costs, and uncontrolled, unmanaged purchases.

4. Life care plans delineate options for maintaining care and needed goods and services within a managed care environment and within a realistic framework for individual needs, family structure and dynamics, and geographic location.

5. Life care plans demonstrate researched costs for care, equipment, supplies, and services, as well as alternate resources to meet individual needs.

H. Benefits of a life care plan may include the following:

1. The life care plan is a tool for case management.

2. It may be used to educate patients and families regarding the need for and outcomes of ongoing monitoring and care.

3. The plan may be used to collaborate among health care providers when providing case managements services in complex cases.

TABLE 17–1

Example of a Life Care Plan for Mr. X, a Patient With a Severe Spinal Cord Injury

CONCLUSION #1: Due to health status, Mr. X will require various medications throughout his life, as prescribed by his treating physicians.*

Current Prescription	Frequency	Outcome	Current Cost**	Comments	Resource/ Reference
Levaquin	250 mg daily	Urinary tract infection controlled/ resolved	$263.95/30 tablets $1,583.70/ year (Anticipate 6 prescriptions per year)	This was a current prescription, 12/2007.	3, 7

NOTE: All the other medications will be listed in the life care plan, including information similar to that described for Levaquin.

---

*Mr. X is a construction worker who sustained a spinal cord injury while on the job after a fall from the roof of a building. Mr. X's treating physician prescribed him multiple medications for anticoagulation prophylaxis, diabetes, hypertension, and perlipidemia. It is reasonable to anticipate that, with appropriate rehabilitation intervention, additional medications relating to improved health with spinal cord injury will be prescribed.

**Costs are based on rates at the time this chapter was written. They vary based on insurance agency, state of patient's residency, and cost of living.

NOTE: This life care plan is neither thorough nor comprehensive. It includes three conclusions as examples for clarification purposes. Ideally, the life care plan addresses all conclusion/problems as well as presents a summary of the patient's medical history, the acute or sub acute treatment and progression prior to the involvement of the life care planner, and a report on the injury if applicable.

TABLE 17–1

Example of a Life Care Plan for Mr. X, a Patient With a Severe Spinal Cord Injury (*continued*)

CONCLUSION #2: Due to functional limitations associated with injury, Mr. X requires specific durable medical equipment to maintain his health, functioning, and safety for the remainder of his life.

Care/Need	Frequency	Outcome	Current Cost	Comments	Resource/ Reference
Manual light-weight wheelchair	Current pre-scription; replace every 5–7 years	Mobility through-out the home and commu-nity	$2,895–$3,400	Currently uses this prescribed equipment	1, 2, 3, 9, 13
Wheelchair mainte-nance	Annual, beginning 2006	Prolong function-ing of equipment	$350	Annual cost of manual chair main-tenance, beginning one year after pur-chase	10, 13
Tire replace-ment (manual chair)	Minimum annual, beginning 2006	Mobility	$42 each	4 tires must be replaced	10, 12
Inner tubes (manual chair)	Minimum annual, beginning 2006	Mobility	$12 each	4 inner tubes must be replaced, depending on tire pre-scribed	10, 12
Jay II low-pressure cushion	Replace every 2–4 years, after wheel-chair pur-chase	Prevent skin break-down	$294–$350	Currently uses a Roho and has had skin break-down	2, 8, 10, 11
Cushion covers	Replace annually		$75/cover (2 covers needed)	Cushion cov-ers are additional cost, but are neces-sary due to inconti-nence.	2, 8, 10, 12

(*continued*)

TABLE 17–1

Example of a Life Care Plan for Mr. X, a Patient With a Severe Spinal Cord Injury (*continued*)

CONCLUSION #2: Due to functional limitations associated with injury, Mr. X requires specific durable medical equipment to maintain his health, functioning, and safety for the remainder of his life.

Care/Need	Frequency	Outcome	Current Cost	Comments	Resource/ Reference
Power wheel-chair	Purchase once at age 60	Mobility throughout the community	$12,000–$15,000 $350–$500 (annual mainte-nance)	Due to endurance and a shoul-der injury, a power chair is anticipated.	1, 2, 5, 9, 10
Hand-held shower	Replace every 10 years	Ease in personal hygiene	$28.40	Bathroom must be accessible.	1, 9
Shower chair	Replace every 7–10 years	Ease in personal hygiene	$695–$972 (list price)	This item can only be used with an accessible bathroom.	1, 11
Reacher	Replace annually	Independent retrieval of items	$57	This item would pro-mote inde-pendence.	6, 11
Sliding board	Replace annually	Ease in transfers	$49	Current prescription	1, 3, 11
Standing frame	Daily use; one time purchase	Promote circulation, cardiac/respiratory/renal function	$2,075	Not able to use in cur-rent resi-dence.	1, 6, 11

CONCLUSION #3: Due to medical diagnosis of a spinal cord injury, Mr. X will require specific medical supplies to maintain health, functioning, and well-being.

Care/Need	Frequency	Outcome	Current Cost	Comments	Resource/ Reference
Intermittent catheter	8 times daily	Bladder drainage	$29/30 catheters $348/year	Currently uses this item. Note: At assessment he stated self-catheteriza-tion 4–5 times daily; 12/21/05, he stated "every two hours."	3, 11

TABLE 17–1

Example of a Life Care Plan for Mr. X, a Patient With a Severe
Spinal Cord Injury (*continued*)

CONCLUSION #3: Due to medical diagnosis of a spinal cord injury, Mr. X will require
specific medical supplies to maintain health, functioning, and well-being.

Care/Need	Frequency	Outcome	Current Cost	Comments	Resource/ Reference
Lubricating jelly	One tube per month	Ease in catheteri-zation and bowel pro-gram	$14/each $168/year	Currently uses this item	3, 11
Bed drainage collection bag	Once per week	Urine collec-tion	$91/20 $273/year	Currently uses this item	3, 11
Chux	Daily	Bed protec-tion	$37/200 $135/year	Currently uses this item	3, 11
Depend	Daily 3–4	Clothing pro-tection from incon-tinence	$13.79/16 $1,101/year	Currently uses this item	3, 7

4. The life care plan offers a mechanism to serve as an information management tool for the complex information generated in catastrophic
   cases or individuals with chronic illness.
5. The life care plan specifies long-term medical, psychological, rehabilitation, and quality needs for the individual's life.

I. Applications for a life care plan are multiple. The life care plan is a preventive plan used for:
   1. Disability management
   2. Elder care management
   3. Discharge planning from health care facilities
   4. Long-term care for children or adults with disabilities

J. A life care plan may be used in litigation to:
   1. Establish long-term needs
   2. Specify costs

K. A life care plan may be used in insurance settings to:
   1. Determine cost exposure
   2. Identify a profile for long-term needs

L. Life care plans include specific information. They must be consistent
   with the clinical needs of the individual. The life care plan must:
   1. Reflect risk factors for complications that may lead to higher costs
   2. Include the quality-of-life needs
   3. Identify the impact of aging on needs

■ DEVELOPMENT OF THE LIFE CARE PLAN

A. Health care professionals in various disciplines may prepare the life care plans. Case managers may prepare the life care plans due to their role in referral, purchase of goods and services, knowledge of psychosocial status, health plans and other insurance carriers, and local resources.

B. Professionals involved in life care planning must have a thorough understanding of the diagnoses, treatment protocols, factors affecting the diagnoses, psychological implications, rehabilitation relating to disability, psychosocial implications, family dynamics, and reimbursement structures and methods.

C. Professionals involved in life care planning must have knowledge of available community resources.

D. Professionals involved in life care planning must be creative in the development of alternative plans and in maintaining fiscal accountability to meet the patient's and family's needs.

E. Professionals involved in life care planning must develop a life care plan that integrates available resources and is preventive, rehabilitative, and curative, if possible, for the individual with catastrophic injury and/or long-term health care needs.

F. Review of records is an initial activity in the development of the life care plan:

1. *Medical records,* both pre- and post-injury or illness, to provide background in diagnosing and treating, and to identify the expected outcomes of care for the individual

2. *School records* to clarify the individual's cognitive and social abilities and behaviors. These may be especially helpful in working with a child or a teenager.

3. *Military records* may define work tasks assigned, performance, and physical capabilities.

4. *Depositions,* if available or appropriate to the case, to provide insight into the patient and family understanding of their situation and perception of their condition and needs.

G. An assessment interview with the patient and family must also be completed so that the life care plan is comprehensive, individualized, and specific to the patient and family needs.

1. If the patient is nonverbal, assessment and observation periods of care and outcomes are critical to accurate understanding of his or her needs.

2. Care providers and/or family members must be included in the interview to clarify needs, define roles and role reversals, and identify stresses and their reasons.

3. Data gathering for the development of the life care plan is necessary and must be comprehensive. It is categorized as follows:

a. History of injury and health, including past medical history and consumption of medications

b. Complications

   c. Current diagnoses
      i. Patient understanding of the diagnoses
     ii. Family understanding of the diagnoses
   d. Treatment plan
      i. Current care
     ii. Future potential care
    iii. Patient and family understanding of the treatment plan
   e. Current status
   f. Functional skills and abilities
      i. Self-care
     ii. Communication
    iii. Cognition
    iv. Behavior
     v. Mobility and physical functioning
    vi. Safety
   vii. Community reintegration
  viii. Household management and safe environment
   g. Risk factors
      i. Psychosocial dynamics
     ii. Health condition–related
    iii. Financial/insurance-related
   h. Psychosocial impact
      i. Viability of the family unit
     ii. Family of choice involvement
   i. Education
      i. Formal/degree(s) held
     ii. Military
    iii. Experiential
   j. Vocational background
      i. Financial status
     ii. Social Security benefits obtained
    iii. Eligibility for Medicaid or Medicare benefits
    iv. Current or previous health insurance plan if any
   k. Medications
      i. Confirm knowledge of why prescribed, schedule of medications intake
     ii. Confirm knowledge of side effects
    iii. Confirm knowledge of proper medications administration and adherence
   l. Medical supplies
  m. Durable medical equipment
   n. Adaptive equipment

o. Accessibility needs

p. Home care/facility care

q. Personal care attendant

4. Observations made during assessments may include the patient's mood, willingness to respond, patient's and family's behavior, voice characteristics, and manner.

H. Collaboration with a treatment team when possible helps to determine projected treatment, actual or potential needs, frequency of care or services, and the probability of future therapeutic or diagnostic interventions.

I. A life care planner/physician team may assess a patient for the collaborative development of the life care plan.

J. Clinical practice guidelines and other types of literature may serve to supplement medical records when a treatment team is not immediately accessible.

K. Community resources and geographically accessible services may be identified through collaboration with community-based programs.

L. Data analysis must be completed to develop recommendations for long-term needs.

1. The life care planner must analyze all the data collected through the assessment and monitoring of the patient's condition, interactions with the patient's family, and collaboration with the treatment team.

2. The life care planner must use the results of the analysis in the development of the treatment plan or life care plan, which includes goals, priorities, and expected outcomes.

3. The life care planner must have a strong clinical knowledge base as well as ability to collect and analyze relevant data to provide for accurate projections of the patient's needs.

4. Data analysis produces a clear presentation of the patient's needs, the necessary goods and services, and the outcomes of implementation of the recommendations.

M. Research in life care planning improves patient care outcomes and allows the provision of quality health care services and treatments.

1. Recommendations for management of the patient's condition as included in the life care plan must be supported by the evidence-based literature, clinical practice guidelines, and/or physician recommendation.

2. Cost research for the purpose of cost effectiveness may be completed by the life care planner through contacting other care providers and health care agencies, bill review, or search of computer databases for durable medical equipment or supplies.

3. Current published data on length of stay, frequency of complications or services, and outcomes of care may be used as adjunct research.

■ COMPONENTS OF THE LIFE CARE PLAN

A. The life care plan should initially specify the records reviewed as a foundation for the plan.

1. A brief summary of the patient's history and injury/illness identifies diagnostics and treatment.
2. Current status defines the patient's ability to participate in routine life activities, functional skills, medications, activities of daily living, complications, and perception of status.
3. The family status should also be addressed, as well as family stressors.

B. Projections within the life care plan are important.

1. Projected medical care identifies both periodic and episodic care activities, both diagnostic and therapeutic, that may be necessary and consistent with the patient's and family's needs and interests.
2. Projected interventions specify necessary treatment or services that are designed to maintain or improve the patient's status, prevent complications, or minimize risk factors.

C. Diagnostic testing may relate to monitoring the patient's condition medically, psychologically, socially, and cognitively. These may include neuropsychological evaluation or vocational assessment.

D. Durable medical equipment and maintenance address mobility needs, physical functioning, community reintegration, and socialization.

E. Supplies are identified to meet individual needs to maintain health.

F. Adaptive equipment promotes independence and well-being. Certain equipment may be essential to enhance the patient's ability to be socially interactive.

G. Medications that are currently prescribed and risks for additional medication use may be noted.

H. Home care or facility care must be included, noting the impact and ability of the family to be involved in care.

I. Transportation needs must also be included. The plan, in this way, provides for the patient's accessibility to the community, medical care and services, recreation, and vocational needs.

J. Accessibility issues and the barrier-free environmental needs of the patient must be noted within the life care plan. Types of necessary home furnishings and accessories may be specified.

K. Vocational needs and services must be addressed, as appropriate, within the plan. Community resources for evaluation, training, and job placement should also be included.

L. Health maintenance services such as counseling, recreation, occupational therapy, and community involvement should be defined within the life care plan.

■ MEDICARE SET ASIDES: A LIFE CARE PLANNING SPECIALTY

A. Medicare Set Asides (MSA) has been mandatory for workers' compensation claims since 2001. It requires documentation that shows the amount of dollars that must be "set aside" for a worker's compensation liability case. These set-aside funds are used for coverage of future medical expenses.

B. An MSA is a document that specifies future injury-related care needs and associated costs. Only Medicare-covered expenses are identified in this document and include:

1. Costs based upon Medicare payments within the beneficiary's state of jurisdiction.
2. Part of a settlement award "set-aside" to pay for future costs that Medicare would have paid.

C. MSA was legislated to protect Medicare from being placed in a role as the primary payer, when it should be in the role as secondary payer and when the primary payer should be the responsibility of another entity.

1. The Medicare Secondary Payer (MSP) statute was created in 1980, to ensure that other insurance carriers covering the individual for payment of medical expenses would be primary payers.
2. The statute was created to prevent shifting of the burden of future expenses for injury-related care from workers' compensation insurance companies or others with responsibility for payment to Medicare.
   a. An MSA considers Medicare's interest when agreement is reached for the future medical needs of the injured individual.
   b. The Center for Medicare and Medicaid Services (CMS) is to be contacted if a workers' compensation claim is going to settlement.
   c. The arrangement for a MSA document is necessary when there is an expectation of enrollment within 30 months of a settlement date on a claim.
   d. The arrangement for a MSA document is necessary when there is anticipation of a greater than $250,000 settlement.

D. Development of an MSA

1. Review of records, which may include the following:
   a. Medical
   b. Billing records
2. Verify eligibility for benefits
   a. Social Security
   b. Medicare
3. Secure a rated age
4. Obtain medical recommendation for ongoing care
   a. Research applicable standards of care
   b. Research clinical practice guidelines
   c. Research evidence-based literature and health outcomes
5. Research a Medicare lien

6. Identify future medical needs
   a. Medicare-covered goods and services
   b. Medicare costs specific to the individual's geographic region

E. Consequences for noncompliance with the statute
   1. Denial of payment for future medical care
   2. Medicare may designate its own allocation
   3. Lawsuit filed against the injured individual, attorney, and/or the insurance carrier

F. The life care planners/case managers may be best to assume responsibility for MSA.
   1. They analyze services rendered compared to the patient's medical diagnosis eliminating any unnecessary costs associated with a claim. By compiling, analyzing, and summarizing extensive amounts of medical data, case managers are able to reduce the amount of time and money spent preparing for the application process of an MSA.
   2. They provide a standardized, objective, organized, and concise projection of current and long-term medical and nonmedical needs, and associated costs for individuals who have experienced catastrophic injury or significant chronic or long-term medical impairment.
   3. They ensure that the MSA includes a complete file review, execution of appropriate medical releases, projection of future medical needs, and submission and tracking of the MSA to the appropriate CMS regional office.
   4. They ensure that the MSA also provides a complete and accurate picture of Medicare's expected future medical exposure, by utilizing Medicare's current reimbursement guidelines in determining eligibility and coverage for future medical treatment.

REFERENCES

Deutsch, P., and Sawyer, H. (1987). Guide to rehabilitation. New York, NY: Matthew Bender and Co., Inc.

International Academy of Life Care Planners (IALCP). (2006a). Scope of practice. Website: *www.internationalacademyoflifecareplanners.com/Default.htm*. Retrieved on March 7, 2006.

International Academy of Life Care Planners (IALCP). (2006b). *Standards of practice for life care planners*. Santa Cruse, CA: Author.

Isom, R., & Marini, I. (2002). An educational curriculum for teaching life care planning. *Journal of Life Care Planning, 1*(4), 239–264.

Kendall, S., & Deutsch, P. (2002). Research methodology for life care planners. *Journal of Life Care Planning, 1*(2), 157–168.

Manley, B. (2003). Workers' compensation settlements with Medicare set-aside arrangements: Problem solving the issues. *Journal of Life Care Planning, 2*(1), 25–32.

McCollom, P., & Weed, R. (2002). Life care planning: Yesterday and today. *Journal of Life Care Planning, 1*(1), 3–7.

Weed, R. (Ed.). (2004). *Life care planning and case management handbook*. Boca Raton: CRC Press.

18

Workers' Compensation Case Management

Deborah V. DiBenedetto

LEARNING OBJECTIVES

Upon completion of this chapter, the reader will be able to:

1. Define terms and acronyms specific to workers' compensation case management.

2. Identify the primary purposes of workers' compensation as a social insurance program.

3. State the impact of workers' compensation laws on the provision of case management services.

4. Identify the need to adapt case management services to comply with state or federal statutory requirements.

5. Describe the market forces in the cost of workers' compensation programs that produced opportunities for skilled case management.

6. List the types of workers' compensation cases typically assigned for medical management and ways to successfully apply case management skills to them.

7. Understand the burden that medical, legal, and financial factors place on the practice of ethical, advocacy-based case management.

8. Identify current business trends that impact the delivery of workers' compensation case management.

IMPORTANT TERMS AND CONCEPTS

Disability Impairment Rating
Evidence-Based Medicine (EBM)
First Report of Injury (FROI)
Functional Ability Testing (FAT)
Functional Capability Examination
  (FCE)
Impairment Rating
Indemnity Payments
Independent Medical Evaluation (IME)
Maximum Medical Improvement (MMI)
Modified Duty
Modified Work
Partial Permanent Disability (PPD)
Partial Temporary Disability (PTD)

Repetitive Stress Injury and
  Cumulative Trauma Injuries
Reserves
Return to Work (RTW)
Scheduled Injury
Second Injury Fund (SIF)
Self-Insured
Social Insurance
Temporary Alternate Work (TAW)
Third-Party Administrator (TPA)
Total Permanent Disability (TPD)
Total Temporary Disability (TTD)
Transitional Work
Vocational Rehabilitation (VR)

■ INTRODUCTION

A. Skillful case management in the field of workers' compensation demands a knowledge and understanding of pertinent terms, practices, and parameters not usually taught in health care settings.

B. It is essential for the case manager practicing in the workers' compensation field of case management to be familiar with the terms used throughout the industry and how to apply them in practice.

C. Review of the history of workers' compensation programs in U.S. business leads to an understanding of today's health care delivery and workers' compensation systems.

D. The industrial revolution in America that began the transformation of the workforce from agrarian to industrial in the late 19th and early 20th centuries spawned the workers' compensation system that is taking us into the 21st century.

  1. Common-law practices held that an employer was responsible for injuries or death to his or her workers only if they were caused by a negligent act.

  2. The injured employees or their survivors had to bring suit to establish that there was negligence on the part of employers. This process was difficult and out of the reach for most employees or family members.

  3. Injured workers' financial and health needs were absorbed by their families or the communities around them.

E. As the workplace became larger and more mechanized, the risk to workers increased. Social reformers recognized the need for legislated

---

NOTE: This chapter is a revised version of what was previously published in the first edition of *CMSA Core Curriculum for Case Management*. The contributor wishes to acknowledge Sharon Brim, as some of the timeless material was retained from the previous version.

standards to protect individual workers and the community as a whole.

F. The first laws passed in the various states merely replaced common law with enacted laws, but the burden remained on the injured worker to prove employer responsibility.

G. In 1911, the first state workers' compensation laws were enacted that established a no-fault system to deal with work-related injuries.

H. Today, all 50 states and several U.S. territories have workers' compensation laws. Federal legislation has been enacted to cover federal workers in several different programs.

■ KEY DEFINITIONS

A. First report of injury (FROI)—This is a formal document completed by the employer—a report of a work-related injury or condition—that begins the process of a workers' compensation claim. The report is filed with the appropriate state jurisdiction and sent to the workers' compensation carrier or third-party administrator (claims handlers for self-insured employers). Workers' compensation systems allow injured workers or their designee to file a report of injury directly with the relevant state or federal workers' compensation board or industrial commission.

B. Functional capacity examination (FCE)—A systematic, objective process of assessing an individual's physical capacities and functional ability to execute tasks (e.g., sedentary, light, medium tasks). The FCE matches human performance levels to the demands of a specific job, work activity, or occupation. The FCE is often used in determining a person's potential for job placement, accommodation, and/or return to work after an injury.

C. Impairment rating—The basis for determining the medical outcome of a workers' compensation claim. Many states require an impairment rating to be based on the findings of a licensed physician using an impairment rating system such as the current issue of the American Medical Association's *Guides to the Evaluation of Permanent Impairment*. The final decision on a disability rating rests with the state or federal workers' compensation board or industrial commission.

D. Indemnity payments—Monies paid as wage replacement when the injured worker is determined to be medically unfit to work. Indemnity payments are based on the worker's usual wage, factored by a formula set by the state that has jurisdiction for the claim.

E. Maximum medical improvement (MMI), maximum medical recovery (MMR)—Terms used to indicate that the injured worker has recovered from injuries to a level at which a physician states that further treatment will not substantively change the medical outcome. If the injured worker has a medically substantiated permanent change to pre-injury health and function, an impairment rating may be done.

F. Permanent partial disability—The designation used to indicate that there is a presumptive or actual decrease in wage-earning capacity due to injury. A benefit is paid according to the severity of impairment in a formula derived by the state. Most states have *scheduled* injuries (benefit paid by a formula based on loss of, or loss of the use of, specific body members) and *nonscheduled* injuries (a benefit is based on the percentage of impairment in a formula computed by the state).

G. Permanent total disability—This evaluation is based on a medical assertion that the injured worker is precluded by the extent of his or her disability from gainful employment. Each state has guidelines on which this designation and subsequent benefits are paid (U.S. Chamber of Commerce, 2005).

H. Reasonable accommodation—Any change in the work environment or in the way a job is performed that enables a person with a disability to enjoy equal employment opportunities. There are three categories of reasonable accommodations—changes to a job application process, changes to the work environment or to the way a job is usually done, or changes that enable an employee with a disability to enjoy equal benefits and privileges of employment (such as access to training).

I. Reserves—The sum of money the insurance company or self-insured funds set aside to pay all costs associated with a claim.

J. Social insurance—Insurance that employers must provide or pay premiums as mandated by law. Social insurance programs include: unemployment insurance, state disability insurance (mandated by NY, NJ, RI, HI, CA, and the commonwealth of Puerto Rico), social security, Medicare, and workers' compensation.

K. Temporary partial disability—Status in which impairment prevents an injured worker from returning to his or her usual job, but the worker can be employed in some capacity. A benefit is paid when the restrictions to work activity result in a decrease of usual wages.

L. Temporary total disability—Status in which indemnity is paid when an injured worker is unable to work in any capacity while treatment continues, with the expectation of recovery and return to employment. In most states, the injured worker receives benefits for the entire time he or she is medically deemed to be unable to work.

M. Vocational rehabilitation—Cost-effective case management services provided by a skilled (preferably certified as a vocational rehabilitation professional or counselor) who is knowledgeable about the implications of medical status/functional ability and vocational services necessary to facilitate an injured workers' expedient return to gainful employment.

■ PRIMARY GOALS OF WORKERS' COMPENSATION PROGRAMS (DIBENEDETTO, 2006)

A. Provide injured workers prompt medical care and wage replacement for the workers, their dependents, or their survivors regardless of responsibility for the injuries

B. Establish a single, primary remedy for workplace injuries to decrease the legal costs and relieve the judicial system of heavy caseloads of personal injury cases

C. Relieve both the public and private sectors from demands on financial and medical services

D. Provide a system for the delivery of workers' compensation benefits and services

E. Promote workplace safety and accident prevention

F. It is imperative to remember that the injuries or illnesses covered under the relevant workers' compensation statute must "arise out of and in the course of employment."

■ UNDERSTANDING THE IMPACT OF WORKERS' COMPENSATION COSTS

A. Workers' compensation is a social insurance program, mandated by law.

B. In 2000, workers' compensation programs covered 126.5 million workers (NASI, 2002).
   1. All states, except Texas, mandate workers' compensation coverage for most private employers.
   2. In Texas, coverage is voluntary, but employers not providing coverage are not protected against injured workers' tort suits.
   3. An employee not covered by workers' compensation insurance is allowed to file suit claiming the employer is liable for his or her work-related injury or illness.

C. Employers are experiencing double-digit inflation with respect to group health care benefits, averaging a 43% increase in 2001 (DiBenedetto, 2002).

D. Smaller employers are also experiencing higher premiums with limited capacity to absorb the costs of medical care. Workers' compensation is also affected by the increase in the delivery of medical care.
   1. Medical care delivered in an unmanaged environment can be up to 2.5 times more costly than caring for the same injury (sustained "off-the-job") under a group health or non-WC plan.
   2. On average, 24% of work-related injuries result in lost time, for an average cost of $19,000 per claim; in a managed care environment, the same claim costs, on average, $13,500.
   3. For employers who channel employees to a managed care environment or preferred provider network, significant cost savings are realized.

E. Workers' compensation medical costs can range from 40% to 60% of a state's workers' compensation experience. This variance can be attributable to factors such as:
   1. Industry mix in each state,
   2. Compensability laws,
   3. Indemnity payments required, and
   4. Use of managed care arrangements (NASI, 2002).

F. Workers' compensation program costs are born by the employer if they "self-fund" or "self-insure" their workers' compensation program, or through purchased insurance policies, all of which must meet state requirements for these types of programs/insurance.

G. Workers' compensation programs for state and federal employees are publicly supported.

H. The cost of workers' compensation insurance and all costs associated with workplace injuries are reflected in the price of goods and services sold by the employer.

I. Besides the direct cost of buying insurance premiums, workers' compensation medical care, and indemnity payments, there are other indirect costs associated with these programs that are included in the total cost of occupational disability:
   1. Accident investigation;
   2. Worker replacement and resultant overtime;
   3. Lost productivity; and
   4. Claim administration (DiBenedetto, 2006).

J. The cost of buying workers' compensation insurance is based on a formula of previous claims, types of workers insured (e.g., clerical personnel have less risk of injury than do truck drivers), and an element calculated by the state based on annual costs (US Chamber of Commerce, 2006).

K. The only factor that can be effectively modified by the employer is the cost associated with the number and severity of workplace injuries.

L. Workers' compensation insurance carriers and self-insured employers have a stake in decreasing costs of claims submitted to them. A competitive marketplace demands that companies sell their products at the lowest possible price; this provides the foundation for managing the cost of risk, and, ultimately, the cost of workers' compensation claims and experience.

M. Many strategies are employed in keeping claims costs low, including loss control, risk management, safety and health programs, and managed care arrangements, including, but not limited to medical case management (see Box 18-1).

■ FITTING THE PIECES TOGETHER: MEDICAL CASE MANAGEMENT IN THE WORKERS' COMPENSATION SYSTEM

A. Medical management processes have been involved in the periphery of workers' compensation programs for a number of years, both medically and vocationally.

B. Societal changes and escalating medical costs have placed a larger burden on employers required to provide workers' compensation coverage for their employees.

C. Case management strategies, as a component of managed care arrangements (see Box 18-1) are used as tools to lower medical costs, improve communication, promote best medical and claim outcomes, and maintain a stable workforce.

BOX 18–1

Characteristics of Managed Care Arrangements in Workers' Compensation

- Use of preferred providers, physician panels, or networks specializing in occupational disability/workers' compensation
- Negotiated fee schedules or, less often, capitated rates for medical care provided
- Evidence-based or state-mandated medical treatment protocols
- Evidence-based disability duration guidelines
- Medical case management
- Aggressive, facilitated, and early RTW
- Quality assurance
- Utilization and medical bill review

Note. DiBenedetto, D. V. (2006) *Principles of workers' compensation and disability case management.* Battle Creek, MI: DVD Associates LLC. Adapted with permission.

D. Case managers working in the workers' compensation field encounter a greater number of stakeholders than in other areas (see Box 18-2).

E. A workers' compensation claim can be a complicated, often protracted process in which case managers can become involved at any time.
   1. The longer the time it takes to assign a case manager to a claim, the situation can mitigate progressive and positive claim and case outcomes.
   2. Case managers assist the injured worker, the provider, employer, carrier/third-party administrator (TPA) in understanding the impact of injury, disability, the workers' compensation system, medical care on health, and productivity, i.e., return to work (RTW).
   3. Case managers are primarily advocates for the injured worker, however, with competing issues and circumstances, the case manager will be an advocate for other stakeholders (such as the carrier/TPA, medical provider, employer, etc.).

F. Workers' compensation laws demand the case management process be adapted to work within that structure.

■ HISTORICAL APPLICATION OF MEDICAL CASE MANAGEMENT IN WORKERS' COMPENSATION

A. Claims processors have attempted to provide some degree of medical management for a number of years using various legal maneuvering to limit overuse of medical services and bring compensation claims to closure.

BOX 18–2
Key Stakeholders in Workers' Compensation

- Employee/injured worker
- Provider (medical, rehabilitation)
- Employer/supervisor
- Human resources/labor relations
- Insurance company/adjuster/TPA
- Family/significant others
- Union representative
- Occupational health case manager
- Vocational/rehabilitation specialist
- Case manager
- Social services/community supports
- Legal advisor/attorney
- Others

Note. DiBenedetto, D. V. (2006) *Principles of workers' compensation and disability case management.* Battle Creek, MI: DVD Associates LLC. Adapted with permission.

B. The services of medical professionals in the claims-handling process were usually limited to catastrophic accidents and other injuries that would severely limit an injured worker's prospects of returning to gainful employment.

C. In the decade between the mid-1980s and the mid-1990s, the costs of workers' compensation exploded in the American industry (Stoddard, Jans, Ripple, & Kraus, 1998).

1. The National Council of Compensation Insurance published data indicating that the nationwide cost of compensation claims was $69 billion, with about 45% of the cost in medical care.

2. Medical costs have tripled in workers' compensation in the early 1990s. Some of the reasons for the escalating medical costs are thought to be:

   a. Health care inflation

   b. Aging of the workforce

   c. Coverage expanding in repetitive-use injuries, stress, psychological injuries, and aggravation of usual diseases of life and coverage of occupational diseases

   d. Cost shifting from other areas of health care

   e. Lack of ability to impose medical utilization standards (Douglas, 1994)

D. Since the 1990s, states have moved toward the implementation of managed care arrangements (see Box 18-1) to address the rising cost of workers' compensation medical care and resultant lost time (DiBenedetto, 2006).

■ KEY STAKEHOLDERS IN WORKERS' COMPENSATION

A. Adapting usual case management techniques and practices to the workers' compensation field requires the practitioner to recognize the responsibilities of the various people and organizations with a role in mediating a work-related injury claim (see Box 18-2).

   1. Employer—Reports claim and monitors claim; may have a risk manager, human resources manager, occupational health, safety, or other representative to assist with managing or coordinating workers' compensation claims and employee RTW.
   2. Claims adjuster/claim examiner—Has the responsibility of investigating the claim, applying laws, and making the first determination about compensability, paying indemnity, paying medical bills, and directing case management. This is also called *adjudicating the claim*.
   3. Attorneys—The plaintiff if retained by the injured worker; the defense for insurance carrier and employer.
   4. Union representative—Can assist in protecting worker's rights and, depending upon negotiated agreements/labor contracts, may also have input regarding RTW, modified duty, or transitional work assignments.
   5. State administrative agency—Body at state level with jurisdiction over workers' compensation claims. These agencies may be called the Workers' Compensation Board, Industrial Commission, or another title.

B. Case managers are key professionals in maintaining open lines of communication among the stakeholders in the workers' compensation arena. The breakdown of these lines of communication may adversely impact the claim; protract worker disability; delay injured worker access to timely medical care; or delay recovery, return to function, and, ultimately, maximal medical improvement and return to pre-injury status (DiBenedetto, 2006).

■ WORKERS' COMPENSATION LAWS THAT DIRECTLY AFFECT CASE MANAGEMENT PRACTICE

A. Laws governing workers' compensation administration are enacted by each state and territorial legislature and administered by state agencies.

B. The U.S. Congress legislates development of regulations for federal workers and all other workers in the District of Columbia. Programs that are also overseen on the federal level include:

   1. Federal Employee's Compensation Act
   2. Federal Employment Liability Act (FELA)
   3. Merchant Marine Act (Jones Act)
   4. Longshore and Harbor Workers' Compensation Act (LHWCA)
   5. Black Lung Benefits Act

C. Laws are written and amended frequently. Because case managers must comply with the laws in order to practice legally and ethically, a source for learning about them is essential. Comprehensive compendia of state and federal laws can be found in:

1. Annual editions of *Analysis of Workers' Compensation Laws,* prepared and published by the U.S. Chamber of Commerce
2. U.S. Department of Labor Website: *www.dol.gov/dol/topic/workcomp*
3. Other Websites as listed at the end of this chapter

D. Each state has its own workers' compensation act. These may vary from one state to another; however, the main aspects of workers' compensation case management tend to be similar.

E. There are specific workers' compensation laws that govern individuals in certain industries such as railroad workers, longshoremen, and federal employees. Some of these laws may be specific to vocational benefits and entitlements of spouses, especially when the situation involves death.

F. The workers' compensation laws function as "no fault" laws and protect the employer from civil lawsuits. However, such laws may vary from one state to another.

G. Workers' compensation laws dealing with claims issues have only a peripheral impact on medical management. However, knowledge of laws creating the medical system has a direct effect on the case manager's ability to accomplish case management goals and objectives (Mullahy and Jensen, 2004).

H. Workers' compensation case managers have a responsibility to be familiar with applicable laws but must exercise caution to avoid the appearance of giving legal advice to key stakeholders, especially injured workers, providers, employers, and adjusters, among others.

I. Arguably the most challenging laws for workers' compensation medical managers are those that dictate the selection and use of health care providers. States may mandate the manner in which providers or medical services can be chosen (US Chamber of Commerce, 2006).

1. The initial choice of a health care provider can be made by:
   a. The injured worker without restriction
   b. The employer or insurance company by:
      i. Directly selecting a provider for the injured worker
      ii. Posting a panel of providers from which the injured worker selects
      iii. Belonging to a medical care organization (MCO) with preferred provider (PPO) lists from which the injured worker may choose
2. State laws also control changes of providers during the course of treatment. These guidelines for changes are quite complex in many states, and the claim handler can guide the case manager.*

---

*A listing of managed care and cost-containment strategies in workers' compensation can be accessed at *www.worklossdata.com.*

   3. State laws may also regulate the use of independent medical examinations (IMEs). These are evaluations generally arranged by the carrier or payer to confirm, rebut, or supplement medical findings offered by the injured worker's chosen physician or other provider.
      a. Regulations might limit the number of such examinations.
      b. There may be a specific time interval required between IMEs.
      c. State regulations can limit the type of practitioner who performs IMEs.
      d. Administrative agencies can require the payer and the injured worker to abide by the findings of specific physicians on a "designated provider" list.

J. State regulations pertaining to the use of health care services by injured workers often reflect efforts to contain medical costs. MCOs for workers' compensation health care providers are allowed or required in a few states.

K. Mandated managed care requirements are available from the state workers' compensation administrative agency (see listing of Websites at the end of this chapter for relevant state and federal links).

L. Guidelines for case managers working for or with an MCO vary by state.
   1. States that do not allow MCOs often have some mechanism for regulating cost-containment efforts by payers.
   2. Use of health care services can be regulated by: type of provider, number of visits, duration of visits, cost of treatment, utilization and peer review, and medical practice parameters.
   3. Precertification, preauthorization, or utilization review is generally required in some states for:
      a. Nonemergency surgery
      b. High-dollar durable medical equipment, diagnostic tests, costly or extensive therapies and procedures (such as MRIs, epidural injections, and work-reconditioning programs)
      c. Treatment for specific diagnoses (such as a second opinion for spinal surgery)
   4. Medical bill reviews and repricing services are allowed in most states. State regulations for utilization review and medical payments indicate whether re-pricing at so-called usual and customary rates (payments are based on a database reflecting standard charges for geographic area) or a fee schedule (published schedule of reimbursement allowed for charges for health care related to on-the-job injury) is allowed. The repricing is based on uniform databases.

M. States (such as CA) mandate the use of evidence-based medical (EBM) treatment protocols (or in FL, that providers be knowledgeable about relevant EBM guidelines) to direct the medical care of injured workers by their providers. The use of EBM tools reduces unnecessary medical care, facilitates positive medical outcomes, and ultimately saves costs.

N. Sources of EBM protocols for workers' compensation medical care includes:

1. American College of Occupational and Environmental Medicine's (ACOEM) *Occupational Medicine Practice Guidelines Evaluation* and *Management of Common Health Problems and Functional Recovery in Workers*, 2nd Edition (also referred to as the *ACOEM Guidelines*)
2. National Guideline Clearinghouse (www.guideline.gov)
3. Official Disability Guidelines (ODG) *Treatment in Workers' Compensation*, which has been accepted by the Federal Agency for Healthcare Research and Quality (AHRQ) for inclusion in the National Guidelines Clearinghouse

O. Almost all states and territories set up second-injury funds for injured workers to assist the injured worker and provide a financial offset for the employer. Conditions covered include:
1. Previously rated permanent impairment resulting from an on-the-job injury
2. Medical disability
3. Diseases that substantially impact recovery from a work-related injury (U.S. Chamber of Commerce, 2006)

P. Vocational rehabilitation as provided by workers' compensation regulations is sometimes coordinated concurrently with medical management.
1. Each state regulates the parameters concerning vocational rehabilitation for injured workers who are unable to return to previous employment.
2. A complete listing of state and territorial programs is available in the annual *United States Chamber of Commerce Analysis and the U.S. Department of Labor* (see end of chapter for list of Websites).

■ PRACTICING THE CASE MANAGEMENT PROCESS WITHIN THE WORKERS' COMPENSATION SYSTEM

A. The entire range of case management practices can be applied in a workers' compensation industry setting. The skills and knowledge described are among those identified as critical for case managers by Chan and colleagues (1999).

B. There are customary requirements for employment as a workers' compensation case manager.

C. The settings in which a case manager might practice these processes are varied.

D. The organization or facility paying for case management services often determines the scope and duration of the requested case management service(s).

E. The case management process as described in Chapter 9 and by many other authors, can be applied to the most frequently encountered workers' compensation claims.

■ MEDICAL CASE MANAGEMENT PROCESSES USED IN WORKERS' COMPENSATION

A. Case finding and targeting

1. "Lost time" or "indemnity" claims (cases in which the injured worker has not returned to work within the time frame that triggers wage replacement benefits) are far more likely to be referred for case management than "medical only" cases, implying the injury has not prevented the injured worker from working at his usual job.

B. Evaluating and assessing

1. Case managers in workers' compensation settings assess the injured workers' needs through claim file and medical record review; direct contact with the injured worker and his or her family, medical providers, employer, and others; and evaluation of current treatment plan and setting for that treatment.

2. Part of the assessment process in workers' compensation case management is to evaluate the extent of injuries, probable treatment plan, expectation of complete recovery, and estimated time out of work.

3. The assessment information is reported to the claims handler so that appropriate reserves can be set. Reserves are the sum of money the insurance company or self-insured funds set aside to pay all costs associated with a claim. This process is an important one for claims handling, and the case manager's assessment can be critical.

C. Planning, identifying, and solving problems

1. Case managers in workers' compensation have the special task of recognizing the problems that have resulted from an on-the-job injury or illness and their ramifications.

2. The payer will generally not address nonoccupational health concerns and/or social problems unless these have a direct impact on the injured worker's recovery from the occupational condition.

3. Workers' compensation laws actually proscribe offering benefits for nonrelated care and activity. Case managers can direct injured workers and their families to appropriate agencies and services.

4. Plans for addressing related problems are written and provided to appropriate parties.

D. Coordinating multiple health care providers

1. In the current workers' compensation atmosphere, there are likely to be a number of health care providers involved.

2. Recognition of state laws governing selection of care providers, including the use of MCOs, is essential.

3. Highly developed communication skills are involved in monitoring health care progress, making recommendations based on it, and then assisting the injured worker in receiving the most effective care available.

E. Utilization and peer review

1. Because workers' compensation laws regulate health care service selection and utilization, the case manager must practice these activities within that framework.

2. The workers' compensation system now contains utilization review (UR) companies and MCOs used by insurance companies, large

employers, and self-insureds. Case managers from these settings often have the responsibility of coordinating UR activities with the cost-containment companies.

3. UR, case management, and workers' compensation networks may seek and obtain URAC accreditation in these areas (see www.urac.org).

F. Precertification, preauthorization determinations

1. In the workers' compensation mosaic of state laws, preauthorization and precertification of procedures, services, and equipment can be mandatory, allowed, or forbidden. Therefore, it is necessary that the case manager be knowledgeable about the requirement in the state with jurisdiction for the claim.

2. MCOs and other cost-containment companies often have the responsibility for the processes in states with an allowance or requirement for them.

3. Because providers of health services and equipment are accustomed to securing preauthorization, a workers' compensation case manager is often requested to make decisions on authorization.

4. The basic premise in all of workers' compensation health care allowance is that payment will be made for services that are "reasonable and necessary" to treat work-related injuries.

   a. The case manager is often called on to evaluate the reasonableness and necessity of various health care providers' services and charges.

   b. This role may also be a source of ethical conflict for the medical case manager: balancing advocacy, cost, access, and the best solution for the injured worker.

G. Negotiation and contracting

1. The payment structure in workers' compensation in almost all states is based on a fee schedule or an acceptance of "usual and customary" costs listed in databases. The case manager must be aware of allowable charges before negotiating prices with health care providers or risk negotiating at higher costs.

2. Some services or equipment that are seen infrequently in dealing with injured workers are considered "off-record" and not on fee schedules or in databases. These items need to be negotiated on a case-by-case basis or through the use of PPOs.

3. When there is no statutory guidance for regulating charges and the selection of health care providers is strictly the injured worker's choice, there is often little incentive for the providers to negotiate for reduced cost or utilization.

4. Establishing a network of providers is part of most case managers' responsibilities, whether on a formal or informal basis. When provider selection is allowed by the payer, there is an increasing trend toward using established workers' compensation PPOs for both health care services and equipment. It is imperative that the MCO/network providers:

   a. Are familiar with the relevant state workers' compensation laws and requirements

      b. Facilitate maximal medical recovery of the injured worker with return to health and productivity/RTW (i.e., applying a "sports medicine model") in a timely manner

      c. Use EBM tools as proscribed by state law, and as a best practice in other jurisdictions

   5. Be familiar with established disability duration guidelines to benchmark expected RTW. Popular disability duration guidelines include:

      a. Official Disability Guidelines (ODG)

      b. The Medical Disability Advisor (MDA)

H. Reporting

   1. Most case management services in the workers' compensation field are performed at the request of the payer in the system (insurance company, TPA, employer), and reporting needs to be concise and clear.

   2. Reporting of all assessment, planning, intervention, and outcome activities documents the value of case management services in facilitating positive outcomes in workers' compensation such as moving the injured worker toward maximal medical improvement and timely return to function and productivity.

   3. All case management reports are part of legal records. In the workers' compensation arena, there is a likelihood that case management reports will appear in litigated cases.

   4. HIPAA[1] confidentiality requirements do not apply in workers' compensation, the evaluation of occupational injuries/illnesses, and other agency reporting or medical surveillance/evaluation (such as OSHA and the Department of Transportation [DOT]).

■ FREQUENTLY ENCOUNTERED REQUIREMENTS FOR WORKERS' COMPENSATION CASE MANAGERS

A. A degree or registration in a health care–related field with a strong clinical background

B. National case management certification (a number of certification programs are considered acceptable)

C. Background in emergency care, occupational health, rehabilitation, or orthopedics

D. Case managers in the workers' compensation arena do not function as lawyers, adjusters, or private investigators. They do not assume responsibility for claims-related activities such as investigation, surveillance, or determination of compensation. However, they are obligated to report acts of fraud.

E. Some states may have strict requirements for becoming a workers' compensation case manager, which may include additional licensure or certification in addition to national credentials.

---

[1]Detailed information on HIPAA and workers' compensation may be found at: *www.hhs.gov/ocr.*

■ MOST COMMON SETTINGS FOR WORKERS' COMPENSATION CASE MANAGERS

A. Insurance companies and workers' compensation carriers

B. TPAs

C. Risk management consulting companies

D. Independent case manager companies:
   1. National companies
   2. Small local companies
   3. Individual case managers

E. Employers
   1. Usually large companies with many employees
   2. May be part of an integrated disability management or total health management program
   3. Workers' compensation, disability case management, and other roles encompass the scope of occupational health nursing.

F. Providers
   1. Occupational medicine practices
   2. Orthopedic or other medical practices treating large numbers of workers' compensation injured workers
   3. Physical medicine and rehabilitation clinics and facilities

G. Government entities
   1. State and local government employees
   2. Large government institutions such as universities and hospitals
   3. State insurance funds
      a. State-funded workers' compensation programs that directly compete with insurance companies writing business within the state (e.g., in CA)
      b. Monopolistic state funds that write workers' compensation insurance exclusively in a state and do not allow competitive insurance (e.g., ND, NV, OH) (Douglas, 1994)
   4. Federal government
      a. Case management conducted through the U.S. Department of Labor
      b. Case managers are usually contracted independent practitioners.
      c. Program started in 1994

H. Managed care organizations (MCOs)

■ SCOPE OF MEDICAL MANAGEMENT IN WORKERS' COMPENSATION SETTINGS

A. Referrals for most case management services come from the payer (self-insured employer, carrier, or TPA); therefore, the payer generally decides the scope of services they are requesting or that may be required.
   1. Internal case managers are those working directly for the payer.

   2. External case managers are those, generally in independent case management companies, from whom the payer purchases case management services.
   3. Case managers with providers and MCOs derive their income from the payer.

B. At present, medical management services are being performed in three different ways:
   1. Telephonic case management (TCM)
      a. In workers' compensation, TCM is restricted to the three-point contact (injured worker, employer, and physician) via telephone calls, faxes, e-mail, other means of electronic communication, and traditional methods of correspondence, such as letters.
      b. TCM allows a case manager to oversee a high volume of open cases from a single location, making it a less costly way to apply medical management services.
      c. Effective TCM requires adequate computer software application designed for the purpose of monitoring medical procedures, physician appointments, therapy schedules, compliance, and the various complexities of workers' compensation medical management.
      d. Anecdotally, case management activities that are performed only through electronic communication are perceived to be less effective in achieving the same level of positive outcomes for injured workers as other forms of case management, but to date, no studies have been performed to verify it.
      e. Relying on TCM for catastrophic and serious workplace injures is of limited value.
      f. Case managers doing solely TCM must be knowledgeable in the case management process and skilled communicators in order to be effective managers and not merely observers and reporters.
   2. Onsite case management
      a. The "traditional" method of workers' compensation case management in which the injured worker is visited in his home setting for an initial assessment, a workplace visit is made, a job analysis is performed, and most physician appointments are attended by the case manager.
      b. Onsite case management performed by an external case manager adds to the cost of file handling.
      c. Internal case managers usually have too large a caseload to perform onsite case management effectively.
      d. Although onsite case management is thought to be effective in producing positive outcomes for injured workers, few studies directly address cost:benefit ratios (Akasbas, Gates, and Galvin, 1992).
      e. Case selection is an important component in measuring the benefit of onsite case management. In general, the more potentially expensive the claim might be, the more cost effective onsite case management can be.

3. Collaborative case management services are an amalgamation of telephonic and onsite activity. They combine techniques of both types of case management to offer appropriate services in the most cost-effective manner.

   a. Insurance carriers and large employers manage cases in this manner.

   b. The Office of Workers' Compensation for federal employees has been established with the Department of Labor's nursing staff coordinating case management activities with field nurses. Although other factors are involved, case costs have decreased dramatically as this program grows.

■ APPLYING THE CASE MANAGEMENT PROCESS

A. The duration and amount of workers' compensation benefits vary depending on the severity of the injured workers' disability.

1. Most workers' compensation cases do not progress to lost time past the initial waiting period. In some cases, only medical benefits are paid. These cases are referred to as *medical only* cases. Medical only cases represent a small amount of benefit payments because these injuries are often minor in nature and do not result in lost time from work.

2. For the period of 1996 to 1998, medical only cases accounted for 76% of reported workers' compensation cases and only 6.2% of benefits paid (NCCI, in NASI, 2002). Therefore, cases involving lost time and cash wage-replacement payments—24% of reported cases—accounted for 94% of benefits paid for cash and medical care combined.

3. The above example demonstrates the Pareto Analysis (also known as the *80/20 rule*) in that 80% of cases generate 20% of cost (medical only cases in this example), and that 20% of cases (lost time/indemnity cases) generate 80% of costs (DiBenedetto, 2006).

4. Most often, it is the lost time indemnity and "catastrophic" cases that are most frequently referred to medical case managers.

B. A workers' compensation claim can be prolonged and complex. A case management referral can occur at any time in that continuum, and the case management process needs to be adapted to meet the needs of the injured worker and the payer at that level. It behooves the payer/carrier/TPA to refer cases as soon as possible for effective case management outcomes.

C. Because relatively few categories of injury cases are referred for case management, the case management process can be modeled to describe the most common types.

1. Catastrophic and serious injury cases

   a. Catastrophic injuries include severe head injuries, spinal cord injuries, severe burns, limb amputation, multiple fractures, and major organ and tissue damage. These cases are the easiest to identify and are usually referred to case management services soon after notice of the injury is received.

    b. Each referral source might have a different definition of what kinds of injuries are deemed serious, such as potential high-dollar loss or potential for severe impairment.

    c. Goals for case management are to ensure high-quality, effective medical care for the injured worker while containing costs and attempting to limit impairment.

2. Case management process model—catastrophic and serious case

    a. Assessment

       i. Begin the assessment immediately after the referral is received. Discuss expectations for case management with the referral source.

      ii. Identify and contact the facility case manager or discharge planner and establish credentials and responsibility.

     iii. Determine the nature and extent of the injuries, current treatment plan, and prognosis.

     iv. Review the chart and all medical records available.

      v. Speak to physicians and other caregivers to understand the injured worker's current status.

     vi. Interview the injured worker and family members.

    vii. Determine the injured worker's understanding of injuries, prognosis, and treatment.

    viii. Identify the strength of the injured worker's support system.

     ix. Identify any critical needs (such as lodging, childcare). The home environment is assessed by establishing where the injured worker lives, with whom, the structure (in case home modification is contemplated), and any safety concerns.

      x. Question the availability of transportation for injured worker visits when appropriate.

     xi. Contact the employer to identify any source of support by employer and coworkers, including options for the injured worker's RTW. During this contact, a rapport should be developed with the employer that will be maintained throughout the case management process.

    b. Analyzing and planning

       i. Determine whether the current setting is appropriate for the injured worker's medical needs and its accessibility for family members. (It is not uncommon for an injured worker to be injured at a remote job site or to be transported to a facility that is a distance from family members.)

      ii. After assessment of the diagnosis and treatment plan and monitoring of medical progress, formulate the expected time frame before discharge.

     iii. Establish whether the injured worker can be dismissed directly to home or will need to be admitted to another facility for a different level of care.

     iv. Determine level of care based on knowledge of home environment and support system.

      v. Cost of home care versus institutional care is a strong factor. If the injured worker needs multiple health care services or is unable to safely perform activities of daily living (ADL), these needs can often be met more economically at a sub-acute or skilled nursing facility.

     vi. The case management plan reflects knowledge of the concurrent plans of medical providers, family members, and the facility case manager. The case management plan deals with health care needs and optimum recovery of function expected, including RTW.

c. Implementing and coordinating

      i. The facility discharge planner is made aware of PPOs, special contracts, and other cost-containment issues at the outset in states where this is allowed.

     ii. If there are no PPOs or other contracts in place, the case manager seeks out appropriate providers for needed services and negotiates the best service at the best price with each of them.

    iii. The case management plan is shared with the injured worker, family, claims handler, employer, medical providers, and hospital discharge planner. The plan is then adjusted until agreement on the plan is reached.

    iv. Coordination with the facility discharge planner is necessary to set up transportation needs, home care providers, durable medical equipment providers, and injured worker appointments for follow-up care.

     v. When the injured worker is not yet ready for discharge to home, but must be transferred to another facility, coordination with the discharging and the admitting facilities is the workers' compensation case manager's responsibility.

     vi. When needs are identified that seem to be outside the scope of workers' compensation coverage, the claims manager/payer is consulted. If it is determined that concurrent medical or social service needs do not arise from the injury and do not significantly impact recovery from injuries, the injured worker or the family and the facility discharge planner are informed. The workers' compensation case manager can provide limited assistance in referring the injured worker and his family to appropriate providers and agencies.

d. Monitoring, evaluating, and reporting of outcomes

      i. The case manager receives and reviews reports from all health care providers.

     ii. If the injured worker is treated in rehabilitation or another extended stay facility, the case manager attends team conferences.

    iii. The case manager maintains contact with the injured worker and family through telephone calls and visits.

     iv. Physician visits are monitored either by attending appointments when treatment decisions are anticipated or through telephonic management procedures.

     v. Medical services are evaluated, coordinated, and changed to meet the goals of recovery of health and function.

     vi. The injured worker's recovery is usually monitored until he or she is stated to be at MMI.

     vii. Assistance is made to return to regular or modified work whenever possible. When a work-related injury results in permanent disability, with ongoing needs for medical care and equipment, the case management plan often includes a life care plan and recommendation for case manager involvement.

3. Prolonged treatment, multiple providers, overuse of service cases

   a. These cases are referred for case management often out of the frustration of the injured worker, the claims handler, or the employer over a lack of case resolution. The case manager is likely to receive this referral later in the claims process.

   b. This category of cases might include:

     i. Prolonged treatment for an injury with unrelated complications

     ii. Development of complex injury sequelae such as regional causalgia (formerly identified as reflex sympathetic dystrophy [RSD]), chronic pain, fibromyalgia, or chronic myofascial syndrome

     iii. Longer-than-expected recovery from injuries without known complications

     iv. Prolonged disability from a minor injury with insufficient medical causation

     v. Inability to communicate successfully with medical providers or a noted lack of clear diagnosis, treatment plan, or work status

     vi. Multiple treatments with physical therapy, chiropractor, and other practitioners without documented progress

   c. Claims-handling issues or litigation may be involved or imminent.

   d. The goals for case management are to determine appropriate and effective medical care, coordinate timely delivery of that care, communicate goals to all stakeholders, and assist in the injured worker's RTW when possible.

4. Injury claims with known barriers to recovery and rehabilitation, "red flag" cases

   a. Claims adjusters recognize that some injured workers have innate or acquired barriers to achieving optimum recovery from injuries and rehabilitation, and refer them to case management.

     i. Injured workers with concurrent disability or disease that may or may not be associated with a work-related incident.

      ii. Injured workers who do not speak or understand English will have difficulty understanding and complying with medical regimens.

      iii. Injured workers with a perceived lack of incentive to comply with medical treatment and RTW.

  b. Goals for case management are to address specified problems, identify achievable solutions for problems, coordinate medical care that will help the injured worker recover from injuries, and assist in the injured worker's RTW.

5. Case management process model—prolonged treatment with complications and complicating factors

  a. Assessment

    i. Discuss case management expectations with the referral source.

    ii. Review the claim file thoroughly.

      1. Understand the mechanism and causation of injury.

      2. Review all medical bills and find matching medical reports.

      3. Determine the treating physician or other practitioner (such as chiropractor) who is directing care.

      4. List all health care providers since the injury.

      5. Identify what medical records are needed to complete a medical record review.

    iii. Interview the employer to gather his or her understanding of injury, treatment, and barriers that are preventing the injured worker from returning to work. Determine the availability of modified work to address activity restrictions.

    iv. Interview the injured worker and the family. If the worker is represented by an attorney, permission is sought from the attorney before directly contacting the injured worker or the family. If the worker is represented and contact allowed, the interview might be scheduled in the attorney's office or in other controlled surroundings.

      1. Determine the injured worker's understanding of the injury; any diagnoses, treatment including medication, barriers to RTW; and additional treatment that he or she feels might be helpful.

      2. Determine whether language or culture is a barrier to understanding medical treatment and the RTW process.

      3. Ask about concurrent medical problems, family dynamics, the home environment, and the potential for job placement if necessary.

      4. Interview the worker and the family to understand whether the prolonged treatment and time off work is meeting some other needs such as caring for children, other family members, or any other financial disincentives to returning to work.

      5. The injured worker or his or her attorney might not allow all questions to be answered.

b. Planning and analyzing

   i. The case management plan focuses on the injured worker achieving the goals of return to optimum health and recovery of function, including RTW.

   ii. Through the detailed review of medical records, the case manager determines the most appropriate provider to achieve these goals.

   iii. The plan will include suggestions for diagnostic procedures to confirm diagnoses, if appropriate (e.g., if a diagnosis of regional causalgia is suspected, electrodiagnostics, three-phase bone scan, and ganglion blocks are standard procedures in this condition).

c. Implementing and coordinating

   i. The case management plan is shared with all stakeholders and revised as needed. Examples of workable communication tools for telephone calls and letters can be found in *The Case Manager's Handbook,* 3rd Edition (Mullahy and Jensen, 2004).

   ii. Communicate with all medical providers to get the injured worker's updated records, along with current diagnosis, treatment plan, and activity restriction, including restrictions for work.

   iii. Ideally, the injured worker (and attorney) will cooperate in trying to achieve the goals of optimum recovery of health and function, but should an adverse reaction occur, the claims adjuster will be consulted.

   iv. Selecting the appropriate provider to help in achieving goals can be accomplished with the cooperation of the injured worker by scheduling a second opinion or a change of physician. If an adverse situation exists, an IME will be scheduled with approval from the adjuster.

   v. Communication with the employer continues, and efforts are made to assist the injured worker in his or her RTW.

   vi. Coordination of the delivery of appropriate medical care continues until there is a physician-issued MMI date.

d. Monitoring, evaluating, and reporting of outcomes

   i. Follow up with the injured worker and employer to evaluate success of medical treatment and return to work.

   ii. If a full duty release is anticipated soon after the injured worker has returned to work on modified duty or shortened hours, monitoring of status will continue until that release.

   iii. A report of case management activity and outcomes will be given to the adjuster.

6. Workplace violence, a growing concern, results in physical and psychological injuries. Most employers will seek assistance from their Employee Assistance Program (EAP) provider, the occupational health professionals, and, for those employees requiring additional medical care or support, the services of a medical case manager.

    i. The sources of workplace violence are varied.

        a. Internal conflicts and disruptions such as assaults, fistfights, labor unrest, disgruntled employees or family members, "horseplay," and arson or bomb

        b. External criminal activity such as aggravated robberies, effect of a fellow worker's homicide, physical assaults outside the workplace (fire personnel, service and delivery employees)

    ii. The workers' compensation aftermath of workplace violence can be very challenging for the medical manager.

        a. Physical injuries that result from gunshots, stabbings, and beatings are often complex and require multiple providers for treatment.

        b. Many workplace violence injuries result in some posttraumatic stress symptoms for the injured worker and other personnel.

        c. The aftereffects of violence complicate the RTW process for the injured worker and his or her family, coworkers, and employer.

    iii. Goals for the case manager are to identify the effects of violence on the injured worker and others; coordinate timely delivery of health care, including psychological support when it is determined to be necessary; and assist in the injured worker's return to work.

7. Case management process model—violence in the workplace—aftermath

  a. Assessment

    i. Medical records are reviewed and providers consulted to determine nature and extent of the injured worker's injuries, treatment plan, and prognosis.

    ii. Review police and newspaper reports, if available.

    iii. The injured worker and family are interviewed.

        a. Determine their understanding of injuries, treatment plan, and prognosis.

        b. Understand family structure and support system.

        c. Assess the injured worker's ability to remember and discuss the details of the injury.

        d. List any preexisting mental and physical health concerns that might affect the injured worker's recovery from injuries.

        e. Identify barriers to recovery of health and function, including signs of posttraumatic stress in injured worker or family members, or both.

    iv. Interview the employer to discuss the events of the injury and determine plans for the injured worker's return to work.

        a. Discuss the impact of the injured worker's injuries on the employer and coworkers.

        b. Identify the employer's ability to modify the injured worker's job for RTW, including changes of hours and addressing safety concerns.

    b. Planning and analyzing
       i. The case management plan focuses on achieving goals of return to optimum health and recovery of function, including RTW.
      ii. Determine appropriate health care providers for physical and psychological care.
     iii. Determine whether posttraumatic stress signs are present; the case management plan includes an opportunity for the injured worker to be evaluated by an appropriate mental health care professional.
     iv. The case management plan is shared with all stakeholders and modified as needed.

    c. Implementing and coordinating
       i. Gather medical records.
      ii. Coordinate all health care provider visits for timely delivery of services.
     iii. Whenever possible, attend physician appointments that will include decision-making activity with the injured worker.
     iv. Communicate with the employer.
        a. Discuss progress of injured worker in return to health and function.
        b. The employer may identify other workers who are having difficulty coping with the episode of workplace violence. An external case manager can offer services only to an employee who has filed a claim. Therefore, the employer needs to be directed toward other resources such as EAPs for these workers.
        c. Address concerns in regard to the injured worker's RTW.
      v. Check on availability for modifications to meet physical restrictions resulting from injuries.
     vi. Implement plan for modification of job duties, task assignments, hours of work, and other workplace concerns in coordination with mental health recommendations if available.
    vii. Facilitate RTW by communicating with appropriate health care providers.

    d. Monitoring, evaluating, and reporting of outcomes
       i. Monitor and review all medical records.
      ii. Communicate with injured worker, providers, and employer until MMI statement is received and the injured worker has returned to optimum functioning.
     iii. A report of case management activity and outcomes is given to the adjuster.

8. Workers' compensation referrals to assist in RTW activities
    a. Regaining all functional activities by an injured worker is important, but the activity most central to the process is RTW.
    b. Studies show that only 50% of injured workers return to their jobs after being off for 6 months, 25% after 12 months, and less than 2% after 2 years (Glass, 2004).

c. The case manager integrates RTW in all assigned cases for workers' compensation medical management unless instructed to do so otherwise. (Note: Because case managers in employer settings usually have employer-specific guidelines and procedures to follow in facilitating an RTW for injured workers, only the role of external case managers is considered here.)

d. Goals of case management are to assess barriers to RTW; communicate with the employer and educate him or her, if necessary, on the positive effects of returning injured worker to work; address medical concerns that may prevent RTW; and coordinate the RTW process.

9. Case management process model—RTW referral

a. Assessment

   i. Discuss case management expectations with referral source.

   ii. Ascertain whether the assignment includes a need for comprehensive interview with injured worker.

   iii. Identify any claims-handling issues involved in the failure of the injured worker to RTW.

      a. Extraneous employment issues

      b. Plaintiff attorney involvement

   iv. Review the claim file thoroughly.

      a. Understand the mechanism and causation of injury.

      b. Review all medical records to determine what restrictions on activity have been identified.

      c. Determine treating physician or other practitioner (such as chiropractor) directing care.

      d. Identify the barriers preventing the injured worker from RTW.

      e. Consider the impact of permanent disability and the need to consider reasonable accommodation under the Americans with Disabilities Act (ADA)

   v. Interview the employer to gather his or her understanding of injury, treatment, and barriers preventing the injured worker from RTW.

   vi. Communication with the employer includes:

      a. A review of the employer's RTW policy

      b. If no formal policy exists, the case manager will ask about usual practices in allowing an injured worker to RTW before being released for full, unrestricted duties.

      c. A discussion about modified or "light" duty

      d. Any union rules affecting RTW

      e. An understanding of the injured worker's preinjury position and essential tasks

      f. Application of ADA requirements for permanent disabilities

   vii. If it is part of the case management assignment, interview the injured worker and the family, if approved by plaintiff attorney of a represented worker.

      a. Determine understanding of injuries and treatment.

b. Identify barriers to RTW.
b. Planning and analyzing
   i. The case management plan focuses on barriers to RTW and possible solutions to these identified problems.
   ii. The case management plan is shared with all stakeholders and is modified as required.
c. Implementing and coordinating
   i. The case manager determines whether the treating physician has identified appropriate activity restrictions, and if not, communicates with the physician to determine specific restrictions.
   ii. The case manager coordinates the medical care identified by the physician as necessary to release the injured worker for work.
   iii. Communication with the employer about the RTW includes:
      a. Education on the positive effect on both the injured worker and the workers' compensation claim process when the worker returns to work as soon as possible (Pimentel, 1995).
      b. An understanding of modifying usual job duties to meet activity restrictions as stated by the treating physician.
      c. Discussion of short-term employment in another job for the employer to meet the stated activity restrictions.
      d. Referral to a claims adjuster to discuss partial temporary payments (PTDs) if wages or hours are less than usual wage.
   iv. The case manager derives from communication with the employer an understanding of the physical activity involved to do the injured worker's usual job.
      a. A job description is requested from the employer.
      b. If no job description is available or if the physical requirements of the job are not detailed, the case manager may opt to conduct a job analysis that will provide the treating physician with a clear idea of the physical abilities necessary to return the injured worker to his or her usual job.
      c. Information included on a job analysis includes (Douglas, 1994):
         i. Job title
         ii. Tools, machines, and equipment used regularly
         iii. The usual work cycle and number of hours worked weekly
   iv. Specific essential physical demands regarding lifting (including amount lifted in pounds), bending, reaching, crawling, climbing, and kneeling
   v. Hours typically spent sitting, standing, and walking
   vi. The frequency each essential function occurs in a workday
   vii. Repetitive activity, including physical action and duration of activity in a work shift
   viii. Environment (temperature, air quality, uneven surfaces for walking)

    ix. RTW options and modifications available

        a. The case manager will recommend using the services of an ergonomic specialist for job analysis and activity recommendations if the physical demands are particularly complex or the RTW issues are critical in the claim-handling process.

        b. The case manager will communicate with the treating physician and present the completed job analysis for review.

        c. If a clear diagnosis is present, appropriate treatment has been rendered, and all barriers for recovery of health and function have been addressed, but the injured worker has not been released for work, the case management plan will include a request for a Functional Capacity Evaluation (FCE).

    x. The FCE objectively identifies the injured worker's current level of functioning and provides the physician objective testing to assist in determining activity restrictions and possible impairment.

    xi. The FCE includes testing the work category the injured person is capable of performing; that is, sedentary, light, medium.

    xii. Specific validation parameters are taken into consideration and are considered useful in measuring submaximal effort or inconsistencies in work abilities.

    xiii. As a result of the FCE, recommendations for activities, such as work hardening or work conditioning, are determined to increase the injured worker's physical capacity and allow less restrictive functioning.

    xiv. When all activity fails to return the injured worker to work, a referral to vocational rehabilitation may be made in accordance with individual state laws. The case manager's involvement with vocational rehabilitation will be directed by paying source.

  d. Monitoring, evaluating, and reporting of outcomes

    i. Follow up with the injured worker and employer to evaluate the success of medical treatment and RTW.

    ii. If a full duty release is anticipated soon after the injured worker has returned to work on modified duty or shortened hours, monitoring of status will continue until that release.

    iii. Vocational rehabilitation is monitored if requested.

    iv. A report of case management activity and outcomes will be given to the adjuster.

10. Cases assigned to a case manager for scheduling IMEs and second opinions

  a. An IME is a frequently used tool to resolve medical issues and questions in a workers' compensation claim.

  b. The scope, content, utilization, and provider used may be proscribed by statute. Specifically, the frequency and number of IMEs and the practitioner used may be regulated by state workers' compensation laws.

    c. Whether the case manager is arranging an IME as a specific task or whether it is part of an ongoing management file, general guidelines are as follows:

      i. IMEs are often a claims-handling maneuver and are coordinated with the claims adjuster or manager to ensure that appropriate goals are set and met.

      ii. Because an IME can be viewed as an adversarial action, a careful explanation of the reasons for scheduling the evaluation is made to the injured worker if direct communication is allowed.

      iii. The selection of the practitioner to do the evaluation is key to the outcome.

      iv. The physician selected (or other practitioner required) will be well qualified and credentialed, usually with board certification in the specialty. The American Board of Independent Medical Examiners (ABIME) has developed standards for the delivery of IMEs and certification of IME providers (*www.ABIME.org*).

      v. Many physicians do not perform IMEs; the ones who do perform them as part of their practices generally have specific guidelines and requirements that must be followed.

      vi. The claims adjuster may have input into selection as part of the overall claim-handling process.

      vii. The communication among stakeholders is vital both for the success of resolving medical questions and as a legal responsibility of the case manager.

      viii. It is essential both as a process component and as a legal responsibility that the case manager gets all accumulated medical records, including x-ray studies, to the independent examiner for review.

      ix. The final case manager task following an IME is to secure a report and provide it to the claims adjuster for distribution; however, the IME is usually directed to the adjuster and the case manager may have to request a copy for her information and case management planning.

■ ETHICAL AND LEGAL CONSIDERATIONS FOR WORKERS' COMPENSATION CASE MANAGERS

    A. Case managers have the responsibility to adhere to established standards of practice and professional codes of ethics, promote the adherence of ethical standards in the workplace, and establish ethical standards in their profession.

    B. Case managers apply ethical standards to their practice.

    C. Legal issues in workers' compensation claims challenge both the practice and the professionalism of case managers.

    D. Case managers must perform within their professional scope of licensure.

    E. Medical case managers (i.e., registered professional and advanced practice nurses) must be licensed in the state in which they deliver medical case management services.

F. In response to interstate practice in today's electronic age and mobile workforces, the National Council of State Boards of Nursing (NCSBN) has developed the "interstate compact." Nurses residing in, and licensed in compact states will have an unrestricted license to practice in states within the compact. Today there are more than 20 states in the compact (see *www.ncsbn.org*).

■ WORKERS' COMPENSATION CASE MANAGERS ARE GUIDED BY ETHICAL PRINCIPLES

A. General ethical principles as defined by a number of ethicists are:
   1. Injured worker advocacy and autonomy
   2. Beneficence versus malfeasance (strive to do good, but do not do harm)
   3. Justice
   4. Truthfulness or veracity

B. Individual case managers develop their own personal ethical guidelines by study and research and have a responsibility to assist others in the profession in establishing ethical standards in the workplace and scope/standards of practice for the profession as a whole (CMSA, 2002).

C. The Commission for Case Manager Certification (CCMC) has published the "Code of Professional Conduct for Case Managers," available online at *www.ccmcertification.org*.

D. Case managers in any practice setting or specialty find themselves in daily struggles to address injured workers' rights while fulfilling responsibilities for which they are paid (Mullahy and Jensen, 2004).

E. Case managers involved in workers' compensation claims practice in an inherently difficult area because there are many stakeholders, often with sharply competing interests.

F. The case managers in workers' compensation communicate established ethical standards as developed by their professional society that guide the practice.

G. Injured worker advocacy and autonomy
   1. Goals for advocating for an injured worker include recommending and coordinating the most effective medical care to treat injuries that will lead to an optimum recovery of function.
   2. The principle of promoting injured worker autonomy is tempered by state laws and claims considerations. However, the case manager communicates to the injured worker rights and responsibilities of all concerned in the coordination and delivery of medical care.
   3. It is imperative that the case manager inform the injured worker when the payer is providing the services and clearly define the expectations of the payer for activity and reporting.

H. Striving for promoting good and preventing harm in workers' compensation case management
   1. Medical management in the workers' compensation system is based on promoting appropriate (preferably EBM) care for the injured worker, working within the laws of the state.

2. A positive outcome for the injured worker in achieving maximum medical improvement and a return to the highest possible level of function, including work, is an application of the principle (Purtillo, 1998).

I. Justice

1. This area is one with the most potential ethical dilemmas for a workers' compensation case manager.

2. The entire workers' compensation system came about as a result of unfair treatment of an injured worker. A primary goal of the present-day system is to promote safety in the workplace.

3. The injured worker has the right to expect confidentiality in the handling of medical records and other personal information; however, workers' compensation laws give access to the records to a number of stakeholders. The use of electronic mail and other Internet communication is opening new areas of concern regarding confidentiality (Purtilo, 1998).

4. As noted earlier, the cost of workers' compensation is borne by the employer and by society as a whole in the price of goods and services. Taxes are used to provide workers' compensation coverage to local, state, and federal government employees. Overuse or abuse of the system by any participant does an injustice to all members of society.

5. Some examples of conflict in the application of the principle of justice are:

   a. The injured worker has an agenda that does not include recovering from his or her injuries and returning to work.

   b. The employer's dealings with the injured worker are not consistent with either the letter or the spirit of employment laws.

   c. The claims handler fails to inform the injured worker of pertinent facts and rights that might affect the outcome of his or her injury claim.

   d. The medical provider overbills or prolongs medical care, treatment, or management of an injured workers' case unnecessarily.

J. Truth or veracity

1. Telling the truth is the underlying principle in nursing and business conduct. Being truthful allows the case manager to gain trust and, therefore, cooperation from the injured worker, the employer, the adjuster, and all medical providers (Mullahy and Jensen, 2004).

2. Telling the truth is the basis for the case manager to be an advocate for the injured worker in a system that has many competing interests.

3. Truthfulness is necessary when medical records are presented to a medical provider for review so that all interests are represented fairly.

■ LEGAL ISSUES FOR THE WORKERS' COMPENSATION CASE MANAGER

A. The case manager's role, while primarily medically focused, is linked to the legal issues in a claim.

1. The case manager has the responsibility of knowing and following state laws dictating medical care providers in a workers' compensation claim.
2. The case manager cannot contact an injured worker directly when he or she is represented by an attorney without permission and needs to abide by the instructions of the plaintiff attorney in matters concerning communication with the injured worker. The case manager should follow company guidelines/policies when dealing with litigated cases.
3. Laws in some states restrict the flow of information between medical providers and the case manager.
4. Failure to adhere to laws can result in penalties against the payer with substantial fines.

B. The case manager is legally accountable to practice case management within the scope of her or his professional license.

C. The case manager has the responsibility of knowing about applicable laws dealing with workers' compensation practice; to fail to do so falls below professional standards (CMSA, 2002).

D. Case law is developing that increases the case manager's accountability for referrals to health care providers when an unanticipated negative event occurs (Guido, 1997).

E. The case manager has a responsibility to report accurately on case management activity and provide the report to appropriate parties.

F. Medical case managers must have the relevant state nursing license to provide case management services (see *www.ncsbn.org*).

■ TRENDS IN WORKERS' COMPENSATION CASE MANAGEMENT

A. The effort to contain costs in workers' compensation claims continues to promote innovative programs.

B. The use of managed care arrangements (see Box 18-1) includes medical case management as an effective means of managing workers' compensation medical care.

C. Outcome-driven quality assessment is a tool for case management practices.

D. The quest for quality and standardization of medical and case management services is evidenced by the development of accreditation programs in workers' compensation and case management (among others) by URAC (see *www.urac.org*).

E. The mandate for EBM, utilization/peer review, and case management are quality elements in workers' compensation medical care.

F. There is a greater awareness of the impact of technology on practice (i.e., the use of the Internet, telephonic services), mobile/virtual workforces, and globalization. This has moved the NCSBN to initiate the interstate compact form of nursing licensure.

■ MEDICAL COST-CONTAINMENT PROGRAMS

A. Managed care companies
1. A number of state legislatures are considering application of additional managed care principles to their workers' compensation systems.
2. Managed care companies are forming to meet current and anticipated needs in the various states.
3. Case management is a vital part of all managed care legislation.

B. Early intervention by case managers
1. Historically, claims by injured workers (except for catastrophic or serious cases) have been referred to case management after the worker fails to respond to medical treatment or is unable to return to work.
2. Today, the trend is to allow both internal and external case managers to become involved soon after the injury is reported (Chan, Leahy, Mc Mahon, Mirch, & DeVinney, 1999).

C. Twenty-four–hour coverage
1. The concept of 24-hour coverage by combined health and workers' compensation insurance or for self-insured employers has long been considered.
2. The basic premise is that health insurance would cover all injuries and illnesses to American workers without regard to causation. Therefore, the resources spent in investigating causation and related health care needs would be saved.
3. Although pilot programs have been tested in several states and by major employers, there is no clear consensus on its applicability for larger populations or how the issue of indemnity is addressed.

■ FEDERAL LAWS AFFECTING WORKERS' COMPENSATION CASE MANAGEMENT

A. The American with Disabilities Act (ADA)
1. The act went into effect on July 26, 1992.
2. The intent was to prohibit employers from discrimination against qualified individuals with a disability in many areas of employment.
3. Nearly 3 years after the law was enforced, the Equal Employment Opportunities Commission (EEOC) reported that 85% of charges received involved existing employees, many of whom reported work-related impairment.
4. Case managers involved in any part of an injured worker's RTW activities are responsible for knowing the basic tenets of ADA.
5. The case manager does not give legal advice concerning protection of injured workers' rights in respect to the ADA, but refers the employer to his or her employment attorney for that advice.
6. The Job Accommodation Network (JAN) is a consulting service that provides information about job accommodations and the employability

of people with disabilities at no charge. It is an excellent resource in RTW and job accommodation planning (see *www.jan.wvu.edu*).

B. The Family Medical Leave Act (FMLA)

1. This act was signed into law in 1993.

2. The intent of the act is to provide employees with an option to take up to 12 weeks of unpaid leave for a serious illness of the worker or a family member with job restoration (or equivalent) guaranteed.

3. Most workers' compensation claimants are eligible for FMLA as a result of their work-related injury, if they meet eligibility requirements.

4. Employees are not obligated to return to work on modified or "light duty" when claiming benefits under the FMLA. However, an injured worker might not be eligible for workers' compensation indemnity payments if he or she does not return to work while claiming FMLA benefits, he or she cannot be dismissed from employment during the 12 weeks of FMLA sanctioned leave.

■ DOCUMENTING QUALITY OF SERVICES BY OUTCOME MEASUREMENTS

A. For legal and ethical protection, the case manager makes referrals to health care providers who offer outcome measurements as proof of their competency. It behooves providers to have the relevant URAC accreditation to demonstrate their commitment to excellence and quality.

B. Case managers document the success of their interventions by the outcomes they achieve.

1. Though there is a great deal of anecdotal evidence of the benefit of case management in the workers' compensation system, there are few objective data to confirm it (Akabas, Gates, and Galvin, 1992).

2. There is not yet general agreement on what data are measured and what measurements are needed to make comprehensive statements about positive outcomes.

3. Private industry is developing common metrics to define the value and consistency of services in the marketplace. These measures, called the Employers Metrics for Productivity and Quality (EMPAC) are meant to be the beginning of standardized metrics to demonstrate value and return-on-investment for employee benefit and workers' compensation programs. (Weblinks to EMPAC measures follow at the end of this chapter).

4. It is estimated that case management activities toward the RTW process can reduce the cost of a claim by 50% (Pimentel, 1995).

5. Case managers can demonstrate cost savings on a workers' compensation case by medical cost avoidance, application of EBM tools and disability duration guidelines, facilitated RTW, saving of lost workdays, and levels of satisfaction among stakeholders (DiBenedetto, 2006).

REFERENCES

Akabas, S., Gates, L., & Galvin, D. (1992). *Disability management.* New York: American Management Association.

Case Management Society of America (CMSA). (2002). *Standards of practice,* 2nd ed. Little Rock, AR: CMSA.

Chan, F., Leahy, M., McMahon, B., Mirch, M., & DaVinney, D. (1999). Foundation knowledge and major practice domains of case management. *The Journal of Care Management, 5*(1), 10–28.

DiBenedetto, D. V., (2002). In Toni Cesta, *Survival strategies for nurses in managed care.* Workers' compensation in managed care, 25, 398–407. St. Louis, Mo: Mosby.

DiBenedetto, D. V. (2006). *Principles of workers' compensation and disability case management.* Battle Creek, MI: DVD Associates LLC. Website: *www.DVDandHaag.com.*

Douglas, J. (1994). *Managing workers' compensation.* New York: John Wiley and Sons.

Glass, L. (2004). American College of Occupational and Environmental Medicine (ACOEM). *Occupational medicine practice guidelines: Evaluation and management of common health problems and functional recovery in workers,* 2nd ed. Beverly Farms, MA: ACOEM Press.

Guido, G. W. (1997). *Legal issues in nursing.* Stamford, CT: Appleton & Lange.

Mullahy, C., & Jensen, D. (2004). *The case manager's handbook,* 3rd ed. Gaithersburg, MD: Aspen Publications.

National Academy Social Insurance (NASI). (2002). Workers' compensation benefits, costs and coverage, 2000 new estimates. Website: *www.NASI.org.*

Pimentel, R. (1995). *The return to work process.* Chatsworth, CA: Milt Wright & Associates.

Purtilo, R. (1998). Rethinking the ethics of confidentiality and health care teams. *Bioethics Forum 14,* 3(4), 29–37.

Stoddard, S., Jans, L., Ripple, J., & Kraus, L. (1998). *Chartbook on work and disability in the United States:* An InfoUse Report available online at http://www.infouse.com/disabilitydata/workdisability. Washington, DC: Institute on Disability Rehabilitation Research.

United States Chamber of Commerce. (2006). *Analysis of workers' compensation laws.* Washington, DC: Author.

SUGGESTED READING

Links to state and federal workers' compensation programs and laws:
U.S. Department of Labor—*www.DOL.gov*
http://www.dol.gov/esa/regs/compliance/owcp/wc.htm
www.workerscompensation.com
www.workcomcentral.com

HIPAA and workers' compensation
http://www.hhs.gov/ocr/hipaa/guidelines/workerscompensation.rtf
http://answers.hhs.gov

Evidence-based treatment and disability duration guidelines
www.guideline.gov
www.odgtreatment.com
www.acoem.org
www.worklossdata.com
www.disabilityduration.com
www.disabilitydurations.com
www.rgl.com

Sources of quality standards for workers' compensation networks, utilization review, and case management
www.urac.org

Other resources/websites:
Case Management Society of America—*www.cmsa.org*
Commission for Case Manager Certification—*www.ccmcertification.org*
EMPAC—*www.empac.org*
Integrated Benefits Institute—*www.ibiweb.org*
Job Accommodation Center—*www.jan.wvu.edu*
National Academy Social Insurance—*www.nasi.org*
National Business Group on Health—*www.wbgh.org*
National Council Compensation Insurance—*www.ncci.com*
National Council State Boards of Nursing—*www.ncsbn.org*

19 Disability and Occupational Health Case Management

Karen N. Provine
Lewis E. Vierling

Upon completion of this chapter, the reader will be able to:

1. Describe the background and perspective of the disability management movement including occupational health.
2. Define important terms and concepts related to disability and occupational health case management.
3. List the driving forces that lead to disability and occupational health case management practice.
4. Describe factors and discuss components that are important to the development and implementation of a disability management or occupational health case management program.
5. Apply the case management process to disability and occupational health case management.
6. State key characteristics of RTW programs and examples of reasonable accommodations.

IMPORTANT TERMS AND CONCEPTS

Americans with Disabilities Act (ADA)
Disability Management
Early Intervention
Employee Assistance Program (EAP)
Ergonomics
Family Medical Leave Act (FMLA)
Functional Capacity Assessment
Functional Job Analysis
Independent Medical Examinations
Integrated Benefits
Integrated Disability Management
Long-Term Disability
Modified Duty
Occupational Health Case Management
Occupational Injury versus Non-
  occupational Injury

Occupational Medicine Practice
  Guidelines
Paid Time Off Arrangements
Reasonable Accommodation
Return-to-Work Program
Short-Term Disability
Third Party Administrators (TPA)
Ticket to Work and Work Incentive
  Improvement Act
Time Loss Management
Transitional Work Duty
Treating Physician
Vocational Rehabilitation
Wellness Program
Workers' Compensation
Workforce Management

■ INTRODUCTION AND BACKGROUND

A. The current disability management programs evolved from the workers' compensation programs.

B. In the 1970s and 1980s, many states reformed their workers' compensation laws because of rising costs. Employers and insurance carriers began to develop cost-effective ways to respond to workers with occupational illnesses and injuries; hence, disability management and occupational health (OH) programs became more common.

C. From the perspective of reducing costs came the implementation of disability management programs, to not only address the needs of those employees, both ill or injured, but also in response to reducing costs and duration of absences from the workplace.

D. By facilitating earlier return-to-work (RTW) activities, the overall cost of disability was not only reduced, but there was also an increase in productivity as well. Gradually, the disability management program expanded to include an integrated approach.

1. Today's integrated disability management programs combine the management of short-term disability (STD), long-term disability (LTD), workers' compensation (WC), and group health benefit programs.

2. The integrated approach streamlines claims handling and reporting, administration, medical management, and RTW activities.

This chapter is a revised version of what was previously published in the first edition of *CMSA Core Curriculum for Case Management*. The contributors wish to acknowledge Lesley Wright, Martha Heath Eggleston, and Deborah V. DiBenedetto as some of the timeless material was retained from the previous version.

3. This integrated approach offers a single medical management plan focusing on the provision of quality, timely, cost-effective medical care and successful return to productive activity.

E. The primary mission of disability management programs is to reduce the financial costs associated with all disabilities in a nonadversarial environment of claims administration. This is accomplished through the development of a coordinated program with the focus on the individual's ability rather than disability.

F. Disability management programs include coordinated access to employer-provided benefit plans and services that impact the employee with a disability. This includes:
   1. WC
   2. Health care including 24-hour medical coverage and managed care
   3. Sick leave
   4. State disability; STD and LTD
   5. Salary continuation, pension and retirement plans
   6. Union plans
   7. Medical leaves of absence
   8. Paid time off (PTO)
   9. Social Security Disability

G. Internal departments that typically have responsibility for the design, administration, and implementation of one or more programs are human resources, risk management, OH, safety, finance, legal, and bargaining units.

H. External sources or departments that may be involved in the disability management program are the WC insurance carriers, health care providers, third party administrators, life insurance carriers, re-insurers, disability carriers, and managed care providers.

I. The expanding recognition that both nonoccupational and occupational disabilities could be managed effectively and efficiently with the support of employers, supervisors, and caregivers gave rise to the managed integrated disability approach.

J. According to the American Association of Occupational Health Nurses (AAOHN), poor employee health costs about $1 trillion annually, so business executives look to OH nurses and case managers to maximize employee productivity and reduce costs through lowered disability claims, fewer on-the-job injuries and improved absentee rates.

K. Through their recognized value to business, OH professionals commonly take a seat at the management table, providing input about staffing issues, budgetary considerations and corporate policies and procedures that positively impact worker health and safety, and thus contribute to a healthier bottom line.

L. The practice of occupational and environmental health focuses on the promotion and restoration of health, prevention of illness and injury, and protection from work-related and environmental hazards.

■ KEY DEFINITIONS

A. Assistive device—Any tool that is designed, made, or adapted to assist a person in performing a particular task.

B. Assistive technology—Any item, piece of equipment, or product system, whether acquired commercially or off the shelf, modified or customized, that is used to increase, maintain, or improve functional capabilities of individuals with disabilities.

C. Capacity—A construct that indicates the highest probable level of functioning a person may reach. Capacity is measured in a uniform or standard environment, and thus reflects the environmentally adjusted ability of the individual.

D. Clinical practice guidelines—These guidelines are voluntary in nature and may be specific to an institution; some are mandated by state WC laws (e.g., Massachusetts), or they may be voluntary (e.g., New York). There are no nationally promulgated clinical guidelines dictating medical care.

E. Disability—Can be defined in different ways, all referring to a lack of or inability to function in a certain aspect of daily living.
  1. A physical or neurological deviation in an individual's makeup. It may refer to a physical, mental, or sensory condition. A disability may or may not be a handicap to an individual, depending on one's adjustment to it.
  2. A diminished function, based on the anatomic, physiological, or mental impairment that has reduced the individual's activity or presumed ability to engage in any substantial gainful activitity.
  3. Inability or limitation in performing tasks, activities, and roles in the manner or within the range considered normal for a person of the same age, gender, culture and education.
  4. Any restriction or lack of ability (resulting from an impairment) to perform an activity in the manner or within the range considered normal for a human being.

F. Disability case management—The process of managing occupational and nonoccupational diseases with the aim of returning the disabled employee to a productive work schedule and employment. It is also known as limiting a disabling event, providing immediate intervention once an injury or illness occurs, and returning the individual to work in a timely manner.

G. Ergonomics—The scientific discipline concerned with the understanding of interactions among humans and other elements of a system. It is the profession that applies theory, principles, data, and methods to environmental design (including work environments) in order to optimize human well-being and overall system performance.

H. Ergonomist—An individual who has (1) a mastery of ergonomics knowledge; (2) a command of the methodologies used by ergonomists in applying that knowledge to the design of a product, process, or environment; and (3) applied his or her knowledge to the analysis, design, test, and evaluation of products, processes, and environments.

I. Functional Capacity Evaluation (FCE)—A systematic process of assessing an individual's physical capacities and functional abilities. The FCE matches human performance levels to the demands of a specific job or work activity or occupation. It establishes the physical level of work an individual can perform. The FCE is useful in determining job placement, job accommodation, or RTW after injury or illness. FCEs can provide objective information regarding functional work ability in the determination of occupational disability status.

J. Handicapped—Refers to the disadvantage of an individual with a physical or mental impairment resulting in a handicap.

K. Handicap—The functional disadvantage and limitation of potentials based on a physical or mental impairment or disability that substantially limits or prevents the fulfillment of one or more major life activities otherwise conisdered normal for that individual based on age, sex, and social and cultural factors, such as caring for one's self, performing manual tasks, walking, seeing, hearing, speaking, breathing, learning, working, etc.

L. Impairment—A general term indicating injury, deficiency or lessening of function. Impairment is a condition that is medically determined and relates to the loss or abnormality of psychological, physiological, or anatomical structure or function. Impairments are disturbances at the level of the organ and include defects or loss of limb, organ, or other body structure or mental function, e.g., amputation, paralysis, mental retardation, psychiatric disturbances as assessed by a physical.

M. Injury—Harm to a worker subject to treatment and/or compensable under workers' compensation. Any wrong, or damages done to another; either done to his or her person, rights, reputation, or property.

N. LTD income insurance—Insurance issued to an employee, group, or individual to provide a reasonable replacement of a portion of an employee's earned income lost through a serious prolonged illness during the normal work career.

O. Mobility—The ability to move about safely and efficiently within one's environment.

P. Nondisabling injury—An injury which may require medical care, but does not result in loss of working time or income.

Q. Nonoccupational disease—Any disease that is not common to, or does not occur as a result of a particular occupation of specific work environment.

R. Occupational disease—Any disease that is common to, or occurs as a result of, a particular occupation of specific work environment.

S. Occupational health case management—The process of coordinating the individual employee's health care services to achieve optimal quality care delivered in a cost-effective manner. It may focus on large-loss cases—that is, high-cost, prolonged recovery—or those with multiple providers and fragmented care.

T. Paid time off (PTO) arrangements—A benefit that provides employee with the right to scheduled and unscheduled time off with pay. Full and part time regular employees accrue PTO based on years of service. PTO days may be used for vacation, personal time, illness or time off to care for dependents. It usually does not include jury duty, military duty, bereavement time for an immediate family member, or sabbatical leave.

U. Partial disability—The result of an illness or injury that prevents an insured from performing one or more of the functions of his or her regular job.

V. Physical disability—A bodily defect that interferes with education, development, adjustment, or rehabilitation; generally refers to crippling conditions and chronic health problems but usually does not include single sensory handicaps such as blindness or deafness.

W. Social Security Disability Income (SSDI)—Federal benefit program sponsored by the Social Security Administration. Primary factor: disability and/or benefits received from deceased or disabled parent; benefit depends on money contributed to the Social Security program either by the individual involved and/or the parent involved.

X. STD income insurance—The provision to pay benefits to a covered disabled person/employee as long as he or she remains disabled up to a specific period not exceeding 2 years.

Y. Time loss management—A proactive process used for the management of employee absenteeism due to sickness and medical leaves. Usually a time loss management program focuses on ensuring employees health, productivity, safety and welfare. It does not aim to prohibit sickness absence; rather, it facilitates a timely return to work.

Z. Vocational assessment—Identifies the individual's strengths, skills, interests, abilities, and rehabilitation needs. Accomplished through onsite situational assessments at local businesses and in community settings.

AA. Vocational evaluation—The comprehensive assessment of vocational aptitudes and potential, using information about a person's past history, medical and psychological status, and information from appropriate vocational testing, which may use paper and pencil instruments, work samples, simulated work stations, or assessments in a real work environment.

BB. Vocational rehabilitation—Cost-effective case management by a skilled professional who understands the implications of the medical and vocational services necessary to facilitate an injured worker's expedient return to suitable gainful employment with a minimal degree of disability.

CC. Vocational rehabilitation counselor—A rehabilitation counselor who specializes in vocational counseling; i.e., guiding handicapped persons in the selection of a vocation or occupation.

DD. Vocational testing—The measurement of vocational interests, aptitudes, and ability using standardized, professionally accepted psychomotor procedures.

EE. Work adjustment—The use of real or simulated work activity under close supervision at a rehabilitation facility or other work setting to develop appropriate work behaviors, attitudes, or personal characteristics.

FF. Work adjustment training—A program for persons whose disabilities limit them from obtaining competitive employment. It typically includes a system of goal-directed services focusing on improving problem areas such as attendance, work stamina, punctuality, dress and hygiene and interpersonal relationships with co-workers and supervisors. Services can continue until objectives are met or until there has been noted progress. It may include practical work experience or extended employment.

GG. Work conditioning—An intensive, work-related, goal-oriented conditioning program designed specifically to restore systemic neuromusculoskeletal functions; e.g., joint integrity and mobility, muscle performance (including strength, power, and endurance), motor function (motor control and motor learning), range of motion (including muscle length), and cardiovascular/pulmonary functions (e.g., aerobic capacity/endurance, circulation, and ventilation and respiration/gas exchange). The objective of the work conditioning program is to restore physical capacity and function to enable the patient/client to RTW.

HH. Work hardening—A highly structured, goal-oriented, and individualized intervention program that provides clients with a transition between the acute injury stage and a safe, productive RTW. Treatment is designed to maximize each individual's ability to RTW safely with less likelihood of repeat injury. Work hardening programs are multidisciplinary in nature and use real or simulated work activities designed to restore physical, behavioral, and vocational functions. They address the issues of productivity, safety, physical tolerances, and worker behaviors.

II. Work modification—Altering the work environment to accommodate a person's physical or mental limitations by making changes in equipment, in the methods of completing tasks, or in job duties.

JJ. Work rehabilitation—A structured program of graded physical conditioning/strengthening exercises and functional tasks in conjunction with real or simulated job activities. Treatment is designed to improve the individual's cardiopulmonary, neuromusculoskeletal (strength, endurance, movement, flexibility, stability, and motor control) functions, biomechanical/human performance levels, and psychosocial aspects as they relate to the demands of work. Work rehabilitation provides a transition between acute care and RTW while addressing the issues of safety, physical tolerances, work behaviors, and functional abilities.

KK. Workers' compensation—An insurance program that provides medical benefits and replacement of lost wages for persons suffering from injury or illness that is caused by or occurs in the workplace. It is an insurance system for industrial and work injury, regulated primarily among the separate states, but regulated in certain specified occupations by the federal government.

■ PERSPECTIVES ON DISABILITY

A. Disability has been defined in a variety of ways for the purposes of programs, policies, and the law.

B. In a recent report by the Cherry Engineering Support Services, Inc., Federal Statutory on Definitions of Disability prepared for the Interagency Committee on Disability Research (2003), it was noted that there are 67 separate laws defining disability for federal purposes.

C. Section 504 of the Rehabilitation Act of 1973 and the Americans with Disabilities Act (ADA) of 1990 have adopted a definition that takes into consideration the individual, the physical surroundings, and the social environment.

1. The *biopsychosocial approach* to disability emphasizes that a disability arises from a combination of factors at the physical, emotional, and environmental levels.
2. The biopsychosocial approach is in sharp contrast to the *illness model,* which approaches disability from the perspective of diagnosing, treating, and discharge.
3. The biopsychosocial approach focuses on the three interrelated concepts cited in 1 and extends beyond the individual.

D. From a legal, benefit, and social program perspective, disability is often defined on the basis of specific activities of daily living (ADLs), work, and other functions essential to full participation in community-based living.

E. To be found disabled for the purposes of Social Security Disability income benefits, the individual must have a severe disability that has lasted, or is expected to last, at least 12 months, and which prevents the individual from working at a "substantial, gainful activity" level.

F. Both Section 504 of the Rehabilitation Act of 1973 and the ADA of 1990 define a person with a disability as someone who:
1. Has a physical or mental impairment that substantially limits one or more "major life activities;"
2. Has a record of such an impairment; or
3. Is regarded as having such an impairment.

■ COMPONENTS OF DISABILITY CASE MANAGEMENT PROGRAMS

A. The Certification of Disability Management Specialists Commission (CDMSC), the only nationally accredited organization that certifies disability management specialists, recently completed a role and functions study tracking the changes in disability management. Three specific practice domains were identified:
1. Disability case management—Involving specific tasks and required knowledge to carry out those tasks related to working with individuals who are ill or injured, or have disabilities.
2. Disability prevention and workplace intervention—Bringing together individual and organizational practice. This "blended" area identifies how tasks and duties within the disability management practice have evolved, with a broader scope of responsibility not only to the individuals served, but also to the programs that serve them.
3. Program development, management, and evaluation—Combining the administrative and managerial tasks that are increasingly becoming the responsibility of disability managers. The emphasis is on designing, implementing, managing, and evaluating programs in line with specific desired outcomes.

B. Disability case management programs highlight the following functions or activities:
1. Performing comprehensive individual case analysis and benefits assessment using accepted practices in order to develop appropriate interventions.

2. Reviewing disability case management intervention protocols using standards of care in order to promote quality care, recovery, and cost effectiveness.

3. Collaborating among stakeholders (e.g., disabled individual, employer, insurer, care provider) using effective communication strategies to optimize functional recovery.

4. Performing worksite/job analyses using observation, interviews, and records review in order to determine the requirements of the job.

5. Developing individualized RTW plans consistent with standard practices and procedures by collaborating with relevant stakeholders in order to facilitate employment.

6. Implementing interventions using appropriate counseling and behavior change techniques in order to optimize functioning and productivity.

7. Coordinating benefits, services, and community resources (e.g., orthotics, prosthetics, FMEs, independent medical exams (IME), durable medical equipment, home care, and vocational rehabilitation) through strategic planning in order to facilitate optimal functioning.

8. Monitoring progress for achievement of targeted milestones through ongoing comparisons with established best-practice guidelines in order to make recommendations, optimize functional recovery, and provide needed follow up.

9. Managing a caseload of clients using evidence-based practice standards and ethical strategies in order to enhance effectiveness and efficiency.

10. Preparing case notes and reports using applicable forms and systems in order to document case activities in compliance with standard practices and regulations.

C. Disability prevention and workplace intervention consists of the following activities or functions:

1. Implementing disability prevention practices (i.e., risk mitigation procedures such as job analysis, job accommodation, ergonomic evaluation, health and wellness initiatives, etc.) through training, education, and collaboration in order to change organizational behavior and integrate prevention as an essential component of organizational culture.

2. Developing a comprehensive transitional work program through consultation with all relevant stakeholders in order to facilitate optimal productivity and value in the workplace.

3. Engaging in an interactive process for job site modification or accommodation, or job task assignment incorporating appropriate resources (e.g., ergonomics and assistive technologies) in order to facilitate optimal functioning in the workplace.

4. Supporting employment practices that align work abilities with essential job functions by serving as a resource for employees and management in order to prevent disabilities and optimize productivity.

5. Recommending strategies to identify ergonomic, safety, and risk factors using available resources (e.g., data and assessment tools) in order to mitigate exposure and improve employee health.

6. Recommending strategies that integrate benefit plan designs and related services (e.g., EAPs, community resources, and medical services) by evaluating and coordinating delivery in order to promote prevention, optimal productivity, quality care, and cost containments.

7. Recommending health and wellness interventions by targeting the specific needs of employees and the organization in order to increase organizational health and productivity while demonstrating measurable value.

D. Disability case management program evaluations consist of the following activities:

1. Analyzing workplace practices (e.g., benefit design, policies and procedures, regulatory and compliance requirements, employee demographics, and labor relations) using a needs assessment to establish baselines and design effective interventions.

2. Developing a business rationale for a comprehensive disability management program using baseline data, best practices, evidence-based research, and benchmarks and incorporating cultural and environment factors to secure stakeholder investment and commitment.

3. Collaborative approach for the development and management of the disability management program by specifying essential procedures and training components consistent with pertinent regulations and identifying appropriate services and metrics in order to offer effective services for stakeholders.

4. Championing individual and organizational behavioral change by assigning responsibility to stakeholders at all levels of the organization in order to achieve strategic outcomes.

5. Procuring internal and external services/resources using commonly accepted selection criteria to maximize consistency and desired program outcomes.

6. Managing service providers using stakeholder-defined performance standards in order to maximize the quality of services and the return on investments.

7. Facilitating the exchange of data and metrics by integrating information systems for disability management programs in order to achieve and report desired program outcomes.

8. Conducting ongoing formative and summative program evaluations using qualitative and quantitative methods to improve process and measure outcomes.

9. Creating disability management performance reports and other communication vehicles targeted to relevant stakeholders using a variety of media in order to promote stakeholder awareness and collaboration.

E. Disability case management is not only an important workplace productivity program but also addresses more advanced workplace productivity concepts. These include:

1. Absence management—addressing unscheduled absences by workers due to illnesses, disability, personal, or other issues.
2. Improving the productivity of employees who are on the job but may not be performing at their maximum potential. This deficient performance can be related to a variety of health, personal, or other issues.

F. Disability managers are a part of a multidisciplinary team involved in integrated benefit practice, productivity enhancement, and health and wellness programs.

G. Increased emphasis on early intervention and job accommodation reduces disability-related costs.
   1. Combined direct and indirect costs of disability and absences, according to recent research, often exceed 20% of a company's payroll—or more than $40 million in annual absence costs for a company employing 5,000 people at an average salary of $40,000 per year.

H. The U.S. Surgeon General, Richard H. Carmona, through the United States Department of Health and Human Services has issued a "call to action to improve the health and welfare of persons with disabilities (2006)." This call to action has four main goals that are consistent with the goals and objectives of a disability case management program:
   1. Increase the understanding, nationwide, that people with disabilities can lead long, healthy, and productive lives.
   2. Increase knowledge among health care professionals and provide them with tools to screen, diagnose, and treat the whole person with a disability with dignity.
   3. Increase awareness among people with disabilities of the steps they can take to develop and maintain a healthy lifestyle.
   4. Increase individuals' accessibility to health care and support services to promote independence for people with disabilities.

■ CHALLENGES TO DISABILITY CASE MANAGEMENT

A. It is important to recognize that from a disability case management perspective the number of workers 55 and older is expected to grow 48% by the year 2008 and that the incidence of disability increases with age.

B. The number of employees with work-limiting disabilities increases with age, particularly in the 50- to 59-year-age group.

C. The U.S. Census Bureau in 2002 reported that approximately one out of ten persons with disabilities has a severe disability. In the prime employable years of 21 to 64, 26% of those individuals with severe disabilities are employed.

D. The aging workforce will demand more services, especially because of the increasing number of people with disabilities. This trend positions disability case management to be a key strategy in prevention and wellness programs.

E. The Society for Human Resource Management (SHRM) released the results of a survey in 2003 related to employers' incentives for hiring individuals with disabilities.

1. The primary focus of the survey was to determine how knowledge-able human resource professionals were regarding various governmental incentives for hiring individuals with disabilities.
2. Of the human resource personnel surveyed, 77% reported not using any incentive program for hiring persons with disabilities.

F. It should be noted that seven different tax credits are available to companies who hire disabled workers. However, fewer than 20% of human resource personnel surveyed reported being "very familiar with any of these tax credits."

G. Research findings from the John J. Heldrich Center for Workforce Development at Rutgers University, New Jersey, indicate that many employers do not provide any training to their employees regarding working with people with disabilities.[1]
1. Less than half (40%) of employers surveyed provided training of any kind to their employees regarding working with or providing accommodations to people with disabilities.
2. The employment environment for people with disabilities has a direct effect on disability management programs.
3. As the population ages and experiences more disabilities, the number of chronic conditions also increases and is associated with higher health care costs. All work places are affected.

H. A survey of 723 companies by Mercer Human Resource Consulting found that many employers have experienced significant increases in the incidence of LTD and STD.[2]
1. During a 2-year period, of the employers who measured the rate, STD incidence rates increased 33% and LTD incidence rates increased 26%.
2. The Department of Labor estimated that 5.5 million individuals were on LTD in 2002, a 62% increase from 1992. The most-cited explanation for this increase was the aging workforce.

■ THE AMERICANS WITH DISABILITIES ACT (ADA)

A. The ADA is both a challenge and a resource in disability management case management.

B. The ADA took effect on July 26, 1992. Title I of the ADA prohibits private employers, state and local governments, employment agencies, and labor unions, from discriminating against qualified individuals with disabilities in job application procedures, hiring, firing, advancement, compensation, job training, and other terms, conditions, and privileges of employment.

C. The overall goal of ADA is to extend maximum opportunities for full community integration to people with disabilities in both public and private sectors of our society.

---

[1]See *http://www.heldrich.rutgers.edu* (John J. Heldrich Center for Workforce Development).
[2]See *http://www.mercerhr.com* (Mercer Human Resource Consulting).

D. The law was enacted to provide a clear and comprehensive national mandate for the elimination of discrimination against individuals with disabilities.

E. The goals of the ADA are as follows:
   1. Equality of opportunity
   2. Full participation
   3. Independent living
   4. Economic self-sufficiency

F. According to the Supreme Court:
   1. An *employer* is a "person engaged in an industry affecting commerce who has fifteen or more employees for each working day in each of twenty or more calendar weeks in the current or preceding calendar year."
   2. An *employee* is defined as "an individual employed by an employer."

G. The Supreme Court has not recognized just any impairment to be a per se disability.
   1. A per se disability or condition, by its very nature, presumably would qualify as a disability.
   2. It is no longer enough for an individual to submit evidence of a medical diagnosis of impairment. The individual must have a case-by-case assessment to prove that a particular or specific impairment is protected under the ADA.
   3. Under the ADA, individuals are protected, not specific disabilities.

H. To be a qualified individual with a disability, the individual must possess the requisite skills, education, experience, and training for the position and be able to perform the essential job functions with or without reasonable accommodation.
   1. Under the definition of disability, the impairment must substantially limit a major life activity.
   2. The impairment may be so severe that the individual with or without reasonable accommodation is unable to participate in the covered activity or, in the case of employment, is not able to perform all the essential job functions.
   3. Another challenge for the employer and employee with impairment may be that individuals with impairment are considered to be a direct threat to either themselves or others in the workplace.
   4. The individual with impairment may not be qualified under the ADA if it can be shown that the individual poses a direct threat to the health and safety of others and to himself or herself, and that the threat cannot be eliminated by modification of policies, practices, procedures, or by the provision of auxiliary aids or services.

I. The Supreme Court has noted that employers are justified in their desire to avoid losing time as a result of sickness; WC claims; excessive turnover from medical, retirement, or death; and the threat of litigation, under state law.

1. Employers are not required to hire individuals who are unable to carry out the essential functions of the job without incurring risk to the health and safety of others and to themselves.

2. The Supreme Court included a provision in its decision that requires employers to assess the individual's current or prospective ability to safely perform the essential functions of the job.

   a. The assessment must be individualized and based on reasonable medical judgment that relies on the most current medical knowledge and the best available objective evidence.

   b. The imminence of risk and severity of harm to the individual also must be assessed.

3. The following four factors are to be considered in deciding whether an individual poses a direct threat:

   a. Duration of the risk

   b. Nature and severity of the potential harm

   c. Likelihood that the potential harm will occur

   d. Imminence of the potential harm

4. The Supreme Court has held that employers must gather substantial information about the employee's work history and medical status.

   a. Employer's requiring that an employee must be "100% healed" before returning to work is considered an ADA violation.

   b. The emphasis should not be whether or not the individuals are 100% healed, but rather whether they pose a direct threat to themselves or others in the workplace.

5. The Supreme Court has also held that an employer is free to decide that physical characteristics or mental conditions that do not rise to the level of a disability are preferable to others. The Court has noted that the employer is free to decide that some limiting, but not substantially limiting impairments, make individuals less suited for a job.

6. Generally speaking, the ADA permits qualification standards that are "job-related" and "consistent with business necessity."

7. In October 2002, the Equal Employment Opportunity Commission (EEOC) issued new enforcement guidelines on reasonable accommodation and undue hardship under the ADA.

   a. The updated guidelines revised the standards for "reasonableness" of an accommodation. Reasonableness is now evaluated on whether or not it is considered not only effective, but also "feasible or plausible" for the typical employer.

   b. Requests for accommodation can be made either verbally or in writing.

      i. In most cases, the employee must request the accommodation before the employer is obligated to respond.

      ii. Requests for accommodation may also come at any time during the employment application process or at different intervals during an individual's employment with the company.

    iii. The employer is obligated to consider each request and engage in an "interactive process" to investigate, assess, and provide reasonable accommodations.

    iv. If the employer is aware that an employee with a disability is experiencing problems in the workplace or is unable to request an accommodation because of mental impairment, the employer is obliged to initiate the process. However, each situation requires a case-by-case assessment.

    v. Examples of reasonable accommodation may include job restructuring, leave of absence, modified or part-time schedules, and reassignment to a vacant position.

    vi. Examples of accommodations that are considered unreasonable include reducing production or performance standards that are not uniformly applied, providing personal use items, changing supervisors, monitoring medications, unwarranted promotion, or eliminating the essential functions of the job.

    vii. If the problem the individual is experiencing as a result of the disability is not related to the actual performance on the job, reasonable accommodation may not be required. For example, a request to transfer to a different work shift may not be considered a reasonable accommodation.

c. Situations may arise in which the employer will need additional information regarding the disability and the employee's level of functioning.

    i. The employee may need to undergo an evaluation by a health care professional.

    ii. In order to be protected under the ADA, the employee is obligated to cooperate with this aspect of the interactive process.

    iii. The employer has the final discretion to choose a reasonable accommodation.

    iv. If an employee refuses to accept the employer's offer of reasonable accommodation, the employee then may not be qualified to remain in the job.

    v. The employee first bears the burden of proof that an accommodation would be considered reasonable. That burden then shifts to the employer to prove that the accommodation would cause an undue hardship.

8. Almost all federal courts, as well as the EEOC, are in agreement that an employer must consider reassigning an employee who is no longer able to perform his or her job because of impairment. There is general agreement on the following points:

a. Reassignment is available only to employees and not to job applicants.

b. Employees on probationary status who have been performing the job satisfactorily may be entitled to reassignment.

c. An employer is not required to create a new position by "bumping" another employee.

    d. An employer is not required to promote an employee as a reassignment. This includes promoting an individual with impairment from a part-time position to a full-time position or hourly to a salaried position.

    e. Employees may only be reassigned to a job that they are qualified to perform and the EEOC and courts agree that reassignment should be considered as a "last resort."

J. The Job Accommodation Network (JAN) is a service of the Office of Disability Employment Policy of the U.S. Department of Labor. JAN's mission is to facilitate the employment and retention of workers with disabilities by providing employers, employment providers, people with disabilities, family members, and other interested parties such as case managers with information on job accommodations.

K. A 2005 survey with employers that used the JAN network, conducted by the University of Iowa's Law, Health Policy, and Disability Center (LHPDC) found that:

    1. In more than half of the accommodations needed by employees and job applicants with disabilities, there was no cost involved. Of the accommodations that did require expenditures, the typical cost by employers was around $600.

    2. Employers experienced multiple direct and indirect benefits after making the accommodations. The top three most frequently mentioned direct benefits were:

        a. The accommodation allowed the company to retain a qualified employee

        b. The accommodation eliminated the cost of training a new employee

        c. The accommodation increased the workers' productivity.

L. Drug and alcohol issues under the ADA

    1. Case managers are oftentimes confronted with how to handle circumstances surrounding the employment of individuals who have a drug and/or alcohol (substance) addiction.

    2. A frequent question case managers raise is, If the individual has been terminated because of conduct related to drug or alcohol addiction, do they have rehire rights under the ADA? Another issue is, Can the organization refuse to rehire the individual following successful rehabilitation?

    3. The ADA protects qualified individuals with drug addiction if they have been rehabilitated. However, the ADA does not protect employees currently engaging in drug and/or alcohol use.

    4. The Courts have ruled that organizations cannot make a rehire decision based solely upon an individual's disability, whether it be drug, alcohol, or other impairment.

    5. If an employer has a neutral no-rehire policy, one that refuses to rehire an employee who was terminated for violating workplace conduct rules, then the policy is considered legitimate, and nondiscriminatory.

      6. While the ADA does not protect an employee or applicant who is currently engaging in drug use, it protects qualified individuals with a drug addiction who have been successfully rehabilitated.

  M. The role of mitigating and/or corrective measures

      1. The Supreme Court has ruled that the use of mitigating measures, such as medications, corrective lenses, prosthetic devices, and the body's ability to compensate for impairment, are to be a part of determining whether an individual has a disability under the ADA.

      2. When assessing an individual, the case manager must consider whether or not the individual is using any mitigating and/or corrective measures. The individual's actual circumstances must be assessed in this process.

      3. The case manager needs to understand that mitigating measures may lessen or eliminate limitations caused by impairment. Both the positive and negative effects of mitigating or corrective measures need to be considered in the assessment process.

  N. Social Security Benefits and the ADA

      1. In a disability case management program, the case manager may be confronted with a situation in which an employee on Social Security Disability Income (SSDI) may seek protection under the ADA.

      2. The Supreme Court has declared that because the qualification standards for social security benefits and the ADA are not the same, that application for receiving social security benefits is not inconsistent with being a qualified individual with a disability under ADA.

      3. The implications of this may be that when individuals on SSDI seek to RTW and identify themselves as qualified to do the essential functions of the job. The conflict is that they have stated in the social security application that they are not gainfully employable.

      4. The Courts have ruled that this is not inconsistent and that the individual may still be able to perform the essential functions of the job with or without reasonable accommodation.

      5. The case manager should be aware that there is a possibility that an individual receiving social security benefits would still be protected under the ADA and would require reasonable accommodation to RTW especially if they are qualified to perform the essential functions of the job.

■ THE TICKET TO WORK AND WORK INCENTIVE IMPROVEMENT ACT: A RESOURCE TO DISABILITY CASE MANAGEMENT PROGRAMS

  A. In November 1999, Congress passed the Ticket to Work and Work Incentive Improvement Act (TWWIIA) to give individuals with disabilities both the incentive and the means to seek employment.

B. The threat of losing health care coverage has been a barrier to competitive employment for many individuals with a disability.

1. It has been noted that 70% of people with disabilities are unemployed.

2. Individuals with disabilities who rely on Medicaid or Medicare for their health coverage have been at risk of losing their coverage if their income or savings exceeds certain limited levels.

3. The TWWIIA addresses the problem of a loss of health care coverage by allowing states to extend coverage under Medicaid to certain workers with disabilities.

   a. The workers are permitted to either purchase Medicaid coverage or extend Medicaid eligibility.

   b. The law extends Medicare hospital insurance coverage for an additional 4½ years to beneficiaries with disabilities who lose their Social Security Disability assistance when they RTW.

4. Thirty-eight states have received grants created under the TWWIIA called *Medicaid Infrastructure Grants*.

   a. The grants enable states to increase services and supports to workers and help others RTW without fear of losing health coverage.

   b. Grants have ranged from $1.5 million to $5.8 million over 4 years.

5. The TWWIIA also created a demonstration program that allows states to receive funding to develop a program that provides Medicaid-equivalent coverage to workers with health conditions that, without medical treatment, would cause them to become disabled. The demonstration will give states the opportunity to evaluate whether providing these workers early access to Medicaid services delays the progression of actual disability.

6. The Ticket to Work and Self-Sufficiency Program is the cornerstone of the TWWIIA and is a key component of the New Freedom Initiative.

   a. The goal of the Ticket program is to give disability beneficiaries the opportunity to achieve steady, long-term employment by providing them with greater choices and opportunities to go to work if they choose to do so.

   b. Under this program, Social Security beneficiaries with disabilities may obtain employment, vocational rehabilitation, or other support services from public and private organizations called *employment networks*.

   c. The employment networks can receive a dollar value for up to 5 years for every eligible individual for whom they provide jobs and/or services (or service coordination) as long as that individual is employed and remains employed according to the program requirements.

■ OTHER RESOURCES FOR DISABILITY CASE MANAGEMENT PROGRAMS

A. The Disability Management Employers Coalition, Inc. (DMEC) is a national organization that focuses on education and training of employers.

1. DMEC promotes an integrated approach to employer programs in disability and health management, absence, and productivity management.
2. DMEC has developed, in association with the Insurance Education Association (IEA), the Certified Professional in Disability Management (CPDM) Program. This program provides training to industry-specific personnel who are involved in the integrated process.

B. The Integrated Benefits Institute, located in San Francisco, California, provides research, discussion and analysis, and date of services to improve integrated benefits programs.

C. The Washington Business Group on Health (WBGH) has taken an active role in educating the industry on disability management. WBGH coordinates an annual national conference on disability management topics.

D. The American Association of Occupational Health Nurses (AAOHN) and the American College of Occupational and Environmental Medicine (ACOEM) provide disability management and RTW services in addition to OH programs for employers.

■ OTHER IMPORTANT DISABILITY LAWS

A. Employment
1. *Section 501, Rehabilitation Act 1973:* Requires affirmative action and nondiscrimination in employment by federal agencies of the executive branch.
2. *Section 503, Rehabilitation Act:* Requires affirmative action and prohibits employment discrimination by federal government contractors and subcontractors with contracts of more than $10,000.
3. *Section 188, Workforce Investment Act:* Prohibits discrimination against people with disabilities in employment service centers funded by the federal government.

B. State and local government programs and services
1. *Americans with Disabilities Act, Title II:* Prohibits discrimination in the provision of public benefits and services (e.g., public education, employment, transportation, recreation, health care, social services, courts, voting, and town meetings).
2. *Section 504, Rehabilitation Act:* Requires that buildings and facilities that are designed, constructed, or altered with federal funds, or leased by a federal agency, comply with federal standards for physical accessibility.

■ INTEGRATED DISABILITY CASE MANAGEMENT STRATEGIES

A. Disability case management should encompass both occupational and nonoccupational disabilities and be fully integrated with STD, LTD, and WC programs.

B. Often, the first groups of benefits to be integrated are STD and WC.

C. The disability case management process should involve establishing clinical guidelines and expectations that can assist with the medical management of disabilities.

D. Employing a managed care network minimizes time lost accessing specialty physicians and treatment providers.

E. Using one source to provide medical equipment, pharmaceuticals, and other supplies can promote efficiency of delivery and cost containment.

F. Having onsite wellness programs benefits all areas of health and disability management.

G. Qualified professionals can create therapeutic RTW protocols as a part of the program. Use of these protocols ensures quality and cost effectiveness.

H. Transitional work and modified-duty programs are essential components of disability case management programs. They are especially effective in returning employees to work and add to the productivity of the work force.

I. Integrated disability case management strategies ensure that injured employees have timely intervention, medical, disability, and RTW management. Integrated disability case management programs often include OH case management as a fundamental component.

■ OCCUPATIONAL HEALTH CASE MANAGEMENT

A. According to AAOHN, occupational and environmental health nursing is the specialty practice that provides for and delivers health and safety programs and services to workers, workers' families, worker populations, and community groups.

B. Whenever case management services are provided to workers, worker populations, or persons whose care is financed by an employer's benefit program, the implications for the individuals' health status and functional recovery must be coordinated with OH and RTW goals and objectives.

C. OH case management involves the management of occupational (WC) disability, nonoccupational disability, and incidental absence from work.

D. OH case management is designed to prevent fragmented care and delayed recovery while facilitating the employee's recovery and appropriate RTW in a full-duty or modified work capacity.

E. OH case management includes the development of preventive systems and the mobilization of appropriate resources for care over the course of the health event.

F. OH case management and medical care is delivered with the ultimate goal of returning the worker to pre-illness or pre-injury function or to the highest level of functioning achievable in the most cost-effective and time-efficient manner.

G. Standards of practice for OH nurses have been established by AAOHN.[3]

---

[3]Standards of practice may be obtained by contacting AAOHN at *www.aaohn.org* or by calling (800) 241-8014.

■ ROLE OF OH CASE MANAGERS

A. The scope and role of the OH case manager providing services vary depending on the nature of the business setting, expectations of the employer, role assignments, and philosophy of the OH program.

B. OH case managers, in collaboration with other providers, such as physicians, play an integral role in determining, facilitating, and expediting the appropriate RTW of employees who are absent from work due to occupational or nonoccupational injuries or illnesses, or both. This also may include the delivery of case management services to the worker's dependents.

C. Case management has generally been an integral component of OH programs but is becoming more formalized as a specialty within the field of practice. The OH scope of practice has expanded today to include:
1. Health promotion
2. Emergency preparedness in response to natural, technological, and human hazards to work and community environments

D. In addition to assessing, planning, directing, coordinating, implementing, managing, monitoring, and evaluating care, the OH case manager establishes or qualifies a provider network, recommends treatment plans, monitors outcomes, and maintains a strong communication link among all the parties (AAOHN, 1996).

E. OH case managers coordinate the proactive efforts of the multidisciplinary health care team to facilitate an individual's health care services from the onset of injury or illness to a safe RTW or an optimal alternative. This may include:
1. Coordinating treatment, follow up, and referrals, as well as emergency care for job related injuries and illnesses
2. Gatekeeping for health services, rehabilitation, RTW, and case management issues
3. Influencing employers' health care quality and cost containment
4. Providing counseling and crisis intervention, developing health education programs, and working with employers to comply with workplace laws and regulations

F. OH case managers may conduct research on effects of workplace exposures, gathering health data, and using this information to prevent injury and illness.

G. OH case managers are most often registered professional nurses or vocational rehabilitation counselors.
1. According to Cesta and Tahan (2003), employers in the OH areas of case management practice, are increasingly requiring a certification in case management as a prerequisite credential for hiring.
2. Professional certifications for OH case managers include:
   a. Certified case manager (CCM)
   b. Certified OH nurse (COHN)

    c. Certified OH nurse specialist (COHN-S)

    d. Certified OH nurse case manager (COHN/CM)

    e. Certified OH nurse specialist/case manager (COHN-S/CM)

    f. Certified disability management specialist (CDMS)

H. OH case managers generally belong to the AAOHN, the Case Management Society of America (CMSA), or a similarly oriented professional organization.

■ KEY CONCEPTS OF OH CASE MANAGEMENT

A. Goals of OH case management programs include (DiBenedetto, 1998, 2000):

1. Facilitating the employee's RTW in a timely manner
2. Assisting employees in navigating the benefit and medical care arenas
3. Minimizing lost time in the workplace
4. Decreasing the cost of lost-time benefit programs such as STD and LTD, salary continuation, and WC
5. Facilitating employers' control of disability issues
6. Improving corporate competitiveness
7. Maximizing use of employer resources
8. Reducing the cost of disability
9. Enhancing employees' morale by valuing their physical and cultural diversity
10. Protecting the employability of the worker
11. Ensuring compliance with relevant laws and organizations, such as the ADA, FMLA, OSHA, and Department of Transportation (DOT)
12. Ensuring the delivery of quality services

B. The American College of Occupational and Environmental Medicine (ACOEM) has developed clinical practice guidelines for potentially work-related health problems in worker populations, entitled *Occupational Medicine Practice Guidelines: Evaluation and Management of Common Health Problems and Functional Recovery in Workers*, 2nd Edition (2004).

C. The Occupational Medicine Practice Guidelines (OMPGs):

1. Are based on the injured workers' presenting complaints
2. Emphasize prevention
3. Emphasize proper clinical evaluation
4. Provide guidance for medical and disability management

D. Guidelines are invaluable as a frame of reference when used in conjunction with other factors of disability, work requirements, values and belief systems, and so forth.

E. Guidelines that are important for OH case management, other than the OMPGs, include the disability duration guidelines (DDGs) and specified recovery guidelines (SRGs).

1. The DDGs help the provider and OH case manager to determine a person's potential for RTW within a given time frame.
   a. A variety of DDGs are available for determining the potential length of a worker's absence due to injury or illness; examples include:
      i. The Medical Disability Advisor
      ii. Occupational Disability Guidelines
      iii. Milliman
2. The SRGs assist by establishing a benchmark or expected time frame during which a worker recovers from his or her disability or injury.
3. Persons with the same diagnosis or medical condition will recover at different rates and be able to RTW within a general time frame; however, recovery is as variable as a person's individuality.

F. Disability and ability to RTW are dependent on the worker's healing or adaptation to illness or injury and the scope of his or her job functions.

G. Functional capacity assessments (FCAs) are used in OH case management programs and by OH case managers to directly measure a person's functional ability to perform specific work-related tasks.
1. An FCA may be requested by the OH professional/case manager, human resources, provider, adjustor, or other key stakeholder.
2. The FCA involves examining an individual as he or she performs activities in a structured setting. It does not necessarily reflect what the person should be able to do, rather what he or she can do or is willing to do at the time of the evaluation.
3. The FCA depends on motivation, cognitive awareness, behavioral factors, and sincerity of effort, all of which have a major impact on the FCA (AMA, 2002).

H. There are three primary tools used in OH case management programs that assist in returning individuals to work and in planning the care and necessary treatments. These are:
1. Functional job analysis that is used to help return the injured worker to his or her pre-injury occupation or job. The job analysis defines job requirements and lists and describes the job's essential and nonessential functions. It should be current and representative of the employee's job responsibilities and should always be shared with the treating physician or provider and the OH case manager to aid in RTW planning.
2. Independent medical examination (IME) that is used to confirm a person's diagnosis, current medical treatment and care, the scope and nature of disability, the potential for permanent disability and impairment, ability to RTW, and medical information and testing outcomes. The IME provider never becomes the treating physician.
3. Second opinion examination (SOE) that also is used to confirm a person's diagnosis, provide more information, and make recommendations for potential treatment options. Often the employee may choose to be treated by the SOE provider.

I. Occupational or vocational rehabilitation services are often used in OH case management as treatment options in addition to the usual medical and physical rehabilitation. The main goal is to restore the employee's function and return him or her to the pre-injury state.

J. Work hardening is also used in OH case management. It is therapy that mimics actual work demands and includes exercises and work-simulated activities that are monitored by professionals to allow the injured worker to gradually build up his or her work task tolerance. Work hardening activities may be provided at the work site under the supervision of physical therapists and the OH case manager (DiBenedetto, 2000).

■ SUCCESS FACTORS FOR OH CASE MANAGEMENT PROGRAMS

A. Know the organization's employee benefits program.[4]
   1. In addition to WC, STD, LTD, and sick pay programs, monetary benefits often can be obtained through life insurance programs, pension programs, retirement, and union and state disability benefits.
   2. This information usually can be accessed through the human resources or benefits departments, which is why members from these disciplines make good RTW program team members.

B. Know the organization's most commonly occurring illnesses and disabilities. Identifying these is beneficial for the safety or OH case manager so that clinical pathways/guidelines or established modified jobs can focus on these frequent disabilities.
   1. If the in-house case manager does not have a medical background, this information can be sought from a medical case manager, OH nurse/case manager, or established primary treating physician.

C. Selecting vendors
   1. Select a network of providers that not only covers tertiary care but that specializes in the core area that the organization predominantly needs.
   2. Maintain a provider database that lists both their addresses and specialties.
   3. Select vendors who are invested in the employees and will assist in the implementation of the RTW program.
   4. If possible, implement a software program that will enhance communications between the organization and its vendors.

D. Education
   1. The case manager, in collaboration with the employer's representative or team, will need to educate all parties involved in the RTW program.

---

[4]Adapted from "Disability case management," by L. Wright, M. H. Eggleston, and D. V. DiBenedetto (2000). In S. K. Powell and D. Ignatavicius (Eds.), *CMSA core curriculum for case management* (pp. 181–194). Philadelphia: Lippincott Williams & Wilkins.

2. Education should begin before implementation so that all divisions associated with the program have become thoroughly acquainted with it and understand their role in its success and purpose.
3. Education should also include the case manager who is managing individuals' care both proactively and after disability.
4. Providing employees with information on the organization's policies and procedures can prepare them in the event of a disability or disease.
5. Proactively providing the access channels, corporate policy, and structure can minimize many of the traditional obstacles that prevent people with a disability from returning to gainful activity.

E. Accessibility
   1. The OH case manager must remain accessible to both the employees and employers.
   2. Delegation is an important skill the case manager can learn. He or she should be prepared to guide employees to the appropriate division to obtain the information they are seeking.
   3. State and federal laws and statutes often have minute changes that can affect individuals' benefits significantly. Although informed OH case managers are aware of much of this information, it is usually best if it is provided by an individual in that discipline—that is, benefits, human resources, or bargaining union.

F. Modified or transitional duty team
   1. Productivity management is the goal driving the RTW program. To maximize productivity management, an organization needs to minimize costs associated with it.
   2. From a disability perspective, costs can encompass "hard dollar" savings by minimizing loss time, training time, and medical costs, or "soft dollar" savings by improving employee morale.
   3. The OH case management team should meet routinely and should be led by the OH case manager.
      a. The OH case manager may often be the primary coordinator of the RTW program.
      b. In other cases, the team may be chaired by representatives of the organization (e.g., human resources and OH).

G. Clinical aspects
   1. The OH case management program may benefit from an assigned precertification program.
   2. Thorough clinical communication and documentation should be made so that administrative personnel can make informed decisions.
   3. An OH case manager with related credentials and experience in occupational illness or injuries, and RTW clinical, vocational, and psychological aspects of injury, disability, and disease would likely be best suited for this position.
   4. An RTW support group would provide avenues for shared experiences and peer assistance.

5. Make available an early intervention program with clear access method.
   a. Many employers have adopted a call-in telephone number or reporting line.
   b. Timely access through one source can minimize lost and delayed reported claims.
   c. It may be of benefit to standardize the intake format so the emergency or treating physicians become familiar with the specific information you need or how to ask for information they need to document the claim appropriately.
6. Implementation of a communications protocol.
   a. Often, losing or displacing employees arises from a lack of communication between the employer and the injured employee.
   b. Traditional WC field case managers have reported that one of their primary obstacles in returning an injured worker back to his or her place of employment is the worker's perception that the employer lacks interest in the worker and does not wish for his or her return—that he or she may somehow now be "labeled."
   c. In-house OH case management programs facilitate effective communication skills and can accomplish this goal.
7. EAPs are excellent resources for OH case managers and can provide confidential counseling services for a variety of needs.
   a. OH case managers need to be aware of other problems that can arise from an individual's disability such as financial difficulties (e.g., reduced income), dependency difficulties (e.g., single parent), or addiction (e.g., prescription drugs).
   b. With the OH case manager's trained ear, the ill or injured employee can be referred to an EAP should concerns arise about his or her emotional well-being.
8. If the organization has the capability, establish an employee wellness program. This program can be in house or can be in partnership with a local facility. Such programs have the capacity to:
   a. Facilitate onsite extended physical and occupational therapy services
   b. Allow a specially devised program to combine both therapy and job functions in the RTW processes
   c. Implement proactive wellness incentives and programs
   d. Coordinate with the wellness program's routine health screens and education on routine aging illnesses and concerns (e.g., high-cholesterol diets, high blood pressure)
   e. Encourage corporate physical activities (e.g., walks, aerobics, softball team) that are designed to provide employees with the recommended weekly exercise regimens.

H. Coordination of program
1. The OH case manager is ultimately the RTW coordinator in the absence of an RTW coordinator at the employer's site.

a. As the RTW coordinator, the case manager maintains regular contact with all key stakeholders:
   i. Injured or sick worker and family
   ii. Treating physician
   iii. Other treatment providers
   iv. Worker's supervisor and management
   v. Medical, OH, and wellness departments
   vi. Human resources and employee benefits
   vii. External case management (as appropriate)
   viii. Claims adjuster or TPA
   ix. Modified or transitional duty team
   x. EAP (as appropriate)

b. Establishing workflow procedures
   i. The OH case manager must be immediately advised that a claim has been filed.
   ii. If the claim warrants specialty care, the case manager can advise of the referral and submit to the treating physician a description of the worker's job functions.
   iii. The case manager should expect from the physician time frames for medical or rehabilitation intervention and estimates on the duration of the worker's treatment and rehabilitation plans; and what, if any, physical limitations may be permanent.
   iv. Important information should be provided to the members of the case management team.

c. The OH case manager:
   i. May assume responsibility for providing the treating physician with a description of a modified duty/job and for authorization to release the employee back to work on either a limited, part-time, or full-time basis
   ii. Communicates the treating physician's projections to the benefits division so that benefits providers can be informed
   iii. Coordinates with the team all activities of the RTW process and plan of care
      (a) Implementation is achieved through supervision, documentation, monitoring, and communication.
      (b) The case manager executes the process and follows it through.
   iv. Documents progress, addresses pitfalls, and consults with administration, precertification, managed care, health care, or any other outside provider who is not part of the internal modified duty team
   v. Assists in the availability of quality care for all people by eliminating providers or participants recognized for acts of abuse or fraud. Having access to all medical files improves

the chances that fraudulent or "laissez-faire" practices are identified

    vi. Promotes effective, intensive medical care to bring about healthy outcomes

  d. The OH case manager's knowledge is instrumental in reporting satisfaction with the providers of service.

  e. The OH case manager has an ethical and professional obligation to ensure that the client—the injured or ill person—receives appropriate, quality medical intervention and is not placed at risk for further injury. Continuity of medical care and its proper sequencing is necessary for promoting the patient's early RTW.

  f. Cost-contained quality medical care can be afforded to all employees who require it by systematically streamlining access to quality care and monitoring standards and progress of care or service provided.

2. Corporate policy

  a. Corporate policy and pressures are frequently focused on productivity and finance.

  b. The OH case manager must sensitively meet the needs of both the employer and the employee when coordinating the RTW program.

  c. Juggling personalities and problems is what effective OH case managers are often recognized for, despite their intensive training within their own discipline. For example, accessing ergonomic specialists who can make work-site accommodations for modified duty or injury prevention programs is an excellent tool for combining productivity management with employee needs.

■ MAXIMIZING WORKFORCE HEALTH AND PRODUCTIVITY

A. Proactive education of the employee in the organization's total benefits program can promote employee morale; reduce lost time, malingering, litigated costs, and training and production costs; and foster a supportive work environment.

B. Workforce management centers on the concept of managing all aspects of occupational disability and proactive health and safety information and training, aggressive management (including case management) of occupational and nonoccupational lost-time cases and effective RTW within the regulatory arena specific to the employer (DiBenedetto, 2000).

C. Workforce management is concerned with (DiBenedetto, 1998):

1. Demographics of the employer's worker populations
2. OH and non-OH management
3. Health and productivity programs, metrics, and outcomes
4. Benefit plan design that augments the needs of the worker population
5. Consideration of work, life, and family impacts on the worker population and the impact on their ability to be at work
6. Integrating benefit programs such as integrated disability management, OH case management, and coordinated RTW programs

D. Transitional Work Duty

1. Transitional work duty (TWD) programs are progressive, individualized, time-limited programs that focus on returning the injured and disabled employee to the original employment site, however with some restrictions.

2. Transitional work allows the injured worker to perform productive work at the workplace under the direction of rehabilitation professionals. The program may include progressive conditioning, on-site work activities, education for safe work practices, work re-adjustment and Job Modification. The costs associated to a transitional work program are rehab costs charged to the surplus fund.

3. TWD programs use structured protocols of "value-added temporary positions" that are focused on RTW. The protocols are carefully designed to be appropriate for the skills, knowledge, and capabilities of the recovering employee so that the work can be accomplished safely.

4. A TWD assignment is temporary in nature and complies with all medical restrictions indicated by the employee's treating physician. It may involve modification of the injured employee's job duties, i.e., tailoring work duties to the injured employee's medical limitations and vocational abilities to maximize recovery, or alternate work that is compatible with the employee's job skills and experience.

5. TWD programs cover all compensable disabling conditions insured under Workers Compensation and are limited to employees with temporary impairments.

6. The TWD assignment is documented by a Transitional Work Plan that is written for a specific period of time (90 calendar days on average). The Plan is signed by the injured employee and the department supervisor or representative.

7. Employees with temporary partial disabilities are eligible for transitional work if they are anticipated to progress in their recovery from an industrial injury or illness and require temporary, short-term modification of their job duties.

8. Employees with restrictions that would permanently prevent them from returning to the job and hours worked at the time of their injury are not eligible for participation in the TWD programs.

9. Employees who participate in TWD programs obtain written medical documentation from their treating physician or health care professional indicating their specific work restrictions.

10. The benefits of a formalized TWD program include the following:
    a. Injured employees return to work sooner than those not provided with transitional work duty opportunities
    b. Claims costs can be reduced
    c. Employees recover faster than those that attempt recovery while at home
    d. Reduced litigation
    e. Avoidance of the time and expense involved in hiring and training replacement workers

    f. Injured employees maintain productivity while dollars pay for actual work

    g. Reduction in fraud

    h. Increased employee morale

■ MODELS OF OH CASE MANAGEMENT

A. OH case management is generally provided by OH case managers and physicians who are familiar with the employee's job tasks, conditions of work, work processes, benefit programs, supervisors, and community providers.[5]

B. OH case managers possess knowledge of medical and vocational aspects of disability, OH and safety practices, relevant work conditions, health promotion, regulatory issues, benefit programs, and RTW requirements.

C. OH case management service delivery models include:

    1. Onsite case management services—Services are provided by the employer's own staff or designee (i.e., vendor) at the actual workplace. These services may involve actual client contact in the workplace, by phone, or through field visits.

    2. Telephonic case management—Services are coordinated through electronic communication. Services may be provided on an interstate or intrastate basis.

    3. Offsite or field case management services—Services are provided outside of the employer's workplace, generally by a TPA, insurance company, or OH case management vendor. In some cases, the employer's OH case managers may conduct field visits to the employee, provider, or carrier to facilitate appropriate case management services and RTW.

    4. OH case management settings include acute care hospitals and systems; corporations; social insurance programs; public and private insurance sectors; fee-for-service, managed care, and case management organizations; government, military, and government-sponsored programs; and provider agencies and facilities.

D. The OH case management process (ABOHN, 2004) consists of the following steps:

    1. Assessment

        a. Establishes criteria and uses case finding and screening to identify workers who are appropriate candidates for OH or disability case management

        b. Conducts comprehensive assessment of employees

        c. Assesses employee's and organization's informal and formal support systems

---

[5]Adapted from "Occupational health case management," by D. V. DiBenedetto (2000). In S. K. Powell and D. Ignatavicius (Eds.), *CMSA core curriculum for case management* (pp. 195–212). Philadelphia: Lippincott Williams & Wilkins.

    d. Assesses community, workplace, and vendor resources

    e. Assesses essential functions of job (physical and mental demands) to facilitate hiring, proper placement, and RTW activities

    f. Identifies gaps that exist in the service continuum

    g. Periodically reassesses the health status of the worker

    h. Assesses the need for health-risk appraisals, for safety, accident prevention, wellness, and health promotion programs

    i. Conducts comprehensive assessment of all disability-related expenses and benefit utilization

    j. Assesses workplace policies on RTW and job accommodations

    k. Identifies legal, labor, and regulatory implications

    l. Assesses disability plans, policies, procedures, and communication links

    m. Identifies roles and responsibilities of the worker, supervisor or manager, case manager, benefits-risk manager, health care providers, TPAs and insurers, and others, as needed

    n. Recognizes challenges to successful outcomes

2. Planning

    a. Reviews worker's goals

    b. Reviews employer's and corporate goals for integrated health management team approach

    c. Prepares analysis and synthesis of all data to formulate an appropriate plan of care

    d. Uses appropriate components of employee benefits plan(s)

    e. Analyzes and synthesizes data to formulate appropriate diagnoses and interdisciplinary problem statements

    f. Plans and balances the needs of the worker's RTW

    g. Coordinates service providers responsible for furnishing services

    h. Participates in special provider arrangements; for example, preferred provider organizations (PPOs), health maintenance organizations (HMOs), point-of-service organizations (POSs), and managed care contractors

    i. Collaborates with community, workplace, and vendor personnel

    j. Develops a plan of care or an RTW plan, including health care and medical treatment goals, through an interdisciplinary and collaborative group process, which includes the employee and his or her caregivers

    k. Participates in development of programs for safety, accident prevention, and health promotion to prevent future occurrence of injury and illness cases

    l. Coordinates administration of case management services among benefit plans, including WC and OH

    m. Applies principles consistent with the ADA in preplacement and ongoing job placement activities

    n. Participates in disability plan design and policy and procedure development

3. Implementation
    a. Links the worker with the most appropriate community resources
    b. Acts as a liaison with health care providers
    c. Coordinates access to quality, cost-effective care and services
    d. Coordinates clinical and medical management of cases
    e. Implements early RTW/modified-duty programs
    f. Facilitates rehabilitation and job accommodation for WC and nonoccupational disabilities and/or injuries
    g. Provides appropriate education for the worker, family, providers, and community resources
    h. Assists the worker in negotiating the health care system
    i. Develops and maintains standards, policies, and protocols to support the case management process
    j. Participates with interagency groups and community agencies to support or represent the case management program
    k. Prepares for legal proceedings
    l. Provides testimony during legal proceedings
    m. Assures confidentiality and complies with established codes of ethics and legal or regulatory requirements
    n. Documents case management activities and outcomes
    o. Participates in public speaking and marketing related to case management services and the programs involved
    p. Functions as an employee advocate and balances the needs of the workplace with the needs of the worker
4. Evaluation
    a. Manages data and information systems for the purposes of research, trend analysis, program modification and evaluation, and continuous quality/performance improvement
    b. Evaluates quality of management efforts, teamwork, and workflow design
    c. Monitors and modifies the RTW plan
    d. Monitors the worker and others to ensure a smooth transition to work and continued progress
    e. Evaluates and monitors the plan of care/RTW plan to ensure its quality, efficiency, timeliness, and effectiveness
    f. Ensures that services are appropriate, cost effective, and supportive of worker independence
    g. Monitors the worker's decision-making abilities regarding choices, utilization of resources, and consequences
    h. Evaluates worker's outcomes to determine case disposition
    i. Evaluates the effectiveness of safety, accident prevention, and wellness/health promotion programs
    j. Evaluates disability-related expenses and programs for program or benefit enhancement and refinement, as well as for areas of duplication

    k. Tracks and evaluates program outcomes periodically for success of case management activities (e.g., reduced cost, reduced accidents, reduced severity, efficiency of process, and customer satisfaction)

    l. Evaluates due diligence of providers and provider networks

    m. Participates in public speaking, marketing, and research related to case management services and the programs provided

■ THE KNOWLEDGE BASE REQUIRED FOR OH AND DISABILITY CASE MANAGERS

A. The following knowledge, skills, and abilities are needed to function effectively as an OH or disability case manager (ABOHN, 2004):

1. Process of case management
2. Rehabilitation principles, e.g., work hardening/conditioning, functional capacity evaluation, worker and workplace
3. Fitness for duty, vocational rehabilitation, e.g., labor market survey, transferable skills analysis
4. Prevention and wellness promotion
5. Federal regulatory programs, e.g., Family Medical Leave Act (FMLA), Employee Retirement Income Security Act (ERISA), Americans with Disabilities Act (ADA), Social Security Insurance (SSI), Consolidated Omnibus Budget Reconciliation Act (COBRA), Department of Transportation (DOT), Occupational Safety and Health Administration (OSHA), U.S. Federal Regulatory, and Ministry of Labor (Canada)
6. State regulatory programs, e.g., WC, statutory disability
7. Liability issues in case management
8. Legal/ethical issues, e.g., confidentiality, privacy (e.g., HIPAA [U.S.] and the protection of health information, PIDA [Canada])
9. Community/governmental agencies and resources
10. Life-care planning concepts
11. Statistical/data analysis, benchmarking, incidence, prevalence, trending, economic analysis
12. Tracking/measuring costs, cost: benefit, return on investment, trends analysis
13. Conflict management skills
14. Employee advocacy, balancing worker/workplace issues, negotiating skills, benchmarking, cost: benefit analysis
15. Oral and written communication skills
16. Decision-making ability
17. Problem-solving ability
18. Adult learning principles
19. Principles of teaching
20. Marketing internal/external
21. Principles of quality improvement, e.g., continuous quality improvement (CQI), total quality management (TQM), International Standards Organization (ISO) 9000, ISO 14,001
22. Protocol development/utilization

23. Understanding of the role and function of case management participants, i.e., human resource personnel, benefits managers, insurance carriers, TPAs, risk managers, safety professionals, line managers, external providers, labor relations, and legal counsel
24. Use of information technology
25. Sociocultural influences
26. Principles of utilization review and precertification
27. Alternative treatment modalities
28. Job analysis
29. Principles of management/utilization of resources
30. System abuse, e.g., fraudulent practices by worker, employer, or vendor
31. Health care delivery systems, e.g., health insurance, managed care models (HMO, PPO, POS)
32. Trends in case management, i.e., disability, WC, rehabilitation, integrated models, etc.
33. Disability plan designs, e.g., STD, LTD, WC
34. Disability terminology and concepts, e.g., IME, second opinion, impairment ratings, deductibles, co-pays, indemnity, reserves
35. Contractual agreements, i.e., with workers, employers, vendors, TPAs, unions
36. Clinical guidelines, clinical pathways, algorithms, standards of care
37. Screening tools, e.g., CAGE, health-risk appraisals, depression screening
38. Role of the case managers on the interdisciplinary team

■ RETURN TO WORK PROGRAMS

A. In OH case management, case managers are not only concerned about ensuring appropriate medical care but must also address, from the initial assessment on the date of injury or illness, the goal of returning an individual to productive work at the earliest possible time in either a transitional, modified, or full-duty capacity.[6]

B. The ultimate goal of OH case management is to assist the ill or injured person to achieve the highest level of medical improvement and to facilitate his or her successful RTW in the most cost-effective and efficient manner.

C. Companies should have in place formal RTW policies and procedures to expedite the injured worker's effective RTW in a timely manner.

D. Employer RTW programs should allow for the following types of work assignments:

---

[6]Adapted from "Occupational health case management," by D. V. DiBenedetto (2000). In S. K. Powell and D. Ignatavicius (Eds.), *CMSA core curriculum for case management* (pp. 195–212). Philadelphia: Lippincott Williams & Wilkins.

1. Full duty
2. Temporary, alternative, or transitional work
3. Modified-duty assignments

E. RTW assignments that focus on "other than full duty" must be reviewed on a regular basis by both the OH case manager and company to ensure the employee is progressing as planned.

REFERENCES

American Association of Occupational Health Nurses (AAOHN). (1996). *Position statement: The occupational health nurse as case manager.* Atlanta, GA: AAOHN.

American Association of Occupational Health Nurses (AAOHN). (2006). Occupational and environmental health nursing profession fact sheet. Website: *http:www.aaohn.org.* Retrieved February 20, 2006.

American Board for Occupational Health Nursing (ABOHN). (2004). *Candidate handbook case management examination.* Hinsdale, IL: ABOHN.

American College of Occupational and Environmental Medicine (ACOEM). (2004). *Occupational medicine practice guidelines: Evaluation and management of common health problems and functional recovery in workers,* 2nd ed. Beverly Farms, MA: OEM Press.

American Medical Association (AMA). (2002). *Guide to the evaluation of permanent impairment,* 5th ed. Chicago: AMA.

Americans with Disabilities Act of 1990, 41 U.S.C., section 12101 *et seq.*

Cesta, T. G., & Tahan, H. A. (2003). *The case manager's survival guide: Winning strategies for clinical practice,* 2nd ed. St. Louis, MO: Mosby.

Cherry Engineering Support Services, Inc. (2003). Federal statutory definitions of disability prepared for the Interagency Committee on Disability Research, United States Department of Health & Human Services, Washington, D.C.

DiBenedetto, D. V. (1999). Benchmarking the effectiveness of integrated disability management strategies. *Total Health Management, 1*(1).

DiBenedetto, D. V. (2000). *Principles of workers' compensation and disability case management course.* Yonkers, NY: DV DiBenedetto & Associates.

The U. S. Equal Employment Opportunity Commission (EEOC). (October 17, 2002) Enforcement Guidance: Reasonable Accommodation and Undue Hardship under the Americans with Disabilities Act. EEOC, notice number 915.002. available on line at *http://www.eeoc.gov/policy/docs/accommodation.html.*

Job Accommodation Network (JAN) (2005), Fact Sheets Series, Workplace Accommodations: Low Cost, High Impact, New Research Findings Address the Cost and Benefits of Job Accommodation for People with Disabilities, available from: *www.jan.wvu.edu.*

Powell, S. K., & Ignatavicius, D. D. (2000). *CMSA core curriculum for case management.* Philadelphia: Lippincott Williams & Wilkins.

United States Department of Health & Human Services. The Surgeon General's call to action to improve the health and wellness of persons with disabilities. Website: *www.surgeongeneral.gov/library/disabilities/calltoaction/factsheetwhatwho.html.* Retrieved March 23, 2006.

SUGGESTED READING

Commission for Case Manager Certification (CCMC). (2005). *Glossary of terms.* Rolling Meadows, IL: CCMC.

Hursh, N., & Rosenthal, D. (2005/2006). Dynamic changes in the field of disability management: Responding to employer needs with broader responsibilities. *Care Management, 11*(6).

Vierling, L. (2002). *Court decisions involving the Americans with Disabilities Act: A resource guide for rehabilitation professionals.* Athens, GA: Elliott & Fitzpatrick, Inc.

Vierling, L. (2005). Courts interpret the Americans with Disabilities Act (ADA). In P. Deutsch & H. Sawyer, *A guide to rehabilitation—annual update.* White Plains, NY: Ahab Press, Inc.

Vierling, L. (2005). Disability legislation and rehabilitation. In D. L. Huber (Ed.), *Disease management: A guide for case managers.* St. Louis, MO: W. B. Saunders, Elsevier, Inc.

chapter 20

Disease Management and Case Management

Suzanne K. Powell
Hussein A. Tahan

LEARNING OBJECTIVES

Upon completion of this chapter, the reader will be able to:

1. Determine the similarities and differences between case management and disease management strategies.
2. Define important terms and concepts relative to disease management.
3. List the driving forces that lead to disease management programs.
4. Discuss important components to building a successful disease management program.
5. Describe factors that are important to the development, design, and implementation of a disease management program.
6. Identify the stages of the case management or disease management process.

IMPORTANT TERMS AND CONCEPTS

"At-Risk" Member
Best Practices
Component Management
   Model
Demand Management

Disease Management (DM)
   Model
Disease State Case Management
   (DSCM)
Disease State Management

Evidence-Based Guidelines/Health Care
Health Plan Employer Data and
  Information Set (HEDIS)
National Committee for Quality
  Assurance (NCQA)
Outcomes Measurement

Population Management
Practice Guidelines
Predictive Modeling
Quality Indicators (QI)
Report Card
Risk Screening

■ INTRODUCTION

A. Case management (CM) as a component of disease management (DM) versus DM as a component of CM

B. CM—Use of an *individual*-based approach; DM—use of a *population*-based approach. Both are multidisciplinary in nature and employ collaborative approaches to care delivery.

C. CM focuses on individual patients and operates across the continuum of care settings or delivery systems.

D. DM focuses on diseases within populations, and operates across the continuum of the disease.

E. DM emerged a little more than a decade ago in response to growing concern about the quality and cost of health care services for groups of individuals with common, chronic, and expensive health conditions such as diabetes, heart failure, and asthma.

F. DM programs target people with chronic illnesses for which long-term management, demand management, health education, health promotion and illness prevention, and close monitoring of symptoms can minimize or prevent acute exacerbations and complications (Huber, 2005).

G. DM programs were first implemented by managed care organizations as a service to their enrollees and employees and as an effort to reduce the expenses incurred in the care of employee with chronic conditions.

H. DM programs employ collaborative practice models of care. These models are multidisciplinary and consist of physicians, nurses, allied health professionals (such as dieticians), and support service providers.

I. According to the Disease Management Association of America (DMAA), DM is defined as "a system of coordinated health care interventions and communications for populations with conditions in which patient self-care efforts are significant" (DMAA, 2006). DM:

1. "Supports the physician or practitioner/patient relationship and plan of care;

2. Emphasizes prevention of exacerbations and complications utilizing evidence-based practice guidelines and patient empowerment strategies; and

3. Evaluates clinical, humanistic, and economic outcomes on an ongoing basis with the goal of improving overall health" (DMAA, 2006).

■ KEY DEFINITIONS

A. Best practices—Practices that have been determined to produce the most favorable outcomes; these practices have been gleaned from comparative quality measurements and are thought of as ideal standards with national or international reputation.

B. Component management model—In this model, the "components" are the various providers that a patient may require along the continuum. Each component, separately and episodically, may strive for cost-effective, quality care.

C. Demand management—"The use of self-management and decision support systems to enable, educate, and encourage people to improve their health and make appropriate use of medical care" (Nash and Todd, 1997, p. 331). Demand management usually involves 24/7 telephonic nurse triage lines.

D. Disease management model—A holistic model of care provision in which all the components are (ideally) working toward the good of the population or of patients with a particular disease state that is mainly chronic and complex in nature, such as heart failure.

E. Disease state management and disease state case management—

1. DM uses a set of prospectively determined interventions with the intent of altering the course of the disease, improving clinical and financial outcomes, as well as quality of life, while reducing health care costs. The goal is preventing exacerbation of illness and reducing of the effects of co-morbidities, thereby avoiding or delaying the onset of acute episodes of illness (Powell, 2000b).

2. DM brings together outcomes research and clinical management of diseases to provide efficient care to patient populations in a continuous quality improvement environment. Furthermore, DM is a continuous process focused on efficiency and is applied to selected patient populations (Nash and Todd, 1997).

3. DM is a comprehensive, integrated approach to care and reimbursement based on a disease's natural course, focusing on clinical and nonclinical interventions when and where they are most likely to have the greatest impact. Ideally, DM prevents exacerbation of a disease and use of expensive resources, making prevention and proactive CM two important areas of emphasis (Rieve, 1998).

4. Disease state case management (DSCM) is a population-based approach that identifies individuals with chronic diseases, assesses their health status, develops a program or plan of care, and collects data to evaluate the effectiveness of the process. DSCM proactively intervenes with treatment and education so that the individual with a chronic disease can maintain optimal function with the most cost-effective and outcome-effective health care expenditure. The goal of DSCM is to manage at-risk populations across the entire continuum of care (Levitt, Startz, and Higgins, 1998).

5. A system of coordinated health care interventions and communications for populations with conditions in which patients' self-care

efforts are significant. A DM program supports provider–patient relationship; emphasizes prevention of exacerbations using evidence-based protocols; and evaluates clinical, humanistic, and economic outcomes on an ongoing basis (Gorski, 2006).

F. Evidence-based guidelines, practice guidelines, practice parameters, and clinical practice guidelines—Defined by the Institute of Medicine as systematically developed statements to assist practitioner and patient decisions about appropriate healthcare for specific clinical circumstances.

G. Evidence-based health care—The purposeful and judicious use of best practices and evidence from systematic research findings in clinical practice.

H. Outcomes management—Seeks to produce desirable outcomes in a clinical setting, and is the application of outcomes research into practice. This involves assessment/measurement of outcomes at one point in time, monitoring and evaluation of same outcomes over time (longitudinal), interpretation of the data, and taking actions that focus on improving the outcomes.

I. Population management—A collaborative approach to identifying, mobilizing, and coordinating services to promote optimum community-based wellness within an identified population.

J. Predictive modeling:
    1. A set of tools used to stratify a population according to its risk of nearly any outcome—ideally, patients are risk stratified to identify opportunities for intervention *before* the occurrence of adverse outcomes that result in increased medical costs (Meek, 2003).
    2. Utilizing practice patterns to identify diagnostic groups or individuals at risk for adverse health events in order to proactively provide assistance with lifestyle changes to avoid, delay, or minimize the adverse health event.

K. Report cards, dashboards, and performance indicators—Reports that include a set of measures that can be used to rate providers, insurers, or health care plans according to their performance along several criteria. Common indicators include mortality rates, cost, rates of specific procedures, rates of hospitalization or emergency department visits for preventable diseases, and consumer satisfaction with care.

■ DRIVING FORCES THAT LEAD TO DISEASE MANAGEMENT PROGRAMS

A. Fragmentation of care
    1. In part due to the "component management model" of health care.
        a. The "components" are the various providers that a patient may require along the continuum, with each component, separately and episodically, striving for cost-effective, quality care.
        b. Usually does not support education or preventive elements through which hospitalizations and emergency care could be reduced

    c. Studies have shown that optimizing any component of care separately from other components often generates higher system-wide costs (Nash and Todd, 1997).

  2. A fragmented and chaotic environment or model of care results in medical errors and compromises patient care and organizational outcomes.

  3. The disease management (DM) model has been used as an antidote to fragmentation of care.

B. Financial pressures

  1. Cost pressures—Disease-specific health care spending

  2. Risk sharing—Financial risk being transferred from the insurance company as the sole payer to the provider sector, thus sharing the risk

  3. Growing concerns over the rising costs of health care services consumed by individuals with chronic illnesses

C. Quality improvement projects showing outcomes of care

  1. Importance of quality improvement projects

    a. Early projects often demonstrated poor quality of care.

    b. Variations of practice patterns for the same disease state or procedure (e.g., prostate cancer or total hip replacement) are an area of concern among providers and health care payers.

  2. Quality improvement projects assist in development of best-practice guidelines.

  3. Best-practice clinical guidelines support strong DM programs. The use of evidence-based guidelines is an integral component of DM programs.

  4. Process and outcomes measurement, evaluation, and management aspects of DM programs enhance quality improvement activities through identifying problems or undesired outcomes to be addressed and improved on.

D. Accreditation and certification programs that help ensure quality of care in DM programs:

  1. The National Committee for Quality Assurance (NCQA)—NCQA's DM accreditation and certification programs

  2. Health Plan Employer Data and Information Set (HEDIS)

  3. Joint Commission on Accreditation of Healthcare Organizations (JCAHO)

  4. Utilization Review and Accreditation Commission (URAC; also known as the American Accreditation Health Care Commission) DM accreditation program

E. Computer systems

  1. Computer and information technology as a driving force in DM

    a. Sophisticated software programs that assist the DM steps of population screening, patient identification, assessment, planning, condition management, and outcomes

    b. Disease-specific decision trees are available and used by telephone triage nurses and demand management companies.

      c. The crucial outcome measurement element that is responsible for continuous improvement in the management of disease would be impossible without sophisticated and integrated computer systems.

F. Informed consumers
  1. Consumers are demanding cost-effective, quality, safe, and error-free health care.
  2. Health care information is relatively easy to acquire.
     a. HEDIS report cards and major magazines compare plans.
     b. Internet users find disease-specific protocols easily.
     c. Pharmacies pass out free literature about disease, health, and prevention.
     d. Prime-time commercials inform the public of drug uses and side effects.
     e. Magazines, newspapers, and television regularly carry information about new treatments for cancer, human immunodeficiency virus (HIV), and other conditions.
     f. Health fairs saturate the public with important topics.
  3. DM programs include routine reporting structures or feedback loops that enhance communication among the varied parties involved including patients and their families, physicians, health plans, support services providers, and others.
  4. The case manager as an informational resource—An important role of the case manager is to ensure that the patients in their charge get the most accurate information for their health and disease prevention.

G. Future driving forces for DM programs—DM programs will continue to exist because of the following conditions:
  1. The continual increase in the aging population, especially the number of elderly with multiple chronic illnesses
  2. Increased demand for reducing variation in the treatment and management of chronic conditions
  3. Popularity of and the need for research-/evidence-based practices and practice guidelines
  4. Acute care setting being the most expensive setting of the health care continuum
  5. Educated consumers and their demand for error-free and best care
  6. Increasing prevalence of chronic conditions

■ COMPONENTS AND PRINCIPLES OF A SUCCESSFUL DISEASE MANAGEMENT PROGRAM

A. Understanding the course of the disease and application of evidence-based practice guidelines
  1. Disease-specific clinical excellence is required in every aspect of management of the chronic disease.

2. Case managers examine relevant data to delineate core issues; examples of data may include cost and quality drivers, causes and patterns of symptom manifestation, etc.

3. Judicious use of primary care physicians and specialists for disease-specific care

4. Prevention of exacerbations of diseases

5. Preventive measures to avoid disease-specific conditions

6. Use of evidence-based practice guidelines to guide interventions and patient education

7. Awareness of complementary and alternative medicine (CAM) as it relates to disease-specific conditions

8. The plethora of clinical trials and other research methods and evidence regarding which treatment modality is best for which condition

9. Available resources from professional organizations and societies (e.g., American Heart Association, National Kidney Foundation), especially those that are disease specific

10. Focus on prevention of disease or complications of disease

B. Identifying patients likely to benefit from intervention; evaluation of members most likely to benefit from a given DM program

1. Predictive modeling—finding the "right" high-risk patients before they get sick, using a set of tools used to stratify a population according to its risk of nearly any outcome (Meek, 2003a, 2003b).

   a. Primary goal of predictive modeling—identification of patients that are appropriate for DM and proactive CM

   b. May include use of self-reported health risk appraisal surveys

   c. Currently uses three main statistical techniques

      i. Rules-based techniques (used by many health plans)

      ii. Various statistical regression techniques to produce predictive models

      iii. Neural network technology—looks for relationships between the desired prediction and factors that are *most* predictive

C. Focusing on diagnosis and treatment of disease, rather than on availability of reimbursement for a given therapy, *and* allocation of resources that support evidence-based treatment of the disease

D. Focusing on prevention—prevention of illness or exacerbation of existing chronic conditions is an essential function of DM.

1. Educational efforts as an important component of preventative care. Patient self-management education may include primary prevention, secondary prevention, and behavior modification

2. Use of demand management as an educational method and as a system to use medical resources wisely

3. Use of CAM modalities for prevention

4. Demand for health promotion and disease prevention as integral aspect of health care. For example, the National Quality Forum and

Center for Medicare and Medicaid Services (CMS) advocate for smoke cessation and counseling as a core measure and a necessary intervention for individuals with pneumonia or heart disease.

E. Increasing patient adherence to medical regimens through education and support groups
   1. Patient educational component should, at the minimum, include
      a. Etiology and progression of the disease—instruction in how to monitor the disease to avoid exacerbation
      b. Precipitating reasons and signs and symptoms of impending problems
      c. Medication timetables, dosages, side effects, what to do about various side effects, etc.
      d. Dietary considerations and other lifestyle modifications such as exercise and weight management
      e. A discussion about adherence to physician and clinic appointments
      f. A specific focus on health prevention such as smoking cessation, activity and exercise, and other healthy lifestyle behaviors
   2. Reimbursement is limited for counseling, support groups, education, and many forms of preventive therapy.
   3. Self-management is essential—empowers and prepares patients to manage their health and health care services

F. Patient management that cuts across all settings
   1. Integration of health care in organizations through:
      a. Mergers
      b. Partnering with other companies
      c. Carve-outs for specific treatments or diseases
   2. The continuum of care must be geographically convenient to provide access to care and preventive services.
   3. Use of case or disease managers throughout the continuum.

G. Use of telemedicine/telemonitoring and telehealth in DM
   1. Programs should begin with well-developed goals and include an evaluation of the program's outcome
   2. Telemedicine—The use of telecommunications technology to provide, enhance, or expedite health care services, as by accessing offsite databases, linking clinics or physicians' offices to central hospitals, or transmitting x-rays or other diagnostic images for examination at another site.
   3. Telehealth—The delivery of health-related services and information via telecommunications technologies.
   4. Increased use of remote/home monitoring devices
   5. Increased use of rural telemedicine
   6. Barriers continue:
      a. Expensive; costs often passed on to consumer
      b. Does not always integrate with current IT systems

H. Establishing integrated data management systems for process and outcome measurements

1. Measuring outcomes is important, because outcomes direct efforts toward change; they show what works and what needs improvement. They also demonstrate the effectiveness of the DM program.

2. Sophisticated software systems that integrate care-based inpatient and outpatient settings are necessary to compile data necessary for a well-developed DM program.

3. Barriers to care

   a. Cost to integrate computer systems across the continuum

   b. Time consuming to input all the details necessary for good data

4. Outcomes of DM programs may include the following:

   a. Decrease in health care expenses for the populations of patients with chronic illnesses

   b. Reduction in avoidable hospitalizations and emergency department visits

   c. Improvement in disease-specific clinical outcomes

   d. Increase in patient satisfaction with care

   e. Improved adherence to clinical practice guidelines

   f. Proactive approach to care delivery

   g. Enhanced access to health care services

I. Routine "feedback loop" where good communication/reporting occurs between patients, physicians, health plans, and ancillary providers, reporting such events as:

1. Changes in condition

2. Results of diagnostic tests

3. Progress towards expected outcomes

4. Barriers to achieving expected outcomes

5. Routine progress reports to primary provider

■ DESIGN AND IMPLEMENTATION OF A DISEASE MANAGEMENT PROGRAM

A. The DMAA has not advocated for a specific conceptual framework for DM models; however, it has identified six main components of a model or program. Full-service DM programs must include all six components. Programs consisting of fewer components are known as DM *support services*. The six components are:

1. Population identification processes;

2. Evidence-based practice guidelines;

3. Collaborative practice models to include physician and support-service providers;

4. Patient self-management education (may include primary prevention, behavior modification programs, and compliance/surveillance);

5. Process and outcomes measurement, evaluation, and management; and

6. Routine reporting/feedback loop (may include communication with patient, physician, health plan, and ancillary providers, and practice profiling) (DMAA, 2006).

B. DM programs are found to perform the following six common functions:
1. Use evidence-based care/practice guidelines that are disease specific;
2. Identify the population with a chronic or complex disease;
3. Stratify the population based on risk state (low, moderate, or severe);
4. Match the intervention with the need of the individual patient or risk group;
5. Educate patients in self-management; and
6. Evaluate the program's processes and outcomes (Welch, Bergsten, Cutler, et al., 2002).

C. Define the target population—decide which diagnosis or diagnoses to target; that is, chronic illnesses such as diabetes, asthma, and heart failure.
1. Consider patient population, case mix index, and location.
2. Evaluate criteria for the selection of conditions; decide which criteria will elicit the most accurate data.
3. Evaluate the organization's current processes and programs that are in place.
4. Criteria commonly used in the identification of a target population/disease entity may include high-cost/high-expense conditions, large volumes, at high-risk conditions, tendency for increased/frequent emergency department visits or hospitalizations, and availability of evidence-based practice guidelines.
5. Determine the procedure for candidate (patient, health plan member, or employee) identification and stratification, enrollment in the program, and follow up.
6. Gillespie (2002) identified the following eight criteria for use in the identification of conditions that may warrant the development of DM programs:
   a. Availability of nationally recognized and agreed-on practice guidelines;
   b. Generally recognized problems in therapy that are documented in the medical literature;
   c. Large practice variations in treatment among clinicians;
   d. Variety of drug treatment for specific conditions;
   e. Large volume of patients with a medical condition whose treatment regimen needs improvement;
   f. Preventable acute events (e.g., emergency department visits and acute hospitalizations), which are often associated with the chronic disease;
   g. Specific outcome indicators that can be clearly defined and measured using standardized measures and that can be improved; and
   h. Potential for cost savings.

7. Common diseases and conditions targeted for DM programs include:
   a. Asthma
   b. Cancer (various types)
   c. Cardiovascular diseases (congestive heart failure, coronary artery disease)
   d. Chronic obstructive pulmonary disease (COPD)
   e. Depression and mental/behavioral health disorders
   f. Diabetes
   g. High-risk pregnancy
   h. HIV or acquired immunodeficiency syndrome (AIDS)
   i. Hypertension
   j. Pain management
   k. Pneumonia and infectious diseases
   l. End-stage renal disease and hemodialysis
   m. Organ transplantation
   n. Premature babies
   o. Sickle cell anemia
   p. Substance/chemical dependency
   q. Frail elderly

D. Organize a multidisciplinary, cross-functional team
   1. Determine the goals, objectives, and expected outcomes for the team and the DM program.
   2. Determine who will be on the team. Include major stakeholders such as: patients and their families, members of the health care team (clinicians such as physicians, nurses, and allied health professionals), support-service providers, performance/quality improvement specialists, health care agency administrators, health plan representatives, finance, marketing, and others as indicated.
   3. Team tasks may include, but not limited to the following:
      a. Examination and evaluation of data
      b. Initial and ongoing training required for team members and for those who will manage and implement the DM program
      c. May require development of clinical pathways, admissions or discharge criteria and orders, proactive treatment plans
   4. Assessment of barriers to a successful DM program
      a. System barriers
      b. Patient or family barriers
      c. Provider barriers
      d. Economic barriers
      e. Regulatory barriers
      f. Lack of necessary technology including communication and information systems

E. Define core components, treatment protocols, and monitoring and evaluation methods
   1. Determine how to monitor and evaluate the outcomes.
   2. Design a continuous approach to quality improvement.
   3. Base the DM program on best practices and current evidence-based practice guidelines.
   4. Consider a well-respected physician "champion" to direct the DM effort; this person would facilitate the medical advisory team.
   5. Focus the intervention protocols on the specific health condition being addressed and target the population most likely to benefit from the intervention.
   6. Understand the course of the disease and incorporate into the program and the treatment protocol.
   7. Ensure that the protocol focuses on prevention and resolution of problems/issues such as symptoms of disease and complications, and increase patient's adherence to medical regimen through health education.
   8. Build the process of maintaining continuity and consistency in care in the protocol of the DM program's processes
   9. Determine goals and objectives.
      a. Organizational goals and objectives
      b. Clinical goals and objectives
      c. Financial objectives
      d. Patient population–related goals
      e. Process and outcomes of care improvement

F. Pilot the program
   1. Initially, conduct the program on a small scale.
   2. Incorporate training when required.

G. Measure the outcomes of the pilot DM program.
   1. Examine
      a. Clinical outcomes—reduction in symptoms of disease, condition is under control (e.g., diabetes control)
      b. Humanistic (quality-of-life) outcomes
      c. Financial outcomes—cost prevention, revenue, return on investment
      d. Process outcomes—utilization of care/resources, adherence to the practice guidelines
      e. Behavioral outcomes—adherence to medical regimen, self-management skills
      f. Member satisfaction outcomes—consumer satisfaction with care
   2. Understand quality indicators as a measurable method of determining outcomes.
   3. Determine whether the pilot DM program was successful.
      a. The program was successful, or
      b. The program requires revisions
   4. Examples of clinical outcomes for specific health conditions are:

a. Heart failure—hospitalizations and readmission rates, use of emergency departments, prescribing of ACE inhibitors/ARBS beta blockers, diuretics and inotropics, weight control, left and right ventricular functions, blood pressure management, and smoking cessation.

b. Asthma—presence/absence of symptoms (shortness of breath, wheezing, dehydration, and insomnia), absenteeism from work or school, air exchange (peak flow), activity level, hospitalizations and readmission rates, and use of emergency departments

c. Diabetes—HbA1c, lipid profile, urine protein level, eye examination and vision, blood pressure management, foot examination and peripheral neuropathy, weight, hospitalizations and readmission rates, and use of emergency departments

H. Implement the DM program and plan continuous quality improvement (CQI) efforts

1. Successful DM programs include a process for outcomes measurement and evaluation.

2. It is important to have an automated outcomes management system in place to simplify the evaluation process, be comprehensive in measuring outcomes, and to optimize cost of evaluation.

3. Findings must be communicated to key stakeholders including administration team, physicians, consumers, employers, and accreditation and regulatory agencies.

4. Findings must also be tied into performance improvement or CQI processes.

■ PREDICTIVE MODELING/RISK STRATIFICATION IN DISEASE MANAGEMENT PROGRAMS

A. A set of tools used to stratify a population, according to its risk, to identify opportunities for intervention *before* the occurrence of adverse outcomes (or deterioration in health condition and disease state) that result in increased medical costs

B. DM programs rely on claims and pharmacy data to find the high-cost, high-utilization individuals of the population and target them for DM interventions.

C. Predictive models are used in three ways (Meek and Citrin, 2005):

1. To predict future costs for a population so that the design of benefit packages, premium levels, deductibles, co-pays, and overall coverage can be specified more accurately for payers

2. To impact providers' behaviors; claims data can be used to examine whether providers are practicing within the clinical practice guidelines and successfully managing patients with chronic illnesses.

3. To manage the health of a population by identifying individuals who are in need of proactive health coaching and care management

D. The primary goal of predictive modeling is to identify individuals in a population who would benefit from care management activities. For example, a health plan may enroll individuals who fall in the top 10% cost group into a DM program to ensure quality of care and to reduce cost.

E. Those who would benefit from a DM program are stratified into three groups of risk (low, moderate, high) and specific interventions are employed relevant to the risk category.

F. Predictive modeling is best when it results in identifying the right *high-risk* individuals before they become *high-cost* individuals who consume the most expensive health care resources. This is best achieved by intervening before acute crisis so that cost can be better managed and the health condition of an individual is kept at the lowest possible risk for deterioration.

G. By employing predictive modeling techniques:
   1. The population can be screened to identify those at risk for illness or deterioration of illness condition;
   2. Those found at risk can be stratified into three groups (low, moderate, high) based on measures of health and well-being;
   3. Intervention can use principles of primary (for those found at risk but experiencing no signs or symptoms of illness), secondary (for those at risk but exhibiting beginning signs or symptoms of illness), and tertiary prevention (for those already experiencing disease conditions that also are perhaps progressive).

H. Care coordination, CM, or care management is implemented based on the need of each risk group. For example, a low-risk group may receive health prevention and promotion services that are basically educational in nature; a moderate-risk group may receive coordinated care in addition to health prevention with a focus on building self-management skills; and a high-risk group may receive integrated care management approach with a focus on building self-management skills and prevention of the need for acute hospitalizations or emergency department visits.

■ THE CASE MANAGEMENT AND DISEASE MANAGEMENT PROCESS

A. Identification of at-risk members
   1. Use criteria to evaluate high-risk members for the chosen disease (e.g., predictive modeling techniques)
   2. Potential sources to identify high-risk members include:
      a. Encounter data
      b. Hospital and outpatient utilization patterns
      c. Pharmacy data
      d. Claims and billing (cost) data
      e. Case manager's knowledge of particular members or population

B. Assessment and evaluation of members and patients
   1. Psychosocial issues
   2. Financial issues
   3. Individual motivational factors
   4. Competency barriers to optimal self-care behavior

5. Disease-specific clinical details
   a. Physical signs and symptoms
   b. Knowledge deficits
6. Assess for severity of target disease state
   a. Priority 1—Patients who have a significant potential for exacerbations and emergency room visits or re-hospitalizations (high risk)
   b. Priority 2—Patients whose needs must be monitored on a regular basis, but can often be managed telephonically (moderate risk)
   c. Priority 3—Patients requiring minimal attention, whose sole need may be education about the disease (low risk)
7. Assess available health care benefits

C. Development and coordination of DM plans
   1. Use of evidence-based practice guidelines
   2. Individualization of the practice guideline to meet the patient's needs
   3. Establish goals and objectives including desired outcomes

D. Implementation of DM plans
   1. Involvement of the patient and family in the DM program and plans
   2. Ongoing monitoring and reassessment of the patient's condition compared to desired outcomes and goals of treatment
   3. Refer to specialists as needed
   4. Arrange for services as indicated by condition and ensure that health education is completed including building of self-management skills

E. Evaluation—outcome measurements
   1. Clinical outcomes
      a. Use of quality indicators
   2. Humanistic (patient and provider satisfaction) outcomes
      a. For patients, *The Health Status Survey (SF-12 or SF-36)* is a patient's self-assessment of perceived quality-of-life issues and has been proved to be a predictive tool that may indicate the member has a potential for a hospital admission in the next 6 to 12 months.
      b. Provider satisfaction tools
      c. Use of quality indicators
   3. Financial outcomes
      a. Use of cost indicators such as resource utilization and cost effectiveness

REFERENCES

Disease Management Association of America (DMAA). (2006). DMAA definition of disease management. Website: *http://www.dmaa.org/definition.html*. Retrieved June 6, 2006.

Gillespie, J. (2002). The value of disease management. Part 3: Balancing cost and quality in the treatment of asthma. *Disease Management, 5*(4), 225–232.

Gorski, L. (2006). Disease management and home care. Presented for Quality Insights of Pennsylvania, February 27, 2006.

Huber, D. (2005). *Disease management: A guide for case managers.* St Louis, MO: Elsevier, Inc.

Levitt, D., Startz, T., & Higgins, R. (1998). Disease state case management in an academic medical center utilizing osteoarthritis-of-the-knee model. *The Journal of Care Management, 4*(5), 45–55.

Meek, J. (2003a). Increasing return on investment potential in care management: Predictive modeling and proactive care, Part I. *Lippincott's Case Management, 8*(4), 170–174.

Meek, J. (2003b). Increasing return on investment potential in care management: Predictive modeling and proactive care, Part II. *Lippincott's Case Management, 8*(5), 198–202.

Meek, J., & Citrin, R. (2005). Predictive modeling and its application to disease and case management. In H. Huber, *Disease management: A guide for case managers* (pp. 21–31). St Louis, MO: Elsevier, Inc.

Nash, D., & Todd, W. (Eds.). (1997). *Disease management: A systems approach to improving patient outcomes.* Chicago: American Hospital Publishing, Inc.

Powell, S. K. (2000b). *Advanced case management: Outcomes and beyond.* Philadelphia: Lippincott Williams & Wilkins.

Rieve, J. (1998). Disease management concerns. *The Case Manager, 9*(2), 34–36.

Welch, W., Bergsten, C., Cutler, C., Bocchino, C., & Smith, R. (2002). Disease management practices of health plans. *The American Journal of Managed Care, 8*(4), 353–361.

SUGGESTED READING

Goldstein, R. (1998). The disease management approach to cost containment. *Nursing Case Management, 3*(3), 99–103.

Joint Commission on Accreditation of Healthcare Organizations (JCAHO). (2003). *Joint Commission disease-specific care certification guide.* Oakbrook Terrace, IL.

Kozma, C., Kaa, K., & Reeder, C. E. (1997). A model for comprehensive disease state management. *The Journal of Outcomes Management, 4*(1), 4–8.

McDonald, A. (2000). Telemonitoring in disease management: A format for successfully facilitating behavior change. *Journal for Case Management, 6*(3), 24–31.

Meek, J., & Citrin, R. (2004). Integrating services for optional proactive care. *Lippincott's Case Management, 9*(5), 232–238.

Minerd, R., & Lee, S. (1997). Using business process reengineering to develop disease management programs. *Inside Case Management, 4*(9), 8–9.

Nash, D. (2002). Disease management: What does the research evidence show? *Drug Benefit Trends, 14*(12), 18–24.

National Committee for Quality Assurance (NCQA). (2006). Website: *http://www.ncqa.org/Programs/Accreditation/DM/dmmain.htm.* Retrieved May 21, 2006.

Owen, M. (2004). Disease management: Breaking down silos to improve chronic care. *The Case Manager, 15*(3), 45–47.

Powell, S. K. (2000a). *Case management: A practical guide to success in managed care.* Philadelphia: Lippincott Williams & Wilkins.

Schofield, G. (1998). Developing a disease management program to improve outcomes and efficiencies. *Health Care Innovations, 8*(1), 11–29.

Utilization Review and Accreditation Commission (URAC). (2006). Disease Management Accreditation Program. Website: *http://www.urac.org/prog_accred_DM_po.asp?navid=accreditation&pagename=prog_accred_DM.* Retrieved May 21, 2006.

Ward, M., & Rieve, J. (1995). Disease management: Case management's return to patient-centered care. *Journal of Care Management, 1*(4), 7–12.

Whitfield, A. (2000). Branching out. *Continuing Care, 19*(5), 24–28.

21 Maternal–Child Case Management

Lori A. Davis

LEARNING OBJECTIVES

Upon completion of this chapter, the reader will be able to:

1. Identify components of maternal–infant case management.
2. Define important terms in maternal–infant case management.
3. Identify specific skills for case managers in maternal–infant case management.
4. Outline essential knowledge areas for case managers in maternal–infant case management.

IMPORTANT TERMS AND CONCEPTS

Betamethasone
Fetal Heart Rate Monitoring
Gestational Diabetes
Health Maintenance Organization (HMO)
Home Uterine Activity Monitoring
  (HUAM)
Hyperemesis Gravidarum
Multifetal Pregnancies

Placenta Previa
Predisposing Factors to Preterm Labor
Preeclampsia
Pregnancy
Premature Rupture of Membranes
  (PROM)
Preterm Birth
Prostaglandin

Tocolytic Therapy
Total Parenteral Nutrition (TPN)
Trimester

Vaginal Birth After Cesarean Section
(VBAC)
Viable

■ INTRODUCTION TO PART I: MATERNAL–INFANT CASE MANAGEMENT

A. Maternal and newborn care are two of the leading health plan expense categories in the United States, accounting for an estimated 27% of hospital admissions, 25% to 33% of hospital costs, and 10% to 49% of health plan costs.

B. Maternal–infant case management is not care management of an individual but of a family unit, more specifically a mother–child unit.

C. In maternal–infant care management, our task begins at conception and continues throughout pregnancy, birth, and the postdelivery phase.

D. The quality of a child's future depends on many factors, not the least of which include the physical and psychological conditions of pregnancy.

E. Identifying women at risk for the development of problems can begin with care from a primary care physician, but often care is not sought until pregnancy is determined. This is where the role of the maternal–infant case manager begins.

■ KEY DEFINITIONS

A. Betamethasone—A steroid given to a pregnant woman to aid in fetal lung development in anticipation of preterm birth.

B. Gestational diabetes—A carbohydrate intolerance that is diagnosed during pregnancy in which the blood sugar levels are elevated. The condition is usually controlled by diet; however, insulin may also be required. The condition usually resolves after delivery.

C. Home uterine activity monitor (HUAM)—A portable and compact monitor that records uterine activity and transmits data via telephone to the perinatal home care provider. Normally, this is not a continuous activity but is done intermittently at frequencies prescribed by the physician or when the mother feels the presence of contractions.

D. Hyperemesis gravidarum—Excessive vomiting during pregnancy; may lead to dehydration and possible starvation.

E. Multifetal pregnancies—A pregnancy of more than one fetus.

F. Placenta previa—A condition in which the placenta is implanted near or covering the cervix, which can result in bleeding and hemorrhage.

G. Preeclampsia—A complication of pregnancy, characterized by increasing hypertension, proteinuria, and generalized edema (toxemia).

H. Premature rupture of membranes (PROM)—Spontaneous rupture of the membranes that occurs more than 1 hour before the onset of labor. The term "premature" here only refers to the relationship with labor and not with gestational age.

I. Preterm birth—A birth occurring before the 37th week of gestation or 21 days before the estimated date of conception (EDC).

J. Preterm labor—Uterine activity accompanying cervical change, occurring between the 20th and 37th week of pregnancy.

K. Prostaglandin—A naturally occurring substance that causes strong contractions of the smooth muscle and dilation of certain vascular beds. It can be used in a gel form to soften the cervix before the induction or in suppository form (as a means of labor induction) for second-trimester pregnancy terminations.

L. Tocolytic therapy—Drug regimen given to decrease uterine activity and arrest the progression of preterm labor. May be given continuously through subcutaneous infusion or orally, although the oral route is usually given a trial before the subcutaneous method.

M. Trimester—Pregnancy is commonly broken down into trimesters: the first, second, and third months equal the first trimester; fourth, fifth, and sixth months are equal to the second trimester; and seventh, eighth, and ninth months are equal to the third trimester.

N. Vaginal birth after cesarean section (VBAC)—Vaginal delivery in a patient who has previously had a cesarean section.

O. Viable—Capable of sustaining life, usually a fetus that is 24 to 28 weeks of gestation; able to sustain life outside of the uterus.

■ ROLE OF THE MATERNAL–INFANT CASE MANAGER

A. The role of a case manager in the scope of maternal–infant health care can be a contributing factor to the well-being of a community.

B. A case management program that functions within the definition of case management as a collaborative process which assesses, plans, implements, coordinates, monitors, and evaluates options and services to meet an individual's health needs through communications and available resources to promote quality, cost-effective outcomes; maternal–infant health care can have a significant impact on the health status, resource utilization, and future health care needs of a community.

C. The outcome of a healthy infant born to a healthy mother integrated successfully to a community with sufficient resources can validate a successful case management program.

D. With the proper tools, defined core competencies, and clinically experienced case managers, a maternal–infant case management program can be developed and implemented.

■ ASSESSMENT

A. When the case manager demonstrates the basic skills of understanding the physiologic and psychosocial events that occur during the antepartum, perinatal, and postpartum phases, performing the next skill of assessment will be logical and well defined to the case manager.

1. The assessment phase allows the case manager to collect data through a series of interviews of the client that can be tied to the knowledge of the basic physiology and psychosocial events of the antepartum, perinatal, and postpartum phases of maternal–infant health care. There are many components of a maternal–infant assessment.

2. Some behavioral components of the assessment process for a maternal–infant case management program should not be disregarded.

3. These behaviors include the competencies of:
   a. Interviewing skills for collecting subjective data for the database
   b. Listening and observation (if face-to-face) skills
   c. Communication and recording skills for a historical database
   d. Sensitivity to preconceived ideas, languages, and cultural barriers
   e. Awareness of the case manager's personal attitudes and beliefs

4. When the case manager demonstrates successful competencies of the so-called soft skills of assessment, the development of the database will allow him or her to assess the needs of the client through the gathering of physical, social, psychological, and historical information.

B. The framework of assessment for a maternal–infant case management program is built around the collection of multiple data elements, both historical and current.

C. Gathering of objective and subjective data should be included in the database collection instrument.

D. Objective data items collected include physician office visit findings, diagnostic and laboratory test results, the client's current health status, family history, psychosocial history, activities of daily living, and review of systems.

E. Subjective data items collected include a client's personal perspective of past history.

F. The subjective and objective data collected allow the case manager to define the perceived issues with the objective findings. This will lead the case manager to the identification phase of any problems, concerns, or interventions, allowing the case manager to begin the planning phase.

■ KNOWLEDGE DOMAINS

A. Five major domains of essential case management knowledge have been identified and recognized as core knowledge areas used by practitioners across the essential activities and functions that constitute case management. These domains are:
   1. Coordination and service delivery
   2. Physical and psychosocial aspects
   3. Benefit systems and cost–benefit analysis
   4. Community resources
   5. Case management concepts

B. A core of any curriculum begins with the understanding and application of the basic components and skills required to apply the knowledge to practice. The defined basic components of a maternal–infant case management program include:

1. Knowledge of the anatomic changes to women that occur during the conception, antepartum, perinatal, and postpartum phases of pregnancy
2. Knowledge of the physiologic changes in women that occur during the conception, antepartum, and postpartum phases of pregnancy
3. Knowledge of fetal development phases during the conception and antepartum period of pregnancy
4. Knowledge of maternal and fetal nutrition
5. Knowledge of the phases of labor and delivery of the birthing process
6. Knowledge of the biologic and behavioral characteristics of the newborn infant
7. Knowledge of newborn nutritional needs
8. Knowledge of the psychosocial components of the childbearing family, including family dynamics, cultural context, and coping skills
9. Knowledge of the various risk factors of the antepartum, perinatal, and postpartum phases of maternal–infant health care
10. Knowledge of the pathophysiology of a high-risk pregnancy, including:
    a. Preeclampsia (toxemia)—occurs in 3% to 6% of all pregnancies
    b. Preterm labor and preterm birth—Between 1993 and 2003, the rate of infants born preterm in the United States increased nearly 12%.
    c. Multifetal pregnancy—increasing occurrence with prevalence of infertility treatment
    d. Gestational diabetes—occurs in 3% to 12% of pregnancies
    e. Hyperemesis gravidarum—occurs in 0.7% to 2.1% of pregnancies
    f. Placenta previa
    g. Other preexisting physical conditions or diseases
11. Previous pregnancies with pathophysiology
12. Medical chronic disease and the effect of those diseases on pregnancy
13. Current pathologic "states" of pregnancy—hypertensive states, hemorrhage, preterm and postterm labor, and age-related conditions
14. Knowledge of social risks to the pregnancy state, including:
    a. Smoking, drug, and alcohol usage
    b. Community support and available resources
    c. Previous psychiatric disease

C. Many of these knowledge domains are developed through clinical experiences in a variety of health care and provider settings. These clinical experiences allow the development of knowledge of various treatment modes and outcomes.

■ CASE MANAGEMENT CONCEPTS

A. The basic concepts of case management, such as planning, monitoring, coordinating, directing, and evaluating the plan for results-oriented, cost-effective services, form a domain of the case management model.

B. In a maternal–infant case management program, the assessment and the formulation of issues, problems, or concerns lead to an individualized plan for the patient.

C. The case manager's ability to create a plan is included as a competency.

D. Planning requires input and agreement from multiple providers, community service agencies, and the client to set mutual goals.

E. To identify the appropriate interventions to reach the mutual goals, the case manager must translate the problem statements into a positive health statement and establish criteria to meet the mutual goals.

F. The health statements tied to possible interventions for the client will lead to the case management plan.

G. The communication, coordination, organizing, and directing of this plan through intervention remain a major function and required competency of a case manager in a maternal–infant case management program.

H. In a maternal–infant case management program, the case manager must plan for the physical, emotional, and psychosocial needs of the pregnant patient.
   1. Pregnancy affects the entire body of a woman and can produce a very different response from one client to another.

I. The assessment and plan of any pregnant patient must be made in the context of the maternal–fetal unit. The areas for planning include:
   1. Preparation and education of the patient on her physical changes and possible requirements
   2. Discussion of financial issues or concerns related to pregnancy and maternal–infant needs
   3. Review of the present and future effect on the patient in the performance of activities of daily living, including nutrition, exercise, travel, personal hygiene, sexual activity, smoking, alcohol, drugs (prescription, over the counter, and recreational), and pets
   4. Outline of emotional changes related to changes of pregnancy from physical factors (e.g., hormone changes and body image) to the additional requirements of a new dependent, financial constraints, and family dynamics
   5. Consideration of psychosocial requirements of the pregnancy, such as changes in housing needs, occupational risks and consequences, religious and cultural practices, marital status, and age

J. The maternal–infant case management plan directs the appropriate interventions to direct the actions needed.
   1. A case manager should include in the maternal–infant plan:
      a. Therapeutic interventions
      b. Teaching and counseling interventions

      c. Monitoring and continued assessment interventions

      d. Referral interventions

K. The maternal–infant case manager directs and organizes the interventions for action.

L. There is coordination of activities, collaboration of resources, and monitoring of results from the interventions.

M. On completion of the activities, the maternal–infant case manager must evaluate the results.

    1. Have the goals been met throughout the pregnancy?

      a. An example of this evaluation may be seen in the attending of physician appointments during the antepartum phase of the pregnancy.

      b. If the client cannot attend the required monthly antepartum visits, the case manager must be aware of this issue and plan accordingly.

      c. The plan may include several contingency items such as child care, transportation options, and financial resources.

      d. Through the case manager process, the case manager will assess and identify this issue, plan for the problem, and direct, monitor, and evaluate the outcomes of attendance at physician's appointments by the client.

      e. This continuous case management process by the case manager for simple to complex problems, concerns, or identified issues will allow for necessary changes in the plan, utilization of appropriate resources, and results-oriented, cost-effective services.

■ PHYSICAL AND PSYCHOSOCIAL ASPECTS

A. Understanding the interrelationships of the physical and psychosocial aspects of the maternal–infant client is a key competency for the case manager.

B. Previous clinical experience in a variety of settings where maternal–infant health care is delivered is a mandatory competency for the maternal–infant case manager.

    1. Competencies include:

      a. Knowledge of the genetic basis of inheritance, including the conception phase and gene transmission within families

      b. Knowledge of embryonic development and fetal maturation, including the various changes in the maternal anatomic systems

      c. Knowledge of a normal pregnancy and the outcomes that result when normal events do not occur

      d. Knowledge of the family-centered approach to maternal–infant care for the support of the mother and infant

      e. Knowledge of the cultural significance of childbearing for a variety of cultures

      f. Knowledge of the developmental tasks and mental processes required for the mother to adapt to the maternal role, from accepting the pregnant state to the mother–child bonding period

C. The maternal–infant case manager's ability to blend the medical, psychological, social, and behavioral knowledge of the pregnant state into an effective plan will benefit the patients, both mother and child.

■ BENEFIT SYSTEMS AND COST–BENEFIT ANALYSIS

A. The outcome of a healthy infant and mother who are integrated into the community, using available and necessary resources that lead to a healthy family, is the goal of a maternal–infant case management program.
   1. Unfortunately, the ideal outcome is not always possible. In the United States in 2003, hospital charges for babies with any diagnosis of prematurity or low birthweight was nearly $18.1 billion.
   2. However, with oversight, compliance, and education, positive pregnancy outcomes remain a viable goal of a maternal–infant case management program.
   3. Additionally, the maternal–infant case management program can be used to differentiate the high-risk patient from the patient with a normal pregnancy.

B. Knowledge of various benefit plans allows the case manager to tie benefits to identified needs.
   1. If there are no benefits available, the case manager will be competent to seek possible alternatives, explore various community resources, or work closely with funding sources for payment of the services needed.
   2. The onset of preterm labor and the delivery of low-birthweight infants have a significant financial impact on health care resources and an emotional impact on the family and community structure.
      a. The family may suffer additional stress if the infant is born prematurely and has congenital defects or develops chronic conditions as a result of prematurity.

C. Benefit analysis is essential for the maternal–infant case manager to provide the highest quality of care within the confines of the mother's resources.
   1. Including a variety of educational and behavioral programs complements the case manager's interactions and enhances the potential for a healthy pregnancy and good outcome.
      a. Examples of this can be demonstrated in
         i. A smoking cessation program
         ii. A work-adjustment program
         iii. A nutrition program for the pregnant woman
         iv. A cost analysis of so-called add-on services, such as home intervention and education to decrease preterm births

D. The easiest way to maximize benefit potential while decreasing expenditures related to pregnancy and birth is through aggressive and consistent use of resources to identify and treat high-risk pregnancies.

■ COMMUNITY RESOURCES

A. A maternal–infant case management program is tied closely to the community.

B. The pregnant patient is encouraged to be involved in the community.

C. A maternal–infant case manager will be competent to:
1. Identify community resources within the neighborhood of the mother
2. Obtain community resource requirements for use by the client
3. Assess every woman for domestic violence, with the ability to provide appropriate counseling and referrals for abuse
4. Determine access to and availability of services for the educational needs of the pregnant patient within the community
5. Evaluate community transportation for access to health care facilities and physician's appointments
6. Determine the employer's involvement in work adaptations for the pregnant worker and the availability of such adaptations
7. Incorporate strategies into the community through educational programs, community volunteer outreach, and community coalitions of persons who seek positive outcomes for future children and families of that community

D. Education of the patient and significant others is another way of increasing the mother's support system and her awareness of ways to ensure a healthy baby.
1. Prenatal education classes are widely produced and available in most areas.
2. Many hospital facilities offer prenatal education as well as childbirth classes for a nominal fee, and often these classes are free.
3. Public health departments offer prenatal education.
4. Many nonprofit organizations within the community offer prenatal education as well.
5. Prepared childbirth classes or Lamaze classes are also offered by many of these groups.
6. For the postdelivery period, there are also centers that offer parenting classes, access to free or low-cost immunizations, car seats, and other services to help ensure a healthy baby.

E. Many HMOs offer prenatal screening and education programs.
1. Although not intended to replace a physician's office visit, prenatal education program, or other health care services, these programs often offer many good booklets, brochures, tapes, and other educational pieces to supplement programs already in place.
2. Many of these programs offer incentives to their plan participants for seeking prenatal care early, keeping monthly or bimonthly visits, or participating in their perinatal wellness program.
3. Incentives are also included for completing either a telephonic or written assessment tool that would help identify mothers at risk.

4. These assessment tools can be useful in obtaining an even more in-depth maternal history and often reveal potential complications or risk factors.

5. Drawbacks to these programs are that health plan participants are already inundated with free educational materials or feel that answering in-depth questions is an invasion of their privacy, even though it would ultimately benefit the pregnancy, mother, and child.

6. Many plan participants enroll in these programs because the incentives can be quite attractive.

   a. Incentives might include coupons or discounts to local stores, car seats, gift baskets, free maid service, etc.

■ COORDINATION AND SERVICE DELIVERY

A. Knowledge of perinatal services available is essential for the provision of services and treatment options.

B. Most often, the birth takes place at a hospital or birthing facility.

1. According to several new laws, both state and federal, length of hospital or facility stay can no longer be mandated or incentivized by third-party payers or facilities for the reduction of health care spending.

   a. These laws mandate that the minimum stay be 72 hours for a routine, uncomplicated vaginal delivery.

   b. The minimum stay following a cesarean section is 96 hours, if it is uncomplicated.

   c. Earlier discharge is possible only if the physician and the mother agree on the discharge decision.

   d. Offering enticements for the mother to leave the hospital early, such as waiving co-payments or deductibles or offering free goods or services, also is not allowed.

   e. These laws were enacted as a direct result of the physician and consumer outcry regarding the movement to discharge mothers and infants within 24 hours after vaginal delivery.

C. When complications arise or a situation becomes high risk, the knowledge of available treatment options becomes key to providing cost-effective, quality care.

1. Complications arising during pregnancy include:

   a. Hyperemesis gravidarum

   b. Preterm labor

   c. Gestational diabetes

   d. Multifetal pregnancies (twins, triplets, or more)

   e. Placenta previa

   f. Preeclampsia

D. Treatment for complications does not always require an extended hospital stay.

1. Some alternatives available that can be used include:
   a. Home uterine activity monitoring (HUAM) for those mothers with preterm labor, multifetal pregnancy, or histories of preterm birth
      i. HUAM—A portable and compact monitor that records uterine activity and transmits data by telephone to the perinatal home care provider.
      ii. HUAM can be done with or without medication (i.e., tocolytics).
   b. Subcutaneous medication therapy can be administered at home for several complications of pregnancy. Examples of subcutaneous medication include:
      i. Metoclopramide (Reglan) therapy for hyperemesis
      ii. Terbutaline pump therapy for preterm labor (usually used after failure of oral tocolytic therapy)
      iii. Insulin pump therapy for diabetes
      iv. Anticoagulant therapy for coagulation disorders
   c. Home nursing visits for administration of injections, nursing assessments, and monitoring, even if provided once daily or several times daily, can be a very cost-effective way of preventing preterm birth and its complications.
   d. There are numerous other specialized perinatal services that can be provided at home safely and cost effectively.
   e. Such services might not be warranted for most patients, but for a mother who is at high risk or on bed rest, they can be the deciding factor in a preterm or full-term delivery.
   f. Examples of other perinatal home services include:
      i. Nonstress testing
      ii. Fetal heart rate monitoring
      iii. Betamethasone therapy
      iv. Dietary analysis
      v. Blood pressure monitoring
      vi. IV hydration therapy for hyperemesis gravidarum
      vii. Total parenteral nutrition (TPN) for severe hyperemesis gravidarum
      viii. Blood testing
   g. Many of the services listed can be provided with electronic equipment that has a modem through which data can be transmitted to a center with trained professionals who can update the physician and alert him or her to potential problems.
   h. Providers of the services listed should be highly experienced and qualified to provide such services.
      i. Not all home health providers are equipped or qualified to take on the responsibility of perinatal care.
      ii. The nurses providing care should have several years of perinatal experience, preferably in labor and delivery, and neonatal and high-risk care, and be well trained to work with the technology at home.

        iii. It is a good idea to know providers for perinatal care before the case manager needs them and be acquainted with the capabilities they have.

   2. Coverage for these types of services is not always available; collaborating with the physician, payer source, and patient is essential.

     a. It is easy to recognize the cost savings that these programs can establish, but home safety and the mother's ability to self-administer or receive therapies at home must also be considered.

     b. The cost savings might not be worth the risk involved; the advantages and disadvantages must be carefully weighed.

     c. A quality perinatal home health provider will also help you make these determinations.

■ PRETERM LABOR AND DELIVERY

A. Because of the prevalence of preterm labor, preterm delivery, and infant mortality and morbidity as a result of prematurity, early diagnosis and treatment is a top priority for the maternal–infant case manager regardless of whether you are a case manager for a health plan or a large birthing facility.

B. In 2003, there were 499,008 preterm births in the United States, representing 12.3% of live births.

C. Premature births account for about 70% of infant deaths—about 28,000 each year.

D. Premature births account for about 50% of neurologic handicaps.

E. Predisposing factors to preterm labor include:

   1. Maternal age under 18 years and over 44 years

   2. Smoking

     a. In 2003, 23.4% of women of childbearing age in the United States reported smoking.

   3. Infections

     a. Chorioamniotis—An inflammatory response in the amniotic membranes, stimulated by organisms in the amniotic fluid, which then becomes infiltrated with polymorphonuclear leukocytes.

     b. Pyelonephritis or kidney infection

   4. Previous preterm birth

   5. Placental problems such as abruptio placentae or placenta previa

   6. Lower socioeconomic status

   7. Uterine or cervical anomalies

   8. Prolonged rupture of membranes (PROM)

   9. Multifetal pregnancy

  10. Previous abdominal surgeries

  11. Chronic maternal conditions or diseases

F. Early detection is the key to preventing preterm birth and prolonging pregnancy.

1. Many preterm births occur not because the treatment of preterm uterine activity is ineffective but because the early warning signs and symptoms are not recognized.
   a. The early warning signs of preterm labor are:
      i. Uterine contractions—Contractions that occur every 10 minutes or more than five contractions in 1 hour.
      ii. Menstrual-type cramps—Such cramps occur in the abdomen just above the pubic bone.
      iii. Pelvic pressure—This sensation may feel as if the baby is pushing down and may come and go.
      iv. Low dull backache—Back pain is often a throbbing feeling.
      v. Increase or change in vaginal discharge
      vi. Pressure or pain in the lower abdomen, lower back, or thighs
      vii. Abdominal cramps similar to severe gas pain, which may occur with or without diarrhea

G. Preventing preterm birth requires an effort by health care professionals at all levels, from the telephone triage nurse to the physician, to educate patients regarding preterm labor.

H. Frequent provider contact through office visits and the telephone is key to keeping lines of communication open with the patient throughout the pregnancy.

I. Risk assessments performed in the first trimester and repeated throughout pregnancy can lead to early diagnosis and treatment of preterm labor.

J. If preterm labor is suspected, immediate treatment, lifestyle alteration, and ongoing education can prolong the pregnancy, particularly if these measures are combined with tocolytic therapies.

K. The goal of treatment for preterm labor is to prolong the pregnancy safely, with the end result being a healthy mother and child.
   1. Treatment options include the following in various combinations:
      a. Bed rest—most common and first step in reduction of contractions, although studies are inconclusive as far as efficacy
      b. Fluid overload
      c. Tocolysis with magnesium sulfate, terbutaline, ritodrine, indomethacin, or calcium channel blockers
      d. Restriction of sexual activity

L. General maturity milestone guidelines according to Creasy (1984):
   1. 24 to 27 weeks at birth—Earliest chance of survival; long-term intensive care is required.
   2. 29 to 32 weeks at birth—Survival rate increases dramatically, but intensive care is still required.
   3. 33 to 37 weeks at birth—Suck–swallow reflex matures, body temperature stabilizes, and lung maturity increases; intensive care may not be requrired
   4. 38 to 40 weeks at birth—Full-term baby

PART II
PEDIATRIC CASE MANAGEMENT

LEARNING OBJECTIVES

Upon completion of this section, the reader will be able to:

1. Define the important terms and concepts relative to pediatric case management.
2. Discuss the important issues related specifically to pediatric case management.
3. Discuss the challenges and opportunities related to pediatric case management and the special issues related to this population.

IMPORTANT TERMS AND CONCEPTS

Apnea Monitor
Bronchopulmonary Dysplasia (BPD)
Caregiver
Communication
Financial Impact on the Family
Home Health Care
Identification of Pediatric Cases with Potential High-Risk Complications
Individuals with Disabilities Education Act (IDEA)

Medically Fragile Child
Neonatal Intensive Care Unit (NICU)
Peripherally Inserted Central Catheter (PICC)
Premature Infants
Prescribed Pediatric Extended Care (PPEC)
Technology-Dependent Child
Very-Low-Birthweight Baby (VLBW)

■ INTRODUCTION TO PART II: PEDIATRIC CASE MANAGEMENT

A. Pediatric case management is care management, not of a child, but of a family unit. You will discover that the issues surrounding the pediatric client encompass the entire family unit of the child.

B. Owing to the availability of advanced medical technologies, emergency medicine, and rapidly expanding medical knowledge, the pediatric population requiring case management has grown exponentially.

C. The primary client focus in this chapter is case management of the technology-dependent or medically fragile child.

1. Twenty million American children experience chronic conditions, and 4 million children suffer from disabling chronic conditions (Newacheck, Stein, and Walker, 1996).

2. With the capabilities within the medical community, we have begun rescuing children who otherwise would have not survived outside of the womb or who would not have survived to realize a cure for their childhood cancer.

3. With these medical miracles comes myriad issues to be resolved if the child is to experience any normalcy in his or her life. Twenty years ago, infants born at 24 weeks' gestation rarely survived. Today, not only do these infants survive, but in many instances they thrive—but not without the assistance of ever-changing health care technology and expertise.

■ KEY DEFINITIONS

A. Apnea monitor—An apnea monitor is used as a warning device to alert the caregiver of a decreased heart rate, decreased depth of respiration, or cessation of respiration. The cardiorespiratory monitor only warns of a problem, it does nothing to correct a problem.

B. Caregiver—The individual who is the parent, responsible party, guardian, or custodian for the pediatric client.

C. Individuals with Disabilities Education Act (IDEA)—A federal law that defines the required educational components that must be available to all individuals with developmental disabilities.

D. Medically fragile child—The child who is medically stable but is fragile as a result of congenital disability, injury, illness, disease, or accident who requires frequent monitoring and treatment for the condition to remain in a state of satisfactory health.

E. Prescribed Pediatric Extended Care (PPEC)—A day care for the medically fragile or technology-dependent child.

F. Technology-dependent child—A child who needs both a medical device to compensate for the loss of a vital body function and substantial and ongoing nursing care to avert death or further disability (U.S. Congress, 1987).

G. Very-low-birthweight baby (VLBW)—An infant weighing less than 1500 g (3 lb, 5 oz).

■ PEDIATRIC CASE MANAGEMENT MODELS

A. The case manager—In case management of the pediatric client, there are often several case managers involved. These may include:
   1. A hospital case manager
   2. The clinic or specialty practice case manager
   3. Home health case manager
   4. A payer source case manager (Deming, 1996)

B. The facility-based and clinic-based case manager
   1. Facility-based and clinic-based case managers often are nurses with advanced degrees or certification in a particular specialty, or social workers (Deming, 1996).
   2. The facility-based case manager is responsible for care coordination while the client is in the facility; this person may have responsibility for a particular unit or floor, whereas other facility-based case

managers may have all discharge planning and case responsibilities for a particular specialty.

3. The clinic-based case manager is often the case manager who will interact with the client for the longest period of time and have the most accurate clinical account of client history for a specific physician. Often, the clinic-based case manager is the one to alert the payer source case manager to changes in the client condition or situation once the child has left the facility.

C. The payer source case manager

1. The payer source case manager is responsible for navigating the client through the health care system and is often the "lead" case manager directing and coordinating care.

2. The payer source case manager is responsible for knowledge of what the health plan allows regarding service, providers, and treatment options covered by the plan. Therefore, this case manager has the ability to interpret and relay the terms of the policy to all other parties.

3. The payer source case manager must have knowledge of the geographic area, providers, and services available within the region.

4. The payer source case manager is often not an expert in pediatric care; therefore, he or she must rely on the expertise of those in the clinic and facility to expound on the particulars of care and treatment for the pediatric patient.

5. Communication is a key function in this role. As important as clinical knowledge is, so is the ability to communicate effectively with all members of the case management team.

D. The home health case manager

1. The child's care at home is extremely important, and the home health case manager must have substantial experience with pediatric care. This case manager (and other professionals in the home) are the eyes and ears to the other team members once the patient has been discharged from the facility and is cared for at home.

2. The home health case manager's ability to assess home and social situations is very important.
   a. Environmental issues are the case manager's responsibility as well.
   b. Home safety is important whether the child is technology dependent or receiving home nursing care alone.

3. Sometimes, home health care companies and home equipment vendors subcontract services to other providers if they cannot immediately meet the home health care needs of the child. As for a case manager from any venue, it is important to know by whom services are being rendered at all times and that the provider is qualified and accredited to provide such services.

■ THE CASE MANAGEMENT TEAM

A. The ultimate goal of the case management team is to provide services that are uninterrupted, coordinated, developmentally and age appropriate, psychologically sound, and comprehensive (White, 1997).

B. The pediatric care management team should include:
1. Case manager or managers
2. Pediatric client
3. Caregiver
4. Primary care physician
5. Specialty physicians
6. Social services
7. Home health care provider
8. Therapists
9. Dieticians
10. Nutritionists
11. Pharmacists
12. School
13. Insurance company or others assuming financial responsibility
14. Anyone else who has an interest in the child's well-being

C. Communication across the entire team is key for a successful outcome. The child may be cared for by multiple physicians at multiple facilities or clinics.
1. Candid discussion with the parents or caregivers of the child is important.
2. Nothing will be resolved easily if decisions are made that do not involve the caregiver in the process.
3. This concept is best illustrated in the following case: A child had a private duty sitter at home. The child spilled a pitcher of red fruit drink while seated on the sofa. The parents had asked previously that he not be given the drink unless he was in the kitchen. The home care company was quick to accept responsibility and resolve the situation. They soon replaced the sofa for the client. It had been documented on the plan of care that the parents did not want him to have fruit drink unless he was in the kitchen. When the home care manager made a follow-up call to the family to evaluate their satisfaction with the problem resolution, he was stunned to find that they were still dissatisfied. The family said that they had received the new sofa and it was nice, but no one had replaced the lost pitcher of fruit drink.

■ THE CHILD

A. Age of the pediatric patient
1. Typically, pediatric case management includes children from birth to 18 years of age.
2. In some instances, there may be a perinatal or maternal–child case manager who works with children who are premature or are still in the neonatal period (the first 30 days after birth).
3. The case management responsibility of those infants would be specific to the institution or corporation policy.

B. Premature infants and those with congenital defects
1. Children requiring case management can have one problem or a multitude of problems. Prematurity and congenital defects account for a large number of children requiring case management.

2. Advanced technology in neonatal intensive care units (NICUs) has increased the number of children who survive, but it also has increased those requiring long-term or even lifetime care.

   a. Over the last 25 years, throughout the industrialized world, survival for the pediatric client has dramatically improved such that about 90% of children with disabilities reach their 20th birthday (O'Shea et al., 1997).

   b. In the 1990s, the survival rate of babies weighing less than 1lb, 10 oz was around 80% (Deming, 1996).

3. Complications of prematurity include bronchopulmonary dysplasia (BPD), necrotizing enterocolitis (NEC), intraventricular hemorrhage (IVH), hydrocephaly, and cerebral palsy.

4. Premature infants often require treatment at home with any of the following home health services: durable medical equipment, infusion services, home therapies, or home health nursing.

5. Many of these children are technology dependent. The technology-dependent child is defined as one who needs both a medical device to compensate for the loss of a vital body function and substantial and ongoing nursing care to avert death or further disability (U.S. Congress, 1987) (Table 21-1).

TABLE 21-1

Summary of Office of Technology Assessment Estimates of the Size of the Technology-Dependent Child Population

Defined Population	Estimated Number of Children
Group I	
Requiring ventilator assistance	680–2000
Group II	
Requiring parenteral nutrition	350–700
Requiring prolonged IV drugs	270–8275
Group III	
Requiring other device-based respiratory or nutritional support	1000–6000
Rounded subtotal (I + II + III)	*2300–17,000*
Group IV	
Requiring apnea monitoring	6800–45,000
Requiring renal dialysis	1000–6000
Requiring other device-associated nursing	Unknown, perhaps 30,000 or more

From U.S. Congress, Office of Technology Assessment (1987). *Technology-dependent children: Hospital v. home care—A technical memorandum, OTA-TM-H-38.* Washington, DC: U.S. Government Printing Office.

6. Examples:
   a. A child who has severe BPD might require an extended hospital stay, oxygen therapy at home, enteral feedings at home, and an apnea monitor.
   b. A child who has lost a large part of his or her intestine owing to NEC might require multiple hospitalizations and surgeries, in addition to home TPN or continuous enteral feedings.
   c. The child who has a moderate degree of cerebral palsy might not require as much "technology" as others but may require a specialized wheelchair, rehabilitation, and perhaps feeding assistance.
   d. All of these situations would require services, skills, and/or equipment that might fall outside the normally covered items under a health plan.
7. A pediatric provider for these services, and the understanding by the payer source of the needs of the child, are absolutely essential.

C. The child with illness and injury
   1. Another group of children to consider are those who have childhood cancer that might require home chemotherapy, frequent hospitalizations, frequent clinic visits, home health nursing, or perhaps a bone marrow or stem cell transplant, requiring extensive communication and coordination of the care management team for an optimum outcome.
   2. One major goal in case management for children is to allow the child to lead the most normal daily life possible. Often this includes coordinating care with the school system or day care center.
   3. Accidents and other illnesses account for another large portion of the home health or rehabilitation services the child may require.
   4. Osteomyelitis is frequently seen in children requiring case management.
      a. Depending on the location of the infection and the susceptibility and sensitivity of the organism, children with osteomyelitis often require home intravenous (IV) antibiotics.
      b. Many children require placement of a central venous catheter or a long-dwelling device such as a peripherally inserted central catheter (PICC).
      c. The duration of care at home can be anywhere from 7 days to several months of IV antibiotic therapy.
   5. Traumatic brain injury
      a. The pediatric population has seen an increase in traumatic brain injury because of the popularity of all-terrain vehicles (ATVs), motorcycles, skateboards, and bicycles.
      b. Children with traumatic brain injuries need to be seen in a comprehensive facility where there is extensive expertise and services specific for the brain-injured child.
      c. The subsequent rehabilitation these children require is also vitally important to optimize the potential for a partial or complete recovery.

■ **THE FAMILY**

A. The family

1. Several indicators should be addressed in assessing the family of the technology-dependent or medically fragile child. It is well documented that family members may experience adverse consequences as a result of the need to focus energy and resources on the child who has a chronic condition. Disposable income, employment, parental health, sibling health and adaptation, and family interaction and support levels are indicators of child health outcomes.

   a. Siblings—ratings of siblings' health status (cognitive, physical, social, and emotional)

   b. Parents—the frequency of occurrence of financially burdensome out-of-pocket expenses for child health care, including premium expenditures; the impact of child health care demands on parental employment (e.g., work out of the house, employment patterns, hours worked, and work loss days); ratings of parents' health status (cognitive, physical, social and emotional)

   c. Family unit—the nature and level of family support provided through the plan (e.g., level of informal care giving, psychological and social support, crisis intervention, respite care) (Newacheck, Stein, and Walker, 1996).

2. As a case manager, you may not always be able to address or impact every issue surrounding your pediatric client; however, you will be able to understand more clearly the behaviors of the client and family when you are aware of the challenges they face and how they react to them.

B. The caregiver

1. When a child is sick or injured, each member of the family, whether nuclear, blended, extended, or foster, is affected to some degree.

2. Establishing the primary caregiver is crucial.

   a. Often the primary caregiver is the child's mother or father.

   b. The primary caregiver is the one who will be responsible for learning all facets of the child's care. This includes learning cardiopulmonary resuscitation (CPR), procedures, treatments, and equipment that might be necessary at home.

3. The case manager should assess the primary caregiver for the willingness and motivation to learn, as well as the ability to learn.

4. The payer source case manager is reliant on the nurses and therapists who have worked with the child and the family to relay this information as well. Home health care professionals are excellent in assessing the abilities of the caregiver; however, it would be prudent to determine caregiver abilities well in advance of discharge.

5. Case management must be performed in cooperation with the child, family, and care management team. In working with the caregiver or parents, it is vitally important to establish rapport with them.

   a. Listening is a sometimes seldom-used but highly needed skill.

b. One unwritten but widely understood rule in the pediatric care industry is "Listen to the mother (caregiver)." The mother or caregiver is with the child most often and knows better than anyone when "something is not right."

c. Never discount what the primary caregiver is telling you about a child. He or she may not have the medical terminology or be the most eloquent in self-expression, but caregivers do very often know their child and what might be necessary.

C. Siblings

1. The siblings of a technology-dependent or medically fragile child are often deeply affected by the circumstances in the home and family. They may feel resentment, loss of attention, anger, fear, and hostility.

2. They show signs of irritability and jealousy as a result of the added attention given to the disabled or ill child. The parent may feel guilty, depressed, or helpless in the situation.

3. Family counseling or individual counseling with the child may be beneficial and could possibly prevent difficulties in the future.

D. Financial impact on the family

1. When a child is ill, the family undergoes stress, not only from the disease or condition itself, but also from the financial impact on the caregiver and family.

2. Family income is significantly lower in families with a child assisted by technology.

3. Reduced income is often seen because the mother is usually the primary caregiver. In homes in which the mother was required to quit work, the loss of income combined with medical expenses and supplies not covered by health insurance can be overwhelming.

■ AFTER HOSPITALIZATION

A. Prescribed Pediatric Extended Care

1. There are specialized day care centers for medically fragile or technology-dependent children in locations across the country, called *Prescribed Pediatric Extended Care* (PPEC). They are few in number, and reimbursement sources have been reluctant to completely or even partially cover the costs associated with this type of day care (Thyen, Kuhlthau, and Perrin, 1999).

B. Home health care

1. There are many home health care companies available in every community, but most often the majority of their patients are elderly adults. However, many agencies that focus on adults employ a few clinicians who have the appropriate pediatric experience to provide basic and sometimes even high-tech care of the child.

a. When being referred to an agency with which you are unfamiliar, you will need to ask regarding their capabilities. When referrals are made to a home health agency for a child, you should specifically ask whether they have pediatric-experienced clinicians available.

    b. Verify the company's ability to provide pediatric equipment. Even a blood pressure cuff small enough for an infant or child might not be available.

2. Most of the same services that you can obtain in the home for adult patients can be provided to the pediatric and neonatal client as well.

3. Today, severely disabled children are cared for at home rather than being institutionalized, as was done in decades past. Most often, the primary caregiver is a parent. It is crucial to know both the capabilities and the limitations of the caregiver.

    a. When the child goes home, it is extremely important for all emergency numbers and plans to be clearly written out and placed in a conspicuous place near the telephone.

    b. The home health care provider and hospital discharge planner or case manager can often screen the parent or caregiver before discharge. Depending on the technology that the child is given, predischarge home health care teaching begins early and the duration of teaching required will vary.

4. The home health care agency caring for the child is responsible for ensuring the safety of the home regarding the home therapy or service provided.

    a. For instance, if a child is discharged with a home ventilator, the home health care agency or home equipment provider would ensure that there were adequate electrical outlets and space for the system in the home. If the home is determined to be inadequate, the provider would notify the physician and hospital immediately.

    b. Determinations should be made before the discharge decision, particularly if the service provided is life sustaining.

    c. Most JCAHO-accredited, state-certified agencies have home safety guidelines and policies to which they must adhere. Sometimes a social worker home visit might be necessary if the situation warrants such assistance.

5. The advantages and disadvantages of home care should be weighed carefully and individually for the medically fragile or technology-dependent child.

    a. Costs of care—the cost of pediatric home health care is relatively the same as that for adult home health care. There are a few companies who sell the service as high-tech or highly specialized, but for the most part, comparable care is available at the usual home health care rates. The cost of home health care is most often significantly less than care provided in the hospital, even for the most high-tech client. If hourly nursing services are required as well, the cost can increase significantly.

    b. Often, the equipment, supplies, and personnel are billed at separate rates. When these costs are combined, the daily rate for home health care in some situations could be higher than the cost of one inpatient day in the hospital. For example, if there is to be 24-hour registered nurse care, with oxygen, a ventilator, multiple medications, therapies, and other ancillary equipment and supplies in the home, carefully evaluate the feasibility of discharge to home health care. This should be evaluated on a case-by-case basis.

c. The advantages to the child are that he or she is in a familiar environment near family and friends. Usually, the child is cared for in his or her own bedroom near toys.

■ IDENTIFYING CASES WITH POTENTIAL HIGH-RISK COMPLICATIONS

A. In the current legal climate, we must be constantly vigilant to the exposure we have as professionals, particularly when children are involved. We concern ourselves first and foremost with the prompt quality care the child receives, but we must also consider each case as if we will be called on to review it in years to come. As case managers, we are increasingly held accountable for the outcome in the cases we manage.

B. With children and obstetric cases, the statute of limitations can be endless in some states. In most states, when children are concerned the statute of limitations is 21 years.

C. Treat each case as if it were the one that you will be scrutinized for in the future. In your work as a case manager, you should always be prepared for an appointment with the legal system.

D. With issues of abuse, neglect, and guardianship, it does not take a medically negligent incident to bring the case into the legal system.

E. Documentation is critical. Many case managers who enter the practice think that perhaps by leaving the clinical bedside, charting and documentation no longer reign supreme. This is a false assumption. As a case manager, documentation is extremely important, not only for communication purposes but also for the legal implications that are present. Document as if you will have no recollection of any event or contact within 5 years. A very basic but common error in documentation is failure to put a complete date on the entry. The year is often left blank. Documentation should always be objective and factual. The case you think is not high risk is often the one that turns out to be so later on.

F. With children, conversations that you have as a case manager with the parent or caregiver are crucial. Records of the times that you telephoned the caregiver(s), whether or not he or she answered, are important. Copies of letters or memos sent to any part of the team should be kept. Notes regarding conversations, home visits, team conferences, calls to physician offices, and voice mail messages you receive are critical information components, even in the simplest of cases.

G. Identifying cases that are considered high risk is a judgment call on the part of the case manager in most instances. Some companies have policies or listings of what they consider to be quality issues or high-risk clients. Many of the types of cases presented in the following list may not be high risk, but it would be prudent to evaluate them and document your findings accurately. A thorough assessment at the beginning of the case management period would also be an asset. Consistent communication with other members of the care management team is also recommended.

   H. Some high-risk pediatric clients or cases include:
   1. Hospital admission longer than 7 to 10 days
   2. Hospital readmission following discharge within 24 to 48 hours
   3. Birthweight of less than 1500 g
   4. Premature birth
   5. Multiple births (twins, triplets, or more)
   6. Neonatal intensive care unit admission
   7. Severe or multiple congenital defects
   8. Normal infant admitted to hospital within 30 to 60 days of birth
   9. Any intensive care admission of a child or neonate
   10. Hospital stay increased owing to nosocomial infection or other complication of hospitalization
   11. Accident involving any provider or facility
   12. Suspected or confirmed child abuse or neglect
   13. More than two hospitalizations within 12 months
   14. Frequent emergency room visits
   15. Cancer
   16. Traumatic brain injury
   17. Multiple physician specialties consulted
   18. Multiple surgeries
   19. Sibling of patient with sudden infant death syndrome (SIDS)
   20. Any child receiving home health care services or home medical equipment
   21. Suspected or known noncompliance with physician orders

■ COST–BENEFIT ANALYSIS

   A. Managed care has made a huge impact on the health care delivery system. Children with chronic illnesses and disabilities are increasingly joining managed care arrangements.

   B. States are actively enrolling Medicaid beneficiaries in managed care plans. By 1994, 40 states were operating or developing Medicaid-managed care plans (Newacheck, Stein, and Walker, 1996). Medicaid programs in many states have been hampered by repeated funding cuts that directly affect patient care. Theoretically, the programs save vital funds for necessary operations by allowing managed care organizations to provide utilization management for this population.

   C. Managed care organizations typically operate by a system of preferred physician networks. Sometimes an independent physician association (IPA) manages the population further. The providers a child might use are further limited, and it is hoped that the primary care physician who manages the care provides only what is absolutely necessary in the way of treatment.

   D. The ideal form of health care is to maintain health and prevent illness; thus, the health maintenance organization (HMO) was developed. Some critics note that the HMO or managed care system limits the availability of expert care, particularly in cases in which pediatric subspecialties are concerned.

E. It is a case manager's role to assist the family and the child in the navigation of this complex system. Whether or not a physician is a participating provider, the affiliation should not impede the quality or availability of necessary pediatric care.

F. Benefit plans do not always allow for the complexity of pediatric case management. As a case manager, it is critical that you carefully weigh the options available and measure them against the benefit plan. Sometimes, services or products are excluded from coverage and there is no "major medical" component to the plan. In instances such as this, a medical decision must be made by the payer about whether it is wise to uphold the policy itself or offer a prudent decision to cover a service based on its potential to prevent medical complications. Issues such as this are confronted daily in case management. Determinations should always be made with the patient's well-being and interest coming first and foremost. In situations like these, the case manager is the client advocate as well as the payer source advocate.

G. Example: Is it cost effective to uphold the denial of disposable medical supplies? What if those disposable medical supplies are central catheter care supplies? Is it not more cost effective in the long run to pay for the catheter supplies than to pay for a potential hospital stay for sepsis if the care is not given? Of course, from a case management point of view the reasonable and prudent decision is to cover the supplies despite what the policy or plan dictates. The client receives quality medical care at home and avoids the possibility of contracting an infection while being hospitalized. The payer source pays a small amount of money to prevent a potential complication of central line care.

■ COMMUNITY RESOURCES

A. Technology-dependent or medically fragile children are living longer and often are outliving their resources. Case managers are constantly in search of ways to help these children, their families, and the community to take better care of them.

B. In establishing a client support system, it is important to interview the family and tap into resources of which they may be unaware, including:
   1. Church and civic groups
   2. Their employer groups
   3. Friends and relatives
   4. Local and national chapters of such organizations (such as The March of Dimes, Cystic Fibrosis Foundation, The American Cancer Society, The American Heart Association, The National Head Injury Foundation, The American Lung Association, Easter Seals, Make-a-Wish Foundation, Candlelighters, SIDS Foundation, United Cerebral Palsy Association, Shriners, Kiwanis, Rotary, Lions, Association for Retarded Citizens, and The Spina Bifida Association)

5. State-sponsored Title V programs can help families obtain specialized medical or rehabilitation services, durable medical equipment and supplies, assistive technology, rehabilitation therapies, and other types of community-based care the child may need. Specific programs vary from state to state, and eligibility for these services is sometimes, but not always, based on financial need. Programs are typically administered through the state maternal and child health agency (American College of Emergency Physicians, 1997).

6. IDEA, a federal law, defines the required educational components that must be available to all individuals with developmental disabilities. Part H of IDEA addresses only early intervention for infants and toddlers from birth to 3 years of age and their families. Although early intervention is federally mandated, it is the responsibility of individual states to set up delivery systems that meet the needs of their youngest citizens (Berger et al., 1998).

7. The children's hospital in your area may also have resources and equipment such as wheelchairs or beds that have been donated to them from children who no longer need them or who are deceased.

REFERENCES

American College of Emergency Physicians, Emergency Medical Services for Children, National Task Force on Children with Special Health Care Needs (1997). EMS for children: Recommendations for coordinating care for children with special health care needs. *Annals of Emergency Medicine, 30,* 274–280.

Berger, S. P., Holt-Turner, I., Cupoli, J. M., Mass, M., & Hageman, J. R. (1998). Caring for the graduate from the neonatal intensive care unit: At home, in the office, and in the community. *Pediatric Clinics of North America, 45,* 701–712.

Creasy, R. K. (1984). Preterm labor and delivery: Disorder of parturition. In R. Creasy & R. Resnik (Eds.), *Maternal–fetal medicine* (pp. 401–448). Philadelphia: W. B. Saunders.

Deming, L. (1996). Planning earlier discharge from the NICU. *The Journal of Care Management, 4,* 13–27.

Newacheck, P. W., Stein, R. E. K., & Walker, D. K. (1996). Monitoring and evaluating managed care for children with chronic illnesses and disabilities. *Pediatrics, 98,* 952–958.

O'Shea, T. M., Klinepeter, K., Goldstein, D. J., Jackson, B. W., & Dillard, R. G. (1997). Survival and developmental disability in infants with birth weights of 501 to 800 grams, born between 1979 and 1994. *Pediatrics, 100,* 982–986.

Thyen, U., Kuhlthau, K., & Perrin, J. M. (1999). Employment, child care, and mental health of mothers caring for children assisted by technology. *Pediatrics, 103,* 1225–1242.

U.S. Congress, Office of Technology Assessment (1987). *Technology-dependent children: Hospital v. home care—A technical memorandum, OTA-TM-H-38.* Washington, DC: U.S. Government Printing Office.

White, P. H. (1997). Success on the road to adulthood: Issues and hurdles for adolescents with disabilities. *Rheumatic Diseases Clinics of North America, 23,* 696–707.

SUGGESTED READING

Abramovici, D., Mattar, F., & Sibai, B. (1998). Conservative management of severe preeclampsia. *Contemporary Obstetrics and Gynecology, 5*(1992), 80–105.

American Academy of Pediatrics, American College of Obstetrics and Gynecology (1992). *Guidelines for perinatal care,* 3rd ed. Washington, DC: American College of Obstetrics and Gynecology.

American Academy of Pediatrics Committee on Fetus and Newborn. (1992). Hospital stay for healthy term newborns. *Pediatrics, 96*(4), 788–790.

American Academy of Pediatrics, Committee on Children with Disabilities (1995). Guidelines for home care of infants, children, and adolescents with chronic disease. *Pediatrics, 96,* 161–164.

Annas, G. J. (1995). Women and children first. *New England Journal of Medicine, 333*(24), 1647–1651.

Beebe, S. A., Britton, J. R., Britton, H. L., Fan, P., & Jepson, B. (1996). Neonatal mortality and length of newborn hospital stay. *Pediatrics, 98,* 231–235.

Beebe, S. A., Britton, J. R., Britton, H. L., Fan, P., & Jepson, B. (1996). Neonatal mortality and length of newborn hospital stay. *Pediatrics, 98,* 231–235.

Braveman, P., Egerter, S., Pearl, M., Marchi, K., & Miller, C. (1995). Problems associated with early discharge of newborn infants—early discharge of newborns and mothers: A critical review of the literature. *Pediatrics, 96*(4), 716–726.

Cavalier, S., Escobar, G., Fernbach, S., Quesenberry, C., & Chellino, M. (1996). Post discharge utilization of medical services by high-risk infants: Experience in a large managed care organization. *Pediatrics, 97,* 693–699.

Couto, J. (2004). Levels of neonatal care. Committee on fetus and newborn [Electronic version]. *Pediatrics, 114,* 1341–1347.

Cowan, M. J. (1996). Hyperemesis gravidarum: Implications for home care and infusion therapies. *Journal of Intravenous Nursing, 19,* 46–58.

Creasy, R. K. Prevention of preterm birth. *Birth Defects, 19*(5), 97.

Diehl-Svrjcek, B. C., & Richardson, R. (2005). Decreasing NICU Costs in the managed care arena. *Lippincott's Case Management, 10*(3), 159–166.

Elliott, J. P., Flynn, M. J., Kaemmerer, E. L., & Radin, T. G. (1997). Terbutaline pump tocolysis in high-order multiple gestation. *Journal of Reproductive Medicine, 42,* 687–693.

Fangman, J. J., Mark, P. M., Pratt, L., Conway, K. K., Healey, M. L., Oswald, J. W., & Uden, D. L. (1994). Prematurity prevention programs: An analysis of successes and failures. *American Journal of Obstetrics and Gynecology, 170*(3), 744–750.

Gabbe, S., Hill, L., Schmidt, L., & Schulkin, J. (1998). Management of diabetes by obstetrician-gynecologists. *Obstetrics and Gynecology, 91,* 643–647.

Giacoia, G. P. (1997). Follow-up of school-age children with bronchopulmonary dysplasia. *Journal of Pediatrics, 130,* 400–408.

Goldberg, A. I. (1995). Pediatric home health: The need for physician education. *Pediatrics, 95,* 928–930.

Gorski, L. (2005). Hospital to home care: Discharge planning for the patient requiring home infusion therapy. *Topics in Advanced Practice Nursing eJournal, 5*(3).

Grady, M. A., & Bloom, K. C. (2004). Pregnancy outcomes of adolescents enrolled in a Centering-Pregnancy program. *Journal of Midwifery & Women's Health 49*(5), 412–420.

Griffin, P. D. M. (1995). *The managed care resource manual for obstetrics.* Marietta, GA: Healthdyne Perinatal Services.

Health Care Finance Administration, Children's Health Insurance Program. Website: *www.hcfa. gov/init/children.htm.* Retrieved September 26, 1999.

Insure Kids Now. Website: *www.insurekidsnow.gov.* Retrieved September 26, 1999.

Ireys, H. T., Grason, H. A., Guyer, B. G. (1996). Assuring quality of care for children with special needs in managed care organizations: Roles for pediatricians. *Pediatrics, 98,* 178–185.

Johnson, K. A., & Little, G. A. (1999). State health agencies and quality improvement in perinatal care. *Pediatrics, 103,* 233–247.

Kogan, M. D., Alexancer, G. R., Jack, B. W., & Allen, M. C. (1998). The association between adequacy of prenatal care utilization and subsequent pediatric care utilization in the United States. *Pediatrics, 102*(1), 25–30.

Kotula, C. (1994). High-risk pregnancy. *Continuing Care, 6,* 15–18.

Kuhlthau, K., Perrin, J. M., Ettner, S. L., McLaughlin, T. J., & Gortmaker, S. L. (1998). High-expenditure children with supplemental security income. *Pediatrics, 102,* 610–615.

Liptak, G. S. (1998). The child who has severe neurologic impairment. *Pediatric Clinics of North America, 45,* 123–144.

Mamelle, N., Segueilla, M., Munoz, F., & Berland, M. (1997). Prevention of preterm birth in patients with symptoms of preterm labor—The benefits of psychological support. *American Journal of Obstetrics and Gynecology, 10,* 947–952.

March of Dimes Birth Defects Foundation. Website: *www.marchofdimes.com.* Retrieved March 6, 2006.

Martin, J. A., Hamilton, B. E., Sutton, P. D., Ventura, S. J., Menacker, F., Munson, M. S. (2003). Births: Final data for 2002. *National Vital Statistics Reports, 52*(10). Hyattsville, MD: National Center for Health Statistics.

Matria Healthcare, Inc. (1996). *Management of preterm labor in a managed care environment.* Marietta, GA: Matria.

Matria Healthcare Inc. (1998). *Managing diabetes in pregnancy in a managed care environment.* Marietta, GA: Matria.

Matria Healthcare Inc. (1999). *Time makes a difference.* Marietta, GA: Matria.

Mendoza, M. E., & Chaves, J. F. (2003). Helping pregnant women cope with smoking cessation. *Topics in Advanced Practice Nursing eJournal, 3*(4).

Naef, R. W. III, Chauhan, S. P., Roach, H., Roberts, W. E., Travis, K. H., & Morrison, J. C. (1995). Treatment for hyperemesis gravidarum in the home: An alternative to hospitalization. *Journal of Perinatology, 15,* 289–292.

Newacheck, P. W. (1996). Children's access to primary care: Differences by race, income, and insurance status. *Pediatrics, 97,* 26–32.

NIH Consensus Development Panel (1995). Effect of corticosteroids for fetal maturation on perinatal outcomes. *Journal of the American Medical Association, 273,* 413–417.

Osberg, J. S., Kahn, P., Rowe, K., & Brooke, M. M. (1996). Pediatric trauma: Impact on work and family finances. *Pediatrics, 98,* 890–897.

Rust, O., Perry, K., Andrew, M., Roberts, W., Martin, R., & Morrison, J. (1997). Twins and preterm labor. *Journal of Reproductive Medicine, 42,* 229–234.

Sala, D. J., & Moise, K. J. Jr. (1990). The treatment of preterm labor using portable subcutaneous terbutaline pump. *Journal of Obstetrical, Gynecologic, and Neonatal Nursing, 19*(2), 108–115.

Scialli, A. R. (1998). High-risk pregnancy: Nausea and vomiting. *Contemporary Obstetrics and Gynecology, 5,* 13–16.

Scholer, S. J. (1997). Predictors of injury mortality in early childhood. *Pediatrics, 100,* 324–347.

Strauss, D., Ashwal, S., Shavelle, R., & Eyman, R. (1997). Prognosis for survival and improvement in function in children with severe developmental disabilities. *Pediatrics, 131,* 712–716.

Toder, D. S., & McBride, J. T. (1997). Home care of children dependent on respiratory technology. *Pediatrics in Review, 18,* 274–280.

Van Cleve, S. N., & Cohen, W. I., (2006). Part I: Clinical practice guidelines with Down syndrome from birth to 12 years. *Journal of Pediatric Health Care, 20*(1): 47–54.

Westbrook, L. E. (1998). Implications for estimates of disability in children: A comparison of definitional components. *Pediatrics, 101,* 1025–1030.

Wilson-Costello, D., Borawski, E., Friedman, H., Redline, R., Fanaroff, A. A., & Hack, M. (1998). Perinatal correlates of cerebral palsy and other neurologic impairment among very low birth weight children. *Pediatrics, 102,* 315–321.

Geriatric Case Management

Linda N. Schoenbeck

Upon completion of this chapter, the reader will be able to:

1. List various methods of identifying high-risk geriatric patients for case management.
2. Assess for and identify common geriatric problems.
3. Assess and identify care needs of the geriatric patient.
4. List available tools to aid in assessment of geriatric patients.
5. Describe comprehensive geriatric assessment and when such assessment is useful.
6. Identify steps of the geriatric placement process.
7. Identify community resources to assist with common problems.
8. List common payment and insurance issues and resources.

IMPORTANT TERMS AND CONCEPTS

Assessment	Elder Depression
Activities of Daily Living (ADLs)	Instrumental ADLs (IADLs)
Altered Mental Status (AMS)	PRA Plus
Comprehensive Geriatric Assessment	Prediction of Repeat Admissions (PRA)
Delirium	Psychological Health Assessment
Dementia	Screening
Elder Abuse	SF-36 and SF-12

■ INTRODUCTION

A. The population that is older than 65 years of age is growing.

B. Just 4% of the population was older than 65 years at the beginning of the century; now the proportion of elderly individuals exceeds 12%.

C. By the year 2030, the older population will be more than double (71.5 million).

D. Eighty-five percent of those over 65 years of age have at least one chronic condition, and many will have multiple conditions, such as hypertension (49.2%), arthritic symptoms (36.2%), and all types of heart disease (31.1%), any cancer (20.0%), and diabetes (15%).

E. In 1997, more than half the older population (54%) reported having at least one disability of some type (physical and nonphysical). Over one third reported at least one severe disability.

F. The fastest growing segments of the population, the oldest old (people greater than 85 years of age), accounted for about 12% of all elderly people in 2000 and is projected to account for 19% by 2040.

G. Expertise in the case management of geriatric patients is critical for case managers owing to:
   1. Numbers of patients seen in this category; and
   2. Diversity of health care delivery sites and services attending to this group

H. Case management of the geriatric patient differs from that of other patient populations.

I. Demographics (2003)
   1. More than 10.5 million Americans (30.8%) older than 65 years of age live alone.
   2. Eighty percent of those living alone are women.
   3. Nearly half of persons aged 75 or older live alone.
   4. Older women, the very old, and the minority elderly population have, on average, the lowest incomes among the older population.
   5. In 2000, 4.5% (1.56 million) of the 65+ population lived in nursing homes.
   6. Functional disability has increased. Almost 76.3% of institutionalized Medicare beneficiaries needed help with three or more activities of daily living (ADLs). Ninety-three percent of all Medicare beneficiaries needed help with one or more ADLs.
   7. About one fourth of all nursing home costs are paid out of pocket by individuals and their families.
   8. Women compose more than two-thirds (71.6%) of the total nursing home population.
   9. Approximately half of all residents are age 85 and older.

J. In the United States, the growing population of elderly people will have enormous effects on the distribution of health care.

■ KEY DEFINITIONS

A. Abuse—The willful infliction of injury, unreasonable confinement, intimidation, or cruel punishment with resulting pain or mental anguish, or the willful depreciation by a caretaker of goods or services that is necessary to avoid physical harm, mental anguish, or mental illness (Abyad, 1996).

B. Multidimensional assessment or comprehensive geriatric assessment (CGA)—A comprehensive assessment that includes evaluation of a patient in several domains: physical, mental, socioeconomic, functional, and environmental status.

C. Neglect—The failure to provide the goods or services that are necessary to avoid physical harm, mental anguish, or mental illness (Abyad, 1996).

D. Pain assessment—A comprehensive assessment of pain in the geriatric patient should include intensity, character, frequency, location, duration, aggravating and alleviating factors, medical history, thorough analgesic medication history and side effects (if any), ADLs, and psychological function. A quantitative evaluation of pain should also be recorded by the use of a standard pain scale. Patients with cognitive, language, or sensory impairments should be evaluated with scales that are tailored for their needs and disabilities (American Geriatrics Society, 1998).

E. Predictor of repeat admissions (PRA)—A valid and reliable tool for identifying high-risk seniors (age 65 years or greater) who have a statistically higher probability of repeat hospital admission; developed by Chad Boult and associates from the University of Minnesota.

F. Screening—The process by which a health care provider institutes specific criteria to select potential recipients of case management. A screening questionnaire can be administered to a defined population of individuals (i.e., new enrollees into a Medicare risk plan) to identify those at high risk for an adverse health event who may be candidates for case management (HMO Work Group on Care Management, 1996).

■ COMMON GERIATRIC PROBLEMS

A. Numerous problems can occur in the geriatric population and are characterized by the following:

1. Frequent occurrence
2. Under-recognition and under-treatment
3. Multiple causes
4. Impact on the individual's ability to function

B. This list is not all-inclusive or comprehensive but represents common issues.

1. The issues above, along with others, are presented to serve as reminders to case managers working with the geriatric population.
2. Many of the issues presented here can manifest themselves in a variety of ways and can also be the precipitating cause of other problems. For this reason, the case manager must be aware of these issues.

3. Many case managers do not see the individuals they are charged with managing, or they do not complete in-depth assessments.

4. Discussing these issues should familiarize the case manager with the key points for each problem so that he or she can appropriately intervene.

5. Regardless of the case management setting, the case manager can ensure that the problems presented here are adequately assessed and the issues addressed appropriately.

C. Altered mental status (AMS)

1. AMS is an umbrella term linked to a variety of other descriptors of mental status, including confusion, delirium, obtundation, stupor, and coma.

2. A great deal of elder assessment depends on the assessment of a person's mental state to some degree (Gallo, Reichel, and Anderson, 1988).

3. Changes in mental status can be very subtle and often go unrecognized.

4. There are several types and causes of cognitive decline; dementia is not the only cause.

5. Case managers who work with geriatric patients should familiarize themselves with the different causes of and risk factors relating to cognitive decline.

6. AMS can be the cause of many other problems identified by case managers:

   a. Nonadherence to treatment plans or medications, or both
   b. Injuries such as falls and burns
   c. Nutritional deficits
   d. Agitation or aggressive behavior
   e. Depression
   f. Social isolation
   g. Fluid and electrolyte disturbances
   h. Infections
   i. Chemical withdrawal
   j. Chemical intoxicants

7. Delirium and dementia can be confused. Although both are AMS, *delirium* is a sudden change in mental functioning and/or acute confusion—*sudden* being the key word. *Dementia* is an *acquired* loss of intellectual functioning that occurs over a long period of time.

8. A baseline assessment of mental status using a standardized tool can help identify and track the progression of mental status.

   a. Standardized tools
      i. There are several tools that test mental status.
      ii. One of the most popular is the Short Portable Mental Status Questionnaire for the Assessment of Organic Brain Disease in the elderly population (Pfeiffer, 1975).

iii. Another popular questionnaire is the Folstein Mini-Mental Status Examination (Folstein, Folstein, and McHugh, 1975).

iv. The confusion assessment method may also be used to determine and distinguish dementia from delirium.

v. Several other tests are available to identify and quantify the presence of cognitive deficits.

vi. The choice of instrument depends on the case manager's practice setting.

vii. The case manager may not be the one who actually administers the test, but he or she should be aware of the availability of the various tools and recommend their use when appropriate.

D. Urinary incontinence

1. Although the urinary system is affected by changes in aging, incontinence should not be thought of as an inevitable part of aging.

2. Assessment for incontinence or the risk of incontinence should be multifaceted and cover the following factors (Miller, 1999):

a. Risk factors influencing elimination, such as prostate surgery

b. Social risk factors such as being able to read bathroom signs when out of the home

c. Signs and symptoms of actual dysfunction, such as leaking urine

d. Whether incontinence is acknowledged. Ask when the problem began, and what has been done about it.

e. Fears about incontinence that include changing activities because of the need to go to the toilet

f. Behavioral signs, such as a urine odor or use of pads

g. Environmental factors that may contribute to incontinence, such as having to go upstairs to use the bathroom

h. Drug side effects

i. Delirium or hypoxia

j. Excessive fluid intake

k. Impaired mobility

l. Physiologic factors—history of prostectomy, atrophic vaginitis, glycosuria

3. Incontinence is often unreported and can have a significant impact on the life and functioning of the older adult.

4. It is important for case managers to assess for and arrange interventions directed at resolving and/or improving the problem.

E. Safety issues

1. Falls

a. Multiple risk factors are associated with falls in the elderly (Miller, 1999).

i. Age-related changes such as:

(a) Vision and hearing changes

(b) Osteoporosis

        (c) Slowed reaction time

        (d) Altered gait

        (e) Postural hypotension

        (f) Nocturia

    ii. Medical problems

    iii. Psychosocial factors such as depression

    iv. Medications

    v. Environmental factors

    vi. Any combination of the abovementioned items

    vii. Fear of falling or post-fall anxiety syndrome are also well recognized as negative consequences of falls

b. The case manager should assess for the presence of the abovementioned risk factors, especially if there is a history of previous falls.

c. As the case manager conducts the overall assessment of the individual, he or she should think about the possibility of falls and whether any of the information collected puts the individual at greater risk.

d. The fall assessment tool should include history of falls, confusion, impaired judgment, mobility status, cooperation, medications, physiological factors that may influence mobility or lack of mobility, mobility aids, to mention a few.

e. Resources are available to help the case manager with the assessment.

    i. The physical therapist can assess the individual's gait and balance.

    ii. A thorough home safety evaluation can identify environmental concerns.

    iii. A thorough history from the primary care physician that includes medications and health conditions can assist with identifying medical risk factors.

f. The case manager should tailor the interventions directed at preventing falls to the specific risk factors.

g. Although creating a safe environment is a good overall intervention, it will not fully address the risk of falls if the medication the person is taking makes him or her dizzy.

2. Elder abuse and neglect

a. As many as one-third of victims unequivocally deny abuse (Abyad, 1996).

b. The prevalence of abuse varies in several studies but ranges between 1% and 10% (Miller, 1999).

c. Victims' characteristics:

    i. Females are at a higher risk owing to the fact that they outlive men and because of gender issues.

    ii. Persons 80 years and older suffer abuse and neglect two to three times more than the older population according to the National Elder Abuse Incidence Study (NCEA, 1998).

     iii. Among known perpetrators of abuse and neglect, the perpetrator was a family member in 90% of cases. Two-thirds of the perpetrators were adult children or spouses (National Elder Abuse Incidence Study, 1998).

     iv. Most elder abuse and neglect takes place at home, not in the nursing home.

     v. Advanced age

     vi. Greater dependency

     vii. Alcohol abuse

     viii. Intergenerational conflict

     ix. Isolation

     x. Internalization of blame

     xi. Provocative behavior

     xii. Past history of being abused

d. Abusers' characteristics:

     i. Alcohol and drug abuse

     ii. Mental illness

     iii. Caregiver inexperience

     iv. History of abuse as a child

     v. Stress

     vi. Economic dependence on elder

e. Families' characteristics:

     i. Caregiver reluctance

     ii. Overcrowding

     iii. Isolation

     iv. Marital conflict

     v. History of past abuse

     vi. Caregiver spouse or companion caring for elder may have some dementia exhibited in abuse or neglect toward the other

f. In assessing elders and creating care plans, it is natural for the case manager to look to the family as a large part of the caregiver equation.

g. It is critical that the case manager evaluate the potential for risk and intervene to reduce and/or eliminate the risk.

h. Some examples of interventions include:

     i. Provide education to the caregiver about each aspect of the expected care.

     ii. Discuss examples of situations in which the behavior of the elder patient causes frustration, anger, or feelings of helplessness in the caregiver. Help the caregiver identify appropriate responses to these feelings.

     iii. Set realistic expectations, and frankly discuss the demands of caring for a dependent individual.

    iv. Provide for direct observation of the home situation and the interaction between the elder family member and the caregivers. A home health nurse or a case manager may be able to identify subtle signs of trouble before it occurs.

    v. Assess the support system of the caregiver, and assist him or her in identification of support groups or respite from caregiver activities.

    vi. Support and encourage the elderly person to continue to be as independent as his or her condition allows.

    vii. Refer the caregiver to marital, substance abuse, or other specialized counseling services.

    viii. Recommend different arrangements for the elderly person. Not every family can successfully provide care for the elder family member.

i. Most states have specific reporting requirements for elder abuse and neglect. Most require reporting by the health care professionals who suspect abuse.

j. The case manager should become aware of both the state and organizational reporting policies for elder abuse and neglect.

k. The case manager can recognize the possibility of elder abuse and neglect through signs such as the following:

    i. Direct reports by the elder of incidents

    ii. A rapid or unexplained decline in the physical condition of the elderly patient

    iii. Malnutrition

    iv. Suspicious injuries or conflicting reports of injury from the patient and the caregiver (Abyad, 1996)

       (a) Lacerations and bruises in multiple states of healing

       (b) Multiple fractures in various states of healing

       (c) Scald burns with demarcated immersion lines and no splash marks, involving the anterior or posterior half of extremity, or to the buttocks or genitals

       (d) Cigarette burns

       (e) Rope burns or marks

       (f) Refusal to go to the same emergency department for repeated injuries

       (g) Evasiveness

l. Many case managers may not see the patient or examine them for these types of injuries.

m. Although most health care professionals are trained to recognize abuse; it is still possible for them to miss the signs.

n. Case managers may be the first to complete the picture and recognize abuse. This is especially true if the caregiver takes the patient to multiple providers and the case manager is the only constant of the health care team.

o. Case managers will want to act as an advocate for the patient and take immediate steps to ensure the patient's safety.

p. Case managers should be aware of state and federal agencies that take reports of elder abuse and neglect—Area Agency on Aging (AOA), Adult Protective Services (APS), and National Domestic Hotline.

F. Elder Depression

1. Depression is underreported and undertreated in the elderly population.

2. Geriatric depression is widespread; at least 16% of patients receiving care in a primary care setting and a higher percentage in hospitals and nursing homes exhibit depression (Reynolds and Kupfer, 1999).

3. Risk factors for depression are family history, alcohol abuse, heart attack or stroke, anxiety disorders, mood disorders, chronic medical illnesses, and personality disorders.

4. Common signs of depression are loss of interest in self-care or following medical advice, trouble sleeping or anxiety, little interest in outside activities, trouble concentrating or remembering things, unexplained aches and pains, change in appetite or weight loss, feeling hopeless about the future, feelings of helplessness, easily irritated or listless, or feeling one is a burden.

5. The five "D's" of depression are disability, decline, diminished quality of life, demand on caregivers, and dementia (Kevorkian, 2005).

6. Depression can be the root cause of many other observed problems in the elderly, such as:

a. Nonadherence to treatment

b. Social isolation

c. Cognitive impairment

d. Malnutrition

e. Alcohol abuse

7. There are tools available to detect unrecognized depression in the geriatric individual.

8. Even though the case manager may not be responsible for the administration of such tests, he or she should be aware of their existence and recommend them as appropriate.

9. The Geriatric Depression Scale (Yesavage and Brink, 1983), developed by Yesavage and colleagues, was used in one geriatric program with good reported success.

10. Case managers using the scale believed that they were able to refer geriatric patients who might be suffering from depression for further evaluation.

11. The Cornell Scale for Depression in Dementia (CSDD) can be used to detect depression in geriatric patients with dementia. It is not an interview tool, but is based on observation and signs and symptoms.

12. The Beck Depression Inventory (Gallo, Reichel, and Anderson, 1988) is another tool for detecting depression. The Beck Inventory is administered by an interviewer but has been adapted for self-administration.

13. Regardless of what tool is used, if any, case managers should be aware of the potential for depression.

14. Appropriate referrals should be arranged if depression (actual or potential) is detected.

G. Constipation

1. Individuals older than the age of 55 are at increased risk for constipation. Constipation affects as many as 26% of elderly men and 34% of elderly women (Schaefer and Cheskin, 1998).

2. The definition of constipation can be described as either functional (straining, hard stools) or rectal outlet delay (anal blockage or prolonged defecation).

3. Other risk factors include (University of Iowa, 1998):
   a. Recent abdominal surgery
   b. Limited physical activity
   c. Inadequate diet, with fiber less than 15 g per day
   d. Intake of medications known to contribute to constipation
   e. History of chronic constipation
   f. Laxative abuse history
   g. Other comorbidities known to cause constipation
   h. Endocrine or metabolic disorders
   i. Neurogenic disorders
   j. Smooth muscle or connective tissue disorders

4. Interventions include diet, exercise, fluid intake, and laxative use, according to the individual situation.

H. Polypharmacy

1. Over 50% of individuals older than the age of 65 years take four or more medications on a routine basis.

2. The normal physiologic changes associated with aging cause the elderly individual to be more prone to medication-related problems.

3. The combination of several medications and the aging process can cause issues in the elderly.

4. All of the problems mentioned earlier in this section can be triggered by medications.

5. Adherence issues increase in proportion to the complexity of the regimen (Council for Case Management Accountability—Hamilton, 1999).

6. A thorough assessment of the individual's prescription and nonprescription medications is essential to the case management assessment of the elderly.

7. Case managers can enlist the aid of the physician or the pharmacist to review the medications used by the older person and can make recommendations for changes.

8. Fifty percent of all medication errors and up to 20% of adverse drug events in the hospital can be attributed to lack of medication reconciliation. Each time a geriatric patient moves from one setting to the other, the case manager should make every effort to review medications with the care team.
9. Case managers should remember to consider medications in relation to other issues presenting in the case.

■ IDENTIFICATION OF HIGH-RISK GERIATRIC PATIENTS

A. A brief history of early identification efforts:
   1. In the early days of case management, cases were identified primarily through diagnostic criteria or through an event such as a workers' compensation injury.
   2. Most of the cases were identified after the diagnosis or event had already occurred.
   3. With the advent of the managed Medicare programs, health maintenance organizations (HMOs) found themselves at financial risk for large populations of geriatric members.
   4. Once a geriatric member became ill, costs were greater and the illnesses were often more severe.
   5. The added burden of comorbidities in this population made interventions by case managers more difficult.
   6. There was an increasing demand for methods to identify geriatric patients before the onset of illness or a major decline in health status. Two reasons propelled the need for earlier identification:
      a. Once a geriatric member became ill, he or she consumed two to four times more resources than a healthy geriatric member. This problem increased costs of care.
      b. The more reactive style of case management that relied on a diagnosis or event did not fulfill the potential for case management impact in this population.
   7. Early efforts at identification and prediction of risks were intuitive and based primarily on the case manager's or medical director's knowledge and experience.
   8. Questionnaires of varying lengths, some up to 12 pages, were mailed to geriatric health plan members, and trigger criteria were established to help identify geriatric patients who were, or could be, at high risk.
   9. There were several pitfalls to the early use of questionnaires:
      a. Intuition has its limits. Some questions that a practitioner believes would be useful in predicting risk are not useful.
      b. Without a specific method of scoring the questionnaires, case managers were left to use their judgment regarding which geriatric members were at risk and should be contacted.
         i. In one informal comparison, one group of case management staff contacted approximately 40% of the members returning

a questionnaire, and another group of staff contacted approximately 6% of the members returning the identical questionnaire.

    ii. The emphasis and focus of the two groups varied significantly and resulted in different rates of follow up.

    iii. There was no way to determine whether either group was actually focusing on the group of patients that could most benefit from case management.

  c. Without a scoring methodology, case managers were still required to review each questionnaire. This did not yield any real efficiency or accuracy in the identification of high-risk geriatric patients.

B. Screening versus assessment

1. It is important to differentiate screening from assessment. Without a clear differentiation of these two concepts, case managers will spend time and resources where they are not necessary.

2. When individuals are identified primarily because of a diagnosis or event, most of those individuals are ultimately deemed appropriate for case management.

3. In the circumstance in which the overwhelming majority of the individuals who are referred to case managers actually need case management, assessment by the case manager is a logical first step.

4. When the goal is to identify individuals who are at risk or in the very early stages of decline, different strategies are necessary.

5. One method of addressing the issues of earlier identification and increasing the objectivity in follow up was the development of screening tools that are valid and reliable in predicting risk.

6. Use the example of a health fair, in which random blood glucose levels are obtained via finger stick. This is illustrative of several key principles of screening:

  a. The screening is aimed at a broad group of individuals to identify as many as possible and as early as possible.

  b. Individuals other than health care professionals can do the screening.

  c. The screening does not positively determine that the individual meets the criteria or diagnosis and requires further assessment by a health care professional.

7. Screening accomplishes the following objectives:

  a. Identifying those geriatric patients who may be at risk before an adverse event without using case management resources

  b. Providing an objective method of determining which members require assessment by a case manager

8. Assessment also differs from screening in several other ways. Unlike screening:

  a. An assessment is reserved for those who have met some initial criteria not broadly applied.

  b. A qualified case manager should perform a comprehensive case management assessment.

    c. An assessment can determine whether the individual actually needs further follow up.

  9. Goals of assessment include:

    a. Collection of data in order to identify problems or issues

    b. Determination of whether the problems or issues identified may be impacted by case management interventions

    c. Creation of an individualized plan of care

C. Development of the Predictor of Repeat Admission (PRA)

  1. The first widely used screening questionnaire was the PRA.

  2. In 1994, Chad Boult and his associates at the University of Minnesota published information on the PRA (Boult et al., 1994).

  3. The PRA was brief (seven questions) and allowed for scoring that placed geriatric members into high-risk, medium-risk, and low-risk groups.

  4. This allowed case managers to focus interventions based on the actual risk of the member being hospitalized.

  5. Although it is efficient and accurate, the original PRA was somewhat unsatisfactory to case managers.

    a. The questions that were used to calculate the risk score did not always correlate with the data case managers used to assess the individual.

    b. The answers to the questions and the score provided the case manager with little information as to where to focus the assessment. For example, were there issues with medication compliance?

  6. The PRA Plus (HMO Work Group on Care Management, 1996) added a set of bridging questions.

    a. The bridging questions were not a part of the scoring.

    b. The questions provided a bridge from the screening of individuals to the assessment of individuals for case management.

    c. Items such as functional status, which allowed the case manager the opportunity to focus on potential problem areas, were added.

D. SF (Short Form) 36—This document is a comprehensive short form with only 36 questions.

  1. It yields an 8-scale health profile, as well as summary measures of health-related quality of life.

  2. SF-36 measures both physical and mental components of health.

    a. Physical component—function, role, bodily pain, and general health

    b. Mental component—mental health, emotional role, social function, and vitality

  3. As documented in more than 4000 publications, the SF-36 has proved useful in monitoring general and specific populations, comparing the burden of different diseases, differentiating the health benefits produced by different treatments, and screening individual

patients. Most widely evaluated generic instrument that is used for the assessment of patient health outcome.

4. Development of the SF-36 health survey and collection of norms for the general U.S. population were supported by grants to the Health Assessment Lab at the Health Institute, New England Medical Center (Boston, Massachusetts) from the Henry J. Kaiser Family Foundation (John E. Ware Jr., principal investigator).

5. The SF-36 is an excellent baseline measure, as is the SF-12 (a shorter version of the SF-36), which can be administered as part of the screening process to allow for comparison of outcomes after case management intervention.

6. In 1996, version 2.0 was introduced to correct deficiencies identified in the original version. The SF-36v2 included improvements such as improvement in instructions; less-ambiguous, improved layout of form; greater compatibility with translations and cultural adaptations; and available in standard (4-week) and acute (1-week) form.

7. SF-12 is a shorter version of the SF-36. It is a single page scannable health survey that documents physical and mental health summary measures. It is useful to general and specific populations.

■ COMPREHENSIVE GERIATRIC ASSESSMENT

A. A small number of geriatric patients should receive a comprehensive geriatric assessment.

B. The assessment is usually conducted by a team of geriatric experts from multiple disciplines and encompasses all aspects of the individual's health and functioning.

C. Usually connected with an academic medical center or veteran's hospital, the assessment is conducted on referral.

D. The elements of the geriatric assessment include:
1. Physical
2. Functional
3. Social
4. Financial
5. Cognitive
6. Nutritional
7. Environmental
8. Medications

E. Geriatric assessment is recommended when there are multiple problems (recognized or unrecognized) and when the current plans are not addressing the identified problems or issues.

F. Caregivers should be a part of the geriatric assessment as they can help the case manager determine specific needs related to the patient, and reflect the stresses experienced by caregivers of geriatric patients.

■ **GERIATRIC ASSESSMENT FOR PLACEMENT OF THE GERIATRIC PATIENT**

A. Functional ability assessment—Activities of Daily Living (ADLs)
   1. Assessment categories:
      a. Bathing
      b. Dressing
      c. Toileting
      d. Transferring
      e. Continence
      f. Feeding
   2. Scoring
      a. The individual receives a point for every function that he or she is able to do independently.
         i. A score of 6 indicates full function.
         ii. A score of 4 indicates moderate impairment.
         iii. A score of 2 indicates severe impairment.

B. Functional ability assessment—Instrumental Activities of Daily Living (IADLs)
   1. Assessment categories focus on the following:
      a. Use of the telephone
      b. Getting to places beyond walking distance
      c. Going shopping for groceries
      d. Preparing own meals
      e. Doing own housework
      f. Doing own handyman work
      g. Doing own laundry
      h. Taking own medication
      i. Managing own money
   2. Scoring
      a. These items can be made gender specific by the interviewer.
      b. The score range is 9 (poor) to 27 (good).
      c. Scores are patient specific only.

C. Psychological health assessment—Folstein Mini-Mental State Examination
   1. Categories of assessment:
      a. Orientation to time, place, and date
      b. Registration: name three objects
      c. Attention and calculation
      d. Recall
      e. Language: repetition, commands, read, and repeat
      f. Draw a clock
      g. Assess level of consciousness

2. Scoring
   a. The score range is 0 (poor) to 30 (good).
   b. Scores are patient specific only.

D. Psychological health assessment—Yesavage Geriatric Depression Scale
   1. The short form addresses various moods with 15 questions.
   2. Scoring is cumulative, based on a "yes or no" response.

E. Physical health assessment
   1. A traditional list of defined diagnoses and symptom complexes
   2. Documentation of the number of days of hospitalization and disability can define the severity of health problems.
   3. May use New York Heart Association Four Point Functional Disability Scale for clarification of degree of disability if the disorder is due to a cardiac problem.
      a. A subjective assessment to determine the severity of congestive heart failure
      b. Scoring system with problem history of last 30 days

F. Fall risk assessment
   1. The fall assessment tool should include history of falls, confusion, impaired judgment, mobility status, cooperation, medications, physiological factors that may influence mobility or lack of mobility, mobility aids, to mention a few.
   2. Case managers should also be aware of previous falls both in the home and at other levels of the health care continuum.

G. Nutritional assessment
   1. Use a nutritional checklist that identifies amount of food eaten on a daily basis, what kinds of food, problems eating certain kinds of food, likes and dislikes, ability to shop, cook, prepare food, and any dental or oral problems.
   2. Be aware of any strange food preferences or only eating one type of food (chocolate cake and cookies). Obesity can also signal a nutritional deficiency.

H. Oral health
   1. Case managers should be aware of any gums, teeth, tongue, or dental pain issues.
   2. Assess, if the geriatric patient has dentures, whether they use them and are they in good repair?

I. Pressure ulcers
   1. Because geriatric patients are always at risk for pressure ulcers due to decreased mobility or immobility, a case manager should use the "Braden Scale for Predicting Pressure Sore Risk."
   2. This tool is not just for the nursing home patient. Geriatric patients have a risk of developing pressure ulcers due to immobility, friction while moving, decreased sensory perception, and poor circulation.

J. Visual acuity

1. Case managers should use the "Snellen Eye Chart" tool to screen for visual acuity.

2. This will help determine the need for referral to an ophthalmologist if visual acuity is worse than 20/40 with glasses. This visual impairment can interfere with ADLs.

REFERENCES

Abyad, A. (1996). Elder abuse: Diagnosis, management, and prevention. *Medical Interface,* October, 97–101.

American Geriatrics Society, Clinical Practice Guidelines. (1998). *The management of chronic pain in older persons: AGS panel on chronic pain in the older person. Journal of the American Geriatrics Society, 46,* 635–641.

Boult, C., Dowd, B., McCaffery, D., et al. (1994). Screening elders at risk for hospitalization. *Journal of the American Geriatrics Society, 42,* 456–470.

Council for Case Management Accountability—Hamilton, G. A. (1999). Patient adherence outcome indicators and measurement in case management and health care. A State of the Science paper.

Folstein, M., Folstein, S., & McHugh, P. (1975). Mini-mental state: A practical method for grading the cognitive state of patients for the clinician. *Journal of Psychiatric Resources, 12,* 189–198.

Gallo, J., Reichel, W., & Andersen, L. (1988). *Handbook of geriatric assessment.* Gaithersburg, MD: Aspen.

HMO Work Group on Care Management, (April, 1996). Identifying high-risk Medicare HMO members. America's Health Insurance Plans, Washington, DC. *Website: http://www.ahip.org/content/default.aspx?bc=38/65/69.*

Kevorkian, R. (May, 2005). Depression in the elderly. *Website:http://www.thedoctorwillseeyounow.com/articles/behavior/depression–12.*

National Center on Elder Abuse (1998). National Elder Abuse Incidence Study. The Clearing House on Abuse and Neglect of the Elderly, Department of Consumers Studies, University of Deleware, Newark, DE.

Pfeiffer, E. (1975). A short portable mental status questionnaire for the assessment of organic brain deficit in the older adult patient. *Journal of American Geriatrics, 23,* 433.

Reynolds, C., & Kupfer, D. (1998). Depression and aging, a look to the future. *Psychiatric Services, 50*(9):1167–1172.

Schaefer, D., & Cheskin, L. (1998) Constipation in the elderly. *American Family Physician, 58*(4):907–919.

University of Iowa. (1998). *Research based protocol, no. 49* (June). National Guideline Clearing House. Website: *www.guidelines.gov.*

Yesavage, J. A., & Brink, T. L. (1983). Development and validation of a geriatric depression screening scale: A preliminary report. *Journal of Psychiatric Research, 17,* 4.

SUGGESTED READING

Administration on Aging and the Older Americans Act. (1999). Aging in America. Website: *http://www.aoa.dhhs.gov/aoa/pages/aoafact.html.*

Administration on Aging. (2004). A profile of older Americans. Administration on Aging, U.S. Department of Health and Human Services.

American Geriatrics Society, British Geriatrics Society, and American Academy of Orthopedic Surgeons Panel on Falls Prevention. (2001). Guidelines for prevention of falls in older persons. *Journal of the American Geriatrics Society, 49,* 664–672.

American Nurses Association and Association of Rehabilitation Nurses. (1986). *Standards of rehabilitation nursing practices.* Silver Spring, MD: American Nurses Association.

Ayello, E. A., & Braden, B. (2002). How and why to do pressure ulcer risk assessment. *Advanced Skin Wound Care, 15*(3), 125–131.

Burke, M., & Walsh, M. (1992). *Gerontological nursing: Care of the frail elderly.* St. Louis: Mosby–Year Book.

Burton, J. Lecture series: Dementia and delirium. Johns Hopkins Medicine. Website: *http://www. hopkinsmedicine.org/gec/series/dementia.html.*

Bushnell, F. K. (1992). Self-care teaching for the congestive heart failure patient. *Journal of Gerontological Nursing, 10,* 27–32.

Carlson, R. (1988). Adult rehabilitation: Attitudes and implications. *Journal of Gerontological Nursing, 14,* 24–30.

Clinical Practice Guidelines. Guidelines abstracted from the American Academy of Neurology's dementia guidelines for early detection, diagnosis and management of dementia. The American Geriatrics Society. Website: *http://americangeriatrics.org/products/positionpapaers/aan_dementia.shtml.*

Flaherty, E. (2000). Assessing pain in older adults. *The Hartford Institute for Geriatric Nursing,* (7).

Gallo, J., & Katz, I. Depression. *The American Geriatric Society. http://www.americangeriatrics.org/ education/forum/depression.shtml.*

Hankes, D. (1984). Self-care: Assessing the aged client's need for independence. *Journal of Gerontological Nursing, 18,* 26–31.

Hoenig, H., et al. (1994). Adult rehabilitation: What do physicians know about it and how should they use it? *Journal of American Geriatrics, 42,* 341–347.

How to translate terminology used by therapists into MDS lingo. (1998). *National Report on Subacute Care, 16,* 5–8.

Kane, R. (1981). *Assessing the elderly: A practical guide to measurement.* New York: Lexington Books.

Lawler, K. (2001). Aging in place, coordinating housing and health care provision for America's growing elderly population. Joint Center for Housing Studies of Harvard University, Neighborhood Reinvestment Corporation.

Merck manual of geriatrics. (1995–1999). Whitehouse Station, NJ: Merck.

Merck manual of geriatrics. U.S. demographics (Chapter 2). Website: *http://www.merck.com/ mrkshared/mmg/sec1/ch2/ch2b.jsp.*

Midelfort, L. (2006). Medication Reconciliation Review. Website: *http://www.ihi.org/IHI/Topics/ PatientSafety/Medication Systems/Tools/Medication+Recon.*

Miller, K. E., Zylstra, R. G., & Standbridge, J. B. (2000). The geriatric patient: A systematic approach to maintaining health. *American Family Physician, 61*(4), 1089–1104.

National Center for Injury Prevention and Control. A tool kit to prevent senior falls. Website: *http://www.cdc.gov.*

National Screening Initiative. (2006). Determine your nutritional health. Ross Products Division of Abbott Laboratories, Inc.

Nyak, M. (1986). Balance in elderly patients: The "get-up and go" test. *Archives of Physical Medicine and Rehabilitation, 67,* 387–389.

Rand Health. (2006). Medical Outcomes Study (MOS), 36-Item Short Form Health Survey Instrument (SF-36). Website: *http://www.rand.org/health/surveys/sf36item/question.html.*

Senior Resource for Aging. (2006). Aging in place. Website: *http://www.seniorresource.com/ ageinpl.htm.*

U.S. Bureau of the Census. (1996). *Statistical abstract of the United States: 1996* (116th ed.). Washington, DC: U.S. Government Printing Office.

U.S. Care. (1999). Glossary of long-term care terms. Website: *http://www.uscare.com/glossary.html.*

U.S. Department of Health and Human Services. (1991). *Aging America: Trends and projections.* Washington, DC: U.S. Government Printing Office.

University of Iowa. (2002). Geriatric assessment tools, assessment tool categories. Website: *http://www.medicaine.uiowa.edu/igec/tools/default.asp.*

Uris, P., & Kearns, J. M. (1990). *Essentials of quality nursing care for the elderly.* Boulder, CO: Western Institute of Nursing.

Wieland, D., & Hirth, V. (2003). Comprehensive geriatric assessment. *Cancer Control, 10*(6).

Mary Rosedale
Becky Bigio

LEARNING OBJECTIVES

Upon completion of this chapter, the reader will be able to:

1. Define behavioral health case management.
2. Discuss the history of behavioral health case management.
3. Compare and contrast different behavioral health case management models.
4. Discuss the diagnosis and treatment of clients commonly referred to case management.
5. Identify and explore challenges in behavioral health case management practice.
6. Discuss behavioral health treatment settings and their impact on the role of the case manager.
7. Identify necessary resources for effective performance of case managers in the behavioral health service settings.

IMPORTANT TERMS AND CONCEPTS

Adverse Consequences
Assertive Community Treatment (ACT)
   Model
Behavioral Health Care

Behavioral Health Case
   Management
Behavioral Health Home Care
Brokerage Model

Diagnostic and Statistical Manual of
   Mental Disorders, 4th edition, text
   revision (*DSM–IV–TR*)
Extended Brokerage Model
Self-Neglect

Severe and Persistent Mental Illness
   (SPMI)
Strengths Model
Substance Abuse
Substance Dependence

■ INTRODUCTION

   A. Behavioral health case management is a strategy for the delivery of
   health care services to all persons with behavioral health disorders, but
   particularly to high-cost, high-volume and high-risk populations (Gage,
   2002; Herrick and Bartlett, 2004).

   B. Behavioral health case management is an essential strategy for producing
   positive outcomes related to hospitalization, quality of life, social functioning, and decreased health care costs (Rosen and Teeson, 2001; Taylor
   et al., 2005).

   C. Case management is especially important in an environment of brief
   inpatient psychiatric hospitalizations, limited access to care, fragmentation,
   and haphazard delivery of community-based behavioral health services.

   D. Recognizing that persons who have multiple episodes of psychiatric
   admissions to the hospital account for the major cost of care, some
   behavioral health insurance plans have shown that 5% of members
   account for 50% of costs, and 20% of members account for almost 80% of
   behavioral health costs (Lave and Peele, 2000; Taylor et al., 2005).

   E. High-volume users of behavioral health care and services are sometimes
   referred to as persons with severe and persistent mental/psychiatric illness.

   F. In the 1950s when it became evident that some World War II veterans
   experienced symptoms of psychiatric illnesses following their return to
   the United States, the Veterans' Administration initiated a model for psychiatric case management.
      1. This model aimed to meet the needs for mental and physical health
      care services as well as for social services (Herrick and Bartlett, 2004).
      2. The concept of the "continuum of care" emerged and a focus on the
      delivery of client-centered, coordinated, comprehensive care took
      hold (Tahan, 1998).

   G. In the 1960s a new worldview held promise that mental illness could be
   better treated in the community rather than in mental institutions and dein-
   stitutionalization was initiated on a broad scale (Krainovich-Miller and
   Gannon-Rosedale, 1999). For many reasons however, the Community
   Mental Health Construction Act of 1963, amended in 1975, was not able
   to implement a model of care that met the needs of persons with severe
   and persistent mental illness.
      1. Although the programs were designed with the concepts of primary,
      secondary, and tertiary prevention, in practice, they were pathology
      focused.

2. While the term *prevention* was used, the actual emphasis was largely monolithic, focusing on medication administration and compliance rather than on providing services that developed the strengths and skills needed for community-based living and reintegration (Krainovich-Miller and Gannon-Rosedale, 1999).

H. The majority of persons with a behavioral health condition, including those with severe and persistent mental illness, live at home with their significant others. Reengineering efforts, including shorter hospitalizations and other managed care initiatives to curtail the rise in health care costs, have contributed to the need for innovative and evidence-based models of case management (Krainovich-Miller and Gannon-Rosedale, 1999).

I. A comparison of expert views concerning intensive case management (ICM), a review of the literature, and meta-analysis investigating the effectiveness of clinical case management (CCM) reveal that case management approaches to care facilitate self-efficacy, reduce symptoms, and decrease total number of hospital days and drop out rates from treatment programs (Ziguras and Stuart, 2000; Rosen and Teeson, 2001; Atai-Otong, 2003).

■ KEY DEFINITIONS

A. Adverse consequences—Conditions that may include failure to fulfill major role obligations, using substances despite obvious physical hazards (e.g., driving under the influence), legal problems resulting from substance use, or recurrent social or interpersonal problems (APA, 2000).

B. Behavioral health care—Evaluation and treatment of psychological and substance dependence/abuse disorders (National Committee for Quality Assurance, 1997).

C. Behavioral health case management—A method of providing cost-effective, quality care (cost, process, experience, and outcomes) by managing the holistic health concerns of clients (individuals, families and groups) who are in need of extensive services. It requires integrating, coordinating, and advocating for complex mental and physical health care services from a variety of health care providers and settings, within the framework of planned behavioral health outcomes (Farnsworth and Bigelow, 1997, p. 319).

D. *Diagnostic and Statistical Manual of Mental Disorders,* 4th edition, text revision *(DSM–IV–TR)*—Manual that describes the various psychiatric, psychological, and substance-related disorders categorically. The *DMS–IV* identifies diagnostic and associated features, differential diagnoses, and incidence and prevalence of disorders, and describes the course of illnesses. The *DMS–IV* codes and terms are compatible with *International Classification of Diseases,* 9th version *(ICD–9–CM)* and 10th version, *(ICD–10–CM)*. This manual promotes a multi-axial system of diagnosis, which includes the clinical disorder that is the focus of treatment, associated personality disorders, general medical conditions, psychosocial and environmental problems, and a global assessment of functioning (GAF) for each patient (APA, 2000).

E. Self-neglect—The result of an adult's inability to perform essential self-care tasks due to physical and/or mental impairments or diminished capacity. The tasks may include providing essential food, clothing, shelter, and health care; obtaining goods and services necessary to maintain physical health, mental health, emotional well-being and general safety; and/or managing financial affairs and adhering to prescribed medications.

F. Severe and persistent mental illness (SPMI)—A diagnosis of nonorganic psychosis or personality disorder that is characterized as prolonged illness or requiring long-term treatment, and operationalized as a two-year or longer history of mental illness or treatment and disability including three of eight specified criteria (NIMH, 1987).

G. Substance abuse—A maladaptive pattern of substance (e.g., alcohol and narcotics) use manifested by recurrent and significant adverse consequences within a 12-month period (APA, 2000). The majority of these patients are diagnosed with schizophrenia or schizoaffective disorder.

H. Substance dependence—A cluster of physiologic, cognitive, and behavioral symptoms caused by repeated self-administration of substances, resulting in tolerance, withdrawal, and compulsive drug-taking behaviors (APA, 2000).

■ BEHAVIORAL HEALTH CASE MANAGEMENT MODELS

A. A major problem with research, training, and clinical application of behavioral health case management is that even when models are specified, they frequently fail to delineate the critical behavioral elements of the interventions or treatments they employ.

   1. It is often unclear what interventions or set of interventions are being compared, whether these behavioral elements are standardized, and how results should be attributed (Chan et al., 2000; Rosen and Teeson, 2001).

B. The following typology illustrates the defining attributes of different behavioral health case management models as well as the overlap and ambiguity.

C. The brokerage model

   1. Entails an individually assigned case manager who assumes case management functions of coordinating care among all involved parties.

   2. The case manager may or may not be a mental health professional.

   3. Some literature suggests that targeted telephonic case management can improve client outcomes (Taylor et al., 2005).

   4. This model has been criticized as a "passive-response" form of case management that involves few interventions other than monitoring and maintaining contact with the client.

   5. There is little evidence-based support for its efficacy (Chan et al., 2000; Rosen and Teeson, 2001).

D. The extended brokerage model

1. Leadership is assumed by mental health professionals who are more actively involved in the patient's assessment and assume some additional direct care responsibilities (Chan et al., 2000).

2. Designed to provide services for persons with SPMI, a psychiatrist often provides clinical leadership for the interdisciplinary treatment team (ITT).

3. Case managers have varied experience (e.g., some are psychiatric nurses, others are social workers).

4. The efficacy of this model has been difficult to evaluate due to lack of standardization (i.e., the heterogeneity of members and interventions in clinical case management and intensive case management programs).

5. Functions of case managers include:

   a. Advocacy

   b. Transportation of consumers to and from treatment sites

   c. Symptom and medication monitoring

   d. Assessment and teaching of skills for community living

   e. Initiating and coordinating referrals and benefits/entitlements

E. The strengths model

1. Differs from the brokerage model in that most services are provided outside an office setting.

2. Training of staff in this model is provided and reflects the broad areas of engagement, strengths assessment, personal planning, and resource acquisition (Marty, Rapp, and Carlson, 2001).

   a. The behavioral elements of engagement include:

      i. Identifying achievements, interests, and aspirations of the client

      ii. Meeting at times and in places that reflect client preference

      iii. Purposeful use of case manager's self-disclosure

   b. Strengths assessment is prioritizing the client's past and present achievements, resources, and future interests versus problematic behavior and crisis response.

   c. Personal planning focuses on the specific, measurable steps toward achieving what the client wants and reflects consumer strengths.

   d. Resource acquisition requires designing activities with the client that increase consumer contact with desired community resources and entitlements.

3. Although a survey of experts in the strengths model of case management concluded that ideal caseloads range from 10 to 20 consumers to case managers (Marty, Rapp, and Carlson, 2001), it is not clear that this ideal is reflected in actual practice.

4. Research on the strengths model has shown consistently positive outcomes related to hospitalization, quality of life, and social functioning, but the strength of the evidence is limited by sampling and methodological problems.

F. The assertive community treatment (ACT) model
  1. The most clearly articulated model; is recognized as an evidence-based practice with more than 25 randomized-controlled trials supporting the following outcomes: it reduces hospital use, increases housing stability, controls psychiatric symptoms, improves quality of life, and is cost effective (Bond et al., 2001; Ziguras and Stuart, 2000; Rosen and Teeson, 2001; Schaedle et al., 2002).
  2. Key elements of the ACT model include:
     a. Team-delivered services
     b. Shared caseloads
     c. An average of 10 consumers to a case manager
     d. Provision of direct services in the community rather than mostly office-based services
     e. Employing brokerage functions
     f. Mobility
     g. Seven-day operation
     h. Capability of responding to crises of all consumers
     i. Having a policy to not close cases
     j. A controlled rate of admitting new clients
     k. Professionally skilled multidisciplinary staff competent in providing psychosocial and pharmacological interventions
     l. Provision of services to a highly and continuously disabled subpopulation of psychiatric service users (i.e., those with SPMI)
     m. Supervision and ongoing training
     n. Team support and debriefing

G. Other models
  1. Include the generalist model (Franklin et al., 1987) and the rehabilitation model (Goering et al., 1988, Antai-Otong, 2003). These are case management models that theoretically differ from the others and lack specification of and standardization of practice.
  2. For example, Atai-Otong's psychosocial rehabilitation model is described as using psychiatric nurses with an intensive case management approach; however, this description is consistent with the extended broker model.
  3. Cox et al. (2003) describe an intensive case management model that, like ACT, uses a multidisciplinary team approach; but, unlike ACT, provides services onsite in a medical center rather than in the community.
  4. Disease management models focus on populations both within hospitals and in the community setting (Herrick and Bartlett, 2004).
  5. Research concerning each of these models has suffered from lack of clear definitions of the providers, services, and set of interventions distinct to each model (Chan et al., 2000).

■ BEHAVIORAL HEALTH CARE CONDITIONS AND THEIR IMPLICATIONS FOR CASE MANAGEMENT

A. According to the American Psychiatric Nurse's Association (APNA) (2000), global projections of mental illness and worldwide increases in the aging population will contribute to a sizable increase in the elder component of society as well as the incidence of chronic illnesses and disability.

B. Behavioral health disorders are projected to account for 11% to 15% of the global disease burden in this century (APNA, 2000).

C. Persons with SPMI frequently have alcohol-related problems as well as physical health problems that require treatment (APNA, 2000).

D. The presence of a psychiatric or substance-related disorder may complicate the diagnosis and/or treatment of general medical conditions.

E. The World Health Organization (WHO) has listed depression, alcohol use, bipolar disorder, schizophrenia, and obsessive-compulsive disorder among the ten leading causes of disability worldwide (APNA, 2000).

F. There exists a growing need for evidence-based behavioral health case management models and interventions.

G. Definitions of the psychiatric disorders cited below are based on criteria from the *Diagnostic and Statistical Manual of Mental Disorders*, 4th edition, text revision (*DSM–IV–TR*) (APA, 2000).

1. Major depressive disorder
   a. Persons with this condition display a depressed mood or loss of interest or pleasure in almost all activities for at least 2 weeks.
   b. Additional symptoms such as weight changes, changes in sleeping patterns, changes in psychomotor activity, persistent feelings of guilt or worthlessness, difficulty concentrating or thinking, impairment of social or occupational role expectations, or suicidal ideation may also be present.
   c. The depressed patient may present for evaluation or treatment following a suicide attempt, and all depressed clients should be considered "at risk" for suicide.
   d. The major depressive patients are diagnosed by a careful interview, including personal and family history.
   e. Alcohol or other substance abuse can mask symptoms of this disorder. Clients may abuse substances in an attempt to "self-medicate" symptoms. A careful history of substance use including nicotine should be taken.
   f. Major depressive disorder can last 6 months or longer if left untreated.
   g. Once the diagnosis has been established, treatment consists primarily of a combination of antidepressant medications and cognitive behavioral therapy (Donohue et al., 2004).
   h. Some clients with severe depression who are not responsive to antidepressant treatment may be acutely treated with electroconvulsive therapy (ECT) on an acute and outpatient basis.

    i. Case management services for this patient population focuses on:

        i. Suicide prevention

        ii. Supporting antidepressant therapy and monitoring for side effects

        iii. Psychotherapy and significant other(s) involvement and education. Some clients find the support and structure of group psychotherapy beneficial, especially if social dysfunction has occurred as a result of depression.

        iv. Education of family members about the illness, treatment, and signs of recurrence.

    j. Case managers should not hesitate to ask patients if they are considering suicide or self-harm.

        i. Patients may demonstrate increased suicide potential by giving away belongings, making a will, saying goodbye to loved ones, or hoarding medications.

        ii. Some patients act on suicidal ideation after initiating treatment for depression, when energy levels begin to improve.

    k. Case managers should be vigilant about the suicide risk in these patients and be watchful of signs that a patient is considering suicide.

2. Alcohol-related disorders

    a. Persons exhibiting alcohol abuse show a maladaptive pattern of alcohol use that results in one or more of the following in a 12-month period:

        i. Failure to fulfill major role obligations at work, school, or home (e.g., repeated absences)

        ii. Recurrent alcohol use in situations where it is physically hazardous (e.g., driving a car)

        iii. Recurrent alcohol-related legal problems (e.g., arrests for disorderly conduct)

        iv. Continued alcohol use despite social or interpersonal problems caused by or worsened by alcohol use (e.g., arguments with spouse, physical fights) (APA, 2000)

    b. Persons with alcohol dependence exhibit:

        i. A physiologic dependence that is characterized by evidence of tolerance (needing more of the substance to produce a desired effect); and

        ii. Withdrawal when administration of the substance is discontinued (a syndrome that may include sweating, tachycardia, hand tremor, insomnia, nausea or vomiting, agitation, anxiety, hallucinations, or grand mal seizures).

    c. Delirium tremens may be considered a more severe form of withdrawal and is considered to be a medical emergency.

    d. Alcohol-related disorders are diagnosed by history, physical examination, and interview.

    e. This condition can go undiagnosed if the patient continues to use alcohol and no withdrawal symptoms are observed.

    f. Over time, patients with this disorder may be increasingly unable to fulfill occupational or social expectations, which may cause distress.

    g. Treatment focuses primarily on alcohol abstinence and an Alcoholics Anonymous (AA) group therapy program (or an equivalent recovery program such as Rational Recovery).

       i. Initially, to elicit their agreement, patients may be asked to contract not to drink for three months so that they can see what abstinence is like and how one's life is affected.

      ii. Patients whose withdrawal symptoms are severe may need to be hospitalized and monitored by expert clinicians during initial alcohol detoxification.

    h. Case managers support the treatment plan as well as provide encouragement to patients and their significant others (who may be referred to support groups such as AA).

    i. Case managers should be alert to the fact that chronic alcohol dependence is associated with social deterioration, decreased tolerance, medical complications of every organ, including liver impairment, which may interfere with the elimination of medications the patient may be on, causing risk for drug toxicity.

3. Bipolar disorder

    a. Persons diagnosed with bipolar disorder experience recurrent episodes of hypomanic or manic episodes, during which they may be hyperactive, hyperverbal, irritable, insomniac, distractible, agitated, grandiose, and experience flight of thoughts and ideas and psychotic symptoms.

    b. Bipolar disorder is diagnosed by careful interview and history.

    c. Patients with bipolar disorder tend to be high risk for suicide or self-harm particularly during periods of high impulsivity or when psychotic symptoms develop.

    d. Treatment focuses primarily on suicide prevention, prescription of mood-stabilizing medication and monitoring of blood levels and for side effects of drugs, and psychotherapy.

    e. Case managers provide support for patients and their significant others who may benefit from support groups such as those provided by National Alliance for the Mentally Ill (NAMI).

    f. Patients may not like the loss of euphoria produced when mood is stabilized and may have difficulty adhering to the treatment regimen.

    g. Some of the medications prescribed for the mood stabilization require that the client submit to regular blood tests; i.e., to monitor blood levels.

    h. The case manager assesses for problems that may lead to nonadherence and addresses these issues proactively with the client and other members of the multidisciplinary team.

4. Schizophrenia

    a. Persons diagnosed with schizophrenia suffer from symptoms that impair functioning and involve disturbances in feelings, thinking, and behavior.

    b. Patients may experience delusions, hallucinations, looseness of associations, social withdrawal, absence of motivation, impoverishment of thought, inappropriate affect, agitation, catatonia, and/or disorientation.

    c. This condition is diagnosed through observation, history, and interview.

    d. Treatment consists of symptom control with antipsychotic medications (greatly improved with the advent of atypical antipsychotic medications), and training in social skills and community-based living.

    e. Adherence should be monitored and addressed by case managers. Some of the antipsychotic medications require blood monitoring to avoid severe side effects (e.g., agranulocytosis).

    f. Patients should be monitored for all side effects including the development of medications-induced movement disorders.

    g. Treatment may involve hospitalization for acute management.

    h. Case managers support the patients' strengths and focus on preventing the conditions most likely to produce relapse including:

        i. Lack of adherence to medication

        ii. Inability to continue outpatient treatment

        iii. Inadequate support in the community

        iv. Inadequate socialization and recreation

        v. The need for ongoing psycho-education (for patients and their significant others)

    i. Case managers advocate for activities and programs that promote healthy lifestyles (e.g., exercise, smoking cessation) and prompt health referrals as these patients often suffer from poor generalized health.

    j. Patients eligible for ACT team should be referred for such case management services. For patients who do not meet ACT criteria, behavioral health home care services may be initiated. Patients and their significant others may additionally be referred to NAMI for support group services.

5. Obsessive-compulsive disorder

    a. Persons suffering from obsessive-compulsive disorder experience recurrent intrusive, obsessive thoughts and repetitive, compulsive behavioral patterns.

    b. If patients attempt to ignore the intrusive thought or to curb compulsive behavior, their anxiety becomes intolerable.

    c. The disorder is diagnosed through interview and history.

    d. Patients often recognize that their behaviors or obsessions are unreasonable but feel powerless to stop them. Distress occurs when these activities and behaviors become excessively time consuming or interfere with the person's ability to function in role-appropriate situations.

    e. Treatment involves medication (typically serotonin reuptake blocking antidepressants or the highly serotonergic tricyclic antidepressant clomipramine). A combination of antidepressants and behavioral therapy are frequently prescribed.

   f. Case management services focus on the here and now, supporting medication treatment, significant other(s) involvement in care, and education.

   g. Some patients may find the support and structure of group therapy beneficial, especially if social dysfunction has occurred.

   h. Patients may be referred to NAMI for support group services.

■ CHALLENGES IN BEHAVIORAL HEALTH CASE MANAGEMENT

A. Preventing self-harm/suicide

   1. Potentially, all patients with psychiatric and substance-related disorders are at risk for suicide.

   2. The most predictive suicide risk is a past history of a suicide attempt.

   3. The most conservative approach is to admit the patient who is at risk for suicide when there is any doubt about his or her safety.

   4. The implications for case management with these patients are the need to develop an effective support system within the family and community to manage emergency situations, and to provide support and safety for the patient.

   5. For suicide assessment protocol a case manager may use, see Appendix A.

B. Preventing violence

   1. Indications of increased risk for violence include:

      a. A recent violent act

      b. Alcohol or substance intoxication

      c. Verbal or physical threats

      d. Presence of a weapon

      e. Patients responding to psychotic thoughts (i.e., command hallucinations)

   2. Patients suffering from disorders that heighten impulsivity (i.e., substance-related disorders, bipolar disorder, disorders affecting the frontal lobe and clients with personality disorders).

      a. These patients may, at times, require crisis intervention in order to protect themselves and others.

      b. The involuntary placement of these patients on locked psychiatric units, when necessary, can increase the patients' anger and aggressive behaviors.

      c. These patients must always be treated in the least restrictive setting necessary to protect themselves and others.

   3. It is important that clinicians, including case managers, carefully question patients' significant others regarding domestic violence.

      a. Abused partners should be referred to domestic violence shelters.

      b. Where child abuse is suspected, clinicians are mandated to report observations to authorities.

C. Reducing self-neglect, including nonadherence to treatment
   1. *Self-neglect* is defined as the result of an adult's inability, due to physical and/or mental impairments or diminished capacity, to perform essential self-care tasks including the following:
      a. Providing essential food, clothing, shelter, and health care
      b. Obtaining goods and services necessary to maintain physical health, mental health, emotional well-being and general safety
      c. Managing financial affairs and adhering to prescribed medications (Abrams et al., 2002)
   2. Relapse of symptoms and return to acute care settings most frequently occur when patients are unable to adhere to treatment or manage their self-care activities while in the community.
      a. Episodes of relapse can be devastating to patients and their significant other(s) who experience a sense of failure and loss of hope.
   3. The implications for case management are to manage the acute phase of illness and treatment, monitor adherence, and proactively investigate problems that may contribute to nonadherence (i.e., side effects, ambivalence about taking medications).
   4. Case managers assist the patients and significant others in reframing the relapse and in maintaining hope as well as realistic expectations about recovery and rehabilitation.
   5. For practical case management approaches for clients with low self-care states, see Appendix B.
D. Treating clients with psychiatric and substance-related diagnoses
   1. Assessment and diagnosis of patients with dual diagnosis (psychiatric and substance-related disorders) can be difficult.
   2. A patient who presents for treatment under the influence of mind-altering substances may not be accurately diagnosed until the effects of the substance have been eliminated.
   3. Until the effects of mind-altering substances are managed/overturned, the patient must be treated symptomatically and conservatively, with the health care staff providing a safe environment while observing for symptoms of psychiatric disorders.
   4. Common dual-diagnosis situations include the patient with generalized anxiety disorder or panic who abuses alcohol to reduce feelings of anxiety, or the depressed patient who uses cocaine to relieve symptoms of depression.
   5. The patient, once accurately diagnosed, must receive treatment for both disorders concurrently.
   6. Many dual-diagnosis treatment programs have been established in ambulatory settings/clinics to meet the needs of these patients.
   7. The psychiatrist (and the case manager) who prescribes anxiolytic medications for a dually diagnosed patient must be aware of the potential for abuse of the medication.
   8. The addictionologist must be cognizant of the "normal" sad affect experienced by some patients who are recovering from alcohol or drug dependence, or both, and be able to distinguish this condition

from an acute mood disorder that may require pharmacologic intervention.

9. All treatment practitioners, including the case manager, must be alert to the potential for suicide in this population.

E. Improving the general health of patients

1. Improving the general health of clients requires the acknowledgment that many patients, particularly those with SPMI, suffer from obesity, a general lack of fitness, poor nutrition, and nicotine dependence.

2. Lack of preventive health services, frequent delays in seeking care, unhealthy lifestyles, and general poor health become an even greater concern as patients age and their chronic illnesses increase.

3. It is vital that case management programs address smoking cessation, health-promotion activities, and timely health-related referrals for patients (Badger et al., 2003).

F. Improving the social functioning of clients' daily lives

1. Improving the social functioning of patients requires that case managers individually tailor treatment plans with the patient to increase sufficiently stimulating, challenging, and interesting daily activities.

2. Additional educational programs and activities to improve functioning and socialization in all areas, including sexual functioning, have been underappreciated in case management models (Badger et al., 2003).

G. Enhancing the client–case manager relationship and care continuity

1. Frequent turnover in staff is a significant problem in case management, and contributes to poor-quality care, recidivism, and high costs in recruiting and retaining case managers (Badger et al., 2003).

2. Establishing a trusting relationship between the patient and case manager as well as working with families as allies in care are key ingredients for success (Yamashita, Forchuk, and Mound, 2005).

3. Efforts to decrease case manager turnover by decreasing or sharing caseloads, providing increased supervision, debriefing and training, and identifying the most effective mix of personnel and interventions for case management are areas that require additional research (Donohue et al., 2004).

H. The above challenges provide an excellent opportunity for behavioral health case managers to make a positive impact on the mental, psychological, social, and physical health of people with psychiatric illnesses and their associated outcomes. These activities should be core to the case manager's job description and responsibilities.

■ TREATMENT SETTINGS AND BEHAVIORAL HEALTH CASE MANAGEMENT

A. Inpatient hospitalization

1. Used for treatment of acute conditions in which patients are in danger of harming themselves or others

2. Also used for the patient who is unable to care for oneself in the community

3. Hospitalization is the most restrictive type of treatment for behavioral health conditions.
   a. It is occasionally used to initiate new medications when the patient must be observed closely for potentially life-threatening side effects.
   b. This treatment modality is used for acute detoxification from substances with which the potential for severe withdrawal symptoms exists.
4. Laws governing involuntary short- or long-term confinement differ from state to state, and case managers must be aware of individual state laws and restrictions.
5. The case manager's role during and following hospitalization entails integrating, coordinating, and advocating for complex mental and physical health care services from a variety of health care providers and settings, within the framework of planned health outcomes (Farnsworth and Bigelow, 1997).
   a. Frequently, one case manager is accountable for the welfare of the patient during the hospitalization and provides support for the client and significant others while moving the client toward a timely discharge (Herrick and Bartlett, 2004).
   b. Psychiatric consultation/liaison nurses have effectively partnered with case managers during unanticipated hospital stays.
   c. Behavioral health critical pathways have been developed and implemented to assure multidisciplinary commitment and coordination of treatment goals (Chase et al., 2000). Case managers must be aware of these pathways and must incorporate them in their practice.

B. Partial hospitalization
   1. This treatment modality involves the patient spending 4 hours or more per day in a structured setting.
   2. Patients in this setting receive milieu therapy, psychoeducation, and individual and group therapies.
   3. Partial hospitalization may be used as an alternative to inpatient hospitalization for the patient who has a strong community support system, is not deemed to be an acute risk, and who requires close supervision of medication effects.
   4. Case management's role in the care of patients who are enrolled in a partial hospital program includes knowledge of how to access emergency treatment for the patient, support and education of client and significant others, and development and implementation of a client-centered aftercare plan.

C. Ambulatory care
   1. Outpatient and intensive outpatient treatment are effective for patients whose conditions can be managed outside of a structured setting.
   2. Individual, group, family, and couples therapy are delivered in this setting.

3. Patients' medications can be monitored effectively on an ambulatory basis once dosages are stabilized.

4. Case management's role in ambulatory care may be minimal. However, it may include patient/family education, counseling, encouragement of adherence to regimen, crisis intervention, as well as maintenance of follow-up care.

5. The case manager and patient should be aware of how to access emergency services if the patient's symptoms should worsen, if he or she experiences suicidal thoughts or impulses, or if intolerable or potentially dangerous medication side effects occur.

D. Home and community-based settings

1. Behavioral health home care is a treatment modality for the delivery of mental health and related physical care within a patient's home setting.

2. Psychiatric nurses are the major providers of psychiatric home care services and function both as direct care clinicians and as case managers who develop, coordinate, implement, and oversee the interdisciplinary treatment plan.

3. Multidisciplinary team members may include the physician (not required to be a psychiatrist), social worker, physical therapist, occupational therapist, and home health aide.

4. Services are covered by Medicare and several other insurances when the following conditions are met:

   a. The patient has a primary psychiatric diagnosis, has been evaluated by a physician, is re-evaluated by the physician every 60 days, requires skilled nursing intervention by a psychiatric nurse, and meets homebound status.

   b. Homebound status for a behavioral health patient means that the patient's psychiatric illness prevents or causes extreme and taxing effort for the client to leave his or her home (Krainovich-Miller and Gannon-Rosedale, 1999).

   c. Behavioral health home care services can be particularly effective in settings where there is limited access to behavioral health clinicians; for example, nonambulatory patients and lengthy distances to travel for behavioral health services.

5. In addition, ACT teams have proven community based.

E. Rural settings

1. To address the limited availability of behavioral health specialists in the rural settings, cognitive behavioral therapy training has been provided to case managers to an eclectic group of psychiatric nurses and clinicians with social work and psychology backgrounds.

2. Services in these settings are similar to those provided in the hospital, ambulatory/clinic, or homecare/community settings.

3. Donoghue et al. (2004) describe ten training modules for assisting case managers to deliver focused psychological strategies in the treatment of depression and anxiety disorders.

F. Drug courts
   1. An innovative model of care that addresses the needs of clients in correctional settings
   2. A setting that provides nonviolent offenders with basic access to physical and mental health care as well as intensive case management led by advanced practice nurses (Naegle, Richardson, and Morton, 2004)

■ ROLES AND FUNCTIONS OF THE BEHAVIORAL HEALTH CASE MANAGER

A. The roles and functions of behavioral health case managers are similar to those who function in other care settings. These may include the following core activities:
   1. Coordination and facilitation of care and treatments
   2. Brokerage of services, especially those needed to keep patients in the community
   3. Patient and family education regarding health condition and treatment
   4. Psychosocial counseling and support including crisis intervention
   5. Transitional planning and actual transitioning of patients from one level of care to the next as well as discharge planning that focuses on discharging patients from the hospital/institution setting
   6. Assessment, monitoring, and evaluation of the patient's condition and response to treatment
   7. Reporting observation findings to other health care providers, especially the psychiatrist
   8. Working closely with insurance company representatives (e.g., case manager), community agencies (e.g., transportation), and other health care providers such as physical and occupational therapy, social work, pharmacy, and so on.
   9. Case managers' activities that are more specific to the behavioral health patient population may include the following:
      a. Patient and family education, counseling, support, and encouragement, especially to enhance adherence to treatment regimen follow-up care
      b. Development and implementation of patient-centered aftercare plans
      c. Responsibility for the welfare of the patient during the hospitalization and support for the patient and significant others while moving the patient toward a timely discharge
      d. Psychiatric consultation and/or liaison with other care providers
      e. Integrating, coordinating, and advocating for complex mental and physical health care services from a variety of health care providers and settings, within the framework of planned health outcomes
      f. Development and implementation of behavioral health clinical pathways and guidelines applying the evidence-based practice principles
      g. Establishing trusting relationships with families to promote families as allies in care

    h. Improving the social functioning of patients' daily lives

    i. Improving the patient's social functioning by individually tailoring treatment plans

    j. Addressing smoking cessation, health promotion activities, and timely health-related referrals

    k. Improving the general health of patients by focusing on issues of obesity, lack of fitness, poor nutrition, and nicotine dependence

    l. Developing an effective support system within the family and community to manage emergency situations, and to provide support and safety for the patient

    m. Prevention of suicide and homicide

    n. Managing the acute phase of illness and treatment, monitoring adherence, and proactively investigating problems that may contribute to nonadherence (i.e., side effects to drugs, ambivalence about taking medications)

    o. Assisting patients and their significant others in reframing relapse, if it occurs, and in maintaining hope as well as realistic expectations about recovery and rehabilitation

    p. Advocating for activities and programs that promote healthy lifestyles such as exercise programs, support groups, and smoking cessation

    q. Identifying problems that may lead to nonadherence and addressing them proactively with the patient and other members of the multidisciplinary team

■ INSURANCE COVERAGE AND FINANCIAL ASSISTANCE

    A. Employer-funded insurance plans, managed care plans, and other types of health insurance plans may offer different benefits for behavioral health care than for other general medical conditions.

    B. The number of behavioral health clinic visits allowed may be limited; or there may be a dollar limitation imposed on the coverage.

    C. The pharmacy benefit or the formulary used by the individual carrier may not include the patient's drug regimen.

    D. The primary implication for the case manager in this type of payment arrangement is to maximize the use of scarce resources.

    E. Most managed care plans require that proposed treatment be "medically necessary and appropriate" for the diagnosis.

    F. Long-term treatment that is not aimed at relieving symptoms, promoting return to premorbid functioning, or affecting the development of a coordinated support and aftercare system may not be approved by the insurance company.

    G. Occasionally, caregivers need respite from the care of a chronically ill patient. The case manager should explore resources to provide such a respite, as well as supportive services and community resources for the caregivers.

■ INTERNET RESOURCES FOR USE BY THE CASE MANAGER

A. Agency for Healthcare Research and Quality (AHRQ) (*www.ahrq.gov*)

B. American Association of Health Plans (*www.aahp.org*)

C. American Psychiatric Nurses Association (*www.apna.org*)

D. Institute for Behavioral Healthcare (*www.ibh.com*)

E. National Alliance for the Mentally Ill (NAMI) (*www.nami.org*)

F. Psychotherapy Finances and Managed Care Strategies (*www.psyfin.com*)

G. American Managed Behavioral Healthcare Association (*www.ambha.org*)

APPENDIX A—SUICIDE PRACTICE PROTOCOL

I. ASSESSMENT

A. Directly inquire about suicidal ideation, intent, and plan and determine degree of suicidal risk (Schwartz and Rogers, 2004).

B. Ideation—determine whether active or passive. Has client expressed ideation to others (Robie et al., 1999)? Older clients may be less likely to express ideation to others.

C. Intent—frequently communicated by giving away possessions, making a will, making funeral arrangements, or similar life-closure activities (Remafedi et al., 1998; Schwartz and Rogers, 2004).

D. Plan—determine whether the client has thought about ways to kill himself/herself; the more lethal the measure and/or more available the means, the higher degree of risk (Robie et al., 1999; Swann et al., 2005).

E. Determine whether the client has made one or more previous suicide attempts/gestures (Robie et al., 1999; Schwartz and Rogers, 2004; Swann et al., 2005).

F. Inquire as to whether the client feels hopeless/helpless about the future (Bai et al., 1997; Robie et al., 1999).

G. Explore recent changes in mood/behavior (Reid et al., 1998; Robie et al., 1999).

H. Conduct mental status specifically evaluating for psychosis (e.g., delusional depression, command hallucinations in schizophrenia, high degree of impulsivity in bipolar disorder) (Reid et al., 1998; Robie et al., 1999; Swann et al., 2005).

I. Evaluate degree of alcohol or substance use including nicotine (Reid et al., 1998; Robie et al., 1999; Schwartz and Rogers, 2004).

J. Determine whether one or more chronic medical conditions exist (Lindberg et al., 1998; Robie et al., 1999; Schwartz and Rogers, 2004).

K. Directly inquire whether client has visited a health care practitioner in past 30 days.

L. Conduct pain assessment and determine if client has painkillers in home or access to overdose quantities (Berger, 1993; McCloskey and Bulacek, 2000).

M. Evaluate the client's current medication regimen:
  1. Research suggests that several cardiac medications and specifically calcium channel blockers have been implicated in depression and increased suicidal risk (Lindberg et al., 1998).
  2. Research indicates that the extrapyramidal effects of antipsychotic medications can increase the risk of suicide (Reid et al., 1998).

N. Evaluate the client's experience of recent loss:
  1. Financial difficulties/loss, interpersonal separation, or altercations associated with risk especially in young–middle adulthood (Bai et al., 1997).
  2. Loss via death of loved one implicated in risk with older adults, particularly widowers (Li, 1995; Robie et al., 1999; Schwartz and Rogers, 2004).

O. Conduct sexual assessment with particular attention to conflicts about sexual orientation in adolescent males. Research suggests that bisexuality/homosexuality is a risk factor among adolescent males (Remafedi et al., 1998).

P. Explore whether the client is a veteran of war and whether he/she was subject to combat, to wounds, and to what extent and how frequently wounded. Research suggests that combat veterans are at exponentially increased risk for suicide based on frequency and extent of wounds incurred (Bullman and Kang, 1996).

Q. Evaluate the presence of the following clinical conditions that are associated with risk:
  1. Major depression (with or without psychotic features) (Bai, 1997; Coren and Hewitt, 1998; Lindberg et al., 1998; Reid et al., 1998).
  2. Schizophrenia (Bai et al., 1997; Reid et al., 1998).
  3. Schizoaffective disorder (Bai et al., 1997; Reid et al., 1998).
  4. Bipolar disorder (Swann et al., 2005)
  5. Substance abuse/dependency (Bai et al., 1997; Remafedi, 1998).
  6. Posttraumatic stress disorder (Bullman and King, 1996).

II. PLAN

A. Enhance the use of client's social supports by encouraging interaction with professionals and significant others (i.e., family meetings, therapist support) (Berger, 1993; Robie et al., 1999).

B. Involve and educate all consented persons in the client's support network about risks; determine their ability to ensure safety in the client's environment (Berger, 1993; Robie et al., 1999).

C. On an ongoing basis, determine whether the client's degree of risk exceeds his/her ability to remain safe (i.e., client refuses to contract and 24-hour supervision is not available) and if that is the case, or there is any question that it is the case, call 911 or otherwise hospitalize the client (Berger, 1993; Robie et al., 1999; Schwartz and Rogers, 2004).

III. INTERVENTION

A. Ensure safety

B. Determine the appropriate level of care in the least restrictive setting (as above) (Berger, 1993; Robie et al., 1999).

C. Remove items that impede safety (i.e., weapons, razors, stockpiles of medications) (Reid et al., 1998; Robie et al., 1999).

D. Tailor suicide prevention to the client's risk factors (i.e., discuss plans for dealing with the specific precipitating factors) (Bai et al., 1997; Remafedi et al., 1998).

E. Treat and manage psychiatric symptoms that may be placing the client at risk of suicide (Bai et al., 1997).

F. Evaluate the medication regimen and explore issues of adherence to determine psychological obstacles and side effects, and make changes as needed (Reid et al., 1995).

G. Provide adequate pain control and treatment of chronic conditions (Berger, 1993).

H. Mediate the use of substances (i.e., encourage AA, NA, smoking cessation) and educate client/significant others about the links with depression.

I. Explore and facilitate the reframing of the client's perceptions about hopelessness and helplessness (Robie et al., 1999).

J. Involve the client and all significant others in care—educating them about risk, illness, ways of coping (Berger, 1993; McCloskey and Bulachek, 2000).

K. Establish follow up (Reid et al., 1999, Robie et al., 1999). Research suggests that young inpatients admitted with depression and suicidal behaviors are likely to attempt suicide shortly after hospitalization (Bai et al., 1997). Mental health follow up on an outpatient basis, through intensive case management or assertive community treatment, cannot be overemphasized (Reid et al., 1998; Robie et al., 1999).

IV. EVALUATION

A. Reassessment of suicide should be an ongoing process—by clients, involved practitioners, and significant others (Robie et al., 1999).

B. Consistent with Joint Commission on Accreditation of Healthcare Organizations (JCAHO) standards, quality improvement should focus on clients who are suicidal or are at risk for suicide and evaluate suicide prevention protocols for assurance of safety, provision of the appropriate and timely treatment, and referral for follow up (Robie et al., 1999).

APPENDIX B—CASE MANAGEMENT APPROACHES FOR PATIENTS WITH LOW SELF-CARE STATES

I. Traditional approaches to clients with low self-care states have shifted from compliance to adherence-focused models.

   A. In the era of compliance, it was typical for providers to lecture, impact by fear, and admonish patients for the various self-neglect or abuse symptoms they demonstrated.

   B. With the advent of the adherence approach to care, the focus has changed to partnering, communicating therapeutically, negotiating, and planning according to the patient's needs and capabilities.

   C. The adherence approach is consistent with the strengths model of case management (Marty, Rapp, and Carlson, 2001).

II. It is important to evaluate the patient globally and consider the accumulation and interaction of medical, psychiatric, social, and physiological aging.

   A. Multidisciplinary team meetings are an important means for sharing perceptions, evaluating the treatment plan, and coordinating this plan with the patient and/or the patient's significant others.

III. Persons exhibiting diminished self-care states have risk factors that include:

   A. Multiple cognitive deficits (e.g., memory impairment, disturbance in executive functioning)

   B. Developmental delays

   C. Sensory impairments

   D. Impaired mobility

   E. Social isolation

   F. Anxiety, phobias, and depression

   G. Psychotic symptoms

   H. Longstanding personality traits that lead to the individual's distress or impairment (Abrams et al., 2002).

IV. Case management of patients with low self-care states begins by:

   A. Assessing the patient's level of self-care using a four-point Likert scale described by Bird et al. (1999):

      1. Level 1—Low risk where the client is attendant to personal hygiene and environment

    2. Level 2—Moderate risk of leading unhealthy lifestyle and choices

    3. Level 3—Severe risk of medical nonadherence

    4. Level 4—Extreme or abusive self-neglect

B. Taking a clear history of the present nonadherence (HPNA) and noting the impact of such behaviors on the patient's quality of life and safety

C. The HPNA questions may include the following:

    1. Section 1

       a. How long has the nonadherence been going on and is it a long-standing or abrupt behavior?

       b. Is it stemming from medical or hygiene domains or both?

       c. Is this "assiduous" stemming from young to mid-adulthood?

       d. Are there cultural considerations that impact the patient's understanding or behavior?

       e. What is the individual's perception of the condition? Does he or she see a problem or feel uncomfortable?

    2. Section 2

       a. Are the patient's medical needs evident and being addressed?

       b. Are the patient's activities of daily living (i.e., eating, bathing) and instrumental activities of daily living (i.e., shopping, housekeeping) needs evident? If so, how are they being addressed?

       c. Is the patient capable of communicating his or her needs and directing care?

       d. Are there cognitive deficits (e.g., memory deficits) and if so, is the patient responsive to the creation of environmental cues (e.g., calendars and notes) and/or verbal reminders?

       e. Is the case management's philosophy of care consistent with what the patient or his/her health care proxy indicates?

    3. Section 3

       a. What are the etiologies or "host domains?" How many are there?

       b. Etiologies or host domains many include the following:

          i. Sensory/functional impairments

         ii. Mental health problems

        iii. Substance abuse problems

        iv. Social-legal problems

         v. Medical co-morbidity

        vi. Health literacy

       vii. Environmental domains

       viii. Social network

        ix. Resource issues

         x. Housing

        xi. Transportation

D. For interventions, consider the following:

    1. Create teams for tailored intervention

2. Access technology that can improve cognitive functions and optimize medical care

3. Address sensory/functional and intellectual impairments

4. Identify resources and housing transition

5. Negotiate to reduce risks of harm as tolerable to the patient

6. Simplify the process whenever possible

E. For the "intractable" self-neglecter, consider the following:

1. Ensure public safety

2. Provide nonjudgmental support

3. Remember that trust is earned and in little ways first

4. Be realistic and be patient

REFERENCES

Abrams, R. C., Lachs, M., AcAvay, G., Keohane, D. J., & Bruce, M. L. (2002). Predictors of self-neglect in the community. *The American Journal of Psychiatry, 159,* 1724–1730.

American Psychiatric Association (APA). (2000). *Diagnostic and statistical manual of mental disorders, text revision* (4th ed.) Washington, DC: APA.

American Psychiatric Nurses Association (APNA). (2000). Scope and standards of psychiatric nursing practice. Washington, DC: APNA.

Antai-Otong, D. (2003). Psychosocial rehabilitation. *Nursing Clinics of North America, 38*(1), 151–160.

Badger, T. A., McNiece, C., Bonham, E., Jacobson, J., & Gelenberg, A. J. (2003). Health outcomes for people with serious mental illness: A case study. *Perspectives in Psychiatric Care, 39*(1), 23–32.

Bai, Y. et al. (1997). Risk factors for parasuicide among psychiatric inpatients. *Psychiatric Services, 48*(9), 1201–1203.

Berger, D. (1993). Suicide evaluation in medical patients: A pilot study. *General Hospital Psychiatry, 15,* 75–81.

Bird, T. D., Nochlin, D., Poorkaj, P., Cherrier, M., Kaye, J., Payami, H., Peskind, E., Lampe, T. H., Nemens, E., Boyer, P. J., & Schellenberg, G. S. (1999). A clinical pathological comparison of three families with frontotemporal dementia and the identical mutations in the tau gene (P301L). *Brain, 122*(4), 741–756.

Bond, G. R., Drake, R. E., Mueser, K. T., & Latimer, E. (2001). Assertive community treatment for people with severe mental illness: Critical ingredients and impact on patients. *Disease Management and Health Outcomes, 19,* 141–159.

Bullman, M., & Kang, H. (1996). The risk of suicide among wounded Vietnam veterans. *American Journal of Public Health, 86*(5), 662–667.

Chan, S., Mackenzie, A., Dominic, T. F., & Leung, J. K. (2000). An evaluation of the implementation of case management in the community psychiatric nursing service. *Journal of Advanced Nursing, 31*(1), 144–156.

Chase, P., Gage, J., Stanley, K. M., & Bonadonna, J. R. (2000). The psychiatric consultation/liaison nurse role in case management. *Nursing Case Management, 5*(2), 73–77.

Coren, S., & Hewitt, P. (1998). Is anorexia nervosa associated with elevated rates of suicide? *American Journal of Public Health, 88*(8), 1206–1207.

Cox, W. K., Penny, L. C., Statham, R. P., & Roper, B. L. (2003). Admission intervention team: Medical center based intensive case management of the seriously mentally ill. *Care Management Journals: Journal of Case Management, the Journal of Long Term Home Health Care, 4*(4), 178–184.

Donoghue, A., Hodgins, G., Judd, F., Scopelliti, J., Grigg, M., & Komiti, A., et al. (2004). Training case managers to deliver focused psychological strategies. *International Journal of Mental Health Nursing, 13*(1), 33–38.

Farnsworth, B. J., & Bigelow, A. S. (1997). Psychiatric case management. In J. Haber, B. Krainorich-Miller and A. McMahon (Ed.), *Comprehensive psychiatric nursing* (5th ed.) 17, 318–331. New York: Mosby Year Book.

Franklin, J., Solovitz, B., Mason, M., Clemons, J., & Miller, G. (1987). An evaluation of case management. *American Journal of Public Health, 77,* 674–678.

Gage, A. (2002). Mental health: Case management in schizophrenia: An integral part of effective treatment. *Disease Management Digest, 6*(6), 4–5, 8–11.

Goering, P., Wasylenki, D., Farkas, M., Lancee, W., & Ballantyne, R. (1988). Improved functioning for case management clients. *Psychosocial Rehabilitation Journal, 12,* 3–17.

Herrick, C. A., & Bartlett, R. (2004). Psychiatric nursing case management: Past, present, and future. *Issues in Mental Health Nursing, 25*(6), 589–602.

Krainovich-Miller, B., & Gannon-Rosedale, M. (1999). Behavioral health home care. In Carol Shea (Ed.), *Advanced practice nursing and psychiatric and mental health care, 15,* 333–354. St. Louis: Mosby.

Lave, J. R., & Peele, P. B. (2000). The distribution of payments for behavioral health care. *Psychiatric Services, 51*(6), 723.

Li, G. (1995). The interaction effect of bereavement and sex on the risk of suicide in the elderly: A historical cohort study. *Social Science and Medicine, 40*(6), 825–828.

Lindberg, G. et al. (1998). Use of calcium channel blockers and risk of suicide: Ecological findings confirmed in population based cohort study. *British Medical Journal, 316*(3), 741–745.

Marty, D., Rapp, C. A., & Carlson, L. (2001). The experts speak: The critical ingredients of strengths model case management. *Psychiatric Rehabilitation Journal, 24*(3), 214–221.

McCloskey, J., & Bulachek, G. (2000). *Iowa intervention project: nursing interventions classification (NIC).* St. Louis: Mosby. pp. 620–621.

Naegle, M., Richardson, H., & Morton, K. (2004). In our community. Rehab instead of prison: Drug courts provide opportunities for nurse practitioners. *American Journal of Nursing, 104*(6), 58–61.

National Committee for Quality Assurance (NCQA). (1997). *Accreditation guidelines for managed behavioral healthcare organizations.* Washington, DC: NCQA.

National Institute of Mental Health (NIMH). (1987). *Towards a model for comprehensive community-based mental health system.* Washington, DC: NIMH.

Reid, W. et al. (1998). Suicide prevention efforts associated with clozapine therapy in schizophrenia and schizoeffective disorder. *Psychiatric Services, 49*(8), 1029–1033.

Remafedi, G. et al. (1998). The relationship between suicide risk and sexual orientation: Results of a population-based study. *American Journal of Public Health, 88*(1), 57–60.

Robie, D. et al. (1999). Suicide prevention protocol. *American Journal of Nursing, 99*(12), 53–57.

Rosen, A., & Teeson, M. (2001). Does case management work? The evidence and the abuse of evidence-based medicine. *Australian and New Zealand Journal of Psychiatry, 35*(6), 731–746.

Schaedle, R., McGrew, J. H., Bond, G. R., & Epstein, I. (2002). A comparison of experts' perspectives on assertive community treatment and intensive case management. *Psychiatric Services, 53,* 207–210.

Schwartz, R. C., & Rogers, J. R. (2004). Suicide assessment and evaluation strategies: A primer for counseling psychologists. *Counselling Psychology Quarterly, 17*(1), 89–97.

Swann, A. C., Dougherty, D. M., Pazzaglia, P. J., Pham, M., Steinberg, J. L, & Moeller, F. G. (2005). Increased impulsivity associated with severity of suicide attempt history in patients with bipolar disorder. *American Journal of Psychiatry, 162*(9), 1680–1687.

Tahan, H. (1998). Case management: A heritage more than a century old. *Lippincott's Nursing Case Management, 3*(2), 55–62.

Taylor, C. E., LoPiccolo, C. J., Eisdorfer, C., & Clemence, C. (2005). Best practices reducing rehospitalization with telephonic targeted care management in a managed health care plan. *Psychiatric Services, 56*(6), 652–654.

Yamashita, M., Forchuk, C., & Mound, B. (2005). Nurse case management: Negotiating care together within a developing relationship. *Perspectives in Psychiatric Care, 41*(2), 62–70.

Ziguras, S. J., & Stuart, G. W. (2000). A meta-analysis of the effectiveness of mental health case management over 20 years. *Psychiatric Services, 51,* 1410–1421.

SUGGESTED READING

Allness, D. J., & Knoedler, W. H. (1998). *The PACT model of community-based treatment for persons with severe and persistent mental illness: A manual for PACT start-up.* Arlington: National Alliance for the Mentally Ill.

Cohen, J. A. (2003). Managed care and the evolving role of the clinical social worker in mental health. *Social Work, 48*(1), 34–43.

Haber, J. (1997). Psychiatric home care. In Judith Haber (Ed.). *Comprehensive psychiatric nursing* (5th ed.) *21,* 366–381. New York: Mosby Year Book.

Kerson, T. S. (2004). Boundary-spanning: An ecological reinterpretation of social work practice in health and mental health systems. *Social Work in Mental Health, 2*(2/3), 39–57.

Lloyd, C., McKenna, K., & King, R. (2005). Sources of stress experienced by occupational therapists and social workers in mental health settings. *Occupational Therapy International, 12*(2), 81–94.

Yang, J., Law, S., Chow, W., Anderman, L., Steinberg, R., & Sadavoy, J. (2005). Best practices: Assertive community treatment for persons with severe and persistent illness in ethnic minority groups. *Psychiatric Services, 56,* 1053–1055.

Complementary and Alternative Medicine

Suzanne K. Powell

Upon completion of this chapter, the reader will be able to:

1. Define concepts and terms relative to complementary and alternative medicine (CAM), including brief descriptions of CAM modalities, along with their indications and contraindications.

2. Identify CAM systems, and the modalities within those systems, that case managers will likely encounter.

3. Describe the current impact of CAM on the health care industry and its potential to change the delivery of health care, including the challenges of CAM integration into the current medical model.

4. Discuss the differences between CAM and allopathic medicine, as well as the areas in which they complement each other.

5. Identify barriers to third-party reimbursement and HMO benefits for CAM, and the CAM modalities most often considered for inclusion.

6. Discuss issues and challenges related to research into CAM modalities.

7. Identify ways in which case management can integrate CAM into treatment plans, and the challenges and opportunities it presents.

IMPORTANT TERMS AND CONCEPTS

Acupuncture
Alexander Technique
Allopathic Medicine
Aromatherapy
Auric Field
Autogenic Training
Ayurvedic Medicine
Bioelectric
Bioelectromagnetic-based
 therapies
Biomedical model
Bioenergy
Bioenergy Therapies
Biofeedback
Complementary and Alternative
 Medicine (CAM)
Chiropractic Manipulation
Craniosacral Therapy
Creative Visualization
Doshas (Vata, Pitta, Kapha)
Feldenkrais Therapy
Flower Essences
Guided Imagery
Hatha Yoga
Herbal Medicine/Herbology

Homeopathy
Hydrotherapy
Hypnosis
Law of Similars
Magnetic Therapy
Meditation
Mind-Body Medicine
Musculoskeletal Therapies
National Institutes of Health (NIH)
Naturopathic Medicine
Neurolinguistic Programming (NLP)
Nutritional Supplementation
Polarity Therapy
Preventive Medicine
Qi
Quantum Healing
Reflexology
Reiki
Relaxation Response
Rolfing
Sound Healing
Structural Integration
Therapeutic Touch
Traditional Chinese Medicine
Yin/Yang

■ INTRODUCTION

A. Definitions (see Table 24-1)
1. Conventional medicine—Medicine practiced in quality-controlled health care, based on evidenced-based practice.
2. Complementary and alternative medicine (CAM)—Any therapeutic intervention not based on conventional, Western, allopathic treatment protocols.
3. Integrative medicine—The incorporation of CAM techniques into the conventional health care delivery system.
4. Complementary medicine and alternative medicine are different (NCCAM, 2006):
   a. *Complementary* medicine is used *together* with conventional medicine. An example of a complementary therapy is using aromatherapy to help lessen a patient's discomfort following surgery.

This chapter is a revised version of what was previously published in the first edition of *CMSA Core Curriculum for Case Management*. The contributor wishes to acknowledge Janice E. Benjamin, as some of the timeless material was retained from the previous version.

TABLE 24–1

Definitions and Foci of Medical Modalities

Type of Medicine Modality	Definition	Focus/Intent	Healing Methods/ Techniques
Conventional medicine	Medicine practiced in quality-controlled health care, based on evidenced-based practice	Illness model that seeks to reverse or halt the progression of a disease or traumatic state	Uses technological and pharmaceutical interventions that have been determined to halt or reverse the condition
Complementary and alternative medicine (CAM)*	Any therapeutic intervention not based on conventional, Western, allopathic treatment protocols	Wellness model based on the balance and integration of the mind, body, and spirit	After a holistic assessment, practitioner chooses the healing modalities based on the premise that the body has an innate ability to heal itself
Integrative medicine	The incorporation of CAM techniques into the conventional health care delivery system	Integrates and uses techniques of both medicine modalities to enhance the effectiveness of therapy	Uses both evidenced-based technological and pharmaceutical interventions, supported by CAM modalities decided on by the practitioner and patient

*NOTE: *Complementary* medicine and *alternative* medicine are different (NCCAM, 2006): *Complementary* medicine is used *together with* conventional medicine. An example of a complementary therapy is using aromatherapy to help lessen a patient's discomfort following surgery.

Alternative medicine is used *in place of* conventional medicine. An example of an alternative therapy is using a special diet to treat cancer instead of undergoing surgery, radiation, or chemotherapy that has been recommended by a conventional doctor.

    b. *Alternative* medicine is used *in place of* conventional medicine. An example of an alternative therapy is using a special diet to treat cancer *instead of* undergoing surgery, radiation, or chemotherapy that has been recommended by a conventional doctor.

B. Brief history of CAM in the United States and the impact of consumer use in bringing CAM into the mainstream of health care delivery

    1. In 1992, as billions of consumer dollars were spent on alternative medicine, the Office of Alternative Medicine's budget increased the CAM budget to $2.0 million and Congress established the Office of Alternative Medicine. Over the next several years, subsequent budget increases occurred (NCCAM, 2005).

        a. Fiscal Year (FY) 1993—$2.0 million

        b. FY 1994—$3.4 million

        c. FY 1995—$5.4 million

        d. FY 1996—$7.7 million

    e. FY 1997—$12.0 million

    f. FY 1998—$19.5 million

  2. In 1999, the National Center for Complementary and Alternative Medicine (NCCAM) became one of the 27 institutes and centers that make up the National Institutes of Health (NIH) and the FY 1999 budget was $50.0 million. Subsequent budgets increased (NCCAM, 2006).

    a. FY 2000—$68.7 million

    b. FY 2001—$89.2 million

    c. FY 2002—$104.6 million

    d. FY 2003—$114.1 million

    e. FY 2004—$117.7 million

    f. FY 2005—$123.1 million

  3. 2006—NCCAM is well-known for research into complementary and alternative healing practices, training CAM researchers, and disseminating authoritative information to the public and professionals.

C. Eisenberg's 1990 and 1993 surveys on consumer use of CAM impacted the health care industry when it clearly determined consumer interest in and use of CAM; subsequent surveys/studies showed the trend in consumer use of CAM rising.

D. Current efforts are being made toward creating integrative medicine and incorporating CAM into the health care delivery system. Training requirements and potential for insurance reimbursement varies from state to state.

E. Theoretical contrasts between CAM and allopathic medicine include:

  1. The biomedical model of cellular pathology as the root of disease compared with the model of a disruption of bioenergetic pathways as the root of disease

  2. Prevention and wellness interventions as the model for treatment compared with acute care interventions and symptom management as the model for treatment

  3. Treatment focused on building the body's own immunity and reparative systems compared with treatment focused on disease processes

F. Broad categories of CAM modalities available in the United States include:

  1. Whole health care systems, which have theoretical foundations, diagnostic guidelines, and treatment protocols for addressing the full range of health care conditions

  2. Mind-body medicine therapies, which effect health through accessing and strengthening the relationship between the mind and body

  3. Musculoskeletal therapies, which work by restoring and maintaining the functions of the body's skeletal and muscular systems

  4. Bioenergy therapies, which work on the bioelectrical and biomagnetic fields of the body

  5. Herbal medicine, which uses whole plants to treat disease and maintain health

  6. Nutritional supplementation, which prescribes megadoses of vitamins and minerals to treat disease and maintain health

■ KEY DEFINITIONS

A. Acupuncture—Acupuncture is a treatment modality based on the concepts of traditional Chinese medicine that involves the placement of very thin, stainless steel needles into specific points on the body with the intention of maintaining or restoring the smooth flow of energy, or Qi, along specific pathways, or meridians, that travel along the surface of the body and enter deep into the body to connect with all the organs. Qi is considered a vital energy necessary for the body to function.

B. Alexander technique—Focuses on restoring a balanced, dynamic posture, or coordination of the head and the spine, by reprogramming neuromotor patterns through repetitive musculoskeletal movements or postures.

C. Aromatherapy—Involves the use of essential oils (extracts or essences) from flowers, herbs, and trees to promote health and well-being (NCCAM, 2006).

D. Auric field—A person's energy body.

E. Ayurvedic medicine—A 5,000-year-old philosophy and system of practice that teaches people how to live in harmony with all aspects of life by caring for themselves on a day-to-day basis. Ayurvedic medicine is deeply rooted in the ancient culture and religion of the Indian continent, and addresses the whole person as body-mind-spirit. The World Health Organization (WHO) supports the use of Ayurvedic medicine and its integration with modern medicine.

F. Bioacoustics—A cross between music therapy and biofeedback. Similar to sound therapy, bioacoustics uses low-based frequency sounds to elicit biological and emotional responses.

G. Bioelectric—Involving the electric phenomena that occur in living tissues (eg, muscles and nerves) *www.spotutah.com/glossary.asp*

H. Bioelectromagnetic-based therapies involve the unconventional use of electromagnetic fields, such as pulsed fields, magnetic fields, or alternating-current or direct-current fields. *http://nccam.nih.gov/health/whatiscam* (2) the magnetic field emanating from living organisms *http://www. biomagnetic.org/magnetic%20vocabulary.html*

I. Biomedical model—(1) Treats disease as a pathology that occurs within the person. The limitation of this model is that it excludes any psychological, social or ecological factors. *www.uwic.ac.uk/shss/dom/newweb/General/ Glossary.htm* (2) The viewpoint that illness can be explained on the basis of aberrant somatic processes and that psychological and social processes are largely independent of the disease process; the dominant model in medical practice until recently *highered.mcgraw-hill.com/sites/0072412976/student view0/chapterl/glossary.html* (3) The biomedical model of medicine, has been around for centuries as the predominant model used by physicians in the diagnosis of disease. The term is used by practitioners of Natural Health, a form of alternative medicine, in contrast to the biopsychosocial model, which incorporates psychological and social factors *en.wikipedia.org/wiki/ Biomedical_model*

J. Bioenergy—Energy generated from renewable biomass, i.e. living plants and plant components *english.forestindustries.fi/glossary/B.html*

K. Bioenergy therapies—Treatment modalities that work on balancing the patient's energy body, sometimes called the *auric field,* and include polarity therapy and therapeutic touch.

L. Biofeedback—Uses technology to provide feedback to patients training to gain conscious control over physiological functions of the body, such as regulation of the heart rate.

M. Chinese medicine—See traditional Chinese medicine.

N. Chiropractic manipulations—Concerned with the relationship of the spinal column and musculoskeletal structures of the body to the nervous system. It is believed that when the spinal column is out of alignment, it interferes with the flow of nerve impulses or messages from the central nervous system. Thus, misalignment can have an impact on every part of the body.

O. Complementary and alternative medicine (CAM)—As defined by NCCAM, a group of diverse medical and health care systems, practices, and products that are not presently considered to be part of conventional medicine. While some scientific evidence exists regarding some CAM therapies, for most key questions remain that are yet to be answered through well-designed scientific studies—questions such as whether these therapies are safe and whether they work for the diseases or medical conditions for which they are used. The list of what is considered to be CAM changes continually, as those therapies that are proven to be safe and effective become adopted into conventional health care and as new approaches to health care emerge (NCCAM, 2006).

P. Conventional medicine—Medicine practiced in quality-controlled health care, based on evidenced-based practice.

Q. Craniosacral therapy—This technique manipulates the bones of the skull to treat a range of conditions, from headache and ear infection to stroke, spinal cord injury, and cerebral palsy. Just as the human body has a rhythm associated with the heart beat and breathing, there is also a rhythm to the ebb and flow of fluid within the cranium and spinal cord generated by subtle pressure changes as fluid enters and exits these spaces.

R. Creative visualization—See guided imagery.

S. Doshas (Vata, Pitta, and Kapha)—The doshas govern psychobiological changes in the body and physiopathological changes.

T. Feldenkrais therapy—This system combines stretching, exercise, and yoga to improve awareness of movement patterns and encourage proper body movement.

U. Flower essences—Flower essences are considered to be a form of "vibrational" medicine. Much like homeopathy, flower essences contain the energetic pattern of a flower, rather than its molecular structure.

V. Guided imagery—Also known as *visualization,* the thought process that invokes an inner mental picture usually using all the senses, which include vision as well as hearing, smell, touch, taste, position, and movement.

W. Hatha Yoga—The yoga of movement and coordinated breath.

X. Health—The WHO's definition of health is a state of complete physical, mental and spiritual well-being, not merely the absence of disease.

Y. Herbology/herbal medicine—The use of whole plants, or parts thereof, for the treatment of disease and the maintenance of good health. It is the oldest form of medicine known and has been practiced for thousands of years.

Z. Homeopathic medicine—A healing technique based on three principles: the Law of Similars, the Law of Infinitesimal Dose, and the Laws of Holism.

AA. Hydrotherapy—Therapies using water for healing.

BB. Hypnosis—An artificially induced state characterized by a heightened receptivity to suggestion; a form of guided imagery.

CC. Integrative medicine—Integrative medicine, as defined by NCCAM, combines mainstream medical therapies and CAM therapies for which there is some high-quality scientific evidence of safety and effectiveness (NCCAM, 2006).

DD. Magnetic therapy—A therapy where magnets or magnetic devices are placed on the skin; thought to prevent or treat symptoms of disease, especially pain.

EE. Meditation—An ancient spiritual practice for achieving spiritual awakening, which works by quieting the incessant, random flow of thoughts through the mind.

FF. Mind-body medicine—The ability of a belief or image held in the mind to directly effect a change in the body on a physical, cellular level is now called mind-body medicine, and includes such practices as meditation, hypnosis, biofeedback, creative visualization, the relaxation response, and autogenic training.

GG. Mindfulness meditation—A form of meditation developed in the traditions of Buddhism and designed to allow the individual to be at peace in any experience in which they find themselves. It requires much focused attention and a nonjudgmental attitude.

HH. Musculoskeletal therapies—Treatment modalities that bring the patient's awareness to body posture and movement, and manipulate the physical body in order to facilitate the flow of blood and energy through the muscles, fascia, and skeletal structures. Therapies include the Alexander technique, the Feldenkrais technique, craniosacral therapy, rolfing, chiropractic manipulation, yoga, massage, and reflexology.

II. Naturopathic medicine—The underlying goal of naturopathic medicine is to strengthen the body's immune system so that it can heal itself. Treatment modalities include the use of western herbs, high dose vitamins, homeopathic remedies, hydrotherapy, counseling, minor surgery, diet and lifestyle changes, detoxification regimens, and physical medicine modalities such as massage.

JJ. Polarity therapy—Promotes the smooth flow of energy along electromagnetic paths around the body by releasing blockages of energy.

KK. Prana—Life force, or energy that occurs throughout the body.

LL. Preventive care—The concept designed to prevent disease, or to detect and treat it early, or to manage its course most effectively. Examples of traditional preventive care include immunizations, Pap smears, mammograms, and cholesterol screening. Alternative therapies such as herbal remedies and various CAM modalities are important forms of preventive care.

MM. Qi—The vital force that runs throughout the body, animating and supporting the function of different organ systems.

NN. Quantum healing—"Quantum healing is healing the bodymind from a quantum level. That means from a level which is not manifest at a sensory level. Our bodies ultimately are fields of information, intelligence and energy. Quantum healing involves a shift in the fields of energy information, so as to bring about a correction in an idea that has gone wrong. So quantum healing involves healing one mode of consciousness, mind, to bring about changes in another mode of consciousness, body" (Chopra, 2006).

OO. Reflexology—Also called *zone therapy*, reflexology is based on the notion that each body part is represented on the hands and feet, where there are believed to be reflex points that can stimulate the glands and organs in the body.

PP. Reiki—A Japanese technique using "laying on hands" for stress reduction, relaxation, and healing promotion. It is based on the idea that an unseen "life force energy" flows through us and is what causes us to be alive. If one's "life force energy" is low, then we are more likely to get sick or feel stress, and if it is high, we are more capable of being happy and healthy.

QQ. Relaxation response—Achieved through mental imagery in a meditative state and activates the body's parasympathetic nervous system; can restore homeostasis and allow the body to heal from the physiological changes that can occur as the result of chronic stress.

RR. Rolfing—A form of deep tissue massage. Rolfers manipulate and stretch the body's fascial tissue in order to release adhesions and relieve restricted muscles and joints.

SS. Sound healing/therapy—Uses vibrational tones to elicit biological and emotional responses to promote healing.

TT. Therapeutic massage—The use of touch to manipulate the soft tissues of the body for the purpose of relieving muscle tension and promoting blood circulation. There are more than 100 styles of massage categorized according to the type of strokes or manipulations used, the depth of the massage, the incorporation of movements with the massage, the body part worked on, and the overall goal of the session.

UU. Therapeutic touch—A form of hands-on healing, although often the practitioner's hands are two to six inches from the patient.

VV. Traditional Chinese medicine (TCM)—A philosophy and practice of medicine based on the theory that health exists when the forces of Yin and Yang are balanced within the body-mind-spirit.

WW. Yin/Yang—The forces that maintain homeostasis in the body-mind-spirit, a balance between catabolism and anabolism, rest and activity, and heat and cold. Yang represents the functional aspect of the body-mind-spirit, and Yin represents the substance of the body-mind-spirit. Examples of Yang energy are heat, agitation, rapid movement, and the daytime. Examples of Yin energy are cold, rest, slow movement, and the nighttime.

XX. Yoga (classical)—Yoga that is organized into eight "limbs" that provide a complete system of physical, mental, and spiritual health. Some of the yogas focus on developing the mind, some on developing the body, and some on developing the deeper inner life of the spirit.

■ ALTERNATIVE WHOLE HEALTH CARE SYSTEMS

A. Four classifications
  1. Traditional Chinese medicine
  2. Ayurvedic medicine
  3. Naturopathic medicine
  4. Homeopathic medicine

B. Traditional Chinese medicine (TCM)
  1. TCM definition of health is a philosophy and practice of medicine based on the theory that health exists when the forces of Yin and Yang are balanced within the body-mind-spirit.
  2. Historical foundation of TCM in the Chinese culture's relationship with nature
     a. The view of humans as the place where Heaven (Yang) and Earth (Yin) come together, so that health is the balance of these forces in the body-mind-spirit
     b. The importance of the patient's relationship to the environment and the seasons, and living in harmony with the changes in nature
  3. Theoretical concepts on which clinical practice is based upon include:
     a. Qi (chi) as bioenergy flow through defined meridians, or pathways, in the body
     b. Yin/Yang and their interrelationships and interplay within the body
     c. The six organ systems (lung, kidney, liver, heart, pericardium, spleen) and their interrelated functions
  4. Modalities used in treatment include acupuncture, herbal medicine, diet therapy, heat, cupping, and massage.
  5. Conditions that can be treated and research supporting the effectiveness of TCM include the National Institutes of Health (NIH) consensus conference outcomes and the recommendations of the WHO.

C. Ayurvedic medicine
  1. A CAM alternative medical system that has been practiced primarily in the Indian subcontinent for 5,000 years. Ayurveda includes diet and herbal remedies and emphasizes the use of body, mind, and spirit in disease prevention and treatment (NCCAM, 2006).

2. Identifying the patient's constitutional type, or dosha, is the basis for maintaining health and designing treatment during illness.
   a. Vata represents the aspects of thinness, dryness, cold, activity, imagination, and the respiratory and circulatory systems.
   b. Pitta represents the aspects of heat, a medium build, strong appetite, emotionality, and the digestive system.
   c. Kapha represents the aspects of heaviness, slow movement, sweet and salty tastes, good memory, and the physical structures of the body.
3. Modalities for clinical treatment include diet, massage, herbs, meditation, yoga, detoxification, and breathing exercises.
4. Considerations for case managers if they are considering use of Ayurveda—have the client/patient:
   a. Tell their health care provider that they are considering or using Ayurveda
   b. Make sure that any diagnosis of a disease or condition has been made by a provider who has substantial conventional medical training and experience with managing that disease or condition.
   c. It is better to use Ayurvedic remedies under the supervision of an Ayurvedic medicine practitioner than to try to treat oneself.
   d. Ask about the practitioner's training and experience.
   e. Find out whether any rigorous scientific studies have been done on the therapies the client/patient is interested in.[1]

D. Naturopathic medicine
   1. Six principles of practice that define naturopathic medicine include:
      a. The body has the ability to heal itself, and treatment is designed to support the innate wisdom of the body.
      b. Treat the underlying cause, rather than just suppress the symptoms.
      c. Do no harm; thus, use only natural means and substances.
      d. Treat the whole person—body, mind, and spirit.
      e. The physician is a teacher to empower the patient.
      f. Prevention is the best medicine.
   2. Naturopathic philosophy of disease cause and progression includes the importance of not suppressing natural body processes such as fever, by which the body attempts to restore homeostasis.
   3. Modalities used in treatment include diet, vitamin/mineral therapy, herbal medicine, hydrotherapy, spinal manipulation, homeopathy, and massage.

E. Homeopathic medicine
   1. Discovery and development of homeopathy was by the German physician, Hahnemann, in the 1700s.
      a. *Provings,* or the testing of substances on healthy persons are used to determine indications for treatment.
      b. Remedies are created based on the results of the provings.

---

[1]See *http://nccam.nih.gov/health/ayurveda/.*

2. Homeopathic remedies work on the energetic body, rather than the cellular body, and stimulate the body's own healing processes.
3. Three principles on which homeopathy are based include:
   a. Law of Similars—"like cures like"
   b. Law of Infinitesimal Doses—the more dilute the homeopathic remedy, the stronger its effect
   c. Law of Holism—treatment directed to the whole person, not just the symptom, is more effective
4. To make a uniquely detailed and thorough assessment and choose an appropriate homeopathic remedy, the practitioner will:
   a. Find the constitutional remedy, or the main remedy that will benefit the patient *most*.
   b. Treat acute versus chronic illness.
   c. Treat psycho-emotional conditions.
5. Current research explaining the mechanisms of action are based on the electromolecular structure of water.

■ MIND-BODY MEDICINE

A. Basic concepts of mind-body medicine and the intimate connections between two concepts
   1. Herbert Benson's work in the early 1970's on the impact of stress on the body, and his discovery of and research on the "relaxation response" include:
      a. Activation of the parasympathetic nervous system to induce relaxation
      b. Comparisons to meditative states and similar physiological changes
   2. Candace Pert's research on the biochemical basis for mind-body medicine and her findings that neurochemical markers found on cells outside of the nervous system allow for pathways of communication between multiple body systems
B. Guided imagery/creative visualization
   1. Directed or self-initiated use of mental images to create change in the patient's health
      a. Engages all the senses in creating a mental image
      b. Patients create images of significance to them, enhancing the process and effect
   2. Conditions that can be treated include pain reduction, reduction in nausea associated with chemotherapy, and reduction of perceived stress.
C. Hypnosis
   1. Guided imagery directed by a therapist to implant a subconscious suggestion that promotes healing on a physical or emotional level
   2. Conditions that can be treated include phobias, insomnia, chronic pain, and depression.

D. Meditation
1. Based on ancient Hindu practices for spiritual awakening by controlling the flow of thoughts through the mind
2. Mindfulness meditation is just one of several styles of meditation, and is used in medical clinics for pain management.

E. Biofeedback
1. The use of technology to reinforce the patient's efforts to regulate the body's autonomic systems through the use of the mind. Biofeedback uses electronic sensors to measure and give "feedback" information to the individual about their bodies. This feedback is linked to processes of which we are ordinarily not aware.
2. In clinical biofeedback, the measured bodily processes are muscle activity, skin temperature, skin conductivity, pulse volume, heart rate, and other physiological data. These signals indicate the degree of relaxation or tension produced.
3. The biofeedback therapist can help teach "self-regulation"—how to alter or change the signals, and thereby, how to correct bodily overreactions.
4. Conditions it can treat include insomnia, asthma, hypertension, irritable bowel syndrome, and migraine headaches.

F. Autogenic training
1. Mental exercises taught to reduce the physiological impacts of stress
2. Unique from other techniques in the very detailed script used to induce relaxation
3. Conditions it can treat include high blood pressure, insomnia, and palpitations.

G. Neurolinguistic programming (NLP)
1. Developed in the 1970s through the study of popular psychotherapy techniques
2. Works to access the mind-body connection through changing the relationships among the patient's nervous system, thought processing, and patterns of behavior
3. A typical session might progress using questioning and suggestions for redefining one's images and thoughts about a health condition.

■ **MUSCULOSKELETAL THERAPIES**

A. A broad category of treatments that bring the patient's awareness to posture and movement, and manipulate the physical body to facilitate the flow of blood and energy throughout the body

B. Alexander technique
1. Developed in the late 1800s in Australia by an actor motivated to restore the loss of his voice
2. The goal of the Alexander technique is to coordinate the functions of the muscle and skeletal systems for maximum efficiency.

C. Feldenkrais therapy
   1. Developed in the 1940s by Moshe Feldenkrais to facilitate his recovery from an injury
   2. The underlying goal is to change dysfunctional postural and movement habits that are contributing to illness or pain.
   3. Two approaches to therapy, with the therapist in the role of teacher in both cases, include:
      a. Group setting (called *awareness through movement*)
      b. One on one (called *functional integration*)

D. Craniosacral therapy
   1. Manipulation of the bones of the skull to treat a range of conditions, including headaches, strokes, ear infections, insomnia, high blood pressure, autism, and chronic pain
   2. Garner Sutherland's technique versus John Upledger's technique
      a. Sutherland's technique was developed in the early 1900s to restore and maintain spinal fluid pressure changes and electromagnetic field patterns.
      b. Upledger's approach was developed in the 1970s to release restrictions in the meningeal tissues and fascia within the craniosacral system.
   3. The overall goal is to release constricted movement or adhesions in order to reduce intercranial pressure.

E. Rolfing/structural integration
   1. Deep tissue massage was developed over a period of 25 years and introduced in the 1950s by Ida Rolf.
   2. Usually offered as a series of 10 sessions to manipulate and stretch the body's fascial tissue in order to release adhesions and relieve restricted muscle and joints

F. Yoga
   1. 2,000- to 4,000-year history in Hindu traditions
   2. Exercises that coordinate movement with breathing, done in a meditative state, in order to balance the nervous and endocrine systems
   3. Benefits include enhanced blood oxygenation, balanced glucose metabolism, stimulation of the immune system, and emotional balance.
   4. Current use of yoga in pain clinics and cardiac rehabilitation clinics
      a. Yoga is believed to reduce pain by helping the brain's pain center regulate the gate-controlling mechanism located in the spinal cord and the secretion of natural painkillers in the body. Breathing exercises used in yoga can also reduce pain. Because muscles tend to relax when you exhale, lengthening the time of exhalation can help produce relaxation and reduce tension.
      b. Cardiac yoga training programs are designed to educate and train certified yoga teachers to work specifically with cardiac patients. Participants learn to adapt basic concepts of yoga and meditation to the special needs of the cardiac patient. Curriculum includes training in the adaptation of yoga postures, breathing, deep relaxation,

and imagery for cardiac patients; understanding heart disease, including risk factors, anatomy and physiology of the heart, and psycho-social factors; designing and implementing a yoga class and discussion group for cardiac patients.

G. Therapeutic massage
   1. Manipulation of soft tissues of the body to relieve muscle tension and promote blood circulation
   2. Contrasting of various styles
      a. Swedish massage, the oldest technique, to promote circulation
      b. Sports massage to improve flexibility and recover from injury
      c. Neuromuscular massage for rehabilitation
      d. Lymphatic massage for detoxification
      e. Esalen massage for inducing meditative states

H. Reflexology
   1. Massage of painful points on the hands and feet to stimulate glands, neuromuscular systems, and organs in the whole body
   2. Proposed mechanisms of action
      a. Stimulation of the nervous system
      b. The microsystem of the hands and feet reflect the body as a whole.
   3. Indications—though empirical studies are lacking, many patients have benefited from reflexology. Conditions treated may include migraine headache, hypertension, menstrual problems, myofascial pain, fibromyalgia, insomnia, and anxiety disorders.
   4. Contraindications include recent surgical removal of a malignant tumor and wounds to hands, feet, or ears.

■ CHIROPRACTIC MANIPULATION

A. History of the chiropractic profession goes back to Hippocrates in ancient Greece; in the United States in 1895, Daniel David Palmer founded the modern profession of chiropractic.

B. Underlying theories for its effectiveness
   1. Spinal column alignment is necessary for proper functioning of the nervous system.
   2. This alignment stimulates the innate intelligence of the body to heal itself.

C. Conditions treated include chronic sinus infections, chronic pain, asthma, and digestive disorders, as well as back, neck, and shoulder pain.

■ BIOENERGY THERAPIES

A. A broad category of therapies that work on balancing the patient's bioenergy and biomagnetic fields to promote healing of the emotional and physical body. According to NCCAM,[2] energy medicine is a domain in CAM that deals with energy fields of three types:

---

[2]See *http://nccam.nih.gov/health/backgrounds/energymed.htm.*

1. *Veritable* energy, which can be measured. Veritable energy employs mechanical vibrations (such as sound) and electromagnetic forces, including visible light, magnetism, monochromatic radiation (such as laser beams), and rays from other parts of the electromagnetic spectrum. They involve the use of specific, measurable wavelengths and frequencies to treat patients.

2. *Putative* energy has not yet been measured. In contrast to veritable energies, putative energy fields (also called *biofields*) have defied measurement to date by reproducible methods. Therapies involving putative energy fields are based on the concept that human beings are infused with a subtle form of energy. This vital energy or life force is known under different names in different cultures, such as *qi* in TCM, *doshas* in Ayurvedic medicine, and elsewhere as *prana, etheric energy, fohat, orgone, odic force, mana,* and *homeopathic resonance*.

3. *Vital* energy is believed to flow throughout the material human body, but it has not been unequivocally measured by means of conventional instrumentation. Nonetheless, therapists claim that they can work with this subtle energy, see it with their own eyes, and use it to effect changes in the physical body and influence health.

B. Polarity therapy
   1. Developed in the 1940s by Dr. Randolph Stone based on his studies of Oriental and Ayurvedic medicine concepts of the body's energy fields
   2. Recognizes that humans have a magnetic field around their body, with a positive and negative pole that can be disrupted (leading to illness) and subsequently restored (leading to healing)
   3. Promotes the smooth flow of energy in the patient's energy field by the therapist placing his/her hands in designated positions on the patient's body so that negative and positive poles are joined
   4. Necessary for the therapist to have a balanced energy field so as not to do harm to the patient

C. Therapeutic touch (TT)
   1. Developed by Dolores Krieger as a tool for health care professionals to do hands-on healing
   2. The goals of TT are to restore balance in the patient's energy field and to promote homeostatic changes in biochemical processes.

D. Reiki (Vitale, 2006)
   1. Means "universal life energy"
   2. Was developed in Japan from techniques described in 3,000-year-old Tibetan scriptures
   3. A Japanese technique using "laying on hands," called an *attunement*
   4. Used for stress reduction, relaxation, and healing promotion
   5. Based on the idea that an unseen "life force energy" flows through us and causes us to be alive. If one's life force energy is low, then we are more likely to get sick or feel stress; if it is high, we are more capable of being happy and healthy.
   6. Knowledge and techniques are passed from masters to students.

E. Quantum healing
   1. Theory developed in the 1990s
   2. Dr. Deepak Chopra brought the theory to the masses.
   3. Definition—"Quantum healing is healing the bodymind from a quantum level. That means from a level which is not manifest at a sensory level. Our bodies ultimately are fields of information, intelligence and energy. Quantum healing involves a shift in the fields of energy information, so as to bring about a correction in an idea that has gone wrong. So quantum healing involves healing one mode of consciousness, mind, to bring about changes in another mode of consciousness, body" (Chopra, 2006).

F. Magnet therapy
   1. Research on the use of magnets to promote healing of bone and to relieve pain is still inconclusive.
   2. Proposed mechanisms of action include:
      a. Improves blood circulation
      b. Affects chemical processes within and between cells
      c. Affects nerve signals
      d. Stimulates acupuncture points
   3. Contraindications or precautions for the use of magnets are rare. One study reported that a small percentage of participants had bruising or redness on their skin where a magnet was worn. Use of magnets is discouraged for the following:[3]
      a. Pregnant women (effects of magnets on the fetus are not known)
      b. People with medical devices such as pacemakers, defibrillators, or insulin pumps (magnets may affect the magnetically controlled features of such devices)
      c. People who use a patch that delivers medication through the skin, in case magnets cause dilation of blood vessels, which could affect the delivery of the medicine. This caution also applies to people with an acute sprain, inflammation, infection, or wound.

G. Sound energy therapy
   1. Also referred to as vibrational or frequency therapy
   2. Includes music therapy as well as wind chime and tuning fork therapy, use of singing, chanting, and percussion instruments to promote healing. In the last two decades, electronic sounds (low-based frequencies) have been used for healing.
   3. The effects of sound on the human body include:
      a. Rhythmic entrainment—occurs when the human body matches its internal rhythms to the tempo of an external rhythm
      b. Resonance—the transmission of vibrations from one medium, such as beating drums, to another, such as the beating of the human heart

---

[3]See *http://nccam.nih.gov/health/magnet/magnet.htm#sideeffect.*

4. The presumptive basis of its effect is that specific sound frequencies resonate with specific organs of the body to heal and support the body.

5. Research—Music therapy has been the most studied among these interventions, with studies dating back to the 1920s, when it was reported that music affected blood pressure. Other studies have suggested that music can help reduce pain and anxiety. Music and imagery, alone and in combination, have been used to entrain mood states, reduce acute or chronic pain, and alter certain biochemicals, such as plasma beta-endorphin levels. These uses of energy fields truly overlap with the domain of mind-body medicine.[4]

H. Flower essences
1. Dr. Edward Bach's work in developing flower essences as a gentler form of healing began in the 1930s in England.

2. Illness is seen as a reflection of imbalance in the energy field of a patient. Dr. Bach felt that harmful emotions are the main cause of disease. He classified various emotions into seven principal categories; these categories were divided further into 38 negative feelings, each of which was associated with a particular therapeutic plant.

3. There are numerous anecdotal reports about successful treatment with Bach flower remedies, but published scientific research is limited.

I. Aromatherapy
1. The effect of the aroma of essential flower oils to stimulate the brain and effect a healing response in the whole body

2. It is important to use food-grade oils.

3. Aromatherapy is a large and unregulated field. Safety concerns include:
a. Essential oils are the steam-distilled volatile compounds 100% derived from a named aromatic botanical source. These concentrated materials are not intended for direct oral consumption. Some oils are toxic, phototoxic, or carcinogenic.

b. Little is currently known about inhalation toxicity, systemic toxicity, genetic effects, or sub-chronic effects of many of the commonly used essential oils.

c. Interactions with medication can occur (as in herbal medicine). Care is suggested if clients take anticoagulant or antidepressant drugs; problems with grapefruit juice, and by inference, grapefruit oil, have been in the media.

d. If taking medication, consult physician

e. Avoid undue exposure to essential oils.

J. Acupuncture
1. Acupuncture is the most prominent therapy to promote qi flow along the meridians.

2. Acupuncture has been extensively studied and has been shown to be effective in treating some conditions, particularly certain forms of pain.

---

[4]See *http://nccam.nih.gov/health/backgrounds/energymed.htm.*

3. The mechanism of action remains to be elucidated. The main threads of research on acupuncture have shown regional effects on neurotransmitter expression, but have not validated the existence of an "energy" per se.

■ HERBAL MEDICINE

A. The use of whole plants for the treatment of disease and the maintenance of health

B. The oldest form of medicine; still the only form of medicine for many cultures

C. Part of TCM, Ayurvedic medicine, naturopathic medicine, and many indigenous medicines

D. Case managers need to keep current on recent research to prevent potential complications from self-prescribed use of herbs, as more consumers use herbal medicine (and many do not report them to their health care practitioner).

E. Quality control of herbal medicines—refers to processes involved in maintaining the quality or validity of a manufactured product.
  1. Without proper quality control, there is no assurance that the herb contained in the bottle is the same as what is stated on the outside label.
  2. Many herbal products are from foreign countries; some countries may also lack quality controls.
  3. Many standardized extracts are currently made in Europe under strict guidelines by members of the European Economic Council (EEC). Included are guidelines for acceptable levels of impurities such as parasites (bacterial counts), pesticides, residual solvents, heavy metals, and product stability.[5]

■ NUTRITIONAL SUPPLEMENTATION AND FUNCTIONAL FOODS

A. Functional foods (International Food Information Council Foundation, 2006)
  1. Functional foods are foods or dietary components that may provide a health benefit beyond basic nutrition. Biologically active components in functional foods impart health benefits or desirable physiological effects.
  2. Consumer interest in the relationship between diet and health has increased the demand for information on functional foods. Rapid advances in science and technology, increasing health care costs, changes in food laws affecting label and product claims, an aging population, and rising interest in attaining wellness through diet are among the factors fueling U.S. interest in functional foods.
  3. Credible scientific research indicates many potential health benefits from food components. Many academic, scientific, and regulatory

---

[5]See *http://www.viable-herbal.com/herbology1/herbs43.htm*.

organizations are considering ways to establish the scientific basis to support claims for functional components or the foods containing them.

    a. FDA regulates food products according to their intended use and the nature of claims made on the package.

    b. Five types of health-related statements or claims are allowed on food and dietary supplement labels:

        i. Nutrient content claims indicate the presence of a specific nutrient at a certain level.

        ii. Structure and function claims describe the effect of dietary components on the normal structure or function of the body.

        iii. Dietary guidance claims describe the health benefits of broad categories of foods.

        iv. Qualified health claims convey a developing relationship between components in the diet and risk of disease, as approved by the FDA and supported by the weight of credible scientific evidence available.

        v. Health claims confirm a relationship between components in the diet and risk of disease or health condition, as approved by FDA and supported by significant scientific agreement.

    c. More credible scientific research is needed.

    d. Consumers must have a clear understanding of, and a strong confidence level in, the scientific criteria that are used to document health effects and claims if functional foods are to deliver their potential public health benefits.

4. Examples in Table 24-2 are not "magic bullets." It is best to include foods from all of the food groups represented on the food guide pyramid.

B. Vitamins, minerals, and trace minerals

    1. Recommended daily allowance (RDA) has been established by the Food and Nutrition Board of the (US) National Academy of Sciences, but is disputed by recent research as too low for many supplements.

    2. Vitamin therapy is used to prevent and treat illness through the use of megadoses; this requires close supervision.

    3. Education and knowledge on current research are needed to prevent potential side effects from improper use.

■ CLINICAL INTEGRATION OF CAM

A. Most-frequently cited consumer reasons for interest in CAM include:

    1. Dissatisfaction with limited allopathic options

    2. Impersonal treatment by medical doctors

    3. Increased research pointing to the benefits of CAM

    4. CAM's emphasis on wellness

    5. Concern with side effects of allopathic treatments

    6. The increased availability of health-related information and options to consumers

TABLE 24–2

Examples of Functional Components

Class/Components	Source*	Potential Benefit
Carotenoids		
Beta-carotene	Carrots, various fruits	Neutralizes free radicals which may damage cells; bolsters cellular antioxidant defenses
Lutein, Zeaxanthin	Kale, collards, spinach, corn, eggs, citrus	May contribute to maintenance of healthy vision
Lycopene	Tomatoes and processed tomato products	May contribute to maintenance of prostate health
Dietary (functional and total) Fiber		
Insoluble fiber	Wheat bran	May contribute to maintenance of a healthy digestive tract
Beta-glucan**	Oat bran, rolled oats, oat flour	May reduce risk of coronary heart disease (CHD)
Soluble fiber**	Psyllium seed husk	May reduce risk of CHD
Whole grains**	Cereal grains	May reduce risk of CHD and cancer; may contribute to maintenance of healthy blood glucose levels
Fatty Acids		
Monounsaturated fatty acids (MUFAs)	Tree nuts	May reduce risk of CHD
Polyunsaturated fatty acids (PUFAs)— Omega-3 fatty acids—ALA	Walnuts, flax	May contribute to maintenance of mental and visual function
PUFAs—Omega-3 fatty acids—DHA/EPA	Salmon, tuna, marine, and other fish oils	May reduce risk of CHD; may contribute to maintenance of mental and visual function
PUFAs—Conjugated linoleic acid (CLA)	Beef and lamb; some cheese	May contribute to maintenance of desirable body composition and healthy immune function
Flavonoids		
Anthocyanidins	Berries, cherries, red grapes	Bolster cellular antioxidant defenses; may contribute to maintenance of brain function
Flavanols—catechins, epicatechins, procyanidins	Tea, cocoa, chocolate, apples, grapes	May contribute to maintenance of heart health
Flavanones	Citrus foods	Neutralize free radicals, which may damage cells; bolster cellular antioxidant defenses
Flavonols	Onions, apples, tea, broccoli	Neutralize free radicals which may damage cells; bolster cellular antioxidant defenses
Proanthocyanidins	Cranberries, cocoa, apples, strawberries, grapes, wine, peanuts, cinnamon	May contribute to maintenance of urinary tract health and heart health

(continued)

TABLE 24–2

Examples of Functional Components (*continued*)

Class/Components	Source*	Potential Benefit
Isothiocyanates		
Sulforaphane	Cauliflower, broccoli, broccoli sprouts, cabbage, kale, horseradish	May enhance detoxification of undesirable compounds and bolster cellular antioxidant defenses
Phenols		
Caffeic acid, ferulic acid	Apples, pears, citrus fruits, some vegetables	May bolster cellular antioxidant defenses; may contribute to maintenance of healthy vision and heart health
Phytoestrogens		
Isoflavones—daidzein, genistein	Soybeans and soy-based foods	May contribute to maintenance of bone health, healthy brain and immune function; for women, maintenance of menopausal health
Lignans	Flax, rye, some vegetables	May contribute to maintenance of heart health and healthy immune function
Polyols		
Sugar alcohols—xylitol, sorbitol, mannitol, lactitol	Some chewing gums and other food applications	May reduce risk of dental caries
Prebiotics/Probiotics		
Inulin, fructo-oligosaccharides (FOS), Polydextrose	Whole grains, onions, some fruits, garlic, honey, leeks, fortified foods and beverages	May improve gastrointestinal health; may improve calcium absorption
Lactobacilli, bifidobacteria	Yogurt, other dairy and nondairy applications	May improve gastrointestinal health and systemic immunity
Soy Protein		
Soy protein**	Soybeans and soy-based foods	May reduce risk of CHD
Sulfides/Thiols		
Diallyl sulfide, allyl methyl trisulfide	Garlic, onions, leeks, scallions	May enhance detoxification of undesirable compounds; may contribute to maintenance of heart health and healthy immune function
Dithiolthiones	Cruciferous vegetables	Contribute to maintenance of healthy immune function

*Source examples are not an all-inclusive list.

**FDA-approved health claim established for component.

Adapted from International Food Information Council Foundation, 2006. Website: *http://www.ific.org/nutrition/functional/index.cfm*. Retrieved July 28, 2006, with permission.

B. Issues related to the integration of CAM and the allopathic model in a clinical setting include:
1. Exploring significant differences between the two
2. Objections by medicine and alternative practitioners to integration
3. Consumer interest in having an integrated medical system
4. Assessing what will be lost or gained with integration of both models—alternative health care and conventional health care

C. Measures necessary for integrating CAM into the health care system include:
1. Acceptance by doctors and hospitals
2. Education of doctors in CAM philosophies and modalities
3. Credentialing of CAM providers
4. Studies of and development of CAM outcomes
5. Insurance coverage of CAM
6. Education of consumers about indications and contraindications of CAM modalities
7. Education of CAM practitioners about maneuvering through the health care delivery system and insurance systems

D. Insurance issues and concerns about the integration and coverage of CAM modalities include:
1. Lack of scientific proof of the efficacy of so many CAM modalities
2. Concern about incurring higher costs rather than saving money
3. Appropriate credentialing of CAM providers to ensure competency
4. Lack of standards and appropriate Current Proceedural Terminology (CPT) codes
5. Problems in establishing standardized fees
6. Motivation for insurance coverage
   a. High consumer demand
   b. Some studies showing CAM to be less expensive
   c. Surveys indicating people attracted to CAM are healthier
   d. Preventive medicine can potentially be cost effective
7. Therapies found to be covered in a survey of 18 health plans were, in order of frequency: chiropractic manipulation, acupuncture, biofeedback, preventive medicine, nutritional counseling, massage therapy, hypnosis, acupressure, homeopathy, and naturopathy.
8. Insurers may consider a specific CAM procedure if:
   a. The procedure can be determined to be medically necessary.
   b. There is evidence in the literature that this therapy has some efficacy.
   c. The CAM provider has licensure or certification in that state and has malpractice insurance.
9. Insurance "red flags" for CAM may include:
   a. There is no evidence that treatment is not tapering after 12 treatments.
   b. The patient displays noncompliant tendencies by not following through with treatment recommendations, but the clinician continues to treat (rather than discharge the patient).

    c. Multiple clinicians are seeing the patient; there is evidence of duplication of services.

    d. A clinician prescribes treatment that has previously been shown to be ineffective.

    e. Preexisting condition(s) are not addressed.

    f. Documentation is not adequate.

    g. Passive treatments are overly used; there is little patient participation. For example, a patient with low back pain uses chiropractic treatment (a passive treatment) for a lengthy period, without results. Physical therapy has not been attempted (an active treatment).

    h. Several concurrent modalities are scheduled for each session (massage, chiropractic, acupuncture).

    i. The diagnosis changes several times.

    j. The clinician submits multiple diagnoses and extensive coding for the same condition.

    k. X-rays (or other diagnostic testing) are performed repeatedly, or are views of areas not included in the initial diagnosis.

E. Research issues

  1. The NCCAM at the NIH is a primary CAM research avenue.

    a. 1992 budget, $2 million; $50 million budget for 1999, representing a 250% increase over 1998; 2005 budget, $123.1 million

    b. More than a dozen medical centers are being supported in conducting research on CAM.

    c. The National Cancer Institute (NCI) has created its own department (Committee on Complementary and Alternative Medicine) to do research on CAM treatments for cancer.

  2. Research is being done with CAM in the areas of geriatrics, HIV/AIDS, asthma, cancer, cardiovascular disease, addictions, pediatrics, allergy and immunologic disorders, women's health, stroke, and pain management through NCCAM budget allocations.

  3. The need continues for unique study designs for research on CAM; some theories about health and illness in CAM cannot be measured with today's models.

    a. Alteration of energy fields by many CAM modalities cannot always be measured with today's technology.

    b. Difficulty remains in measuring, and thus researching, effects of preventive medicine.

    c. The impact of thoughts in mind-body medicine is difficult to measure.

  4. CAM providers often object to the current double-blind, placebo-controlled model for research because it is too impersonal, does not take into account the whole person, and does not appreciate the value of a "placebo" effect in treating disease.

  5. The November 11, 1998 issue of the *Journal of the American Medical Association* was wholly devoted to research on CAM; this and many other movements indicate that mainstream medicine is ready to take CAM seriously.

6. With consumer interest and willingness to pay out of pocket, there is a strong financial incentive to do research on and integrate CAM into mainstream medicine.

F. Legal issues
1. How to assign liability when there are no standards for practice for many CAM modalities
2. Determining a medical facility's liability if it does not offer a CAM modality that has some research showing its effectiveness
3. Credentialing of CAM providers (similar to allopathic providers) should:
   a. Meet state licensing requirements
   b. Meet clinical experience requirements
   c. Require specialty certification (where applicable)
   d. Include a site visit
   e. Prescribe minimum malpractice insurance levels
   f. Involve commitment to continuing education in appropriate discipline
   g. Require biennial reaccreditation
4. Regulatory areas should include:
   a. Safety guidelines
   b. Education requirements
   c. Licensure/certification
   d. Research protocols
   e. Insurance coverage

G. The Milbank Memorial Funds Report offers recommendations to ensure successful integration of CAM into conventional medicine (Milbank Memorial Funds Report, 1998).
1. Consumers need to keep well informed of benefits and risks of CAM modalities.
2. Physicians need to keep well informed about CAM treatments and research.
3. Physicians incorporating CAM into their practice need to advise their patients of their changing role.
4. CAM practitioners need to allow for scientific scrutiny.
5. Medical educators need to keep themselves and their students current on the latest CAM research.
6. Health plans need to clarify their decisions regarding coverage of CAM and be more involved in evaluating the benefits of CAM.
7. State licensing boards need to be more accountable for the regulation of all health care providers, including CAM providers.

■ IMPLICATIONS FOR CASE MANAGERS

A. The process for integration of CAM into a treatment plan
1. Identify who originated the request for a CAM intervention.

2. Clarify the rationale and expectations for the requested treatment and its potential to impact on patient outcomes.
3. Educate the patient and the medical team about the specific modality being considered.
4. Locate appropriate resources and reliable CAM practitioners.

B. Challenges and opportunities for case managers
   1. Lack of availability of practice guidelines and standards of practice for CAM practitioners
   2. Lack of scientific evidence originating in the United States supporting the efficacy of most CAM modalities
      a. European medical professions demonstrate efficacy of many CAM modalities because CAM has been part of accepted medical practice for many years.
      b. NIH and NCCAM is a reliable resource for case managers with questions about scientific evidence for CAM.
      c. Insurance companies often identify lack of research evidence as an obstacle to coverage.
   3. Finding a reliable source for understanding the indications and contraindications for CAM
      a. National associations exist for most CAM modalities and can provide information.
      b. Literature searches and Internet searches can generate information for making a more informed decision.
      c. CAM research centers are increasing, and the NCCAM is now generating good research on efficacy.
   4. Locating credentialing guidelines and services for CAM providers
      a. State licensing boards set standards for their practitioners and can provide lists of qualified providers.
      b. Check with the insurance plan or HMO offering CAM coverage, as they may have credentialing guidelines for their provider list.
      c. More independent credentialing services are being created to address this need, but these services can vary from state to state.
      d. Standards set by Oxford Health Plans include meeting licensing or certification requirements, undergoing a site visit, having minimal malpractice coverage, and committing to continuing education.
   5. Locating or creating outcome measures for evaluating treatments with CAM
      a. Work closely with CAM providers and use their expected outcomes based on professional standards and experience.
      b. Check with national associations to see what outcome measures they may have developed for that profession.
      c. Do a literature search and determine what outcomes can reasonably be expected for your patient when using a specific CAM modality.
   6. Facilitating acceptance of CAM by insurance companies, physicians, and other health care providers

    a. Be well informed about the efficacy and limitations of the CAM modality you and the patient are considering.

    b. Contact other case managers or health plans with supporting evidence of successful use of CAM.

    c. Support your patient in his or her efforts to seek support from other health care team members and in applying for coverage.

7. Educating CAM providers about managed care and insurance concepts

    a. Think about writing an article for the state or national association newsletters for CAM associations.

    b. Become a consultant for CAM providers in your area.

    c. Keep yourself well informed and current on research on CAM so that you can constructively exchange information with CAM practitioners in your area.

8. Educating consumers about the indications and contraindications of using CAM

    a. First, keep yourself well informed and current on research in this area.

    b. Understand that alternative and natural is not always better, especially in emergent or acute situations.

    c. Encourage the patient to become well informed.

    d. Once you have educated yourself, teach a class at a local community college; develop handouts for your patients.

    e. Familiarize yourself with CAM providers in your area.

9. Educating consumers about insurance coverage issues

    a. Clarify what type of CAM coverage the patient's insurance company or plan offers.

    b. If a patient is fully committed and informed about a specific modality, direct him or her to the appropriate channels for appealing a decision regarding coverage of that modality.

10. Identifying which of the many CAM modalities are appropriate for each patient

    a. Stay current on research in this area.

    b. Ask the CAM provider thorough questions and be sure you are comfortable with his or her role in caring for the patient.

    c. Consult national associations for CAM.

C. Discussion points between the patient and practitioner regarding the incorporation of CAM into their treatment care plan

1. Ask the patient to identify his or her principal symptoms, to better understand which CAM modality is appropriate.

2. Have the patient maintain a symptom diary to track outcomes.

3. Discuss the patient's preferences, level of knowledge, and expectations.

4. Review issues of safety and efficacy.

5. Identify a licensed or certified provider, using national associations as resources.

6. Provide key questions for the alternative therapy provider to use during the initial consultation.

      7. Schedule a follow-up visit or telephone call with the patient to review the treatment plan.

      8. Follow up to review the response to treatment after a reasonable period of time.

      9. Provide documentation.

D. The case management process and CAM

    1. Case selection

      a. Many patients are referring themselves to CAM. Note that some studies have concluded that only about 40% of people who use CAM tell their physicians.

      b. Many physicians are making themselves knowledgeable and are referring patients to CAM.

      c. As personal knowledge increases, the case manager can identify when a CAM modality might offer a better outcome, target the consumer's education, and increase patient empowerment.

    2. Assessment/problem identification (also see "Discussion points between the patient and practitioner regarding the incorporation of CAM into their treatment care plan," above)

      a. Identify all modalities, herbs, or supplements currently used by the patient (see Table 24-3 for a sample CAM assessment tool).

      b. Identify the primary care provider's support for and knowledge of CAM.

      c. Identify community providers, their educational level, licensing requirements, and credentialing status.

      d. Clarify insurance benefits and what, if any, the patient is willing to pay out of pocket.

      e. Proceed with assessment and problem identification as with any case management patient, including the patients' expectation of how much the therapy may help.

    3. Development and coordination of the case management plan

      a. Identify the patient's expectations and level of knowledge.

      b. Review issues of safety and efficacy. Most patients do not read outcome research; *advise patients that the absence of documented toxicity for herbs, supplements, or chemical preparations does not equal safety.*

      c. Coordinate with other members of the health care team.

      d. Document clinical encounters, conversations that lead to treatment decisions, refusal of any treatments and the ensuing discussion (among other issues).

      e. Assist the patient/client in articulating questions. For example:

        i. Is the provider's belief in the effectiveness of the therapy based on clinical experience with similar patients?

        ii. What will the therapy include?

        iii. How much time will pass (or how many treatments) before the patient and practitioner have decided that the treatment is or is not helping?

        iv. What is the cost per session? Is there insurance assistance?

TABLE 24–3
A Sample CAM Assessment Tool

Do you take any herbal supplements?

- ☐ Which ones?
- ☐ In what dose?
- ☐ How often?
- ☐ What is the reason(s) for taking this herb?
- ☐ What results have you seen so far?

Do you take any nutritional supplements?
(Make a checklist of those that are commonly encountered.)

- ☐ Vitamins/minerals (please list)
- ☐ Supplements for weight loss
- ☐ Supplements for sleep
- ☐ Supplements for digestion
- ☐ Supplements for arthritis
- ☐ Supplements for pain
- ☐ Other (this list can be quite long)
(Ask for further explanation of anything listed.)

Have you seen any of the following CAM providers? Why? When? What were the results?

- ☐ Acupuncturist
- ☐ Ayurvedic physician
- ☐ Chiropractor
- ☐ Herbalist
- ☐ Homeopathic physician
- ☐ Hypnotherapist
- ☐ Massage therapist/reflexologist/rolfer
- ☐ Musculoskeletal practitioner (e.g., Feldenkrais, Alexander technique)
- ☐ Naturopathic physician
- ☐ Traditional Chinese medicine (TCM) practitioner

From *Advanced case management: Outcomes and beyond*, by Powell, S.K. (2000). Philadelphia: Lippincott Williams & Wilkins. Adapted with permission.

    v. What are the potential side effects (if any)?

    vi. Will the CAM provider communicate diagnostic findings, therapeutic plans, and follow up with the primary care physician?

    vii. (If appropriate) Are there any recommendations that directly conflict with the conventional physician's treatment plan, such as the postponement of surgery in a potentially treatable malignant cancer?

4. Implementation of the plan

    a. Assess the answers to the questions above.

    b. Maintain communication with the CAM provider and request regular reports.

    c. Have the patient maintain a symptom diary to evaluate changes of symptoms in his or her response to treatment.

    d. Provide regular reports to the primary care provider.

5. Evaluation and follow up

a. Realize that sometimes CAM modalities show a slower response rate than do allopathic interventions.

b. Document all contacts and outcomes.

c. After a set period of time (6–8 weeks), ask, Has there been any improvement? If positive outcomes have been observed, then there is anecdotal evidence that the treatment (or the CAM practitioner) may be beneficial for similar patients in the future. If there are no positive outcomes, the physician and patient may need to reevaluate what options exist (see "Have the patient maintain a symptom diary," below).

6. Have the patient maintain a symptom diary

a. To be used for baseline assessment and to evaluate subsequent alternative (or conventional) therapeutic interventions

b. Prior to any therapy, the patient should be given a template for a symptom diary and taught how to use it.

c. Discuss important points to note in the diary.

d. The issues that are important to note in the diary will depend on the condition being treated and the CAM provider chosen. For example:

i. If the condition is back pain, a 1 to 10 scale is recommended, where 1 equals no back pain and 10 equals the worst pain imaginable. The patient should also record exercises done at home and in therapy, visits involving CAM therapies (chiropractic, massage, acupuncture, etc.) and the response to the therapies.

ii. If, however, a homeopathic physician is recommended for depression, the diary would be used quite differently. Mood scales may be used in place of pain scales. And the homeopathic physician will likely ask about dreams remembered; these should also be noted in the diary.

REFERENCES

Chopra, D. Website: *http://www.healthy.net/scr/interview.asp?Id=167*. Retrieved December 15, 2006.

International Food Information Council Foundation. (2006). Website: *http://www.ific.org/nutrition/functional/index.cfm*. Retrieved July 28, 2006.

Milbank Memorial Fund Report. (1998). *Enhancing the accountability of alternative medicine*. New York: Milbank Memorial Fund.

National Center for Complementary and Alternative Medicine (NCCAM). (2006). Website: *http://nccam.nih.gov/health/whatiscam/*. Retrieved July 28, 2006.

Powell, S. K. (2000). *Advanced case management: Outcomes and beyond*. Philadelphia: Lippincott Williams & Wilkins.

Vitale, A. (2006). The use of selected energy touch modalities as supportive nursing interventions: Are we there yet? *Holistic Nursing Practice, 20*(4), 191–196.

SUGGESTED READING

Burton Goldberg Group. (1997). *Alternative medicine: The definitive guide*. Tiburon, CA: Future Medicine Publishing.

Eisenberg, D., Kessler, R., & Foster, C. (1993). Unconventional medicine in the United States: Prevalence, costs, and patterns of use. *New England Journal of Medicine, 328*(4), 246–252.

Gerber, R. (1996). *Vibrational medicine*. Santa Fe, NM: Bear & Co.

The integrative medicine consult: The essential guide to integrating conventional and complementary medicine [monthly newsletter]. Website: *www.onemedicine.com.*

Jonas, W. B., & Levin, J. S. (1999). *Essentials of complementary and alternative medicine.* Philadelphia: Lippincott Williams & Wilkins.

Lambert, C. (2002). The new ancient trend in medicine: Scientific scrutiny of "alternative" therapies. *Harvard Magazine,* 104(4). Website: *http://www.harvardmagazine.com/on-line/030221.html.* Retrieved February 19, 2006.

Parkman, C. (2004). Regulatory issues in CAM. *The Case Manager,* 15(6), 26–29.

CAM RESOURCES

NCCAM Clearinghouse
Toll-free in the United States: 1-888-644-6226
International: 301-519-3153
TTY (for hearing disabled callers): 1-866-464-3615
E-mail: info@nccam.nih.gov
NCCAM Website: *nccam.nih.gov*
Address: NCCAM Clearinghouse, P.O. Box 7923, Gaithersburg, MD 20898-7923
Fax: 1-866-464-3616
Fax-on-demand service: 1-888-644-6226

The NCCAM Web site (*nccam.nih.gov*) includes publications, information for researchers, frequently asked questions, and links to other CAM-related resources.

NIH Office of Dietary Supplements (ODS)
Website: *ods.od.nih.gov*
Telephone: 301-435-2920
E-mail: ods@nih.gov
Fax: 301-480-1845
Address: 6100 Executive Blvd., Bethesda, MD 20892-7517

The ODS, whose mission is to explore the potential role of dietary supplements to improve health care, promotes the scientific study of dietary supplements through conducting and coordinating scientific research and compiling and disseminating research results. ODS provides all its public information through its Website. One of its services is the International Bibliographic Information on Dietary Supplements (IBIDS) database, at *ods.od.nih.gov/databases/ibids.html.*

CAM on PubMed
Website: *www.nlm.nih.gov/nccam/camonpubmed.html*

CAM on PubMed, a database accessible via the Internet, was developed jointly by NCCAM and the National Library of Medicine (NLM). It contains bibliographic citations to articles in scientifically based, peer-reviewed journals on CAM. These citations are a subset of the NLM's PubMed system that contains over 12 million journal citations from the MEDLINE database and additional life science journals important to health researchers, practitioners, and consumers. CAM on PubMed displays links to publisher Websites; some sites offer the full text of articles.

ClinicalTrials.gov
Website: *clinicaltrials.gov*

ClinicalTrials.gov provides patients, family members, health care professionals, and members of the public access to information on clinical trials for a wide range of diseases and conditions. The NIH, through its National Library of Medicine, has developed this site in collaboration with all NIH Institutes and the U.S. Food and Drug Administration. The site currently contains more than 6,200 clinical studies sponsored by NIH, other federal agencies, and the pharmaceutical industry in over 69,000 locations worldwide.

Effectiveness of Case Management

Quality and Outcomes Management

Michael B. Garrett

Upon completion of this chapter, the reader will be able to:

1. Define outcomes.
2. List reasons why outcomes management is important.
3. Describe the common categories of outcomes.
4. List the characteristics of effective outcome measures.
5. Describe methods of incorporating outcomes measurement into practice.
6. Identify key issues in reporting outcomes.
7. Identify case management outcome measures.

Clinical Practice Guidelines
Outcome Indicator
Outcome Measures
Outcomes
Outcomes Management
Outcomes Measurement
Process

Process Measures
Quality
Reliability
Risk Adjustment
Structure
Structure Measures
Variation

■ INTRODUCTION

A. Today's health care consumers are demanding that they receive full value for their health care dollars. Health care executives and other personnel meet customers' expectations by focusing on improving the quality of the services they provide and by ensuring that the customer experience is desirable and rewarding. At the same time, health care executives recognize that a focus on quality care is the best way to ensure that revenues equal or exceed expenses. Focusing on quality, according to Cesta and Tahan (2003), allows health care organizations to achieve many objectives, some of which are:

1. Efficiently and effectively using scarce health care resources
2. Meeting the needs of the customers
3. Enhancing customer and staff satisfaction
4. Providing compassionate, ethical, and culturally sensitive care
5. Ensuring that patients are safe and that the environment of care is conducive to safety
6. Ensuring professional performance by health care providers

B. For several years, case managers have used outcome information from providers to make decisions about patient care activities, including referrals to specialty services and providers. Case managers are now being called on to measure and report outcomes of case management services to the public, federal and state agencies, accreditation agencies, providers of services, administrators of health care organizations, as well as payers.

1. Although there have been numerous anecdotal descriptions of case management outcomes, objective, scientific evidence is sparse.
2. Several issues have contributed to the lack of valid, reliable outcomes data. These include:
   a. Inconsistent definitions of case management and the interventions performed by case managers
   b. Inconsistent methods of measurement. For example, one group calculates cost savings using one method, whereas another group calculates cost savings a different way.
   c. Organizations maintaining their methods of measuring outcomes as proprietary to their program and process
   d. The initial acceptance of case management as a tool to reduce costs reduced the need for case managers to define, document, and measure carefully the results of their activities except via cost savings.

■ KEY DEFINITIONS

A. Administrative and management processes—The activities performed in the governance and management systems of a health care organization.

This chapter is a revised version of what was previously published in the first edition of *CMSA Core Curriculum for Case Management*. The contributor wishes to acknowledge Sherry Aliotta, Nancy Claflin, and Patricia M. Pecqueux, as some of the timeless material was retained from the previous version.

B. Benchmarks—Gold standards or ideal practices established by the leaders or toughest competitors in the field; used by others to measure their performance continuously with these leaders (Powell, 2000).

C. Care delivery processes—The support activities utilized by practitioners and all suppliers of care and care products to get the product/service to the patient.

D. Clinical practice guidelines—Systematically developed statements to assist practitioner and patient decisions about appropriate health care for specific clinical circumstances (Institute of Medicine, 1990).

E. Clinical processes—The activities of health care practitioners with and for patients/families, and what patients do in response.

F. Direct case management outcomes—The measurement or results of those activities and interventions that are within the scope of the case manager's practice and control.

G. End health system outcomes—Those performance indicators measured for the health care system overall; include the following: cost of care, quality of care, and health status and clinical outcomes achieved.

H. External validity—The degree to which the results of a study can be generalized to settings or samples other than the one studied (Polit and Hungler, 1989).

I. Information flow—The creating and transporting of facts, knowledge, and data that make for informed decisions. The sharing of data between providers, health care teams members, with payers, or with patients and their families.

J. Internal validity—The degree to which it can be inferred that the experimental treatment or independent variable, rather than uncontrolled extraneous factors, is responsible for observed effects on the dependent variable (Polit and Hungler, 1989).

K. Materials flow—The movement of equipment and supplies.

L. Outcomes—The end results of care—adverse or beneficial—as well as gradients between; the products of one or more processes. Outcomes used as indicators of quality are states or conditions of individuals and populations attributed or attributable to antecedent health care (Donabedian, 1992). Another way of describing an outcome is as a measurable individual, family, or community state, behavior, or perception that is measured along a continuum and is responsive to nursing interventions (Moorhead et al., 2003). Classifications of outcomes may include clinical, functional, financial/cost, experience perceived.

M. Outcomes management—A technology of patient experience designed to help patients, payers, and providers make rational medical care–related choices based on their better insight into the effects of these choices on the patient's life (Ellwood, 1988).

N. Patient flow—The movement of patients from one place to another, from one level of care to another, or from one care setting to another.

O. Process—The procedures, methods, means, or sequence of steps for providing or delivering care and producing outcomes (Brown, 2005). They are sequentially related steps intended to complete a task and produce specific outcomes (Goonan, 1993).

P. Process measures—Used primarily to determine the degree to which the process is being executed as planned. For example, "The number of patients receiving a case management assessment within 24 hours of admission to a hospital setting."

Q. Quality—The degree to which health services for individuals and populations increase the likelihood of desired health outcomes and are consistent with current professional knowledge (Institute of Medicine, 1990).

R. Reliability—The degree of consistency or accuracy with which an instrument measures the attribute it is designed to measure (Polit and Hungler, 1989).

S. Risk adjustment—A process for introducing an allowance for factors that would introduce bias; taking into consideration multiple factors that contribute to an end result. For example, in one health plan, Medicare-aged patients may be counted as 1.5 patients when establishing caseload numbers. This "risk adjustment" (counting one person as if he or she were one and a half) is meant to account for the additional time that these more-complex patients require from a case manager or a health care delivery system.

T. Standards of care—Measures that define the type of care/service and desired outcome that the patient can expect from the health care encounter (Healthcare Quality Certification Board).

U. Standards of practice—Measures that establish an acceptable level of performance that is expected of health care practitioners (Healthcare Quality Certification Board).

V. Structure—The arrangement of a care system, a part of a system, or elements that facilitate care; the care "environment"; evidence of the organization's ability to provide care to patients (Brown, 2005). Examples include staff qualifications, staffing levels, work environment, technology resources, policies and procedures, equipment, table of organization and reporting structure, and types of services provided.

W. Variation—Deviation, divergence, or difference in results from an assumed or usual standard that is usually selected at the initiation of a quality/outcome management program. Variation can also be defined as the stability (or lack thereof) in a process. If the process has a large amount of variation (instability), it is more difficult to manage than a process with only a slight degree of variation (Powell, 2000).

■ DEFINING OUTCOMES MANAGEMENT AND MEASUREMENT

A. Avedis Donabedian described a quality paradigm from which information can be drawn for inferences about the quality of care (Donabedian, 1966).

1. His paradigm holds that there are three key factors in determining quality: structure, process, and outcome.

2. Structure leads to process, which leads to outcome.

3. These factors represent complex sets of events and factors.

4. How each relates to the other must be clearly understood before quality measurement and assessment begins.

5. Causal relationships may be understood between these factors, but they are considered as probabilities, not certainties.

B. When selecting outcome measures, we are attempting to determine in advance the potential effects, side effects, or consequences of our actions.

C. Outcomes measurement can assist in the demonstration of value by validating:

1. What is effective;

2. What is not effective;

3. The costs of an intervention; and

4. Whether the cost of the intervention is substantiated by the return on the investment.

D. The centerpiece and underlying ingredient of outcomes management is the tracking and measurement of the patient's clinical condition, functional ability, and well-being or quality of life.

E. Outcomes management is a common language of health outcomes that is understood by patients, practitioners, payers, health care administrators, and other stakeholders.

F. This requires a national reference database containing information and analysis on clinical, financial, and health outcomes, estimating:

1. Relationships between medical interventions and health outcomes

2. Relationships between health outcomes and money spent/cost of care

G. Outcomes management is dependent on four developing technologies:

1. Practitioner reliance on standards of care and evidence-based guidelines in selecting appropriate interventions

2. Routine and systematic measurement of the functioning and well-being of patients along with disease-specific clinical outcomes, at appropriate time intervals

3. Pooling of clinical and outcome data on a massive scale

4. Analysis and dissemination of results (outcomes) from the segment of the database pertinent to the concerns of each decision maker

H. One of the typical results from analysis is the detection of variation. Variation is typically measured through an outcomes management program. Variation is neither good nor bad in itself. Further analysis is required to determine what the causation is for the variation. The goal of outcome management is not to eliminate variation but to reduce it in order to produce and sustain stability in processes.

I. There are two types of variation:

1. Common cause variation—Also called *random* variation. This is variation due to the process itself. It is produced by interactions of the variables in the process. Process redesign may be required if this type

of variation needs to be redesigned through a quality improvement initiative.

2. Special cause—Variation that is assignable to a specific cause or causes. It is not part of the usual process, but rather is due to particular circumstances. A focused review of the process needs to be conducted in order to conduct root cause analysis and for potential corrective actions to be taken.

J. Once variation is detected, a variety of quality improvement strategies, techniques, and methods can be used to improve outcomes and decrease variation. Examples may include:

1. Six Sigma—A business strategy focusing on continuous improvement; a disciplined approached in process improvement that addresses the elimination of defects in care or to reduce their occurrence.

2. Lean—A methodology focused on reducing lead time by the elimination of waste and non-value-added processes of care.

3. Human Factors—A scientific discipline focused on understanding interactions among humans and other systems elements in order to optimize human well-being and overall system performance.

■ RATIONALE FOR OUTCOMES MANAGEMENT

A. Measuring outcomes allows us to base improvement on measurement. Without effective outcomes measurements, a health care organization will be unable to objectively track improvements or declines in performance.

B. Measurement of outcomes provides information that allows us to determine whether the results of the process or intervention yield the desired return on investment. It also provides a method for demonstrating value of a process to consumers and other stakeholders. With appropriate outcomes data, stakeholders can be educated regarding the value or potential value of the process or intervention.

C. The ability to verify positive outcomes provides a powerful rationale for a service. Outcomes measurement allows us to determine which processes and interventions are effective and which are not, thereby identifying opportunities for improvement.

D. The combination of outcomes management with case management in an overall model (Wojner, 2001) enables providers to improve clinical practice and individual performance by highlighting opportunities to:

1. Enhance care

2. Stimulate the use of science-based interventions and treatment options

3. Conduct systematic evaluation of overall program effectiveness

E. An outcomes measurement program (Lloyd, 2004) is designed to improve quality by:

1. Shifting the focus away from anecdotal evidence to objective data

2. Enhancing our understanding of the variation that exists in a process

3. Monitoring a process over time

    4. Revealing the effect of a change in a process

    5. Providing a common frame of reference

    6. Providing a more accurate basis for prediction

F. The disease management industry through the Disease Management Association of America (DMAA, 2004), has identified three reasons for undertaking evaluation of outcomes.

    1. Business processes—Creating the framework to conduct interprogram evaluation with analyses that are not structured according to ideal research conditions.

    2. Academic research—Designed prospectively and use randomized control trial study design.

    3. Desire-to-inform policy—Conducted at a national or local level to compare different systems, structures, and approaches.

G. There are a number of clinical and administrative reasons for developing and implementing an outcomes management program, including:

    1. Meeting or exceeding regulatory, accreditation, and contractual requirements

    2. Meeting or exceeding requirements of standards of care and standards of practice

    3. Improving the accountability of health care providers to patients, families, and other stakeholders

    4. Improving the financial performance of the organization

    5. Improving the desirability of the health care organization to employees, pccr organizations, payers, and other stakeholders

    6. Mitigating risk by demonstrating compliance with state-of-the art health care quality guidelines

    7. Evaluating and improving performance in comparison to peers and national standards

    8. Meeting or exceeding individual and organizational ethical principles and values and compliance with such related standards

■ CHARACTERISTICS OF EFFECTIVE OUTCOME MEASURES

A. For an outcome measure to be effective, it must be:

    1. Valid—The effect seen is actually related to the intervention and is not a random occurrence.

    2. Reliable—Measuring what it is actually intended to measure

    3. Not easy to manipulate; as objective and quantifiable as possible

    4. Comprehensive—Covering most or all aspects of the process being measured

    5. Dynamic—The measure can change to reflect changes in practice.

    6. Flexible—If an outcome measure can demonstrate outcomes for more than one process or be used to demonstrate multiple outcomes, this is a positive attribute.

    7. Cogent—The outcome measure must make sense to the user.

B. The National Quality Measures Clearinghouse has identified the following desirable attributes of performance measures:

1. Importance—Relevance to key stakeholders, strategic plan and strategic initiatives, and financial impact
2. Scientific soundness—Clinical logic and properties of reliability, validity, stratification, and understandability
3. Feasibility—The explicit specification of the measure, including the numerator and denominator as well as the availability of the data

C. The American Academy of Family Physicians (AAFP, 2006) defined the desirable attributes of performance measures for health care as follows:

1. Grounded in science
2. Substantial potential for improvement
3. Severity and prevalence
4. Substantial impact
5. Relevant
6. Improve value
7. Influences on outcomes

D. Four factors have been identified (Goonan, 1993) that influence the degree to which health care services achieve desired health outcomes:

1. Disease process and severity
2. Processes of care
3. Patient compliance/adherence
4. Random and unidentified variances

E. The nursing outcomes classification (Moorhead, 2003) identifies three main influences that influence nursing outcomes:

1. Patient characteristics, such as diagnosis, prognosis, education level, socioeconomic status, and understanding of disease process
2. Nurse characteristics, such as type of licensure, education level, knowledge, skills, and abilities
3. Systems characteristics, such as medical services, community resources, and benefits programs

■ OUTCOME MEASURES SELECTION AND DEVELOPMENT

A. In order to have valid and reliable measures, Brown (2005) suggests using certain key principles in selecting and developing performance measures.

1. Identify and organize teams to select or develop appropriate measures.
2. Identify and understand organization functions and key processes.
3. Identify factors explaining potential or expected variation in performance.
4. Identify the measurement purpose and intended use—improve quality, accountability, and research.

5. Inventory relevant measures/data currently available.
6. Ascertain measures already available in reference databases to measure the objective.
7. Define each measure conceptually and operationally.
8. Ensure that each measure possesses the desirable attributes, such as reliability and validity.
9. Document an information set—measure statement, definition of the measure and other terms, rationale for choice, dimensions of performance being assessed, definition of patient populations included, and reference for collection specifications.

B. In order to better organize and categorize the development and implementation of outcomes indicators, Advocate Health Care developed the Indicator Development Form, which has been widely used in the measurement field. This form is divided into three major parts:
1. Part I—Identification of an indicator. To identify an indicator, one must examine and/or determine the following:
   a. Processes and outcomes the indicator measures
   b. Rationale for the indicator
   c. Name of the indicator
   d. Identification of the teams to which the indicator applies
   e. Identification of the objectives the indicator satisfies
   f. Dimensions of excellence the indicator is designed to measure
   g. Literature references for the indicator
2. Part II—Indicator development and data collection. It is necessary to describe the following to maintain clarity of the indicator and its use, and to prevent confusion from occurring:
   a. Operational definition
   b. Description of the data collection plan
   c. Data collection sampling requirements
   d. Baseline data for the indicator
   e. Target or goal for the indicator
3. Part III—Indicator analysis and interpretation. For effective use and interpretation of findings related to the indicator, one must be proactive in designing the analysis and interpretation processes/activities. This may include descriptions of:
   a. The analysis plan, including the statistics to be used (e.g., descriptive, analysis of variance)
   b. Graphs that will be used
   c. Data reporting plan, including who will receive the results and how often they will receive the results

C. Common categories of outcome indicators
1. There are four broad categories of indicators that are typically used for outcomes. These are:
   a. Clinical—morbidity, mortality, improvement in clinical signs and symptoms, and absence of complications

    b. Functional—activities of daily living (ADLs), instrumental activities of daily living (IADLs), ability to return to work or school, maintaining a healthy life style

    c. Financial—costs of care, savings, cost per year/per episode/per case, cost of job-related injuries, recidivism

    d. Satisfaction—patient/family, physician, staff, referral source

D. Using Donabedian's quality paradigm, there are three categories for measuring quality—structure, process, and outcomes (Donabedian, 1966).

E. Outcome measures also have been identified by Lighter and Fair (2000) to fall into one of several categories, including costs of expenditures, health status, complication rates, mortality, and satisfaction with care or outcomes.

F. For the nursing profession, a group of researchers at the University of Iowa (Moorhead et al., 2003) have developed the Nursing Outcomes Classification (NOC), which is a taxonomy of standardized nursing-sensitive patient/client outcomes.

    1. The taxonomy includes outcomes that:

        a. Nursing can affect

        b. Apply to an individual recipient of nursing care

        c. Apply to a lay caregiver of an individual

        d. Describe states and behaviors

        e. Encompass the entire continuum of care

        f. Provide a consistent measure of patient/client and lay caregiver status

    2. NOC is a three-level classification system currently composed of 7 domains, 29 outcome classes, and 260 outcomes. The seven health domains in the NOC include:

        a. Functional health

        b. Physiologic health

        c. Psychosocial health

        d. Health knowledge and behaviors

        e. Perceived health

        f. Family health

        g. Community health

G. There have been initial discussions about creating a framework for classifying social work outcomes.

    1. One social work expert (Mullen, 2001) has suggested that the dimensions to be included in a health and mental health social work outcomes measurement framework should include the following variations by:

        a. System level—clinical, program, and system

        b. Geographical unit—local, municipality, region, nation, group of nations

        c. Outcomes measurement questions asked—efficacy, efficiency, quality, equity

          d. Effects sought across a continuum of possibilities—mortality, physiologic, clinical events, generic or specific health-related quality-of-life measures, composite measures of outcomes, and time

    2. The purpose of this outcomes measurement program is performance measurement and management or outcomes research.

H. The disease management industry has recognized that interventions can affect many outcomes simultaneously (DMAA, 2004). Thus, disease management programs gather data from a number of areas, including:

    1. Clinical outcomes—processes and health status outcome measures

    2. Utilization measures—economic or nonmonetary measures, including resource consumption, service and/or pharmaceutical utilization, and "utility"

    3. Financial outcome measures—return on investment (ROI) and net savings

    4. Humanistic factors—patient satisfaction, measures of social functioning and ADLs, provider satisfaction, functionality, and quality-adjusted life years

    5. Quality measures—standardized indicators of quality care promulgated by nationally recognized entities

    6. Indirect measures—productivity measures

    7. Intangible metrics—provider performance measures

I. Cesta and Tahan (2003) broadly classified outcomes into two categories; those that have an effect on the health care organization and those that have an effect on the patient/consumer of health care services.

    1. Outcomes that affect the organization are those that are not directly related to the patient's health. Examples may include patient satisfaction, staff satisfaction, turn-around time of tests and procedures or results, cost per case, length of stay, and interdisciplinary communication.

    2. Outcomes that affect the patient's health tend to be more clinical in nature. They are not directly related to the health care organization. Examples may include prevention of complications in patient's condition, improvement of signs and symptoms of a disease, physical functioning/functional status, and well-being and quality of life.

■ CASE MANAGEMENT SPECIFIC OUTCOMES

A. There have been some generally accepted goals identified for the implementation of case management programs, regardless of the practice setting, health care professional who assumes the role of the case manager, organizational model of case management, or geographical location (Cohen and Cesta, 2001). These include:

    1. Expanding the scope of services provided to the population

    2. Increasing access to health care services

    3. Reducing the cost of health care services

    4. Improving outcomes of the care delivered

    5. Improving the overall quality of care

B. The Council for Case Management Accountability (CCMA) was formed in 1996 by the Case Management Society of America (CMSA) in response to a growing demand for accountability in health care through outcomes reporting.

1. The CCMA sought opinions from numerous stakeholders regarding case management outcomes and identified the following direct outcomes of case management:

   a. Patient/client knowledge

   b. Patient/client involvement in care

   c. Patient/client empowerment

   d. Improved adherence

   e. Improved coordination of care

2. The CCMA developed the "dimensions of accountability," which provide a framework for linking the core functions of case management (assessment, planning, facilitation, evaluation, and advocacy) to the direct outcomes of case management and the end outcomes of the health system, including:

   a. Improved health status

   b. Increased quality of care

   c. Decreased costs

C. Because case management practice occurs in a variety of settings and systems by professionals from a range of health and human services disciplines, it is particularly challenging to develop standardized outcomes metrics. Using the quality paradigm, listed below are some suggested outcomes indicators for case management practice:

1. Structure—in case management practice examples include:

   a. Percentage of case managers who are certified in case management

   b. Average caseload size per case manager

   c. Ratio of case managers to supervisor

   d. Accreditation status of program/organization

2. Process—in case management practice examples include:

   a. Percentage of cases with documentation of physician collaboration

   b. Percentage of cases with a written care plan

   c. Average number of days from referral date to first contact with patient

   d. Average number of days from referral date to care plan

   e. Average number of case management hours per case

   f. Percentage of cases with documentation of consent from patient/client

3. Outcomes—in case management practice examples include:

   a. Percentage of cases with patient able to appropriately self-manage

   b. Percentage of patients who are adherent to care/treatment plan

   c. Percentage of patients/clients who are satisfied or very satisfied

   d. Percentage of physicians who are satisfied or very satisfied

   e. Average length of hospital stay

   f. Rate of readmissions/rehospitalizations

   g. Percentage of patients/clients with adverse events (e.g., development of pressure ulcer, nosocomial infections, exacerbation of pain, etc.)

   h. Average health service costs per case

   i. Percentage of patients/clients who returned to work

■ INCORPORATING OUTCOMES MEASUREMENT INTO CASE MANAGEMENT PRACTICE

A. Build outcome measures into any new intervention, process, or program.

   1. Consider the goals that led to the intervention, process, or program.

   2. List the problems you are trying to solve.

   3. Describe exactly what you want to improve.

B. List the method you will use to determine whether you have reached your goal.

   1. Describe what things will occur when you have achieved the desired outcome (e.g., no patients will be rehospitalized in the first 60 days after discharge for the same or a related diagnosis; or, Mrs. Smith will schedule doctor's appointments at least one time per month and keep the scheduled appointments).

   2. Be as specific and as descriptive as possible.

C. Determine how you can measure that achievement using different research designs.

   1. Before-and-after comparison—for example, how many appointments were scheduled and kept before case management; or, before case management 90% of patients returned to the hospital within 60 days past discharge, and after case management rehospitalization within 60 days occurred with only 20% of patients.

   2. Randomized comparison—for example, a group of patients who are statistically similar is chosen. The group is randomly assigned to one of two groups before the intervention is tested. One group receives the intervention, and the other group does not receive the intervention. The two groups are compared and the impact of the intervention is evaluated.

   3. Comparison groups; for example, compare a group of patients receiving an intervention with a statistically similar group of patients who do not receive the intervention. This differs from the randomized comparison in that the groups may not have been selected in advance of the comparison, and the groups may have differing reasons for why an intervention was not given.

   4. Other methods of measuring impact include:

     a. Comparison with established benchmarks (e.g., recommendations for hemoglobin A_1C testing in diabetics).

     b. Progress toward an established goal. (This could include increasing or decreasing a particular measurement. For example, admissions for congestive heart failure patients have declined 15%, and we expect to reach our goal of 45% reduction in 3 months.)

D. Identify the best reporting method.

1. Use of a database can allow you to report in multiple ways and from multiple perspectives.

2. Depending on their needs, different perspectives are requested by different people.

3. If you are unable to show the results in a way that will allow your audience to identify the value of the results to them or to those for whom they are responsible, your results may not receive the attention they deserve.

4. Identify people who are the stakeholders in the process.

   a. When establishing a report, it is important to know who will be receiving the report and why the report is needed.

   b. Determine what you know or understand about the stakeholders in order to gain insight into the problem from their perspective. For example, physicians may need to know which of their patients have not had a recommended test or treatment in order to ensure that the patient gets the needed service, and the unit manager may want to know the test or treatment that is most frequently missed in order to examine interventions that may be used to remind practitioners to complete the service.

5. Make sure your report addresses the needs of the stakeholders.

6. Become familiar with the use of graphs, charts, and diagrams that will provide an interesting and illustrative visual representation of the data.

E. Ask and answer the "so what?" question.

1. Quantify or describe the impact or final outcome of the process.

2. If you increased or improved something, what changed other than the process? For example, if the patient keeps all of his or her doctor's appointments, what happens as a result? If readmissions decline, were costs decreased or were patients more satisfied?

F. Think in terms of quantifying and measuring.

1. Instead of describing and explaining, think of objective ways to count or measure the event.

2. Collect baseline measurements to use as a comparison for improvement. It is difficult to judge progress without recording your starting point.

3. Ask yourself how you will know whether your plans or programs are working and how you can demonstrate that success to others.

G. Learn how to use databases and other computer programs.

1. Databases can store information in a format that allows it to be retrieved in various ways.

2. This flexibility allows the case manager to look at all of the available information in several ways:

      a. Sorted by different factors such as age, diagnosis, and interventions

      b. Sorted by common factors, such as all those with "x, y, and z"

      c. Sorted by different elements, such as all those with "x, but not y or z"

   3. Looking at the data in different ways can help identify outcomes or suggest other areas for study.

H. Review statistical principles.

   1. Know the key statistical tools to be used in simple comparisons.

   2. Familiarize yourself with the methods of critically reading and evaluating research papers and findings.

I. Review the continuous quality improvement (CQI) processes and tools.

   1. Develop an understanding of key CQI principles.

   2. Be familiar with CQI tools for process improvement

■ KEY ISSUES IN OUTCOMES REPORTING

A. Varying definitions—For effective comparisons, definitions need to be exact. Even if there are similarities, minute differences can alter the results of a comparison.

   1. For example, compare a Granny Smith apple with a Red Delicious. Both are apples, but evaluation would reveal distinct differences.

   2. For case management to compare outcomes across the industry, definitions must be precise.

B. Varying methodologies—In addition to definitions, the methods for calculating and reporting results must be consistent. It is impossible to complete a valid comparison of results if the methodology used to determine the results is different.

C. Sharing of outcomes methodologies—Some organizations believe that the definitions, methodologies, and reporting practices are proprietary to them. For this reason, they do not wish to share these details with the industry at large.

   1. In order to create an opportunity for the growth of outcomes methodology and reporting, organizations on the forefront of case management should gain recognition for setting the standard in outcomes methodology rather than for being the only one with good outcomes methodology.

REFERENCES

American Academy of Family Physicians (AAFP). (2006). AAFP criteria for performance measures. Website: *http://www.aafp.org/x18919.xml*. Accessed March 11, 2006.

Brown, J. A. (2005). *The healthcare quality handbook: A professional resource and study guide*. Pasadena, CA: JB Quality Solutions.

Cesta, T. G., & Tahan, H. A. (2003). *The case manager's survival guide: Winning strategies for clinical practice*, 2nd ed. St Louis, MO: Mosby.

Cohen, E. L., & Cesta, T. G. (2001). *Nursing case management: From essentials to advanced practice applications*. St. Louis, MO: Mosby.

Disease Management Association of America (DMAA). (2004). *Disease management program evaluation guide.* Washington, DC: DMAA.

Donabedian, A. (1966). Evaluating the quality of medical care. *Milbank Memorial Fund Quarterly, 44*(3), 166–206.

Donabedian, A. (1992). The role of outcomes in quality assessment and assurance. *Quality Review Bulletin, 11,* 356–360.

Ellwood, P. M. (1988). Outcomes management: A technology of patient experience. *New England Journal of Medicine, 319*(18), 1549–1556.

Goonan, K. (1993). *Clinical quality and total quality management.* Juran Institute.

Institute of Medicine. (1990). Medicare: A strategy for quality assurance. *1,* 21.

Lighter, D. E., & Fair, D. C. (2000). *Principles and methods of quality management in health care.* Gaithersburg, MD: Aspen.

Lloyd, R. (2004). *Quality health care: A guide to developing and using indicators.* Sudbury, MA: Jones & Bartlett.

Moorhead, S., Johnson, M., & Maas, M. (2003). *Nursing Outcomes Classification (NOC),* 3rd ed. St. Louis, MO: Mosby.

Mullen, E. J. (2001). *Outcomes measurement: A social work framework for health and mental health policy and practice.* New York: Columbia University School of Social Work.

Polit, D. F. (1989). *Essentials of nursing research: Methods, appraisal and utilization,* 2nd ed. Philadelphia: Lippincott.

Powell, S. (2000). *Advanced case management: Outcomes and beyond.* Philadelphia: Lippincott Williams & Wilkins.

Wojner, A. W. (2001). *Outcomes management: Applications to clinical practice.* St. Louis, MO: Mosby.

SUGGESTED READING

Case Management Society of America (CMSA). (2002). *Standards of practice for case managers.* Little Rock, AR: CMSA.

Johnson, M. (1998). Overview of the Nursing Outcomes Classification (NOC). *On Line Journal of Nursing Informatics, 2*(2).

Juran, M. J., & Godfrey, A. B. (1999). *Juran's quality handbook,* 5th ed. New York: McGraw-Hill.

Mullen, E. J., & Magnabosco, J. (1997). *Outcomes measurement in the human services.* Washington, DC: National Association of Social Workers.

Rieve, J. A. (1997). Benchmarking and using outcomes data. *Case Manager,* July/August, 55–62.

Legal Issues in Case Management Practice

Lynn S. Muller

LEARNING OBJECTIVES

Upon completion of this chapter, the reader will be able to:

1. Understand a wide range of legal terms and identify sources for additional legal research.
2. Gain an appreciation for the interaction of conflicting areas of law and ethical practice.
3. Discuss the role of the case manager in relation to the legal community.
4. Understand patients' rights and case managers' responsibilities.

IMPORTANT TERMS AND CONCEPTS

Advocate	Conflict of Interest
Agent	Contract
Battery	Contribution
Breach	Damages
Breach of Contract	Decision
Case Law	Defendant
Causal Connection	Deposition
Civil Law	Discovery
Codify	Duty
Common Law	Expert Witness

Fundamental Right	Opinion
Harm	Proximate Cause
Informed Consent	Remedy
Intentional Tort	Res Judicata (Latin term meaning
Interrogatories	"a thing [already] adjudicated")
Joint Liability	Several Liability
Law	Standard of Care
Lawyer	Statutory Law
Liability	Subpoena
Liable	Tort
Malpractice	Verdict
Medical Malpractice	Waiver
Negligence	Witness

■ INTRODUCTION

In our litigious society, case managers are concerned with an ethical-legal conflict in which they want to provide quality case management services, obey the law, meet licensing requirements and regulations, please their employers or contractors, and still act as an advocate for their patients. The good news is that it is possible. Legal issues affecting case management are interwoven in the complex matrix that is case management practice. Just as each patient is an individual who presents with uniquely different life experiences, expectations, and outcome potential, so the interplay of the law is unique and will affect decision making. Case managers have recognized the need for greater understanding in this area, but must always be mindful of the parameters of practice. It is knowing those parameters of practice or "knowing your sandbox" that reduces liability (Garner, 1996) exposure for the case manager.

■ KEY DEFINITIONS (GARNER, 1996)

A. Advocate—A person who assists, defends or pleads . . . for another.

B. Agent—One who is authorized to act for or in place of another.

C. Battery—In tort law (civil law), an intentional and offensive touching of another.

D. Breach of contract—Violation (failure to perform) a contract obligation.

E. Breach—Violation or infraction of a law or obligation. A failure on one's part to conform to the standard required.

F. Case law—The collection of reported cases that form the body of jurisprudence within a given jurisdiction.

This chapter is a survey of legal issues and could not possibly contain all relevant law. Please refer to the federal or state agencies, or both, under which you practice for laws and regulations governing professional licensing, workers' compensation, automobile liability, available benefits, and so on. Public and university libraries are a good source for such information. You may also contact the local offices of elected officials to request copies of state and federal legislation.

G. Causal connection—The relationship between cause and effect.

H. Civil law—The law of civil or private rights.

I. Codify/codification—The process of compiling, arranging, and systematizing the laws of a given jurisdiction into an ordered code.

J. Common law—The body of law derived from judicial decisions and opinions, rather than from statutes or constitutions. Also known as *case law.*

K. Conflict of interest—A real or seeming incompatibility between one's private interests and one's fiduciary duties.

L. Contract—A set of promises, for breach of which the law gives a remedy, or the performance of which the law in some way recognizes as a duty.

M. Contribution—The right to demand that another, who is jointly responsible for a third party's injury, supply part of what one is required to compensate a third party.

N. Damages—Monetary compensation for loss or injury to person or property.

O. Decision—A court's (judge's) ruling in a case.

P. Defendant—The party being sued in a civil lawsuit.

Q. Deposition—A witness' out-of-court testimony that is reduced to a writing, usually by a court reporter, for later use in court or for discovery purposes.

R. Discovery—The act or process of finding and learning something that was previously unknown. (Each state's court rules govern the discovery process.)

S. Duty—An obligation recognized by the law, requiring a person to conform to a certain standard of conduct, for the protection of others against reasonable risks.

T. Expert witness—A witness qualified by knowledge, skill, experience, training, or education to provide scientific, technical, or other specialized opinions about the evidence or a fact issue.

U. Fundamental right—(1) A right derived from natural or fundamental law. (2) Fundamental rights as enumerated by the Supreme Court, including the right to vote, interstate travel, along with various rights of privacy.

V. Harm—Actual loss or damage resulting from the actions or inactions of another.

W. Informed consent—(1) A person's agreement to allow something to happen, made with full knowledge of the risks involved and the alternatives. (2) A patient's intelligent choice about treatment, made after a physician discloses whatever information a reasonably prudent physician in the medical community would provide to a patient regarding the risks involved in the proposed treatment.

X. Intentional tort—A tort committed by someone acting with general or specific intent; examples are battery, false imprisonment, and trespass. May also be termed a *willful* tort and is distinguished from negligence.

Y. Interrogatories—A numbered list of written questions submitted in a legal context, usually to an opposing party in a lawsuit as part of discovery.

Z. Joint liability—Liability shared by two or more parties.

AA. Law—(1) A set of rules that order human activities and relations. (2) The collection of legislation and accepted legal principles; the body of authoritative grounds of judicial action.

BB. Lawyer—One who is designated to transact business for another; a legal agent.

CC. Liability—The quality or state of being legally obligated or responsible.

DD. Liable—(1) Legally obligated or responsible. (2) To have a duty or burden.

EE. Malpractice—Negligence or incompetence on the part of a professional. Professional negligence.

FF. Medical malpractice—A tort that arises when a doctor (or other health professional, including registered nurses, dentists, or social workers) violates the standard of care owed to a patient and the patient is injured as a result (often shortened to "med mal").

GG. Negligence—(1) The failure to exercise that standard of care that a reasonably prudent person would have exercised in the same situation. (2) A tort (civil wrong) grounded in this failure.

HH. Opinion—The court's (a judge's) written statement explaining its decision in a given case, including statements of fact, points of law, rationale, and dicta.

II. Plaintiff—The party who brings a lawsuit in a civil action.

JJ. Proximate cause—A cause that directly produces an event and without which the event would not have occurred.

KK. Remedy—The enforcement of a right or the redress of an injury, usually in the form of monetary damages that a party asks of a court.

LL. Res judicata (Latin term meaning "a thing [already] adjudicated")—An issue that had been definitively settled by judicial decision.

MM. Several liability—Liability that is separate and distinct from another's liability, so that the plaintiff may bring a separate action against one defendant without joining the other liable parties.

NN. Standard of care—In the law of negligence, the degree of care that a reasonable person would exercise.

OO. Statutory law—The body of law derived from statutes rather than from constitutions or judicial decisions.

PP. Subpoena—A court order commanding the appearance of a witness, subject to penalty for noncompliance.

QQ. Tort—(1) A civil wrong for which a remedy may be obtained, usually in the form of damages. (2) Breach of a duty that the law imposes.

RR. Verdict—A jury's findings or decision on the factual issues of a case.

SS. Waiver—(1) To voluntarily relinquish or abandon. Waiver may be expressed or implied (by one's actions). A person who is alleged to have waived a right must have had both knowledge of the existing right and intention to relinquish it. (2) Waiver may also refer to the document by which a person relinquishes a right.

TT. Witness—(1) One who sees, knows, or vouches for something. (2) One who testifies under oath or affirmation, either orally or by affidavit or deposition.

■ BACKGROUND

A. Legal basics—Understanding the law is much like learning a new language. It is especially important to learn legal terms, because some legal terms are words that have other meanings in common or medical usage.

The legal system is divided into two major categories, criminal and civil law. Civil law is the law that applies to private rights, as opposed to the law that applies to criminal matters. Civil law is the body of law that permits an individual who believes that he or she has been wronged to sue another and recover damages (dollars). The purpose of tort law is to adjust losses, to compensate one person because of the actions of another. Criminal Law is public law that deals with crimes and their prosecution. Substantive criminal law defines crimes, and procedural criminal law sets down criminal procedure. A tort is a civil or personal wrong, as compared with a crime, which is a public wrong.

B. Intentional torts—Intentional torts include assault, battery, false imprisonment, and trespass. These terms are often confused because they also exist in criminal law. When they are used in criminal law, they are defined by statute (laws passed by the legislature) and can vary from state to state. Each intentional tort represents a direct interference with a person's physical integrity or right to property. Personal freedom is a fundamental right. One does not waive a fundamental right, such as personal integrity, automatically, but a person must be aware that he or she possesses the right and can intentionally relinquish it.

Informed consent is a good example of a knowing and voluntary waiver of rights in the medical setting. In the absence of such a waiver of rights, a person touching or keeping another in a clinic, hospital, or any place he or she chooses not to be may be liable for assault, battery, or false imprisonment. Informed consent is a statutorily created right, given to potential recipients of medical treatment. Many states have enacted a "Patient's Bill of Rights" (Box 26-1). When a law exists, such as a Patient's Bill of Rights in one setting (e.g., the hospital setting), the health practitioner

BOX 26–1

Bill of Rights for Hospital Patients

• •

Every person admitted to a general hospital as licensed by the State Department of Health and Senior Services pursuant to P.L. 1971, c. 136 (C. 26:2H-1 et al.) shall have the right:

a. To considerate and respectful care consistent with sound nursing and medical practices, which shall include being informed of the name and licensure status of a student nurse or facility staff member who examines, observes or treats the patient;

b. To be informed of the name of the physician responsible for coordinating his diagnosis, treatment, and prognosis in terms he can reasonably be expected to understand. When it is not medically advisable to give this information to the patient; it shall be made available to another person designated by the patient on his behalf;

c. To receive from the physician information necessary to give informed consent prior to the start of any procedure or treatment and which, except for those emergency situations not requiring an informed consent, shall include as a minimum the specific procedure or treatment, the medically significant risks involved, and the possible duration of incapacitation, if any, as well as an explanation of the significance of the patient's informed consent. The patient shall be advised of any medically significant alternatives for care or treatment; however, this does not include experimental treatments that are not yet accepted by the medical establishment;

d. To refuse treatment to the extent permitted by law and to be informed of the medical consequences of this act;

e. To privacy to the extent consistent with providing adequate medical care to the patient. This shall not preclude discussion of a patient's case or examination of a patient by appropriate health care personnel;

f. To privacy and confidentiality of all records pertaining to his treatment, except as otherwise provided by law or third party payment contract, and to access to those records, including receipt of a copy thereof at reasonable cost, upon request, unless his physician states in writing that access by the patient is not medically advisable; to give this information to the patient, it shall be made available to another person designated by the patient on his behalf;

g. To expect that within its capacity, the hospital will make reasonable response to his request for services, including the services of an interpreter in a language other than English if 10% or more of the population in the hospital's service area speaks that language;

h. To be informed by his physician of any continuing health care requirements which may follow discharge and to receive assistance from the physician and appropriate hospital staff in arranging for required follow-up care after discharge;

BOX 26–1

Bill of Rights for Hospital Patients (*continued*)

• •

i. To be informed by the hospital of the necessity of transfer to another facility prior to the transfer and of any alternatives to it which may exist, which transfer shall not be effected unless it is determined by the physician to be medically necessary;

j. To be informed, upon request, of other health care and educational institutions that the hospital has authorized to participate in his treatment;

k. To be advised if the hospital proposes to engage in or perform human research or experimentation and to refuse to participate in these projects. For the purposes of this subsection "human research" does not include the mere collecting of statistical data;

l. To examine and receive an explanation of his bill, regardless of source of payment, and to receive information or be advised on the availability of sources of financial assistance to help pay for the patient's care, as necessary;

m. To expect reasonable continuity of care;

n. To be advised of the hospital rules and regulations that apply to his conduct as a patient;

o. To treatment without discrimination as to race, age, religion, sex, national origin, or source of payment; and

p. To contract directly with a New Jersey licensed registered professional nurse of the patient's choosing for private professional nursing care during his hospitalization. A registered professional nurse so contracted shall adhere to hospital policies and procedures in regard to treatment protocols and policies and procedures so long as those policies and procedures are the same for private duty and regularly employed nurses. The registered professional nurse shall not be considered an agent or employee of the hospital for purposes of any financial liabilities, including, but not limited to, state or federal employee taxes, workers' compensation payments or coverage for professional liability.

N.J.S.A. 26:2H-12.8

can reasonably assume that the policy established in that law may apply to a setting not articulated specifically. In other words, if a case manager finds himself or herself in the field setting or on the telephone and in a decision-making dilemma and, to complicate the matter, the patient is very argumentative and difficult, the case manager must be cognizant of the statutory language that states, " [A patient (client) has a right] to considerate and respectful care consistent with sound . . . practices, which shall include being informed of the name and licensure status of a . . . staff member who . . . observes or treats the patient" (see Box 26-1). There is no doubt that a case manager is making observations about a patient, whether on the telephone or at arm's length. Even if there is no statute directly on point regarding case management practice, you can assume that a court will use existing law as a basis for an alternative practice setting for as much as is practical. This is how new laws are developed.

C. Negligence—For a lawsuit to be successful in negligence, there are four required elements. These elements are commonly referred to as duty, breach, cause, and harm. All four of the elements must be proven and the burden of proof is on the plaintiff. Lots of duty and an obvious breach of such duty are not sufficient without also establishing the causal connection to the harm claimed (Keeton & Prosser, 1984). Proof of damages (harm) is an essential element to a negligence case. Negligence is sometimes referred to as simple negligence as compared with malpractice or professional negligence. The standard of proof for a simple negligence case is that of a reasonably prudent person.

The concept of negligence is based on the idea that there can be a generally uniform standard of human behavior. The simplest example of this is that when one drives a car, there is a generally accepted expectation that each person will operate the vehicle in a reasonably prudent and careful manner. Each time that there is a motor vehicle accident, it is likely that one or more persons deviated from the reasonably prudent person's standard and liability may attach. However, state statutes may limit or expand one's ability to bring a cause of action, a lawsuit. So-called "no fault" insurance is an example of such a limitation, particularly when there is an express limitation on one's ability to sue for certain personal injuries (N.J.S.A. 39:6B, *et seq*).

D. How cases are decided—What we refer to as "the law" is a combination of legislated rules—statutory law and case law. Case law is the compilation of common law. Common law, with its historical roots dating back to 12th-century England, provides the foundation for the collection of decisions, the result of various lawsuits. Such decisions are outcomes of particular cases and are either jury verdicts or judges' decisions. Judges' decisions may be verbal, on the record, or in the form of a written opinion. *Res judicata* is the legal term explaining that today's law is based on decisions that came before. Once an issue on a particular set of facts has been decided, there is no reason to relitigate the same issue. For example, it has already been decided that if a surgeon excises the left limb when the informed consent clearly states the right limb, the surgeon is liable and has committed the tort of battery. Whether a new case relates to ears, legs, arms, or breasts, the court will rely on the existing law relating to battery and professional negligence, also known as malpractice. Therefore, today most cases that are heard in court are not reported. A reported case is one that can be found in an official reporter. There are state as well as federal reporters. When entered into a reporter, the case is printed and becomes part of the ever-growing body of case law. It is important to remember that what we hear on the news, no matter the source, is simply news (and oft-times entertainment), not admissible evidence at trial.

E. Professional negligence and malpractice—Each of us comes to case management with education and experience from a profession. We are often licensed in that underlying profession. In fact, such licensure is one of the qualifications for a person seeking to become a case manager. It is critical that the case manager maintains current licensing requirements and updates his or her knowledge each year in both the field of case management and the underlying profession. The standard by which any case manager will be judged remains one derived from an external authority, such as a governmental standard. If you are a nurse, this standard is derived from the Nurse Practice Act. (Each state has a nurse practice act of one variety or another [N.J.S.A. 45:11–23, *et seq*]).* Nurse practice acts provide broad statements defining nursing practice, delineating the educational and other requirements for licensure and renewal, and giving notice to the public of the sort of behaviors that can be expected from a nurse and what unacceptable practices might subject a nurse to disciplinary review or sanctions. When these laws were drafted, the concept of managed care had not been thought of by the legislatures. For a copy of any state's nurse practice act, contact the board of nursing in that state.

Each profession develops a standard for itself through a complicated process of interaction with other professions, professional journals, meetings, and networking with colleagues and the development and refining of educational programs for the profession. In the developing world of new names and new roles, the law has not caught up with these rapid changes. Over time, hundreds of separate standards and comments become the "standard practice" (Eddy, 1982). Each profession has an obligation to monitor itself.

Today, although the legal community knows of case management and case managers, that does not mean they have a complete understanding of the role of the case manager and the standard of practice. The trend appears to be for inclusion of case managers as potential defendants in malpractice lawsuits. The most prevalent areas are workers' compensation cases where case managers have an active role in service and product selection and in hospital case management. That is not to say that there are many successful suits where case managers have been held liable. Such cases are rare. Most malpractice lawsuits settle, prior to trial, in whole or in part.

F. Burden of proof—In the case of professional liability (malpractice), the law requires that an expert witness be engaged to establish the accepted standards of practice. Such experts base their opinions and their testimony on their knowledge, education, and experience. State and federal rules of evidence require that a patient claiming that a professional is responsible for his or her injuries and damages use a "like-kind" expert witness to prove his or her case (Fed. R. Evid. 703, 704, N.J.S.A. 2A:84A-2, *et seq*). In other words, if the case manager who is being sued is a nurse, then it is necessary for another nurse case manager to act as the expert

---

*For a centralized list of links to many states' Nurse Practice Acts, see: *http://www.ncsbn.org/ regulation/nursingpractice_nursing_practice_acts.asp.*

witness. If the case manager on trial were a social worker by education, the expert would have to be a social worker. The plaintiff cannot proceed or be successful in a lawsuit unless a causal relationship is established between the harm claimed, the duty of the case manager, and an alleged breach of such duty. It is not enough to have a generally experienced nurse testify against a nurse in a unique role; rather, case managers require a nurse case manager expert, utilization review nurses require a utilization review expert, and social workers require a social worker case manager expert. Expert witnesses must be knowledgeable and up to date in their field; familiar with texts, journals, and the relevant accepted standard of practice; and are often published authors.

G. Affidavit of merit—In many states, it is now necessary to file an affidavit of merit on the filing of a malpractice lawsuit (N.J.S.A. 2A:53A-27).[1] This is a safeguard for the defendant, the purpose of which is to eliminate lawsuits filed without a genuine cause of action against a professional (licensed) person. In New Jersey, for example, this was part of major tort reform legislation. A person who wishes to bring a negligence or malpractice action against a licensed person must submit the affidavit within 60 days from a neutral-licensed person. This independent person must state that the services were not acceptable, and the law requires that the person providing the affidavit be a qualified expert (N.J.S.A. 2A:53A-27). The only exception to the affidavit requirement is in those cases in which the defendant (licensed professional) failed to provide necessary records that would reveal malpractice (N.J.S.A. 2A:53A-27). In a recent case, an affidavit prepared by an independent expert was found to be sufficient when the author (expert) submitted his *curriculum vitae*, delineating education, experience specific to the defendant's practice, and scientific presentation and papers he had authored (*Wacht v. Farooqui*, 1998). One interesting variation on the affidavit requirement is in the Commonwealth of Massachusetts, where "Every action for malpractice . . . against a provider of health care shall be heard by a tribunal consisting of a single justice of the Superior Court [trial court], a physician licensed to practice medicine in the commonwealth . . . and an attorney authorized to practice law in the commonwealth, at which hearing the plaintiff shall present an offer of proof and said tribunal shall determine if the evidence

---

[1]Affidavit required in certain actions against licensed persons. In any action for damages for personal injuries, wrongful death, or property damage resulting from an alleged act of malpractice or negligence by a licensed person in his profession or occupation, the plaintiff shall, within 60 days following the date of filing of the answer to the complaint by the defendant, provide each defendant with an affidavit of an appropriate licensed person that there exists a reasonable probability that the care, skill, or knowledge exercised or exhibited in the treatment, practice, or work that is the subject of the complaint fell outside of the acceptable professional or occupational standards or treatment practices. The court may grant no more than one additional period, not to exceed 60 days, to file the affidavit pursuant to this section, on a finding of good cause. The person executing the affidavit shall be licensed in this or any other state; have particular expertise in the general area or specialty involved in the action, as evidenced by board certification or by devotion of the person's practice substantially to the general area or specialty involved in the action for a period of at least five years. The person shall have no financial interest in the outcome of the case under review but this prohibition shall not exclude the person from being an expert witness in the case. (N.J.S.A. 2A:53A-27.)

presented if properly substantiated is sufficient to raise a legitimate question of liability appropriate for judicial inquiry or whether the plaintiff's case is merely an unfortunate medical result" (Gen. Laws Massachusetts, Part III, Title II, Ch. 231, §60B). The hearing occurs within fifteen days of the defendant's answer (response to the initiation of a lawsuit). There are similarities and differences between the two approaches. The affidavit of merit must contain the same offer of proof as the hearing, but must be sworn by a similar practitioner. The burden then falls upon the health care provider defendant to challenge the content of the affidavit. The Massachusetts hearing method places the facts before three professionals, who act as independent and impartial appraisers, and if they are not satisfied that the claim is meritorious it will be dismissed immediately and end the suit. These methods are a special protection that modern law provides to health professionals. Their purpose is to avoid dissatisfied or unhappy patients from bringing frivolous lawsuits and ruining a professional's career, where no malpractice has occurred.

H. Liability exposure for case managers—Case managers must be aware of what the law says about case management practice. Because many case managers come from a scientific discipline, with finite rules and measurable answers, it is difficult sometimes to understand the fluid, fact-driven dynamic that is the law. Now case managers have been recognized by some courts as potential defendants.

Until there are more reported cases in which case managers have either been found to be liable or relieved from liability, or states create statutes controlling case management practice, the profession must rely on its own developing standards.

In 1995, the New Jersey Supreme Court held that a health maintenance organization (HMO) was liable for the contribution toward the malpractice of a physician they hired as an independent contractor (*Dunn v. Praiss*, 1995). Logically it would follow that a case manager performing telephonic or field case management services for an HMO, who deviates from the "accepted standards of practice," could be held liable for his or her actions. In addition, the HMO could share in that liability. This is known as *joint* liability.

In an Alabama case, the allegation by a plaintiff/employee, "that the nurse [case manager] was more concerned with saving money than with the employee's recovery," was found to be insufficient to support a claim (*Reid v. Aetna Casualty & Surety Co.*, 1997). In this case, the client was offered a variety of choices for the treatment of pain management and the provider chosen was also the least expensive. In addition, there was an allegation of fraud on the part of the defendant or insurance carrier, in that they had suppressed the following material information (among other things)—"that the nurse [case manager] was not acting as a registered nurse with the normal professional obligations toward the worker [client]" (*Reid v. Aetna Casualty & Surety Co.*, 1997). The court held that even if that were true (and made no finding that it was true), there was no evidence that the actions of the case manager caused any harm to the patient. "It is undisputed that Aetna hired [a case management company] to perform medical case management, that the [case manager] was employed as a registered nurse . . . and that she worked on the client's case." Although the patient claimed that the case manager "prevented her from undergoing beneficial treatments," she failed to offer proof of such alternative beneficial treatments, and the case was dismissed (*Reid v. Aetna Casualty & Surety Co.*, 1997).

It is very important to note that in the concurring opinion, another judge in this case stated the following—"My objection to this practice is not so much that the insurance carriers are employing these nurses [case managers] but that the [case managers] are usually not forthcoming in revealing the existence, nature, and purpose of their employment. Thus, injured employees are presented with [case managers] who appear to be assisting them, when in actuality the [case manager] might be testifying in court using information gained through the employee's trust in them" (*Reid v. Aetna Casualty & Surety Co.*, 1997).

Case managers should recognize this case as a "red flag." It is one example of a court that had a bad experience with case management. The majority of case managers are forthcoming about who they are, who employs them and why they are meeting with the client/patient. This case supports the need for case managers to clarify these issues at the first and subsequent meetings with the patient. Once the case manager has disclosed this information to the patient, any information obtained by the case manager about the patient's illness, injury, prior history, work history, present income, and source of income can be freely shared with the relevant parties. These may include the physician (as is needed for proper treatment), the payer source, and, in some limited circumstances, the employer.

■ CONTRACTS

A. Contract basics—In the discussion of torts and negligence, you learned that a duty is a legally recognized obligation for which a remedy may be sought in the event of breach of that duty. Contract is another example of a source of duty. When a contract is formed, it creates one or many legal obligations for which damages may be available, in the event of a breach of contract. A lawsuit based on contract is a separate and distinct cause of action.

B. Elements of contract—There are three elements to a valid or binding contract: offer, acceptance, and consideration.

1. Offer—A promise to do or refrain from doing something in exchange for a promise, an action, or refraining from action. An offer is demonstrative of one's (*offeror*—the one who makes the offer) willingness to enter into a contract. The offer must be made known to the *offeree* (one to whom the offer is made) at the time of contract formation.

2. Acceptance—Once the offer has been made, acceptance is a voluntary act of the one who is given a contract offer. That person, by his or her action or promise, exercises his or her consent and willingness to enter into agreement and a legal relationship, known as a contract.

3. Consideration—Something of value. A contract must be supported by a benefit or believed benefit to the parties.

C. The case manager and contract—A simple example of contract creation is the following: You are an independent case manager. You receive a telephone call from XYZ Insurance, asking you to provide case management services for Mr. Smith. In addition, XYZ offers you a fee if you visit Mr. Smith and submit a report. There are several ways to bind you to this contract. The first is to simply say, "Thank you, I'll do it." The second is to do what is requested and submit the report. The problem arises when you make a telephonic contact with Mr. Smith, submit the report anyway, and later XYZ discovers your "breach." In other words, you failed to perform the entire contract (including an onsite visit to Mr. Smith) as requested and accepted the fee. This is the foundation for contract litigation. Questions would be asked, such as "Was there a meeting of the minds at the time of contract formation?" "When was the contract formed?" "Was the information contained in the report so complete that the contract was substantially performed, and what is the value of the report and services rendered?" (Williston Contracts, 1957).

There are entire courses on this subject. What is important for the case manager to know is that your words and your actions are very important as you perform your day-to-day work. You have entered a phase of your professional life in which your words are central to the creation of obligations. You may be an agent of your employer or the purchaser of case management services, or both. Your actions and your words may effectively bind (obligate) the payer (insurance company, employer, or health benefits provider) to provide disability benefits, medical expenses, and services or any other service or benefit that you include in your verbal or written report. This concept should not intimidate you but rather aid you in your assessment and recommendations.

Please note: In today's case management practice, the relevant contract may exist without you ever seeing it. The trend today is for payers (either third party administrators for self-insured companies, or insurance carriers themselves) to offer full-service wellness programs. This can occur as part of an employment scenario or as a benefit through a health plan. More and more, case management is a "product" offered in those contracts.

■ THE CASE MANAGER AND THE LEGAL COMMUNITY

Throughout your career, you have used a variety of resources to increase your knowledge. Attorneys are another source of valuable information. A case manager is an advocate for the client.[2] When you share a client with his or her lawyer, many of your goals should be the same. In a personal injury case, the attorney wants his or her client to receive any and all necessary services to improve their medical and physical condition. So do you. The difference is that the case manager has an obligation to accomplish the delivery of medically necessary services in a cost-effective and efficient manner. In general, the attorney does not become concerned with the expense to the payer but simply wants the client's needs to be met. These goals are not inconsistent; in fact,

---

[2]Client—The individual who is ill or disabled who collaborates with the case manager to receive services (CMSA, 2002).

there are times when the attorney can be of assistance to the case manager. If you share a client with a lawyer, and that client is uncooperative in some way, a telephone call or short note to his or her attorney may go a long way.

When the case manager learns that a client is represented by a lawyer, the case manager has an obligation to contact that attorney, identify himself or herself and for whom he or she is working, the purpose in wanting to meet or communicate with the client, and generally what the case manager's goals are.[3] If you present yourself by saying, "I represent your client's automobile policy carrier and I'm here to save money," that will be the last conversation you have with the client or the attorney. However, if you say or write, "I am a case manager working for XYZ Insurance, your client's automobile carrier. I have been asked to meet with your client to assess present and future needs and to facilitate the delivery of those services. I plan on meeting with your client on Tuesday. I look forward to communicating with you," the result should be far more to your liking. Both statements are true, and both statements have the same ultimate goal—cost-effective case management. Remember, there are times when presentation counts. When the case manager communicates with a lawyer, the telephone call should be outlined in advance (a simple note to yourself will do) and written notes or faxes should be presented in a professional manner. Attorneys practice the art of persuasion. Case managers are capable of being persuasive without being combative. If you can cultivate the lawyer as an ally, it can do much to accelerate the progress of your case and ultimately contribute to a successful case outcome.

A. The case manager and litigation—There are times when the case manager is called as a witness in a patient's case. The case manager will receive a subpoena. There are two types of subpoenas, asking for one of two things—either an appearance by the case manager at a deposition or court (*subpoena ad testificandum*), or the submission of records (*subpoena duces tecum*) kept by the case manager relating to a client—or both. In most jurisdictions (states), interrogatories, which are written questions and answers under oath, are served only on parties to an action. Therefore, the only time the case manager may receive them is in the event of a lawsuit against the case manager as an individual. Even if the case manager is an expert witness, most states' discovery rules would not include interrogatories. In some states, attorneys have been serving "subpoenas" on their own letterhead and failing to name a person to whom the subpoena is directed. These are "fishing expeditions" and are frowned on. In one state, legislation enacted a law sanctioning attorneys for misuse of this tool. A lawful subpoena must name an individual (which can be a corporation), request records only, and comply with Health Insurance Portability and Accountability Act (HIPAA) requirements. (It is sufficient for the subpoena to state Custodian of Records, XYZ Hospital, or other entity.)

1. HIPAA and requests for information—With the advent of the HIPAA privacy laws, even a subpoena must be accompanied by a HIPAA-

---

[3]Note: In some states, particularly in the case of workers' compensation, an attorney cannot keep the case manager from meeting with the patient. Please refer to your practice state for this information.

compliant authorization. The only exception to the HIPAA authorization requirement is a court order, signed by a judge. Subpoenas, although they look like and are official court documents, are signed by the clerk of the court (or in most cases, the clerk's name is signed by the lawyer, an approved practice under the rules of court). If a subpoena is served upon you and is not accompanied by an authorization, that authorization must be requested and obtained. Unless you are an independent case manager, the first response to a subpoena should be a call to your company's legal department for further instructions.

2. Investigational subpoenas—In the event of an investigation based on a HIPAA complaint, an administrative law judge or the secretary of Health and Human Services (HSS) issues an investigational subpoena. This document may be very general in nature and seeks not only records, but also to identify individuals. Once identified, those individuals have a right to counsel (USC §160.504). Parties in the HIPAA complaint process may request that the administrative law judge issue subpoenas (USC §160.542).

B. The case manager as witness—More and more, the legal community is recognizing the case manager as a valuable source of information. There are two general categories of witnesses.

1. The first is the *fact* witness. In this case, you would simply be asked to speak about things that you had seen or heard. In other words, you might be asked to describe the condition of the patient as you observed her on a particular date, the treatment that you observed and documented, and to identify records previously made by you. Most likely, you would be appearing on behalf of the patient, as plaintiff, in a civil lawsuit. It is also possible that the defendant insurance carrier in a civil case may also use the case manager as a fact witness. This is nothing to fear. Most attorneys will invest time and prepare you before you testify. All you have to do is tell the truth, which you would do without preparation.

In Louisiana, a case manager's determination was used to ascertain whether a claimant's injury was work related. The claimant alleged that the case manager's assessment was not sufficient "investigation of the claim." The case was decided in favor of the employer, who retained the services of the case manager and held that the case manager's visit, assessment, and recommendations did constitute "reasonable effort" to ascertain an employee's exact medical condition [668 So.2d 1161 (La. App. 5 Cir)].

2. The *expert* witness is used when specialized information is required. Case managers are well qualified to provide such information to the court. In a liability lawsuit, the expert witness does not speak to the specific facts of a case because he or she would not be one of the persons involved in direct care. An expert witness is expected to be impartial. He or she may discuss items such as standards of practice, trends in an industry, educational background, and criteria for entry to a profession. Case managers have been used to clarify procedure and define case management process and practice.

In an unreported New York case, an insurance carrier was joined in a lawsuit initiated by a home care provider. After providing more than $65,000 of home care to a cancer patient, the carrier rejected the claim on the death of the patient. When the home care provider received the case, they immediately and repeatedly contacted the representative of the insurance company. The initial claim was sent to a "nurse approver," a non-medically trained person, then on to a "nurse reviewer" who was a registered nurse. The reviewer forwarded the claim to the "medical management center," where a nurse would review the claim again, with additional documentation. When the claim was denied at this level, it was sent to a "medical director," a physician, for final determination. Initially, the court dismissed the case. However, a case manager with particular expertise in health benefit contract analysis (Krul, 1998) reviewed the contract under which the patient had received home care services. She discovered that the contract required case management and found that the insurance carrier had breached the contract by failing to provide the requisite case management services. The case returned to the New York Superior Court. With the sworn testimony of the case manager, the court found in favor of the home care company, thereby relieving the grieving family of the $66,000 burden. At any step of the approval process, it would have been simple for a case manager to assess the case and discuss the possibility of giving the patient a hospice classification with the physician. This would have triggered another contract obligation, and 100% of the home care would have been covered without the expense and aggravation of litigation.

■ FREQUENTLY ASKED QUESTIONS

A. *I am a new case manager. My boss gave me a caseload immediately. I've been in the clinical setting for years. How can I be a case manager overnight?* There once was a day when you were a new nurse, social worker, or other health professional. The difference is that as a new case manager, you have been developing the necessary skills from the first day of your education and clinical practice in your primary profession. Unless and until your state has enacted a statute or regulation under your licensing structure, there is no legal restriction regarding representing yourself as a case manager.

It is critical that you never forget your professional roots, because the law is slow in developing. In the event that you are sued for malpractice, the basis of that allegation would go first to your primary profession, as case management certification (e.g., CCM) is a dependent credential. For example, if you were a nurse, any action brought against you for work as a case manager would be a suit for nursing malpractice.

B. *The insurance carrier who assigned my latest patient wants me to ask the patient questions about "how the accident happened and who might be at fault."* *Can I do this?* Difficult questions call for complex answers, and this question is actually several questions. When your employer (whether it is an insurance carrier or intermediary) asks you to collect liability information, you are going outside the scope of practice. Your obligation is to collect information relevant to a patient's injuries or illness. A case management client is "the individual who is ill or disabled who collaborates with the case manager to receive services." There is nothing contained in the definition of a patient that would indicate that your role, as you collaborate with that individual, is to collect facts or evidence pertaining to liability.

Note: Having been fully informed of your role, including your duty to report relevant information to the carrier, should the patient volunteer information about the accident or onset of the illness, you can and should deliver that information to the appropriate party. It is important that you relate such information accurately and factually, without editorial or judgmental overtones. Using an example of a soccer injury, when that information is reported, it should simply be written, "Client reports playing soccer on the Sunday immediately preceding the reported accident date." This gives the carrier the information it needs to investigate the report further. (See the discussion of the Alabama case in the section on liability exposure for case managers.)

Insurance investigators are in the business of delving into the history and details of an injury or illness. They have various resources available to them, such as surveillance, photographs, and telephone and personal canvassing. None of those investigative tools falls within the role of the case manager.

C. *How can I honestly advise the patient, upon initial contact, whom I represent and why we are meeting (whether in person or by telephone)?* Honesty is always the best policy. If you are an "in-house" case manager, you should tell the patient that you are a case manager from XYZ Insurance, the company handling his or her claim. If you are employed by a case management company, simply modify the answer, "I am a case manager working for ABC Case Management Services, and in your case, we are working for XYZ Insurance, the company handling their claim."

The reason why this is so important is seen in the potential conflict between confidential information and the duty of the case manager to disclose information to the insurance company. Both of these obligations can exist simultaneously but require the case manager to be clear, particularly on the first patient contact.

D. *What if a patient/client tells me things that may affect his or her coverage under the insurance program through which I was hired?* This is not a new dilemma, merely an old one in a new environment. In your clinical experience, you were required to take patient histories on a regular basis, no matter what your underlying professional background. It is not unusual for a patient in the clinical setting to say, "I'm going to tell you something, but it's just between us." In the clinical setting, the response would be, "I appreciate your feeling comfortable enough to share that information, but I must report it to your physician, because it may affect his diagnosis. Would you prefer telling him yourself?"

In the role of case manager, the scenario is much the same. Typically a patient will say, "I told my boss I fell at work, but I'm telling you that I was injured playing soccer on Sunday. It will be our little secret." The response is similar to that in the clinical setting. "Remember at our first visit I explained that I was hired by the workers' compensation carrier. I also told you then that I have an obligation to report relevant information to them, and I will be passing this along." Do not apologize. It is your job.

E. *What if the patient asks me to keep something "off the record?"* Same answer as in D.

F. *What if I observe something that indicates that the patient is working?* Same answer as in D. Once you have fully informed the patient of who you are, who employs you, and the purpose of your visit, you can and will report all relevant information that you observe.

G. *What if I see or smell illegal drugs in a patient's home?* Case managers must be very careful not to be judgmental in their observations and assessments. The case manager is not a law enforcement person; however, such substances may impact the potential recovery of the patient. The case manager should remove himself from the situation as quickly as possible and report only true and accurate facts (what you observed) to the supervision. You would not want to accuse someone of something as serious as drug use and learn later that your olfactory sense had misled you. Do not guess.

H. *What if I see my patient abuse a child or parent in my presence?* Most states now require medical and educational professionals to report actual acts of child or elder abuse that take place in their presence. Know your state's law on the subject. Contact your state board of medicine, nursing, social work, or other professional body to obtain such information. Again, do not guess. When it is necessary to report such information, the result will be an intrusive and long-term investigation by the appropriate state agency.

I. *What if my patient asks me to change a dressing?* As a case manager, it is not appropriate to perform "hands-on" care, even if you have the education and training to do so. The case manager's role is to coordinate and facilitate medically necessary treatment; therefore, it would be appropriate to contact the home care provider, physician, or family, depending on the circumstances of the particular case.

J. *What do I do if I walk into a medical emergency in a patient's home?* You should be familiar with the "Good Samaritan Act" where you practice.[4] When you enter someone's home as a case manager, you are not there to act as a "hands-on" nurse or other practitioner. It would be appropriate to respond to the best of your ability, based on your education and experience.

---

[4]N.J.S.A. 2A:62A-1. Emergency care (commonly known as the Good Samaritan Act)—Any individual, including a person licensed to practice any method of treatment of human ailments, disease, pain, injury, deformity, mental or physical condition, or licensed to render services ancillary thereto, or any person who is a volunteer member of a duly incorporated first aid and emergency or volunteer ambulance or rescue squad association, who in good faith renders emergency care at the scene of an accident or emergency to the victim or victims thereof, or while transporting the victim or victims thereof to a hospital or other facility where treatment or care is to be rendered, shall not be liable for any civil damages as a result of any acts or omissions by such person in rendering the emergency care.

A recent revision of one state's law provides that "anyone [including RNs, LVNs (aka:LPNs), MDs, etc] who in good faith renders emergency care at the scene of an accident or emergency to the victim . . . shall not be liable for any civil damages as a result of any acts or omissions by such person in rendering the emergency care" (N.J.S.A. 2A:62A-1). The purpose of such legislation is to encourage knowledgeable licensed persons to act, rather than shy away in fear of being sued. There have been incidents where a client has described symptoms over the telephone that would lead the case manager to believe that a heart attack or other serious medical emergency is in progress; in many cases, the best answer is call "911."

K. *My supervisor edits all my reports. I feel like I'm back in high school. Is that OK?* It is important that the product—your report—be presented in a clear, concise, and professional manner. Stylistic and grammatical changes are simply a matter of taste and not a problem. The problem occurs when another changes the substance of your report, particularly if this change is without your knowledge.

Example: You make an observation about a patient and report that he or she has improved significantly since your last contact. You recommend a reduction of services to telephonic case management, with an anticipated closure in 30 to 45 days. The reviewer changes that information to read, "minimal improvement noted" and changes your recommendation from closing the file to "two to three more visits required to monitor progress."

Several things have happened here. First, the report is no longer your professional opinion, based in observation and assessment, but rather is a misrepresentation. It may go so far as to be considered fraud and places you, as well as the employer, in the position of having committed fraud on an insurance company. States vary on the consequences of this kind of action, but certainly the reviewer is risking the company and your presumably good reputation. If the problem is discovered, the company would not hire you again. Not all legal consequences are settled in court. Because litigation is costly, the cost-effective response would be to change case management service providers. Depending on the severity of the fraud, it could result in a lawsuit in which the company would be a named defendant.

L. *What is the significance, if any, of signing my reports?* If reports are signed, the writer should sign them. It is common practice for the report to be submitted in either a rough form, on a floppy disk, or in some instances entered directly into a company computer network. All of these methods still permit editing, revision, and the temptation for the editor to fall to the temptation described above in K. If you are the last person to review a report before submission to the carrier or another person who has purchased the case management services, then you certainly can sign it. On the other hand, if you are in a situation in which you do not get to see the final product before mailing, that too should be indicated on the report. Such methods as, "dictated but not read," alert the reader that the author of the report might not have seen the final product.

There is no magic in the signature itself. It is merely another indication that the author is submitting a completed project. In the ideal situation, the report should be submitted, edited, and returned to the author for review and signature. Should the report end up on the court case, no doubt the author will be held to the contents. Therefore, in a litigious environment one should diplomatically work toward a policy that best protects your integrity.

M. *My employer does not pay for continuing education (CE) or make it available in-house. Do I still have to attend CE programs?* As the field of case management grows and is better recognized by the law, practitioners will be expected to have up-to-date information. To reduce your liability exposure, it is important to read, discuss, and earn CE credits. It is anticipated that as states codify case management practice and as state law regulates other professions, CE will be required. If you are to become a certified case manager (CCM) or other certified professional, CE credits are required and necessary to maintain your credential.

If you were ever called as a fact or expert witness in a case relating to your case management practice, one of the first questions you would be asked is, "Do you have any special training or certification, and do you have any continuing education in the field of case management?"

N. *Is there any value in belonging to a professional organization?* The benefits of belonging to a professional organization, such as Case Management Society of America (CMSA), are immeasurable. Such membership becomes a legal issue, as CMSA is your primary source for reliable case management practice information and guidelines. This is evidenced by the revised standards of practice. CMSA is a leader in the case management industry and works constantly to improve and standardize the practice. As a member, you will receive educational opportunities, practice updates, policy statements, and opportunities to interact with other members of the profession, and be part of the development of the standards of practice and the profession.

O. *Can I refuse to see a patient?* The simple answer is, "yes." The real question is "why?" Patient assignments and services can never have a discriminatory basis. If you sense a potential conflict of interest, this should be reported to your supervision and a decision should be made as to whether another case manager would be more appropriate for the assignment. The difficulty occurs when there are personality conflicts. This is best dealt with through consistent professional contacts with the patient and does not become a legal issue.

P. *Do I have to go back to that patient's home?* Your duty to provide services should never place you in personal or professional danger. If you have been exposed to a danger in a patient's home, the neighborhood, or work environment, there are alternative ways of obtaining necessary information. Such genuine fears should be reported to your supervisor and documented, if appropriate.

Remember: do not be judgmental in your report writing. A smart attorney will use this information to demonstrate that you had some prejudice in your decision making in areas in which the patient is concerned. Describe what you see but do not characterize the information. For example, "The patient was dressed in pajamas when I arrived at his home at 1:30 PM. I asked him three times to turn off the television before I could begin the interview." This description simply tells the reader what you saw and what happened. "The patient appeared lazy. It was early afternoon, he was still in his pajamas and appeared more interested in the soap opera he was watching than in anything having to do with his recovery." This description is your opinion of why the patient presented in a particular way, which may be based on your life experience and not that of the patient. Be cautious.

Q. *What if I refer a patient to a provider and that provider commits malpractice? Could I be liable?* Each health (and other) professional is responsible for his or her own actions. Cost-effective medical care is an essential part of case management. Identifying the highest-quality service or product for the lowest price is consistent with one's professional obligations and ethical duty. When, however, price alone dictates your professional decision making, liability may follow. When you are placed in a position to make a referral, you should not do so blindly. What is the source of your referral? Is it a provider that your coworkers have been very pleased with, or is it simply the lowest price you can find? Are you able to procure an identical product or one that performs as well or simply a lesser product?

This problem has become complicated with the increase of hospital case management. Case managers are finding themselves torn between directives to stay "in network"—or, in some cases, referring only to facilities or vendors owned by large hospital corporations—and identifying the best quality, most cost-effective service. For the most part, these are ethical dilemmas; however, they can translate into liability exposure for the case manager if the referrals are made without investigation and cost-benefit analysis. If there is one area where courts have either ruled or given opinions regarding case management practice, it is this. Case managers have an affirmative duty to know the cost and quality of the services before making referrals.

Make a reasonable inquiry to determine what will be provided for the dollars spent. Sometimes, a dollar saved in the short term can represent long-term expense. It may also expose the decision maker to unnecessary risk. Potential liability rests with whether you acted within the scope of your profession and accepted standards of practice (CMSA, 2002).

R. *I live and work in an east coast state and my employer requires that I contact clients who live in a west coast state. I'm not licensed in that west coast state. Is that a problem?* Yes, the law that controls the relationship (or telephonic communication) between the case manager and the patient/client is the law in the state where the client is, not where the nurse is located or where the employer is based, even in workers' compensation cases.

In the United States today, a professional may practice only in the state or states in which he or she is licensed and in good standing. Therefore, a nurse must be licensed in the state where the patient/client is. Each nurse's practice is controlled by the law in the state(s) where he/she is licensed—typically, by the Nurse Practice Act of that state. The advent of the Nurse Licensure Compact places nurses on notice that interstate practice is only recognized in those states that have passed legislation, rules, and regulations adopting the compact (24 Del. Laws c. 19A,

TABLE 26–1
Nurse Licensure Compact States

Compact States	Implementation Date
Arizona	7/1/2002
Arkansas	7/1/2000
Delaware	7/1/2000
Idaho	7/1/2001
Iowa	7/1/2000
Maine	7/1/2001
Maryland	7/1/1999
Mississippi	7/1/2001
Nebraska	1/1/2001
New Hampshire	1/1/2006
New Mexico	1/1/2004
North Carolina	7/1/2000
North Dakota	1/1/2004
South Carolina	2/1/2006
South Dakota	1/1/2001
Tennessee	7/1/2003
Texas	1/1/2000
Utah	1/1/2000
Virginia	1/1/2005
Wisconsin	1/1/2000

Compact states pending implementation: **New Jersey, 1/2007**
Please note that although New Jersey and South Carolina have enacted the Nurse Licensure Compact, these states have not yet *implemented* (passed into law) the compact. On April 25, 2005, the states of Iowa and Utah agreed to mutually recognize APRN licenses. No date has been set for the implementation of the APRN Compact.
  If you are seeking compact licensure, please contact your state board of nursing for primary state of residence requirements.
  From: National Council of State Boards of Nursing, Inc., (NCSBN). Website: *http://www.ncsbn.org.* Last updated 2/2/2006.

§1901A). The compact permits nurses whose home state is in the compact to practice in any other compact state. In the absence of such law, a nurse must be licensed in each and every state in which he/she practices. With less than half the states included in the compact, the majority of nurses are left having to be licensed in each and every state in which they practice nursing (see Table 26-1).

In December 2005, CMSA took an official position on this issue and incorporated their position in the *CMSA's Standards of Practice for Case Management* (revised 2002), which clearly states that: "The case manager practices in accordance with applicable local, state, and federal laws. The case manager has knowledge of applicable accreditation and regulatory statutes governing sponsoring agencies that specifically pertain to delivery of case management services."

1. CMSA encourages case managers and case manager employers to work aggressively with the state boards of nursing to encourage

compliance and entry into the National Council of State Boards of Nursing (NCSBN) as compact states so that appropriate multistate nursing licensure might continue appropriately and cost effectively.
2. Alternatively, CMSA encourages the enactment of federal legislation mandating the recognition of nurse licensure in all states.
3. CMSA has added its name to the growing list of those organizations supporting and endorsing the nurse compact. (A copy of the CMSA Position Paper can be obtained through its Website, *www.cmsa.org*.)

REFERENCES

668 So.2d 1161 (La. App. 5 Cir.)
Black's law dictionary. (1966). St. Paul: West Publishing Co.
Case Management Society of America (CMSA). (2002). *Standards of practice for case management*, rev. ed. Little Rock, AR: CMSA.
Dunn v. Praiss, 139 N.J. 561 (1995).
Eddy, J. (1982). Clinical policies and the quality of clinical practice. *New England Journal of Medicine*, 343.
Fed. R. Evid. 703, 704, N.J.S.A. 2A:84A-2, et seq.
Keeton, W. P. (1984). *Prosser and Keeton, the law of torts*, 5th ed. St. Paul: West Publishing.
Krul, R. (1998). Personal communication.
N.J.S.A. 2A:53A-27.
N.J.S.A. 2A:62A-1.
N.J.S.A. 39:6B, *et seq.*
N.J.S.A. 45:11–23, *et seq.*
Reid v. Aetna Casualty & Surety Co., et al., 692 So.2d 863 (Alabama App. 1997).
Wacht v. Farooqui, 312 N.J. Super. 184, 711 A.2d 405 (App. Div. 1998).
Williston Contracts §1(3d ed. 1957), Restatement 2d, Contracts §2; See Muller, L. (1998) Provider contracts: What case managers need to know. *The Journal of Care Management, The Official Journal of The Case Management Society of America*, 4, 5.

Ethical Issues in Case Management Practice

John Banja

Upon completion of this chapter, the reader will be able to:

1. Differentiate ethics from morality and from law.
2. List and define key ethical terms.
3. Describe the goals of ethical theories and ethical principles.
4. Characterize four ethical theories and four ethical principles.
5. List ethical responsibilities particularly affecting case managers.
6. Discuss strategies for maintaining ethical behavior in case management.

Advocacy
Autonomy
Beneficence
Client
Code of Professional Conduct for
   Case Managers
Competence
Confidentiality
Conflict of Interest

Deontologism
Dignity
Ethical Dilemma
Ethics
Impartiality
Justice
Moral Character
Morality
Nonmaleficence

Normative Guidelines   Values
Unprofessional Behavior   Veracity
Utilitarianism   Virtue Ethics

■ INTRODUCTION

A. Changes in the American health care delivery system such as the increased number of managed care organizations, the need for authorizations for services prior to care provision, and the demands for cost effectiveness, patient safety, and quality of care, have resulted in a rising number of ethical concerns for health care professionals including case managers.

B. These changes have also resulted in the expectation that the case manager, as a patient advocate, will prevent ethical conflicts from occurring—or at least address them when they arise—and reduce their impact on health care outcomes, the experience of the patient/family, the providers of care, and others.

C. Ethical theories attempt to explain what it means to act ethically by defining:
   1. Key ethical terminologies and concepts
   2. Offering proofs or arguments that explain or justify actions as ethical
   3. Describing the four familiar ethical theories or models:
      a. Virtue ethics
      b. Deontologism
      c. Utilitarianism
      d. Contractualism (Beauchamp and Childress, 2001; Banja, 2003)

D. Ethical principles derive from ethical theories and constitute important values that inform or serve as guidelines for ethical conduct.

E. There are six common ethical principles case managers must be aware of and must incorporate into their practice. These include:
   1. Autonomy
   2. Nonmaleficence
   3. Beneficence
   4. Justice (Beauchamp and Childress, 2001)
   5. Veracity
   6. Distributive justice

F. Ethical ambiguity or ethical conflict occurs when an ethical guideline that might inform behavior is absent, unclear, or controversial. It also happens when guidelines or principles conflict with each other; that is, when satisfying one principle—such as honoring a client's right to make

---

This chapter is a revised version of what was previously published in the first edition of *CMSA Core Curriculum for Case Management*. The contributor wish to acknowledge Patricia M. Pecqueux as some of the timeless material was retained from the previous version.

his or her own decisions—collides with another principle—such as working to provide a benefit rather than a harm for the client (Banja, 1999).

G. Ethics and law share certain similarities and differences (Lo, 2000).

1. Both ethics and law are concerned with right behavior and sustaining a social order where people can settle their differences reasonably and respectably.

2. Law sets only a minimally acceptable standard of conduct and, through enforced regulation (e.g., fines, licensure suspension or revocation, or imprisonment), can insist that its rules and regulations are followed.

3. A violation of an ethical rule (e.g., respect for a patient's inherent dignity) need not necessarily result in a legal sanction.

4. Whereas law tolerates minimally acceptable behavior, ethics aspires to ideal behavior or focuses on the right or best decision in a situation.

5. Controversies exist over certain laws being unethical (e.g., capital punishment), and whether certain illegal acts might sometimes be ethical (e.g., active euthanasia).

H. Codes of ethics, such as the Code of Professional Conduct for Case Managers advocated for by the Commission for Case Manager Certification (CCMC), attempt to:

1. Protect the public interest by providing guidance to the profession's members on what constitutes ethical conduct and on the level of conduct required from the profession's members (or certificants or licensees).

2. While such codes of conduct can be helpful, their primary shortcoming consists in their brevity and their inability to analyze the complex and multifactorial nature of many ethical dilemmas (CCMC, 2004; Lo, 2000).

I. Advocacy is essential in the ethical case manager's practice. It can be accomplished through a process that promotes client's rights and functional independence through education, resource and service facilitation, and informed decision making (CCMC, 2004).

■ KEY DEFINITIONS

A. Advocacy—Acting on behalf of those who are not able to speak for or represent themselves. It is also defending others and acting in their best interest (CCMC, 2005).

B. Advocate—The individual or groups involved in advocacy activities.

C. Autonomy—A form of personal liberty whereby an individual possesses sufficient mental ability to determine his or her behavior in accordance with a plan chosen and developed by himself or herself (CCMC, 2004).

D. Beneficence—Promoting the other's good or taking steps that further the other's legitimate interests (CCMC, 2004).

E. Client—The individual to whom, or on whose behalf, a case manager provides services (CCMC, 2004).

F. Code of Professional Conduct for Case Managers—A document consisting of principles, rules of conduct, and standards for professional conduct, as well as procedures for processing complaints, that the CCMC offers by way of providing ethical guidelines for case managers (CCMC, 2004).

G. Competence—The domain of skills, behaviors, practices, obligations, and responsibilities that are defined and bounded by the professional's training and qualifications, licensure(s), or certification(s) (Banja, 2006).

H. Confidentiality—A nondisclosure responsibility that connotes refraining from divulging client information to individuals who have neither a need nor a right to know it (Jonsen, Siegler, and Winslade, 2002).

I. Conflict of interest—A set of conditions in which professional judgment concerning a primary interest, such as a patient's welfare or the validity of research, tends to be unduly influenced by a secondary interest, such as financial gain (Thompson, 1993).

J. Contractualism—A model for resolving ethical dilemmas, usually bearing on the distribution of benefits, that looks to a formal agreement among the principles where the ethical rules and principles and procedures for settling disputes have been settled and adopted (Banja, 2003).

K. Deontologism—Popularized by Immanuel Kant (1724–1804), an ethical theory that is grounded in reason and bases decisions on the moral acceptability of the principles that are used to resolve a dilemma; the best principles are the ones that have the widest applicability (to similar cases) and that are done from a sense of obligation (Beauchamp and Childress, 2001).

L. Dignity—A characteristic of human beings that explains their inherent value and their enjoying fundamental rights.

M. Ethical dilemma—A situation wherein the ethically correct course of action is unclear; usually arises due to lack of clarity regarding which ethical principle is appropriate to apply, or because multiple ethical principles are in conflict (Banja, 1999).

N. Ethics—A word that can refer to the literature of moral philosophy; the development of a virtuous character; or the analysis of principles, rules, or language that characterize an action or judgment bearing on human welfare as right or good, or wrong, harmful, evil, beneficial, burdensome, etc. (Beauchamp and Childress, 2001).

O. Impartiality—Treating others similarly; making decisions that do not discriminate against individuals or groups on the basis of irrelevant differences such as ethnicity, race, age, gender, or lifestyle (Jansen, 2003).

P. Justice—Providing someone with his or her right or due; providing what a person is owed; treating another fairly (Beauchamp and Childress, 2001).

Q. Moral character—A habituated response or repertoire of responses to situations bearing on human welfare (Beauchamp and Childress, 2001).

  R. Morality—A term that refers to conduct that represents the customs or conventions that define people's moral behavior. Unlike ethics, which tends to be critical and analytical toward beliefs, customs, and social conventions, morality is simply the compendium of a society's sensibilities bearing on acceptable versus unacceptable behavior (Lo, 2000).

  S. Nonmaleficence—Refraining from harming; preventing harm from occurring; or, if only harm can occur from an inevitable act or decision, ensuring that the least amount of harm occurs (Beauchamp and Childress, 2001).

  T. Normative guidelines—Guidelines that are nationally accepted and considered or looked upon as common standards. In relation to ethics, they inform ethical behavior.

  U. Privacy—Protecting or securing sensitive information against persons who have no right to it (Lo, 2000).

  V. Publicity—The act of making decisions based on standards and rules that are not only available publicly but also accessible by those influenced by the decisions (Jansen, 2003).

  W. Unprofessional behavior—Behavior that unreasonably deviates from norms, guidelines, standards, and ethical codes that inform professional behavior.

  X. Utilitarianism—An ethical theory popularized by John Stuart Mill (1806–1873), that recommends as right actions the ones that produce the greatest amount of happiness for the greatest number of people (Beauchamp and Childress, 2001).

  Y. Values—Ascriptions of worth, commonly articulated as standards, goals, or attitudes (Banja, 1997).

  Z. Veracity—The act of telling the truth, or the truthfulness of one's behavior.

  AA. Virtue ethics—Popularized by Aristotle (384–322 B.C.), an approach to moral behavior that emphasizes the development of good character by education and training that concentrates on developing virtuous habits, dispositions, and sensibilities (Beauchamp and Childress, 2001).

■ ETHICAL DECISION MAKING AND THE CASE MANAGER

  A. Case managers are expected to act based on case management–related ethical principles and professional codes as well as those of their original profession or specialty, such as the American Nurses Association's Code of Ethics, the National Association of Social Workers' Code of Ethics.

  B. Examples of case management–Specific ethical principles can be found in the CCMC's Code of Professional Conduct for Case Managers and the CMSA's statement on case management ethics.

  C. Ethically competent case managers are able to:
    1. Act in ways that protect or advance the best interests of their patients;
    2. Be accountable for their practice;

3. Act as effective patient advocates;

4. Mediate ethical conflicts when they occur or prevent their occurrence;

5. Recognize the ethical dimension of their practice (Taylor, 2005); and

6. Abide by their professional code of conduct and ethical principles.

D. Taylor (2005) describes a process for ethical decision making that case managers may apply in their handling of patient care issues. This process is especially important in situations that present potential for ethical conflicts and includes the following steps:

1. Assessment—Gathering and documenting pertinent medical and nonmedical information

   i. Medical may include information about the patient's health condition, past medical history, and any treatment regimens.

   ii. Non-medical information addresses the patient's and family's situation including its characteristics: financial, social, values, beliefs, interests, guardian, including the names of persons who have the authority to make decisions and responsibility for the consequences.

   iii. Pay special attention to factors creating or fueling conflict.

2. Diagnosis—Identifying ethical issues and differentiating ethical problems (e.g., termination of life support measures) from those that are nonethical (e.g., shortness of breath)

3. Planning—identifying goals and desired outcomes. This also includes listing and exploring options and courses of actions that are likely to resolve the ethical issue/conflict.

4. Implementation—putting the course of action into effect and assessing the consequences. This may require calling for an ethics consult from the clinical or organizational ethics committees.

5. Evaluation—critiquing the decision, goals, and course of action, including the consequences.

■ ETHICAL THEORIES

A. Ethical theories try to explain, usually at a very abstract level, how right action or goodness should be understood. Ethical theories generate principles and reasons that help individuals arrive at an ethically appropriate course of action (Beauchamp and Childress, 2001).

B. There are four major ethical theories case managers must be familiar with and must incorporate into their practice. These are:

1. Deontologism—A theory that recommends doing one's "duty" as morally obligatory.

   a. *Duty* might be understood as what any reasonable person would consistently do in that situation or in others like it such that the client's welfare is respected and maintained; or duty might be defined in terms of ethical standards, codes, or regulations.

   b. The first two principles of the Code of Professional Conduct for Case Managers (CCMC, 2004) are deontological: "Certificants will place the public interest above their own at all times" (Principle 1). "Certificants will respect the rights and inherent dignity of all of their clients" (Principle 2).

2. Utilitarianism—A theory that defines "right action" as that which produces the most happiness or benefits for the most people. A common example of utilitarian reasoning is determining how to allocate scarce health care resources, such as in organ transplantation, triage situations, or determining coverage or benefits in a health insurance plan.

3. Virtue ethics—An ethical model that bases action on what a reasonable person would do who acts prudently and in accordance with the laws, regulations, and ethical standards of her/his society or profession. Some prominent virtues among health care professionals including case managers might be caring, faithfulness, justice, beneficence, nonmaleficence, humility, courage, practical wisdom, and subordinating one's self-interest to caring for others.

4. Contractualism—An ethical model that derives from the marketplace. It seeks to define values and principles, especially as they might affect the distribution of benefits (or property and resources), as a result of negotiation or contract. The distribution of coverage under a private insurance policy is an example, where one might argue that what the insured is entitled to are the benefits he or she has purchased in the contract, i.e., the health insurance policy (Banja, 2003).

■ ETHICAL PRINCIPLES AND DECISION MAKING

A. Ethical *theory* is often presented in an abstract and formal way. It provides a broader perspective or framework for ethical practice and decision making. However, it occasionally is not helpful in informing real-life dilemmas, which can be extremely complex. Therefore, it is necessary for case managers to apply ethical *principles* for more realistic and practical application to their decision making.

B. Four ethical principles have derived from the work of Beauchamp and Childress (2001) that are much discussed and are often helpful in assisting persons (e.g., case managers) in doing what ethics requires. Each principle can be read as a professional duty or as a right the patient or client enjoys. These are:

1. Autonomy—An ethical principle that connotes individual liberty, individual rights, self-determination, my "being my own person," personal inviolability, and antipaternalism.
   a. In medicine, a frequent demonstration of autonomy is the patient's right to refuse treatment.
   b. In case management, an instance of autonomy would be the patient's right to refuse case management services or to choose a treating or evaluating physician.

2. Nonmaleficence—An ethical principle that is fundamental to health care ethics in that the professional is obligated "to do no harm." Case management examples of harming patients would be where the case manager loses objectivity and writes reports that bias the treating

health care professional or the payer (insurer) for health care services against the patient.

3. Beneficence—An ethical principle that obligates the health professional to do as much good as possible. Problems with achieving beneficence occur when the case manager differs with the client as to what constitutes the client's best interest, e.g., a return to work versus collecting unemployment benefits for as long as possible.

4. Justice—An ethical principle requiring that the patient/client receives what he or she is owed, or be treated fairly. Problems with justice occur when the client's policy language regarding benefits is unclear, or when the client demands services the case manager believes are excessive, or when the case manager believes the client is noncompliant and finds it difficult to advocate for him or her.

C. The Four-Quadrant Model can be used for ethical decision making by case managers. This model is a method popularized by Jonsen, Siegler, and Winslade (2002) that helps in identifying and grouping ethically important aspects of a case.

1. The model, however, does not resolve cases nor does it prioritize which ethical elements in a case merit the most attention or weight. The case manager must still exercise critical thinking and judgment.

2. The four quadrants or groups are:

a. Medical indications, which include the answers to the following questions:

   i. What is the patient's medical problem and history?

   ii. Diagnosis and prognosis?

   iii. Is the problem acute, chronic, critical, emergent, incurable, or reversible?

   iv. What are the goals of treatment?

   v. What are the probabilities of success?

   vi. What is the plan in case of therapeutic failure?

   vii. How can the patient be benefited and how can harm be prevented?

b. Patient preferences, which include answers to the following questions:

   i. Is the patient mentally capable and legally competent?

   ii. If competent, what are the patient's preferences for treatment?

   iii. Has the patient been informed of benefits and risks?

   iv. Has he or she given consent?

   v. If incapacitated, who is the appropriate decision maker?

   vi. Is the patient's surrogate or proxy making decisions as the patient would wish (which is ethical) or as the surrogate prefers (which is unethical)?

   vii. Has the patient expressed prior preferences, such as by an advance directive (e.g., living will, durable power of attorney for health care)?

   viii. Is the patient's right to choose being respected to the greatest extent possible in ethics and law?

    c. Quality of life, which includes answers to the following questions:
      i. What are the prospects, with or without treatment, for a return to a normal life?
      ii. What physical, mental, and social deficits is the patient likely to experience if the treatment succeeds?
      iii. Are there biases that might prejudice the professional's evaluation of the patient's quality of life?
      iv. Is the patient's present or future condition such that his or her continued life might be judged undesirable?
      v. Is there any plan or rationale to forego treatment?
      vi. Are there plans for comfort and palliative care?
    d. Contextual features, which include answers to the following questions:
      i. Are there family issues, financial and economic factors, or religious or cultural factors that might unjustly influence treatment decisions?
      ii. Are there legal issues or clinical trials (research) involvement that might compromise the patient's welfare?
      iii. Is there any conflict of interest on the part of the providers or the institution?

D. CMSA has summarized the following ethical principles in its statement on ethical case management practice (CMSA, 1996).
  1. Case managers must adhere to the code of ethics of their profession of origin; that is, nursing, social work, rehabilitation counseling, and so on.
  2. Case management practice must be guided by the principles of autonomy, beneficence, nonmaleficence, justice, and veracity. It also must preserve the dignity of the client and family.
  3. Case managers foster the client's autonomy, independence, and self-determination.
  4. Case managers support the client and family in their self-advocacy and self-direction, and in their options and decisions related to health care services and treatments.
  5. Case managers must not discriminate based on social or economic status, personal attributes, or the nature of the health problem. They must show respect for the individual and deal with their clients with dignity and fairness.
  6. Case managers refrain from doing harm to others and emphasize quality outcomes.
  7. Case managers must advocate for their clients to receive needed care and promote access to services, especially when they are rare or limited.

E. CCMC has identified several values of case management practice (CCMC, 2004).
  1. Case management is a means for achieving client wellness and autonomy through advocacy, communication, education, and services facilitation.
  2. Case managers must recognize the dignity, rights, and worth of all individuals.

3. Case managers must commit to quality outcomes, appropriate use of resources, and empowerment of clients and their families.

4. Case management practice must be guided by the principles of autonomy, beneficence, nonmaleficence, justice, veracity, and distributive justice.

5. Case management practice focuses on achieving quality outcomes and facilitates the individual's ability to reach optimal level of wellness and functional capability; thus, everyone benefits—the individuals being cared for and their support system, the health care delivery system, and the various reimbursement systems.

F. CCMC has also identified several rules of conduct for case managers (CCMC, 2004). These are written in terms of violations that result in sanctions up to revocation of certification (the CCM credential). Case managers must avoid these violations at all times.

1. Intentionally falsify an application or other documents.

2. Conviction of a felony that involves moral turpitude.

3. Violation of the code of ethics governing the original profession of the case manager (i.e., nursing, rehabilitation counseling).

4. Loss of primary professional credential (i.e., nursing, social work).

5. Violation or breach of the guidelines of professional conduct.

6. Failure to maintain eligibility requirements once certified.

7. Violation of the rules and regulations governing the taking of the certification examination.

■ ETHICAL RESPONSIBILITIES PARTICULARLY AFFECTING CASE MANAGERS

A. Ethical conflicts can arise despite a case manager's best intentions and efforts (Tahan and Stolte-Upman, 2006).

B. The case manager must advocate for his/her clients and ensure that their needs are comprehensively addressed, service options are provided, and access to resources that meet their individual needs and interests is also made possible (CCMC, 2004).

C. According to CCMC (2004) and Tahan and Stolte-Upman (2006), important ethical responsibilities for case managers may include the following:

1. Advocacy—Ensuring that client's needs are reasonably and justly met. The case manager must never handle or neglect a case in a grossly negligent fashion; i.e., in a manner that fails to meet the case management standard of care and practice.

2. Unprofessional behavior—The case manager must maintain honesty and desist from acts of fraud, deceit, discrimination, or sexual intimacy with a client.

3. Representation of practice—Practicing within the boundaries of competence and never misrepresenting the case manager's role or competence to clients.

4. Conflict of interest—Ensuring that secondary interests (especially bearing on financial gain) do not compromise the case manager's primary responsibility of client advocacy.
   a. Although some conflicts of interest might be ethically manageable, they should be fully disclosed to all parties affected by them.
   b. If, after full disclosure, an objection is made by any party, the case manager should attempt to manage the objection; if all fails, withdrawal from further participation in the case is necessary.
5. Reporting misconduct—Case managers who are aware of ethical violations committed by other case managers should report that knowledge to the appropriate party or to the CCMC if the alleged violator is a certificant. All such reports must be based in fact and not be malicious or unwarranted.
6. Description of services—Case managers should provide information to clients about the services offered, the risks that might be associated with those services, alternatives to services, and the client's right to refuse services.
7. Termination of services—Case managers should provide written notification of service discontinuation to all parties involved in a case consistent with applicable statutes, regulations, and guidelines.
8. Objectivity—Case managers will refrain from imposing their personal (e.g., political, philosophical, cultural) values on their clients; they will respect their clients rights, liberties, and autonomy; they will provide care as dictated by professional case management standards. Case managers will also be objective in reporting the results of their professional activities to third parties and avoid exerting any undue influence on the decision-making process.
9. Disclosure—Case managers who perform services at the request of a third party must disclose their dual relationship, and their role and responsibilities in it, at the outset of establishing a relationship with the client.
   a. Case managers are also ethically required to inform clients who are receiving services that any information obtained through the case management relationship might be disclosed to third parties (e.g., health care providers, third party payers, etc.) who have a legal or ethical right or need to know it.
   b. Disclosure should be limited only to what is necessary and relevant, except in instances to prevent the client from 1) committing acts likely to result in bodily harm, either to the client or to others, and 2) committing criminal, illegal, or fraudulent acts.
10. Records—Case managers must maintain records in a manner designed to ensure privacy; i.e., to protect and secure the information from individuals who have no right to it.
11. Solicitation—Case managers should refrain from rewarding, paying, or compensating anyone who directs or refers clients to them for case manager services.

■ STRATEGIES FOR MAINTAINING ETHICAL BEHAVIOR

A. It is important for health care organizations and administrators of case management programs to consider the implementation of an ethics group, patient services, or professional advisory committee charged to address ethical conflicts or dilemmas as they arise.

1. The group, which presumably can be comprised of persons who are known for their expertise, professional integrity, and for maintaining ethical and legal standards, can be convened for hearing ethical issues and offering ethical recommendations.

2. The group can also initiate ethics roundtables or informal meetings to discuss ethical and professional issues and concerns (Banja, 1999).

B. It is important for case managers to understand the types of ethical conflicts they may face and how to handle them.

1. Jansen (2003) differentiates between two types of ethics consults that one could translate into the need for two types of ethics groups or committees; these are clinical and organizational.

   a. *Clinical* ethics committees—usually handle ethical conflicts that are clinical in nature and related to the medical treatment. Examples of these conflicts are:

      i. End of life matters and termination of care

      ii. Lack of understanding by patient/family of the medical treatment

      iii. Conflicts between patient, family, and provider regarding decisions made (or that need to be made) about best treatment and options

   b. *Organizational* ethics committees—usually handle ethical conflicts that pertain to an organization's behaviors as they relate to the individuals represented by that organization (including patients, health care providers, and other employees), the community served by the organization, and other organizations with which it interacts and collaborates. Examples of these conflicts are:

      i. Utilization management and allocation of resources

      ii. Denial of services

      iii. Delays in care

      iv. Conflicts of interest

2. Jansen (2003) also identified five subcategories of ethical conflicts. These are:

   a. Health care business such as cost shifting, billing practices, resource allocation, and financial interests

   b. Societal and public health considerations such as antidumping issues, public disclosure of medical errors, and discrimination

   c. Health care advertising such as making unrealistic promises and endorsing specific medical products or service agencies

   d. Scientific and educational issues such as clinical trials and education of providers

   e. General business practices such as relationships with vendors, employees, payers, and other outside agencies

C. Case managers must remember that being able to justify an act as ethical is crucial. They should therefore be able to analyze the reasons for their behaviors and decisions and ask themselves whether or not those reasons can withstand public or professional scrutiny (Banja, 1999).

D. Case managers should pay careful attention to their own moral feelings.
   1. Often the first symptom of an ethical dilemma is an affective one, as in, "This situation makes me professionally uncomfortable. What I'm doing (or being asked to do) doesn't feel right."
   2. Ethical behavior and ethical learning tend to be associated with particular feelings about right and wrong.
   3. The case manager who experiences moral anxiety or distress should have some mechanism to have it addressed (Tahan and Stolte-Upman, 2006); for example, seeking the assistance, guidance, or counsel of ethics groups/committees.

E. Case managers should attend conferences on ethics and/or keep abreast of the case management ethical literature.

F. Whether they are certified or not, case managers should be familiar with the CCMC's Code of Professional Conduct for Case Managers just as they should be familiar with the ethical code of their profession and licensing organization such as those of nursing, social work, rehabilitation counseling, and so on.

G. Case managers should examine the literature available in libraries, on the Internet, and at various state chapters of case management professional organizations/societies. They also should access the ethical resources available from these professional organizations/societies either online or during annual conferences; for example, the CMSA's online resources and annual conference.

H. Case managers should review the ethical codes and standards regularly— perhaps each time the case manager renews his or her certification or licensure requirements (Tahan and Stolte-Upman, 2006).

I. Case managers may seek advisory opinions from the CCMC regarding ethical dilemmas. Such activities are important for case managers to ensure compliance with ethical codes and principles.

J. Case managers may request a change of assignment from a supervisor, especially in cases that present ethical distress or conflict (Tahan and Stolte-Upman, 2006).

K. Case managers should work within the case management scope of practice and professional guidelines. They should examine their job description for consistency with applicable ethical standards and modify it as necessary.

L. Case managers should maintain professional objectivity and ethical astuteness in creating records and documentation. The case manager must recognize the admissibility of certain of these documents in litigation and she/he must realize that documentation is a direct reflection of one's ethical sensibilities and behaviors (Tahan and Stolte-Upman, 2006).

REFERENCES

Banja, J. (1997). Values, function, and managed care: An ethical analysis. *Journal of Head Trauma Rehabilitation, 12*(1), 60–70.

Banja, J. (1999). Ethical decision-making: Origins, process, and applications to case management. *The Case Manager, 10*(5), 41–47.

Banja, J. (2003). Antifoundationalism and morality by contract: The case of managed care. In O. Ferrell, S. True, & L. Pelton, *Rights, relationships & responsibilities, Vol 1* (pp. 73–86). Kennesaw, GA: Kennesaw State University, Michael Coles College of Business.

Banja, J. (2006). Case management and the standards of practice. *The Case Manager, 17*(1), 21–23.

Beauchamp, T., & Childress, J. F. (2001). *Priniciples of biomedical ethics*, 5th ed. New York: Oxford University Press.

Case Management Society of America (CMSA). (1996). CMSA statement regarding ethical case management practice. Little Rock, AR: CMSA.

Commission for Case Manager Certification (CCMC). (2004). *Code of professional conduct for case managers with standards, rules, procedures and penalties*. Rolling Meadows, IL: CCMC.

Commission for Case Manager Certification (CCMC). (2005). *Glossary of terms*. Rolling Meadows, IL: CCMC.

Jansen, L. A. (2003). Ethical issues in case management. In T. G. Cesta & H. A. Tahan, *The case manager's survival guide: Winning strategies for clinical practice*, 2nd ed. (pp. 324–335). St Louis, MO: Mosby.

Jonsen, A. R., Siegler, M., & Winslade, W. J. (2002). *Clinical ethics: A practical approach to ethical decisions in clinical medicine*, 5th ed. New York: McGraw-Hill.

Lo, B. (2000). *Resolving ethical dilemmas: A guide for clinicians*. Philadelphia: Lippincott Williams & Wilkins.

Tahan, H. A., & Stolte-Upman, C. (2006). *Code of professional conduct for case managers: Establishing standards for ethical practice*. Rolling Meadows, IL: CCMC.

Taylor, C. (2005). Ethical issues in case management. In E. L. Cohen & T. G. Cesta, *Nursing case management: From essentials to advance practice applications*, (pp. 361–379). St Louis, MO: Elsevier Mosby.

Thompson, D. (1993). Understanding financial conflicts of interest. *New England Journal of Medicine, 329*(8), 573–575.

SUGGESTED READING

Cesta, T. G., & Tahan, H. A. (2003). *The case manager's survival guide: Winning strategies for clinical practice*. St. Louis, MO: Mosby.

Cohen, E. L. & Cesta, T. G. (2005). *Nursing case management: From essentials to advanced practice applications*, 4th ed. St. Louis, MO: Elsevier Mosby.

Powell, S. K. (2000). *Case management: A practical guide to success in managed care*. Philadelphia, PA: Lippincott Williams & Wilkins.

Powell, S. K. (2000). *Advanced case management: Outcomes and beyond*. Philadelphia, PA: Lippincott Williams & Wilkins.

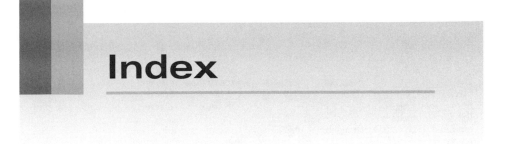

Index

Note: Page numbers followed by *f* indicate figures; those followed by *t* indicate tables.